DESK REFERENCE

MW00651642

Coders' Desk Reference for ICD-10-PCS Procedures

Clinical descriptions with answers to your toughest ICD-10-PCS coding questions

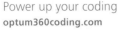

Power up your coding
optum360coding.com

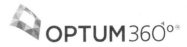

OPTUM360°®

Optum360 Notice

The *Coders' Desk Reference for Procedures (ICD-10-PCS)* is designed to be an accurate and authoritative source regarding coding and every reasonable effort has been made to ensure accuracy and completeness of the content. However, Optum360 makes no guarantee, warranty, or representation that this publication is accurate, complete or without errors. It is understood that Optum360 is not rendering any legal or other professional services or advice in this publication and that Optum360 bears no liability for any results or consequences that may arise from the use of this book.

Acknowledgments

Marianne Randall, CPC, *Product Manager*

Karen Schmidt, BSN, *Technical Director*

Karen Krawzik, RHIT, CCS, AHIMA-approved ICD-10-CM/PCS Trainer, *Clinical Technical Editor*

Anne Kenney, BA, MBA, CCA, CCS, *Clinical Technical Editor*

Peggy Willard, CCS, AHIMA-approved ICD-10-CM/PCS Trainer, *Clinical Technical Editor*

Stacy Perry, *Manager, Desktop Publishing*

Lisa Singley, *Project Manager*

Tracy Betzler, *Senior Desktop Publishing Specialist*

Hope M. Dunn, *Senior Desktop Publishing Specialist*

Katie Russell, *Desktop Publishing Specialist*

Kate Holden, *Editor*

Our Commitment to Accuracy

Optum360 is committed to producing accurate and reliable materials.

To report corrections, please visit www.optum360coding.com/accuracy or email accuracy@optum.com. You can also reach customer service by calling 1.800.464.3649, option 1.

Copyright

Property of Optum360, LLC. Optum360 and the Optum360 logo are trademarks of Optum360, LLC. All other brand or product names are trademarks or registered trademarks of their respective owner.

© 2018 Optum360, LLC. All rights reserved.

Made in the USA
ISBN 978-1-62254-446-2

Karen Krawzik, RHIT, CCS, AHIMA-approved ICD-10-CM/PCS Trainer

Ms. Krawzik has expertise in ICD-10-CM, ICD-9-CM, CPT/HCPCS, DRG, and data quality and analytics, with more than 30 years' experience coding in multiple settings, including inpatient, observation, ambulatory surgery, ancillary, and emergency room. She has served as a DRG analyst and auditor of commercial and government payer claims, as a contract administrator, and worked on a team providing enterprise-wide conversion of the ICD-9-CM code set to ICD-10. More recently, she has been developing print and electronic content related to ICD-10-CM and ICD-10-PCS coding systems, MS-DRGs, and HCCs. Ms. Krawzik is credentialed by the American Health Information Management Association (AHIMA) as a Registered Health Information Technician (RHIT) and a Certified Coding Specialist (CCS) and is an AHIMA-approved ICD-10-CM/PCS trainer. She is an active member of AHIMA and the Missouri Health Information Management Association.

Anne Kenney, BA, MBA, CCA, CCS

Ms. Kenney has expertise in ICD-10-CM/PCS, ICD-9-CM, DRG, and CPT coding. Most recently she has been developing content for ICD-10-CM and ICD-10-PCS applications. Her prior experience in a major teaching hospital includes assignment of ICD-9-CM codes and DRGs, CPT code assignments, and determining physician evaluation and management levels for inpatient, emergency department, and observation cases. Ms. Kenney is an active member of the American Health Information Management Association (AHIMA) and the Minnesota Health Information Management Association (MHIMA).

Peggy Willard, CCS, AHIMA-approved ICD-10-CM/PCS Trainer

Ms. Willard has 18 years of experience in the healthcare field. Her expertise is in ICD-10-CM and ICD-10-PCS, including in-depth analysis of medical record documentation, ICD-10-CM/PCS code and DRG assignment, as well as clinical documentation improvement (CDI). In recent years Ms. Willard has been responsible for the creation and development of several products for Optum360 Coding Solutions that are designed to assist with appropriate application of the ICD-10-CM and ICD-10-PCS coding systems. She has several years of prior experience in Level I adult and pediatric trauma hospital and inpatient rehabilitation facility (IRF) coding, specializing in ICD-9-CM diagnosis and procedural coding, with emphasis in conducting coding audits, and conducting coding training for coding staff and clinical documentation specialists. Ms. Willard is an AHIMA-approved ICD-10 CM/PCS trainer and is an active member of the American Health Information Management Association (AHIMA) and the Minnesota Health Information Management Association (MHIMA).

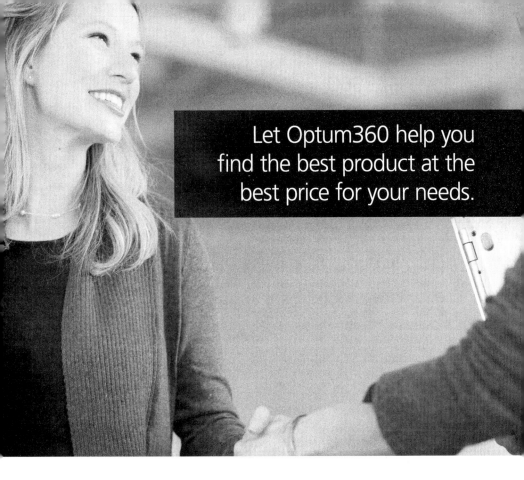

Let Optum360 help you find the best product at the best price for your needs.

Optum360® can help you drive financial results across your organization with industry-leading resources that cut through the complexity of medical coding challenges.

The Price Match Program* is an example of one of the ways in which we can impact your bottom line — to the positive. We're committed to providing you with the best quality product in the market, along with the best price.

Let us help you find the best coding solution, at the best price.

Contact your Medallion representative directly or call Customer Service at 1-800-464-3649, option 1.

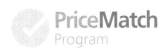

*Some restrictions and exclusions apply.
Visit optum360coding.com/pricematch to learn more about the conditions, guidelines and exclusions.

© 2018 Optum360, LLC. All rights reserved. WF621697 SPRJ5186 4/18

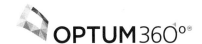

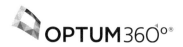
OPTUM360°®

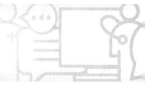

Optum360 Learning

Education suiting your specialty, learning style and schedule

Optum360® Learning is designed to address exactly what you and your learners need. We offer: Several delivery methods developed for various adult learning styles; general public education; and tailor-made programs specific to your organization — all created by our coding and clinical documentation education professionals.

Our strategy is simple — education must be concise, relevant and accurate. Choose the delivery method that works best for you:

eLearning

- **Web-based** courses offered at the most convenient times
- **Interactive**, task-focused and developed around practical scenarios
- **Self-paced** courses include "try-it" functionality, knowledge checks and downloadable resources

You've worked hard for your credentials, and now you need an easy way to maintain your certification.

Instructor-led training

On-site or remote courses built specifically for your organization and learners
- Providers
- CDI specialists
- Coders

Webinars

Online courses geared toward a broad market of learners and delivered in a live setting

NO MATTER YOUR LEARNING STYLE, OPTUM360 IS HERE TO HELP YOU.

Call 1-800-464-3649, option 1, and mention promo code **LEARN19A.**

Visit optum360coding.com/learning.

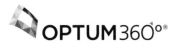
OPTUM360°®

Optum360® has the coding resources you need, with more than 20 specialty-specific products. You can view our selection of code books at **optum360coding.com.**

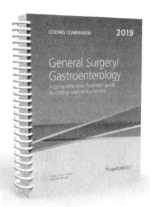
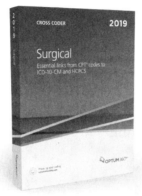
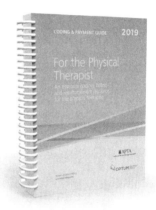

Coding Companions

Comprehensive and easy to use, these guides include 2019 CPT®, HCPCS and ICD-10-CM code sets specific to your specialty. Each procedure code includes both official and lay descriptions, coding tips, terminology, cross-coding to common ICD-10-CM and relative value units.

Coding and Payment Guides

These all-inclusive specialty resources consolidate the coding process. Our guides are updated with specialty-specific ICD-10-CM, HCPCS Level II and CPT® codes sets, Medicare payer information, CCI edits, helpful code descriptions and clinical definitions.

Cross Coders

These resources provide the crosswalks that billing and coding staff need to link CPT® codes for various specialties to the appropriate ICD-10-CM and HCPCS Level II codes so you code it right the first time.

SPECIALTIES INCLUDE:

Radiology
Surgical
Anesthesia Services
Behavioral Health Services
Dental Services
Laboratory Services
Physical Therapist
Cardiology/Cardiothoracic/Vascular Surgery
ENT/Allergy/Pulmonology
General Surgery/Gastroenterology
Neurosurgery/Neurology

OB/GYN
Ophthalmology
Orthopaedics: Hips & Below
Orthopaedics: Spine & Above
Plastics/Dermatology
Podiatry
Primary Care/Pediatrics/Emergency Medicine
Urology/Nephrology
OMS
Medical Oncology/Hematology Services

CPT is a registered trademark of the American Medical Association.   © 2018 Optum360, LLC. All rights reserved. WF626533 04/18

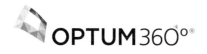

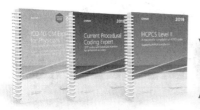

RENEW THIS BOOK
SAVE UP TO 25%
ON 2019 EDITION CODING RESOURCES.*

ITEM #	TITLE INDICATE THE ITEMS YOU WISH TO PURCHASE	QUANTITY	PRICE PER PRODUCT	TOTAL
		Subtotal		
	(AK, DE, HI, MT, NH & OR are exempt)	Sales Tax		
	1 item $10.95 • 2–4 items $12.95 • 5+ CALL	Shipping & Handling		
		TOTAL AMOUNT ENCLOSED		

Save up to 25% when you renew.*

PROMO CODE: RENEW19A

 Visit **optum360coding.com** and enter the promo code above at checkout.

 Call **1-800-464-3649, option 1,** and mention the promo code above.

 Fax this order form with purchase order to **1-801-982-4033.** *Optum360 no longer accepts credit cards by fax.*

 Mail this order form with payment and/or purchase order to: **Optum360, PO Box 88050, Chicago, IL 60680-9920.** *Optum360 no longer accepts credit cards by mail.*

Name

Address

Customer Number   Contact Number

◯ CHECK ENCLOSED (PAYABLE TO OPTUM360)

◯ BILL ME ◯ P.O.# _____

Telephone

Fax

Email

Optum360 respects your right to privacy. We will not sell or rent your email address or fax number to anyone outside Optum360 and its business partners. If you would like to remove your name from Optum360 promotions, please call 1-800-464-3649, option 1.

*Save 25% when you order on optum360coding.com; save 20% when you order by phone, fax or mail. Save 15% on AMA, OMS and custom fee products. Offer excludes digital coding tools, data files, workers' comp, the Almanac, educational courses and bookstore products.
© 2018 Optum360, LLC. All rights reserved. WF626234 SPRJ5188

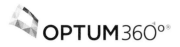

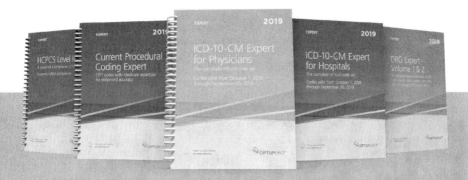

Keep your go-to coding resources up to date

Stay current and compliant with our 2019 edition code books.
With more than 30 years in the coding industry, Optum360® is proud to
be your trusted resource for coding, billing and reimbursement resources.
Our 2019 editions include tools for ICD-10-CM/PCS, CPT®, HCPCS, DRG,
specialty-specific coding and much more.

SAVE UP TO 25% ON ADDITIONAL CODING RESOURCES

Visit us at optum360coding.com
and enter promo code **FOBA19ED**
to save 25%.

Call 1-800-464-3649, option 1,
and be sure to mention promo
code **FOBA19ED** to save 20%.

CPT is a registered trademark of the American Medical Association.

Excludes custom fee and bookstore items, data files, online coding tools and educational courses. Cannot be combined
with any other offer. Offer not valid for Partner or Medallion accounts.
© 2018 Optum360, LLC. All rights reserved. WF621697 SPRJ5185

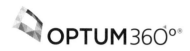

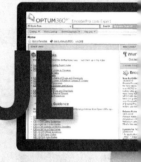

CODING TOOLS THIS

POWERFUL

ARE BUILT FOR **CODING PROFESSIONALS**

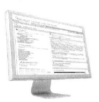

EncoderPro.com for physicians and payers

Quickly and easily access the content from more than 30 code and reference books — and coding guidelines from Medicare and Optum360® — in one dynamic solution. This includes CPT®, HCPCS Level II, ICD-10-CM and -PCS and ICD-9-CM code set content. Boost productivity and first-pass payment.

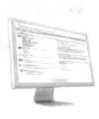

RevenueCyclePro.com for facilities

Simplify your research efforts with reference data compiled in one comprehensive, online problem-solving tool. This comprehensive tool includes access to ICD-10 code sets, ICD-9 to ICD-10 mapping information, crosswalks, updated Medicare LCD and NCD policies, revenue codes, UB-04 billing tips and an enhanced APC calculator. Maximize your coding compliance efforts and minimize rejected and denied claims. Increase efficiency across the entire hospital revenue cycle.

SCHEDULE A DEMO TODAY

 CLICK
optum360coding.com/onlinetools

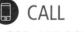 **CALL**
1-800-464-3649, option 1

CPT is a registered trademark of the American Medical Association.
© 2018 Optum360, LLC. All rights reserved. WF593285 03/18

Contents

© 2018 Optum360, LLC

© 2018 Optum360, LLC

© 2018 Optum360, LLC

Stress Test, Cardiac (Myocardial Perfusion Scan)(Cardiovascular Stress Test) 439
Extracorporeal or Systemic Assistance and Performance **440**
Balloon Pump, Intra-aortic (IABP) 440
Bypass, Cardiopulmonary 441
Cardioversion and Defibrillation, External 441
Hemodialysis 442
Oxygen Therapy, Supersaturated 443
Oxygenation, Extracorporeal Membrane (ECMO) 444
Oxygenation, Hyperbaric, Wound 444
Performance, Extracorporeal Hepatic (Liver Dialysis) 445
Removal, Carbon Dioxide, Extracorporeal (ECCO₂R)
(Respiratory Dialysis) 445
Ventilation, Mechanical, Assistance (Respiratory) 446
Ventilation, Mechanical, Performance (Respiratory) 447
Extracorporeal or Systemic Therapies **448**
Oxygenation, Hyperbaric (Decompression) 448
Perfusion, Respiratory Donor Organ (EVLP) (ex-vivo lung perfusion) 449
Pheresis 450
Phototherapy 451
Therapy, Shock Wave, Extracorporeal (ESWT), Musculoskeletal (Orthotripsy) 452
Ultrasound, Therapeutic 453
Osteopathic **454**
Manipulative Treatment, Osteopathic 454
Other Procedures **456**
Acupuncture 456
Assistance, Computer 457
Assistance, Robotic 458
Collection, Cerebrospinal Fluid from Indwelling Device 459
Chiropractic **460**
Manipulation, Chiropractic, Mechanically Assisted 460
Ancillary **461**
Imaging **461**
Angiography, Cardiac (Coronary Arteriography) (Angiocardiography) 461
Arteriography, Renal (Renal Angiography) (Angiography, Renal Arteries) 462
Echocardiography, Intracardiac 463
Echocardiography, Transesophageal (TEE) 464
Endoscopic Retrograde Cholangiopancreatography (ERCP) 465
Fluoroscopy 466
MRI, Fetal, Central Nervous System 467
Ultrasonography, Fetal 468
Ultrasound, Intravascular, Coronary Arteries (IVUS) 469
Ventriculography, Cardiac 470
Videofluoroscopy, Esophageal (Modified Barium Swallow) 471
Nuclear Medicine **472**
Adenosine Sestamibi Planar Scan, Heart Muscle (Technetium) 472
Cisternography, Cerebrospinal Fluid Flow Imaging 473
Scan, Pulmonary, Ventilation and Perfusion 474
Radiation Therapy **475**
Brachytherapy, Prostate 475
Oncology Treatment, Hyperthermia 476
Radiation Therapy, External Beam 477
Radiation Therapy, Plaque Radiation, Eye 478
Radiation Therapy, Stereotactic Radiosurgery, Brain 479
Radiation Therapy, Superficial Dermatologic 480

© 2018 Optum360, LLC

Illustrations

© 2018 Optum360, LLC

Introduction

Coding is a complicated business. It is not enough to have a current copy of an ICD-10-PCS book—coders must have a firm enough grasp of medical terminology, anatomy, and surgical techniques to be able to translate procedure descriptions in medical records into detailed codes. ICD-10-PCS guidelines state that the physician is not responsible for changing the common procedure terminology he or she uses to document procedures so that it better matches terminology used in the coding system. Rather, the burden is on the coder, who must interpret physicians' procedure descriptions and reflect them in the appropriate ICD-10-PCS codes. The *Coders' Desk Reference for Procedures (ICD-10-PCS)* addresses this challenge.

This book provides coders, coding managers, medical staff and health care professionals, payers, educators, and students with comprehensive, clear descriptions of procedures. The goal is to enrich users' clinical understanding of surgical procedures and how they relate to the way ICD-10-PCS classifies procedures. The result is improved coding confidence so that code selection becomes more accurate and efficient. The coding guidance in *Coders' Desk Reference for Procedures (ICD-10-PCS)* is based on the official version of the ICD-10 Procedure Coding System (ICD-10-PCS), effective October 1, 2018. (Please note that this procedure coding reference is intended to be used with an official ICD-10-PCS code book.)

This desk reference is organized by common procedure nomenclature used in the hospital setting, which is linked to the related root operation tables. The procedures are described in layman's terms, translated to ICD-10-PCS root operation terminology, and the corresponding root operation tables are identified.

Detailed descriptions using terminology coders see in medical documents, together with coding clarification and guidance and important instruction regarding ICD-10-PCS conventions, make *Coders' Desk Reference for Procedures (ICD-10-PCS)* an unparalleled guidebook to code selection.

Important Message: Not all categories, subcategories, or procedures have been represented in this first edition of the *Coders' Desk Reference for Procedures (ICD-10-PCS)*. Additional procedures not part of the 2019 edition will gradually be incorporated into future editions.

ICD-10-PCS Overview

ICD-10-PCS Code Structure

ICD-10-PCS has a multiaxial, seven-character, alphanumeric code structure. Each character contains up to 34 possible values. Each value represents a specific option for the general character definition. The 10 digits Ø–9 and the 24 letters A–H, J–N, and P–Z may be used for each character. The letters O and I are not used so as to avoid confusion with the digits Ø and 1.

An ICD-10-PCS code is the result of a process rather than a single fixed set of digits or alphabetic characters. The process consists of combining semi-independent values from among a selection of values, according to the rules governing the construction of codes. A code is derived by choosing a specific value for each of the seven characters. Based on details about the procedure performed, values are assigned for each character specifying the section, body system, root operation, body part, approach, device, and qualifier. Because the definition of each character is also a function of its physical position in the code, the same letter or number placed in a different position in the code has a different meaning.

The seven characters that make up a complete code have specific meanings that vary for each of the 17 sections of the manual. Procedures are divided into sections that identify the general type of procedure (e.g., Medical and Surgical, Obstetrics, Imaging). The first character of the procedure code always specifies the section. The second through seventh characters have the same meaning within each section but may mean different things in other sections. In all sections, the third character specifies the general type, or root operation, of procedure performed (e.g., Resection, Transfusion, Fluoroscopy), while the other characters give additional information such as the body part and approach.

ICD-10-PCS Index

Codes may be found in the index based on the general type of procedure (e.g., Resection, Transfusion, Fluoroscopy), or a more commonly used term (e.g., appendectomy). For example, the code for percutaneous intraluminal dilation of the coronary arteries with an intraluminal device can be found in the ICD-10-PCS index under "Dilation" or a synonym for dilation (e.g., "Angioplasty"). The index then specifies the first three or four values of the code or directs the user to see another term.

The user can use the alphabetic index to locate the appropriate table containing all the information necessary to construct a procedure code. The PCS tables should always be consulted to find the most appropriate valid code. Coders may choose a valid code directly from the tables; they do not have to consult the index before proceeding to the tables to complete the code.

Introduction

Main Terms

The alphabetic index reflects the structure of the tables. The index:

- Is based on the value of the third character
- Contains common procedure terms
- Lists anatomic sites
- Uses device terms

The main terms in the alphabetic index are root operations, root procedure types, or common procedure names. The index provides at least the first three or four values of the code, and some entries may provide complete valid codes. However, the user should always consult the appropriate table to verify that the most appropriate valid code has been selected.

For the Medical and Surgical and related sections, the root operation values are used as main terms in the index. The subterms under the root operation main terms are body parts. For the Ancillary section of the code tables, the main terms in the index are the general type of procedure performed.

The second type of term in the index uses common procedure names, such as "appendectomy" or "fundoplication." These common terms are listed as main terms with a "see" reference noting the PCS root operations that are possible valid code tables based on the objective of the procedure.

Use Reference

The index also lists anatomic sites from the Body Part Key and device terms from the Device Key. These terms are listed with "use" references, which are additional references to the terms located in the appendix keys. The term provided is the body part value or device value to be selected when constructing a procedure code using the code tables. This type of index reference does not direct the user to another term in the index, but provides guidance regarding character value selection. Therefore, "use" references generally do not refer to specific valid code tables.

ICD-10-PCS Code Tables

ICD-10-PCS contains 17 sections of code tables organized by general type of procedure. Each table is composed of rows that specify the valid combinations of code values. In most sections of the coding system, the upper portion of each table contains a description of the first three characters of the procedure code. In the Medical and Surgical section, for example, the first three characters contain the name of the section, the body system, and the root operation performed. The four columns in the table specify the last four characters. In the Medical and Surgical section, they are labeled body part, approach, device and qualifier, respectively. Each row in the table specifies the valid combination of values for characters 4 through 7. All seven characters must be specified to form a valid code.

Note that the code must be constructed with a combination of values within the same row of the table. A combination of values from different rows of the same table will result in an invalid code.

How to Use *Coders' Desk Reference for Procedures (ICD-10-PCS)*

Coders' Desk Reference for Procedures (ICD-10-PCS) is divided into convenient sections for easy use. The basic format of the book provides clinical coding support with illustrations, narratives, and other resources that help the user work from the medical record. The book begins with special chapters that provide detailed information on coding guidelines and conventions relating to ICD-10-PCS procedure coding, as well as common abbreviations, acronyms, and symbols, eponyms, and surgical terms found in the medical record. It then follows the organization of ICD-10-PCS, looking at procedures and their associated ICD-10-PCS root operation tables. Due to the significant expansion of the number of ICD-10-PCS codes, it is impossible to include a description of every procedure. Included are representative examples of procedures, organized by section and subsection.

List of Illustrations

This is a list of illustrations by procedure name with a cross-reference to the appropriate page.

ICD-10-PCS Official Guidelines for Coding and Reporting 2019

For the new coder, and even for the veteran, this chapter provides an overview and detailed instructions on ICD-10-PCS coding guidelines and conventions.

ICD-10-PCS Root Operation Definitions

This resource is a compilation of all root operations in the Medical and Surgical-Related sections of the ICD-10-PCS manual. It provides a definition and in some cases a more detailed explanation of the root operation to better reflect its purpose or objective. Examples of related procedures may also be provided.

Abbreviations, Acronyms, and Symbols

The medical profession has its own shorthand for documentation. Here, acronyms, abbreviations, and symbols commonly seen on operative reports or medical charts are listed for easy reference.

Procedure Eponyms

In the medical record, procedures are often documented by their common name or eponym (such as Billroth's operation I). Eponyms honor the developer of a procedure or test but do little to clarify what the procedure is. ICD-10-PCS does not cross-reference eponyms even though they are commonly noted in

© 2018 Optum360, LLC

medical documentation. Our editors have researched the procedure eponyms in the volume 3 index of the ICD-9 book and identified the associated ICD-10-PCS three- and sometimes four-character tables. The three-character description references the root operation and body system; the four-character description specifies the root operation and body part, when applicable.

Surgical Terms

Operative reports contain words and phrases that not only communicate the importance and urgency of surgery, but also describe the techniques. The *Coders' Desk Reference for Procedures (ICD-10-PCS)* glossary of surgical terms includes the terms operative reports most commonly use to describe techniques and tools.

Procedures

The first section of the desk reference, Medical and Surgical, contains the majority of procedures typically reported in an inpatient setting.

The next section is Medical and Surgical-Related sections, with subsections as listed below:

- Obstetrics
- Placement
- Administration
- Measurement and Monitoring
- Extracorporeal Assistance and Performance
- Extracorporeal Therapies
- Osteopathic
- Other Procedures
- Chiropractic

Next is the Ancillary section, which contains subsections for Imaging, Nuclear Medicine, and Radiation Therapy. Codes in these sections contain character values for contrast, modality qualifier, and equipment.

Last is the New Technology section, which contains codes identifying procedures requested via the new technology application process, and codes that capture new technologies not currently classified in ICD-10-PCS.

This section may include medical and surgical procedures, medical and surgical-related procedures, or ancillary procedures that are currently designated as new technology.

Alphabetic Index

The "Alphabetic Index" enables the user to look up a procedure by principal procedure or keyword, such as "Bypass," followed by descriptive terms, such as "Extracranial-Intracranial." *"See also"* notes are cross-referenced terms within the desk reference that provide additional information.

Format

The *Coders' Desk Reference for Procedures (ICD-10-PCS)* organizes the procedures first by section (Medical Surgical, Medical Surgical-Related, Ancillary, etc.), then by subsection, and then alphabetically by procedure name, using common procedure nomenclature. Use the "Alphabetic Index" to look up a procedure by the term, procedure, or keyword. Use *"see also"* references to identify descriptions of other procedures that may provide additional information.

Each procedure is linked to the related root operation table or tables, including the pertinent body system and root operations. Depending on the procedure, there may also be references to body part, approach, device, and qualifier. Except for the root operation table references, this book provides no character values or complete codes. The ICD-10-PCS code book tables should always be consulted to find the complete, most appropriate valid code.

Following is a brief explanation of the elements on a sample page. Each procedure is different, and not all elements are included in every procedure. The structure may differ slightly in the Medical and Surgical-Related and Ancillary sections from the Medical and Surgical section. For example in some sections, instead of Approach, the value will be specified as Duration, or instead of Device, the value will be Substance.

Introduction

Graft, Skin, Split-Thickness (STSG)

Body System **1**
Skin and Breast

PCS Root Operation **2**
Replacement

Root Operation Table **3**
ØHR   Skin and Breast, Replacement

Body Part **4**
Refer to the ICD-10-PCS tabular list for a
complete list of body parts.

Approach **5**
External

Device **6**
Autologous Tissue Substitute
Nonautologous Tissue Substitute

Qualifier **7**
Partial Thickness

Description **8**
The skin consists of two layers, the epidermis and
dermis. A split-thickness skin graft (STSG) includes the
epidermis and part of the dermis. The thickness of the
graft depends on the donor site and the needs of the
patient. Depending on how much of the dermis is
included, a STSG may be thin, intermediate (medium),
or thick. STSG is used to cover a large skin defect or
injury, often in cases of deep or extensive burns, to
provide coverage and promote healing. It may be
placed as a meshed (with slits or cuts) or a sheet
(whole) graft. Skin harvested from one location and
grafted to another on the same individual is termed an
Autologous Tissue Substitute. Tissue bank grafts and
skin substitute products are reported as
Nonautologous Tissue Substitute.

Under appropriate anesthesia, the physician takes a
dermal autograft from one area of the body and grafts
it to an area in need of repair. This procedure is
performed when direct wound closure or adjacent
tissue transfer is not possible. A dermal skin graft is
harvested by first raising a split-thickness skin graft
0.010 to 0.015 inches in depth with a dermatome, but
not removing it. The dermatome is adjusted to remove
the desired graft, and a second pass is made over the

newly created donor site at that depth to remove a
dermal layer autograft.

9

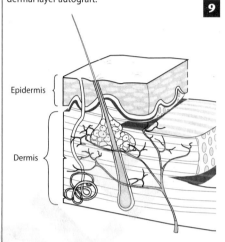

Epidermis

Dermis

The graft may then be used for grafting with or
without meshing by passing it through a meshing
device. Meshing the graft allows the graft surface area
to be expanded up to nine times the donor site surface
area. This may be indicated in large wounds such as
major burns. The recipient wound bed is prepared for
grafting using saline irrigation and debridement of any
nonviable tissue and contaminants. Once the recipient
site has been prepared, the graft is placed over the
wound bed, dermal side down. The graft is then
secured in place by suturing the graft to the
surrounding wound bed with absorbable sutures. A
nonadherent dressing is applied. Negative-pressure
wound therapy (NPWT) with a vacuum-assisted
closure (VAC) device may be applied to enhance
healing.

10

Focus Point
*Debridement done as preparation of the wound bed for
the graft is not reported separately unless the
debridement includes layers deeper than skin level.*

Focus Point
*The harvesting of an autograft from a different
procedure site is coded separately, according to
guideline B3.9.*

Coding Guidance **11**
AHA: 2014, 3Q, 14

© 2018 Optum360, LLC

Within each section, procedures are arranged alphabetically. Using common terminology in the medical record, narratives describing common procedures helps the user select the appropriate ICD-10-PCS table, body system, body part, approach, device, qualifier, etc.

1. Body System

This refers to the general physiological system or anatomical region involved.

2. PCS Root Operation

The PCS Root Operation describes the objective of the procedure.

3. Root Operation Table

Each procedure is linked to the related root operation table or tables, including the pertinent body system and root operations.

4. Body Part

This defines the body part or specific anatomical site where the procedure is performed. In some instances, a list of potential body parts may be too large to include the full list for a given procedure. In these cases, the user is referred to the ICD-10-PCS code book table as follows:

Example:

Body Part
Refer to the ICD-10-PCS tabular list for a complete list of body parts.

If a body part applies only to a specific root operation in the same document, the specific term is shown in parentheses.

Example:

Body Part
Coronary Artery (Bypass)

5. Approach

This defines the applicable approach value for the techniques used to reach the procedure site.

6. Device

Depending on the procedure performed, there may or may not be a device left in place at the end of the procedure. Applicable devices for the specific procedure are included here. Not all procedures include devices; this element may be omitted or referenced with the value "No Device."

If a device applies only to a specific root operation in the same document, the specific term is shown in parentheses.

Example:

Device
Intraluminal Device (Dilation)

7. Qualifier

A qualifier specifies an additional attribute of the procedure, if applicable. If there is no specific qualifier applicable to the procedure, this section may be omitted or reflected with the value "No Qualifier."

If a qualifier applies only to a specific root operation in the same document, the specific term is shown in parentheses.

Example:

Qualifier
Diagnostic (Excision)

8. Description

Each entry in the desk reference includes a description of the condition being treated or the reason the procedure is performed, followed by an explanation of the procedure, including the types of approaches and details of the procedure steps. If more than one root operation applies to the procedure, a separate description is provided for each root operation.

Example:

Repair
The root operation Repair involves restoring the body part, in this case the inguinal region, inguinal canal, or inguinal triangle to its normal anatomic structure and function. Use the root operation Repair when the inguinal hernia repair is accomplished without the use of a tissue graft or synthetic substitute such as mesh.

Supplement
The root operation Supplement involves repair of the inguinal hernia with the use of biological or synthetic material, such as a tissue graft or mesh. The tissue graft or synthetic material is used to reinforce or augment the muscles and fascia in the inguinal region.

9. Illustration

Illustrations help users better understand the anatomical nuances associated with specific codes and reinforces appropriate code selection. The illustrations usually include a labeled anatomical view and may include narrative that discusses specific procedures or anatomic sites. Most are simplified schematic representations. In many instances, some detail is eliminated to make a clear point about the anatomic site that is the focus of the depiction.

10. Focus Point

Focus Points help the user clarify coding problems and issues that may come up.

Some Focus Points highlight the differences when more than one root operation may apply for similar terms. Key procedure terms differentiating the root operations are identified to ensure that the correct root operation is selected.

Refer to the Focus Points for coding clarification and guidance, and important instructions regarding ICD-10-PCS conventions and guidelines.

11. Coding Guidance

The American Hospital Association's *Coding Clinic for ICD-10-CM and ICD-10-PCS* references are included to help the user master correct coding practices. These identify procedure coding issues and provide answers on how to code them properly, based on a given patient's situation.

AHA coding references first identify the year of the publication, followed by 1Q, 2Q, 3Q, or 4Q indicating the quarter, followed by the page number in AHA's *Coding Clinic for ICD-10-CM and ICD-10-PCS*.

© 2018 Optum360, LLC

ICD-10-PCS Official Guidelines for Coding and Reporting 2019

Narrative changes appear in **bold** text.

The Centers for Medicare and Medicaid Services (CMS) and the National Center for Health Statistics (NCHS), two departments within the U.S. Federal Government's Department of Health and Human Services (DHHS) provide the following guidelines for coding and reporting using the International Classification of Diseases, 10th Revision, Procedure Coding System (ICD-10-PCS). These guidelines should be used as a companion document to the official version of the ICD-10-PCS as published on the CMS website. The ICD-10-PCS is a procedure classification published by the United States for classifying procedures performed in hospital inpatient health care settings.

These guidelines have been approved by the four organizations that make up the Cooperating Parties for the ICD-10-PCS: the American Hospital Association (AHA), the American Health Information Management Association (AHIMA), CMS, and NCHS.

These guidelines are a set of rules that have been developed to accompany and complement the official conventions and instructions provided within the ICD-10-PCS itself. The instructions and conventions of the classification take precedence over guidelines. These guidelines are based on the coding and sequencing instructions in the Tables, Index and Definitions of ICD-10-PCS, but provide additional instruction. Adherence to these guidelines when assigning ICD-10-PCS procedure codes is required under the Health Insurance Portability and Accountability Act (HIPAA). The procedure codes have been adopted under HIPAA for hospital inpatient healthcare settings. A joint effort between the healthcare provider and the coder is essential to achieve complete and accurate documentation, code assignment, and reporting of diagnoses and procedures. These guidelines have been developed to assist both the healthcare provider and the coder in identifying those procedures that are to be reported. The importance of consistent, complete documentation in the medical record cannot be overemphasized. Without such documentation accurate coding cannot be achieved.

Conventions

A1. ICD-10-PCS codes are composed of seven characters. Each character is an axis of classification that specifies information about the procedure performed. Within a defined code range, a character specifies the same type of information in that axis of classification.

Example: The fifth axis of classification specifies the approach in sections Ø through 4 and 7 through 9 of the system.

A2. One of 34 possible values can be assigned to each axis of classification in the seven-character code: they are the numbers Ø through 9 and the alphabet (except I and O because they are easily confused with the numbers 1 and Ø). The number of unique values used in an axis of classification differs as needed.

Example: Where the fifth axis of classification specifies the approach, seven different approach values are currently used to specify the approach.

A3. The valid values for an axis of classification can be added to as needed.

Example: If a significantly distinct type of device is used in a new procedure, a new device value can be added to the system.

A4. As with words in their context, the meaning of any single value is a combination of its axis of classification and any preceding values on which it may be dependent.

Example: The meaning of a body part value in the Medical and Surgical section is always dependent on the body system value. The body part value Ø in the Central Nervous body system specifies Brain and the body part value Ø in the Peripheral Nervous body system specifies Cervical Plexus.

A5. As the system is expanded to become increasingly detailed, over time more values will depend on preceding values for their meaning.

Example: In the Lower Joints body system, the device value 3 in the root operation Insertion specifies Infusion Device and the device value 3 in the root operation Replacement specifies Ceramic Synthetic Substitute.

A6. The purpose of the alphabetic index is to locate the appropriate table that contains all information necessary to construct a procedure code. The PCS Tables should always be consulted to find the most appropriate valid code.

A7. It is not required to consult the index first before proceeding to the tables to complete the code. A valid code may be chosen directly from the tables.

A8. All seven characters must be specified to be a valid code. If the documentation is incomplete for coding purposes, the physician should be queried for the necessary information.

ICD-10-PCS Official Guidelines for Coding and Reporting 2019

A9. Within a PCS table, valid codes include all combinations of choices in characters 4 through 7 contained in the same row of the table. In the example below, ØJHT3VZ is a valid code, and ØJHW3VZ is *not* a valid code.

Section:	Ø	Medical and Surgical
Body System:	J	Subcutaneous Tissue and Fascia
Operation:	H	Insertion Putting in a nonbiological appliance that monitors, assists, performs, or prevents a physiological function but does not physically take the place of a body part

Body Part	Approach	Device	Qualifier
S Subcutaneous Tissue and Fascia, Head and Neck **V** Subcutaneous Tissue and Fascia, Upper Extremity **W** Subcutaneous Tissue and Fascia, Lower Extremity	**Ø** Open **3** Percutaneous	**1** Radioactive Element **3** Infusion Device	**Z** No Qualifier
T Subcutaneous Tissue and Fascia, Trunk	**Ø** Open **3** Percutaneous	**1** Radioactive Element **3** Infusion Device **V** Infusion Pump	**Z** No Qualifier

A10. "And," when used in a code description, means "and/or," **except when used to describe a combination of multiple body parts for which separate values exist for each body part (e.g., Skin and Subcutaneous Tissue used as a qualifier, where there are separate body part values for "Skin" and "Subcutaneous Tissue").**

Example: Lower Arm and Wrist Muscle means lower arm and/or wrist muscle.

A11. Many of the terms used to construct PCS codes are defined within the system. It is the coder's responsibility to determine what the documentation in the medical record equates to in the PCS definitions. The physician is not expected to use the terms used in PCS code descriptions, nor is the coder required to query the physician when the correlation between the documentation and the defined PCS terms is clear.

Example: When the physician documents "partial resection" the coder can independently correlate "partial resection" to the root operation Excision without querying the physician for clarification.

Medical and Surgical Section Guidelines (section Ø)

B2. Body System

General guidelines
B2.1a. The procedure codes in the general anatomical regions body systems can be used when the procedure is performed on an anatomical region rather than a specific body part (e.g., root operations Control and Detachment, Drainage of a body cavity) or on the rare occasion when no information is available to support assignment of a code to a specific body part.

Examples: Control of postoperative hemorrhage is coded to the root operation Control found in the general anatomical regions body systems.

Chest tube drainage of the pleural cavity is coded to the root operation Drainage found in the general anatomical regions body systems. Suture repair of the abdominal wall is coded to the root operation Repair in the general anatomical regions body system.

B2.1b. Where the general body part values "upper" and "lower" are provided as an option in the Upper Arteries, Lower Arteries, Upper Veins, Lower Veins, Muscles and Tendons body systems, "upper" or "lower" specifies body parts located above or below diaphragm respectively.

Example: Vein body parts above the diaphragm are found in the Upper Veins body system; vein body parts below the diaphragm are found in the Lower Veins body system.

B3. Root Operation

General guidelines
B3.1a. In order to determine the appropriate root operation, the full definition of the root operation as contained in the PCS Tables must be applied.

B3.1b. Components of a procedure specified in the root operation definition and explanation are not coded separately. Procedural steps necessary to reach the operative site and close the operative site, including anastomosis of a tubular body part, are also not coded separately.

Examples: Resection of a joint as part of a joint replacement procedure is included in the root operation definition of Replacement and is not coded separately.

© 2018 Optum360, LLC

Laparotomy performed to reach the site of an open liver biopsy is not coded separately. In a resection of sigmoid colon with anastomosis of descending colon to rectum, the anastomosis is not coded separately.

Multiple procedures
B3.2. During the same operative episode, multiple procedures are coded if:

a. The same root operation is performed on different body parts as defined by distinct values of the body part character.

   Examples: Diagnostic excision of liver and pancreas are coded separately.

   Excision of lesion in the ascending colon and excision of lesion in the transverse colon are coded separately.

b. The same root operation is repeated in multiple body parts, and those body parts are separate and distinct body parts classified to a single ICD-10-PCS body part value.

   Examples: Excision of the sartorius muscle and excision of the gracilis muscle are both included in the upper leg muscle body part value, and multiple procedures are coded.

   Extraction of multiple toenails are coded separately.

c. Multiple root operations with distinct objectives are performed on the same body part.

   Example: Destruction of sigmoid lesion and bypass of sigmoid colon are coded separately.

d. The intended root operation is attempted using one approach, but is converted to a different approach.

   Example: Laparoscopic cholecystectomy converted to an open cholecystectomy is coded as percutaneous endoscopic Inspection and open Resection.

Discontinued or incomplete procedures
B3.3. If the intended procedure is discontinued or otherwise not completed, code the procedure to the root operation performed. If a procedure is discontinued before any other root operation is performed, code the root operation Inspection of the body part or anatomical region inspected.

Example: A planned aortic valve replacement procedure is discontinued after the initial thoracotomy and before any incision is made in the heart muscle, when the patient becomes hemodynamically unstable. This procedure is coded as an open Inspection of the mediastinum.

Biopsy procedures
B3.4a. Biopsy procedures are coded using the root operations Excision, Extraction, or Drainage and the qualifier Diagnostic.

Examples: Fine needle aspiration biopsy of fluid in the lung is coded to the root operation Drainage with the qualifier Diagnostic.

Biopsy of bone marrow is coded to the root operation Extraction with the qualifier Diagnostic.

Lymph node sampling for biopsy is coded to the root operation Excision with the qualifier Diagnostic.

Biopsy followed by more definitive treatment
B3.4b. If a diagnostic Excision, Extraction, or Drainage procedure (biopsy) is followed by a more definitive procedure, such as Destruction, Excision or Resection at the same procedure site, both the biopsy and the more definitive treatment are coded.

Example: Biopsy of breast followed by partial mastectomy at the same procedure site, both the biopsy and the partial mastectomy procedure are coded.

Overlapping body layers
B3.5. If the root operations Excision, Repair or Inspection are performed on overlapping layers of the musculoskeletal system, the body part specifying the deepest layer is coded.

Example: Excisional debridement that includes skin and subcutaneous tissue and muscle is coded to the muscle body part.

Bypass procedures
B3.6a. Bypass procedures are coded by identifying the body part bypassed "from" and the body part bypassed "to." The fourth character body part specifies the body part bypassed from, and the qualifier specifies the body part bypassed to.

Example: Bypass from stomach to jejunum, stomach is the body part and jejunum is the qualifier.

B3.6b. Coronary artery bypass procedures are coded differently than other bypass procedures as described in the previous guideline. Rather than identifying the body part bypassed from, the body part identifies the number of coronary arteries bypassed to, and the qualifier specifies the vessel bypassed from.

Example: Aortocoronary artery bypass of the left anterior descending coronary artery and the obtuse marginal coronary artery is classified in the body part axis of classification as two coronary arteries, and the qualifier specifies the aorta as the body part bypassed from.

B3.6c. If multiple coronary arteries are bypassed, a separate procedure is coded for each coronary artery that uses a different device and/or qualifier.

Example: Aortocoronary artery bypass and internal mammary coronary artery bypass are coded separately.

ICD-10-PCS Official Guidelines for Coding and Reporting 2019

Control vs. more definitive root operations

B3.7. The root operation Control is defined as, "Stopping, or attempting to stop, postprocedural or other acute bleeding." If an attempt to stop postprocedural or other acute bleeding is **initially** unsuccessful, and to stop the bleeding requires performing a more definitive root operation, such as Bypass, Detachment, Excision, Extraction, Reposition, Replacement, or Resection, then the more definitive root operation is coded instead of Control.

Example: Resection of spleen to stop bleeding is coded to Resection instead of Control.

Excision vs. Resection

B3.8. PCS contains specific body parts for anatomical subdivisions of a body part, such as lobes of the lungs or liver and regions of the intestine. Resection of the specific body part is coded whenever all of the body part is cut out or off, rather than coding Excision of a less specific body part.

Example: Left upper lung lobectomy is coded to Resection of Upper Lung Lobe, Left rather than Excision of Lung, Left.

Excision for graft

B3.9. If an autograft is obtained from a different procedure site in order to complete the objective of the procedure, a separate procedure is coded.

Example: Coronary bypass with excision of saphenous vein graft, excision of saphenous vein is coded separately.

Fusion procedures of the spine

B3.10a. The body part coded for a spinal vertebral joint(s) rendered immobile by a spinal fusion procedure is classified by the level of the spine (e.g. thoracic). There are distinct body part values for a single vertebral joint and for multiple vertebral joints at each spinal level.

Example: Body part values specify Lumbar Vertebral Joint, Lumbar Vertebral Joints, 2 or More and Lumbosacral Vertebral Joint.

B3.10b. If multiple vertebral joints are fused, a separate procedure is coded for each vertebral joint that uses a different device and/or qualifier.

Example: Fusion of lumbar vertebral joint, posterior approach, anterior column and fusion of lumbar vertebral joint, posterior approach, posterior column are coded separately.

B3.10c. Combinations of devices and materials are often used on a vertebral joint to render the joint immobile. When combinations of devices are used on the same vertebral joint, the device value coded for the procedure is as follows:

- If an interbody fusion device is used to render the joint immobile (alone or containing other

material like bone graft), the procedure is coded with the device value Interbody Fusion Device

- If bone graft is the *only* device used to render the joint immobile, the procedure is coded with the device value Nonautologous Tissue Substitute or Autologous Tissue Substitute

- If a mixture of autologous and nonautologous bone graft (with or without biological or synthetic extenders or binders) is used to render the joint immobile, code the procedure with the device value Autologous Tissue Substitute

Examples: Fusion of a vertebral joint using a cage style interbody fusion device containing morsellized bone graft is coded to the device Interbody Fusion Device.

Fusion of a vertebral joint using a bone dowel interbody fusion device made of cadaver bone and packed with a mixture of local morsellized bone and demineralized bone matrix is coded to the device Interbody Fusion Device.

Fusion of a vertebral joint using both autologous bone graft and bone bank bone graft is coded to the device Autologous Tissue Substitute.

Inspection procedures

B3.11a. Inspection of a body part(s) performed in order to achieve the objective of a procedure is not coded separately.

Example: Fiberoptic bronchoscopy performed for irrigation of bronchus, only the irrigation procedure is coded.

B3.11b. If multiple tubular body parts are inspected, the most distal body part (the body part furthest from the starting point of the inspection) is coded. If multiple non-tubular body parts in a region are inspected, the body part that specifies the entire area inspected is coded.

Examples: Cystoureteroscopy with inspection of bladder and ureters is coded to the ureter body part value.

Exploratory laparotomy with general inspection of abdominal contents is coded to the peritoneal cavity body part value.

B3.11c. When both an Inspection procedure and another procedure are performed on the same body part during the same episode, if the Inspection procedure is performed using a different approach than the other procedure, the Inspection procedure is coded separately.

Example: Endoscopic Inspection of the duodenum is coded separately when open Excision of the duodenum is performed during the same procedural episode.

© 2018 Optum360, LLC

Occlusion vs. Restriction for vessel embolization procedures
B3.12. If the objective of an embolization procedure is to completely close a vessel, the root operation Occlusion is coded. If the objective of an embolization procedure is to narrow the lumen of a vessel, the root operation Restriction is coded.

Examples: Tumor embolization is coded to the root operation Occlusion, because the objective of the procedure is to cut off the blood supply to the vessel.

Embolization of a cerebral aneurysm is coded to the root operation Restriction, because the objective of the procedure is not to close off the vessel entirely, but to narrow the lumen of the vessel at the site of the aneurysm where it is abnormally wide.

Release procedures
B3.13. In the root operation Release, the body part value coded is the body part being freed and not the tissue being manipulated or cut to free the body part.

Example: Lysis of intestinal adhesions is coded to the specific intestine body part value.

Release vs. Division
B3.14. If the sole objective of the procedure is freeing a body part without cutting the body part, the root operation is Release. If the sole objective of the procedure is separating or transecting a body part, the root operation is Division.

Examples: Freeing a nerve root from surrounding scar tissue to relieve pain is coded to the root operation Release.

Severing a nerve root to relieve pain is coded to the root operation Division.

Reposition for fracture treatment
B3.15. Reduction of a displaced fracture is coded to the root operation Reposition and the application of a cast or splint in conjunction with the Reposition procedure is not coded separately. Treatment of a nondisplaced fracture is coded to the procedure performed.

Examples: Casting of a nondisplaced fracture is coded to the root operation Immobilization in the Placement section.

Putting a pin in a nondisplaced fracture is coded to the root operation Insertion.

Transplantation vs. Administration
B3.16. Putting in a mature and functioning living body part taken from another individual or animal is coded to the root operation Transplantation. Putting in autologous or nonautologous cells is coded to the Administration section.

Example: Putting in autologous or nonautologous bone marrow, pancreatic islet cells or stem cells is coded to the Administration section.

Transfer procedures using multiple tissue layers
B3.17. The root operation Transfer contains qualifiers that can be used to specify when a transfer flap is composed of more than one tissue layer, such as a musculocutaneous flap. For procedures involving transfer of multiple tissue layers including skin, subcutaneous tissue, fascia or muscle, the procedure is coded to the body part value that describes the deepest tissue layer in the flap, and the qualifier can be used to describe the other tissue layer(s) in the transfer flap.

Example: A musculocutaneous flap transfer is coded to the appropriate body part value in the body system Muscles, and the qualifier is used to describe the additional tissue layer(s) in the transfer flap.

B4. Body Part

General guidelines
B4.1a. If a procedure is performed on a portion of a body part that does not have a separate body part value, code the body part value corresponding to the whole body part.

Example: A procedure performed on the alveolar process of the mandible is coded to the mandible body part.

B4.1b. If the prefix "peri" is combined with a body part to identify the site of the procedure, and the site of the procedure is not further specified, then the procedure is coded to the body part named. This guideline applies only when a more specific body part value is not available.

Examples: A procedure site identified as perirenal is coded to the kidney body part when the site of the procedure is not further specified.

A procedure site described in the documentation as peri-urethral, and the documentation also indicates that it is the vulvar tissue and not the urethral tissue that is the site of the procedure, then the procedure is coded to the vulva body part.

B4.1c. If a procedure is performed on a continuous section of a tubular body part, code the body part value corresponding to the furthest anatomical site from the point of entry.

Example: A procedure performed on a continuous section of artery from the femoral artery to the external iliac artery with the point of entry at the femoral artery is coded to the external iliac body part.

Branches of body parts
B4.2. Where a specific branch of a body part does not have its own body part value in PCS, the body part is typically coded to the closest proximal branch that has a specific body part value. In the cardiovascular body systems, if a general body part is available in the correct root operation table, and coding to a proximal

ICD-10-PCS Official Guidelines for Coding and Reporting 2019

ICD-10-PCS Official Guidelines for Coding and Reporting 2019

branch would require assigning a code in a different body system, the procedure is coded using the general body part value.

Examples: A procedure performed on the mandibular branch of the trigeminal nerve is coded to the trigeminal nerve body part value.

Occlusion of the bronchial artery is coded to the body part value Upper Artery in the body system Upper Arteries, and not to the body part value Thoracic Aorta, Descending in the body system Heart and Great Vessels.

Bilateral body part values

B4.3. Bilateral body part values are available for a limited number of body parts. If the identical procedure is performed on contralateral body parts, and a bilateral body part value exists for that body part, a single procedure is coded using the bilateral body part value. If no bilateral body part value exists, each procedure is coded separately using the appropriate body part value.

Examples: The identical procedure performed on both fallopian tubes is coded once using the body part value Fallopian Tube, Bilateral.

The identical procedure performed on both knee joints is coded twice using the body part values Knee Joint, Right and Knee Joint, Left.

Coronary arteries

B4.4. The coronary arteries are classified as a single body part that is further specified by number of arteries treated. One procedure code specifying multiple arteries is used when the same procedure is performed, including the same device and qualifier values.

Examples: Angioplasty of two distinct coronary arteries with placement of two stents is coded as Dilation of Coronary Artery, Two Arteries with Two Intraluminal Devices.

Angioplasty of two distinct coronary arteries, one with stent placed and one without, is coded separately as Dilation of Coronary Artery, One Artery with Intraluminal Device, and Dilation of Coronary Artery, One Artery with no device.

Tendons, ligaments, bursae and fascia near a joint

B4.5. Procedures performed on tendons, ligaments, bursae and fascia supporting a joint are coded to the body part in the respective body system that is the focus of the procedure. Procedures performed on joint structures themselves are coded to the body part in the joint body systems.

Examples: Repair of the anterior cruciate ligament of the knee is coded to the knee bursa and ligament body part in the bursae and ligaments body system.

Knee arthroscopy with shaving of articular cartilage is coded to the knee joint body part in the Lower Joints body system.

Skin, subcutaneous tissue and fascia overlying a joint

B4.6. If a procedure is performed on the skin, subcutaneous tissue or fascia overlying a joint, the procedure is coded to the following body part:

- Shoulder is coded to Upper Arm
- Elbow is coded to Lower Arm
- Wrist is coded to Lower Arm
- Hip is coded to Upper Leg
- Knee is coded to Lower Leg
- Ankle is coded to Foot

Fingers and toes

B4.7. If a body system does not contain a separate body part value for fingers, procedures performed on the fingers are coded to the body part value for the hand. If a body system does not contain a separate body part value for toes, procedures performed on the toes are coded to the body part value for the foot.

Example: Excision of finger muscle is coded to one of the hand muscle body part values in the Muscles body system.

Upper and lower intestinal tract

B4.8. In the Gastrointestinal body system, the general body part values Upper Intestinal Tract and Lower Intestinal Tract are provided as an option for the root operations Change, Inspection, Removal and Revision. Upper Intestinal Tract includes the portion of the gastrointestinal tract from the esophagus down to and including the duodenum, and Lower Intestinal Tract includes the portion of the gastrointestinal tract from the jejunum down to and including the rectum and anus.

Example: In the root operation Change table, change of a device in the jejunum is coded using the body part Lower Intestinal Tract.

B5. Approach

Open approach with percutaneous endoscopic assistance

B5.2. Procedures performed using the open approach with percutaneous endoscopic assistance are coded to the approach Open.

Example: Laparoscopic-assisted sigmoidectomy is coded to the approach Open.

External approach

B5.3a. Procedures performed within an orifice on structures that are visible without the aid of any instrumentation are coded to the approach External.

Example: Resection of tonsils is coded to the approach External.

© 2018 Optum360, LLC

B5.3b. Procedures performed indirectly by the application of external force through the intervening body layers are coded to the approach External.

Example: Closed reduction of fracture is coded to the approach External.

Percutaneous procedure via device
B5.4. Procedures performed percutaneously via a device placed for the procedure are coded to the approach Percutaneous.

Example: Fragmentation of kidney stone performed via percutaneous nephrostomy is coded to the approach Percutaneous.

B6. Device

General guidelines
B6.1a. A device is coded only if a device remains after the procedure is completed. If no device remains, the device value No Device is coded. In limited root operations, the classification provides the qualifier values Temporary and Intraoperative, for specific procedures involving clinically significant devices, where the purpose of the device is to be utilized for a brief duration during the procedure or current inpatient stay. **If a device that is intended to remain after the procedure is completed requires removal before the end of the operative episode in which it was inserted (for example, the device size is inadequate or a complication occurs), both the insertion and removal of the device should be coded.**

B6.1b. Materials such as sutures, ligatures, radiological markers and temporary post-operative wound drains are considered integral to the performance of a procedure and are not coded as devices.

B6.1c. Procedures performed on a device only and not on a body part are specified in the root operations Change, Irrigation, Removal and Revision, and are coded to the procedure performed.

Example: Irrigation of percutaneous nephrostomy tube is coded to the root operation Irrigation of indwelling device in the Administration section.

Drainage device
B6.2. A separate procedure to put in a drainage device is coded to the root operation Drainage with the device value Drainage Device.

Obstetric Section Guidelines (section 1)

C. Obstetrics Section

Products of conception
C1. Procedures performed on the products of conception are coded to the Obstetrics section. Procedures performed on the pregnant female other than the products of conception are coded to the appropriate root operation in the Medical and Surgical section.

Example: Amniocentesis is coded to the products of conception body part in the Obstetrics section. Repair of obstetric urethral laceration is coded to the urethra body part in the Medical and Surgical section.

Procedures following delivery or abortion
C2. Procedures performed following a delivery or abortion for curettage of the endometrium or evacuation of retained products of conception are all coded in the Obstetrics section, to the root operation Extraction and the body part Products of Conception, Retained.

Diagnostic or therapeutic dilation and curettage performed during times other than the postpartum or post-abortion period are all coded in the Medical and Surgical section, to the root operation Extraction and the body part Endometrium.

New Technology Section Guidelines (section X)

D. New Technology Section

General guidelines
D1. Section X codes are standalone codes. They are not supplemental codes. Section X codes fully represent the specific procedure described in the code title, and do not require any additional codes from other sections of ICD-10-PCS. When section X contains a code title which describes a specific new technology procedure, only that X code is reported for the procedure. There is no need to report a broader, non-specific code in another section of ICD-10-PCS.

Example: XW04321 Introduction of Ceftazidime-Avibactam Anti-infective into Central Vein, Percutaneous Approach, New Technology Group 1, can be coded to indicate that Ceftazidime-Avibactam Anti-infective was administered via a central vein. A separate code from table 3E0 in the Administration section of ICD-10-PCS is not coded in addition to this code.

Selection of Principal Procedure

The following instructions should be applied in the selection of principal procedure and clarification on the importance of the relation to the principal diagnosis when more than one procedure is performed:

1. Procedure performed for definitive treatment of both principal diagnosis and secondary diagnosis

ICD-10-PCS Official Guidelines for Coding and Reporting 2019

a. Sequence procedure performed for definitive treatment most related to principal diagnosis as principal procedure.

2. Procedure performed for definitive treatment and diagnostic procedures performed for both principal diagnosis and secondary diagnosis.

   a. Sequence procedure performed for definitive treatment most related to principal diagnosis as principal procedure

3. A diagnostic procedure was performed for the principal diagnosis and a procedure is performed for definitive treatment of a secondary diagnosis.

a. Sequence diagnostic procedure as principal procedure, since the procedure most related to the principal diagnosis takes precedence.

4. No procedures performed that are related to principal diagnosis; procedures performed for definitive treatment and diagnostic procedures were performed for secondary diagnosis

   a. Sequence procedure performed for definitive treatment of secondary diagnosis as principal procedure, since there are no procedures (definitive or nondefinitive treatment) related to principal diagnosis.

© 2018 Optum360, LLC

ICD-10-PCS Root Operation Definitions

ICD-10-PCS Root Operation Definitions

Ø Medical and Surgical

ICD-10-PCS Value			Definition
Ø	Alteration	Definition:	Modifying the anatomic structure of a body part without affecting the function of the body part
		Explanation:	Principal purpose is to improve appearance
		Examples:	Face lift, breast augmentation
1	Bypass	Definition:	Altering the route of passage of the contents of a tubular body part
		Explanation:	Rerouting contents of a body part to a downstream area of the normal route, to a similar route and body part, or to an abnormal route and dissimilar body part. Includes one or more anastomoses, with or without the use of a device.
		Examples:	Coronary artery bypass, colostomy formation
2	Change	Definition:	Taking out or off a device from a body part and putting back an identical or similar device in or on the same body part without cutting or puncturing the skin or a mucous membrane
		Explanation:	All CHANGE procedures are coded using the approach EXTERNAL
		Example:	Urinary catheter change, gastrostomy tube change
3	Control	Definition:	Stopping, or attempting to stop, postprocedural or other acute bleeding
		Explanation:	The site of the bleeding is coded as an anatomical region and not to a specific body part
		Examples:	Control of post-prostatectomy hemorrhage, control of intracranial subdural hemorrhage, control of bleeding duodenal ulcer, control of retroperitoneal hemorrhage
4	Creation	Definition:	Putting in or on biological or synthetic material to form a new body part that to the extent possible replicates the anatomic structure or function of an absent body part
		Explanation:	Used for gender reassignment surgery and corrective procedures in individuals with congenital anomalies
		Examples:	Creation of vagina in a male, creation of right and left atrioventricular valve from common atrioventricular valve
5	Destruction	Definition:	Physical eradication of all or a portion of a body part by the direct use of energy, force, or a destructive agent
		Explanation:	None of the body part is physically taken out
		Examples:	Fulguration of rectal polyp, cautery of skin lesion
6	Detachment	Definition:	Cutting off all or a portion of the upper or lower extremities
		Explanation:	The body part value is the site of the detachment, with a qualifier if applicable to further specify the level where the extremity was detached
		Examples:	Below knee amputation, disarticulation of shoulder
7	Dilation	Definition:	Expanding an orifice or the lumen of a tubular body part
		Explanation:	The orifice can be a natural orifice or an artificially created orifice. Accomplished by stretching a tubular body part using intraluminal pressure or by cutting part of the orifice or wall of the tubular body part.
		Examples:	Percutaneous transluminal angioplasty, internal urethrotomy

Ø   Medical and Surgical (continued)

ICD-10-PCS Value		Definition
8	Division	**Definition:** Cutting into a body part, without draining fluids and/or gases from the body part, in order to separate or transect a body part
		Explanation: All or a portion of the body part is separated into two or more portions
		Examples: Spinal cordotomy, osteotomy
9	Drainage	**Definition:** Taking or letting out fluids and/or gases from a body part
		Explanation: The qualifier DIAGNOSTIC is used to identify drainage procedures that are biopsies
		Examples: Thoracentesis, incision and drainage
B	Excision	**Definition:** Cutting out or off, without replacement, a portion of a body part
		Explanation: The qualifier DIAGNOSTIC is used to identify excision procedures that are biopsies
		Examples: Partial nephrectomy, liver biopsy
C	Extirpation	**Definition:** Taking or cutting out solid matter from a body part
		Explanation: The solid matter may be an abnormal byproduct of a biological function or a foreign body; it may be imbedded in a body part or in the lumen of a tubular body part. The solid matter may or may not have been previously broken into pieces.
		Examples: Thrombectomy, choledocholithotomy
D	Extraction	**Definition:** Pulling or stripping out or off all or a portion of a body part by the use of force
		Explanation: The qualifier DIAGNOSTIC is used to identify extractions that are biopsies
		Examples: Dilation and curettage, vein stripping
F	Fragmentation	**Definition:** Breaking solid matter in a body part into pieces
		Explanation: Physical force (e.g., manual, ultrasonic) applied directly or indirectly is used to break the solid matter into pieces. The solid matter may be an abnormal byproduct of a biological function or a foreign body. The pieces of solid matter are not taken out.
		Examples: Extracorporeal shockwave lithotripsy, transurethral lithotripsy
G	Fusion	**Definition:** Joining together portions of an articular body part rendering the articular body part immobile
		Explanation: The body part is joined together by fixation device, bone graft, or other means
		Examples: Spinal fusion, ankle arthrodesis
H	Insertion	**Definition:** Putting in a nonbiological appliance that monitors, assists, performs, or prevents a physiological function but does not physically take the place of a body part
		Explanation: None
		Examples: Insertion of radioactive implant, insertion of central venous catheter
J	Inspection	**Definition:** Visually and/or manually exploring a body part
		Explanation: Visual exploration may be performed with or without optical instrumentation. Manual exploration may be performed directly or through intervening body layers.
		Examples: Diagnostic arthroscopy, exploratory laparotomy

ICD-10-PCS Root Operation Definitions

© 2018 Optum360, LLC

Ø Medical and Surgical (continued)

ICD-10-PCS Value		Definition
K	Map	Definition:	Locating the route of passage of electrical impulses and/or locating functional areas in a body part
		Explanation:	Applicable only to the cardiac conduction mechanism and the central nervous system
		Examples:	Cardiac mapping, cortical mapping
L	Occlusion	Definition:	Completely closing an orifice or lumen of a tubular body part
		Explanation:	The orifice can be a natural orifice or an artificially created orifice
		Examples:	Fallopian tube ligation, ligation of inferior vena cava
M	Reattachment	Definition:	Putting back in or on all or a portion of a separated body part to its normal location or other suitable location
		Explanation:	Vascular circulation and nervous pathways may or may not be reestablished
		Examples:	Reattachment of hand, reattachment of avulsed kidney
N	Release	Definition:	Freeing a body part from an abnormal physical constraint by cutting or by use of force
		Explanation:	Some of the restraining tissue may be taken out but none of the body part is taken out
		Examples:	Adhesiolysis, carpal tunnel release
P	Removal	Definition:	Taking out or off a device from a body part
		Explanation:	If a device is taken out and a similar device put in without cutting or puncturing the skin or mucous membrane, the procedure is coded to the root operation CHANGE. Otherwise, the procedure for taking out a device is coded to the root operation REMOVAL.
		Examples:	Drainage tube removal, cardiac pacemaker removal
Q	Repair	Definition:	Restoring, to the extent possible, a body part to its normal anatomic structure and function
		Explanation:	Used only when the method to accomplish the repair is not one of the other root operations
		Examples:	Colostomy takedown, suture of laceration
R	Replacement	Definition:	Putting in or on biological or synthetic material that physically takes the place and/or function of all or a portion of a body part
		Explanation:	The body part may have been taken out or replaced, or may be taken out, physically eradicated, or rendered nonfunctional during the REPLACEMENT procedure. A REMOVAL procedure is coded for taking out the device used in a previous replacement procedure.
		Examples:	Total hip replacement, bone graft, free skin graft
S	Reposition	Definition:	Moving to its normal location, or other suitable location, all or a portion of a body part
		Explanation:	The body part is moved to a new location from an abnormal location, or from a normal location where it is not functioning correctly. The body part may or may not be cut out or off to be moved to the new location.
		Examples:	Reposition of undescended testicle, fracture reduction
T	Resection	Definition:	Cutting out or off, without replacement, all of a body part
		Explanation:	None
		Examples:	Total nephrectomy, total lobectomy of lung

ICD-10-PCS Root
Operation Definitions

Ø   Medical and Surgical (continued)

ICD-10-PCS Value			Definition
V	Restriction	Definition:	Partially closing an orifice or the lumen of a tubular body part
		Explanation:	The orifice can be a natural orifice or an artificially created orifice
		Examples:	Esophagogastric fundoplication, cervical cerclage
W	Revision	Definition:	Correcting, to the extent possible, a portion of a malfunctioning device or the position of a displaced device
		Explanation:	Revision can include correcting a malfunctioning or displaced device by taking out or putting in components of the device such as a screw or pin
		Examples:	Adjustment of position of pacemaker lead, recementing of hip prosthesis
U	Supplement	Definition:	Putting in or on biological or synthetic material that physically reinforces and/or augments the function of a portion of a body part
		Explanation:	The biological material is non-living, or is living and from the same individual. The body part may have been previously replaced, and the SUPPLEMENT procedure is performed to physically reinforce and/or augment the function of the replaced body part.
		Examples:	Herniorrhaphy using mesh, free nerve graft, mitral valve ring annuloplasty, put a new acetabular liner in a previous hip replacement
X	Transfer	Definition:	Moving, without taking out, all or a portion of a body part to another location to take over the function of all or a portion of a body part
		Explanation:	The body part transferred remains connected to its vascular and nervous supply
		Examples:	Tendon transfer, skin pedicle flap transfer
Y	Transplantation	Definition:	Putting in or on all or a portion of a living body part taken from another individual or animal to physically take the place and/or function of all or a portion of a similar body part
		Explanation:	The native body part may or may not be taken out, and the transplanted body part may take over all or a portion of its function
		Examples:	Kidney transplant, heart transplant

ICD-10-PCS Root Operation Definitions

© 2018 Optum360, LLC

Root Operation Definitions for Other Sections

1   Obstetrics

ICD-10-PCS Value			Definition
2	Change	Definition:	Taking out or off a device from a body part and putting back an identical or similar device in or on the same body part without cutting or puncturing the skin or a mucous membrane
		Explanation:	None
		Examples:	Replacement of fetal scalp electrode
9	Drainage	Definition:	Taking or letting out fluids and/or gases from a body part
		Explanation:	None
		Examples:	Biopsy of amniotic fluid
A	Abortion	Definition:	Artificially terminating a pregnancy
		Explanation:	None
		Examples:	Transvaginal abortion using vacuum aspiration technique
D	Extraction	Definition:	Pulling or stripping out or off all or a portion of a body part by the use of force
		Explanation:	None
		Examples:	Low-transverse C-section
E	Delivery	Definition:	Assisting the passage of the products of conception from the genital canal
		Explanation:	None
		Examples:	Manually-assisted delivery
H	Insertion	Definition:	Putting in a nonbiological appliance that monitors, assists, performs, or prevents a physiological function but does not physically take the place of a body part
		Explanation:	None
		Examples:	Placement of fetal scalp electrode
J	Inspection	Definition:	Visually and/or manually exploring a body part
		Explanation:	Visual exploration may be performed with or without optical instrumentation. Manual exploration may be performed directly or through intervening body layers.
		Examples:	Bimanual pregnancy exam
P	Removal	Definition:	Taking out or off a device from a body part, region or orifice
		Explanation:	If a device is taken out and a similar device put in without cutting or puncturing the skin or mucous membrane, the procedure is coded to the root operation CHANGE. Otherwise, the procedure for taking out a device is coded to the root operation REMOVAL.
		Examples:	Removal of fetal monitoring electrode
Q	Repair	Definition:	Restoring, to the extent possible, a body part to its normal anatomic structure and function
		Explanation:	Used only when the method to accomplish the repair is not one of the other root operations
		Examples:	In utero repair of congenital diaphragmatic hernia

ICD-10-PCS Root
Operation Definitions

1 Obstetrics (continued)

ICD-10-PCS Value			Definition
S	Reposition	Definition:	Moving to its normal location, or other suitable location, all or a portion of a body part
		Explanation:	The body part is moved to a new location from an abnormal location, or from a normal location where it is not functioning correctly. The body part may or may not be cut out or off to be moved to the new location.
		Examples:	External version of fetus
T	Resection	Definition:	Cutting out or off, without replacement, all of a body part
		Explanation:	None
		Examples:	Total excision of tubal pregnancy
Y	Transplantation	Definition:	Putting in or on all or a portion of a living body part taken from another individual or animal to physically take the place and/or function of all or a portion of a similar body part
		Explanation:	The native body part may or may not be taken out, and the transplanted body part may take over all or a portion of its function
		Examples:	In utero fetal kidney transplant

2 Placement

ICD-10-PCS Value			Definition
Ø	Change	Definition:	Taking out or off a device from a body region and putting back an identical or similar device in or on the same body region without cutting or puncturing the skin or a mucous membrane
		Examples:	Change of vaginal packing
1	Compression	Definition:	Putting pressure on a body region
		Examples:	Placement of pressure dressing on abdominal wall
2	Dressing	Definition:	Putting material on a body region for protection
		Examples:	Application of sterile dressing to head wound
3	Immobilization	Definition:	Limiting or preventing motion of a body region
		Examples:	Placement of splint on left finger
4	Packing	Definition:	Putting material in a body region or orifice
		Examples:	Placement of nasal packing
5	Removal	Definition:	Taking out or off a device from a body part
		Examples:	Removal of stereotactic head frame
6	Traction	Definition:	Exerting a pulling force on a body region in a distal direction
		Examples:	Lumbar traction using motorized split-traction table

ICD-10-PCS Root Operation Definitions

© 2018 Optum360, LLC

3   Administration

ICD-10-PCS Value			Definition
Ø	Introduction	Definition:	Putting in or on a therapeutic, diagnostic, nutritional, physiological, or prophylactic substance except blood or blood products
		Examples:	Nerve block injection to median nerve
1	Irrigation	Definition:	Putting in or on a cleansing substance
		Examples:	Flushing of eye
2	Transfusion	Definition:	Putting in blood or blood products
		Examples:	Transfusion of cell saver red cells into central venous line

4   Measurement and Monitoring

ICD-10-PCS Value			Definition
Ø	Measurement	Definition:	Determining the level of a physiological or physical function at a point in time
		Examples:	External electrocardiogram(EKG), single reading
1	Monitoring	Definition:	Determining the level of a physiological or physical function repetitively over a period of time
		Examples:	Urinary pressure monitoring

5   Extracorporeal Assistance and Performance

ICD-10-PCS Value			Definition
Ø	Assistance	Definition:	Taking over a portion of a physiological function by extracorporeal means
		Examples:	Hyperbaric oxygenation of wound
1	Performance	Definition:	Completely taking over a physiological function by extracorporeal means
		Examples:	Cardiopulmonary bypass in conjunction with CABG
2	Restoration	Definition:	Returning, or attempting to return, a physiological function to its original state by extracorporeal means
		Examples:	Attempted cardiac defibrillation, unsuccessful

6   Extracorporeal Therapies

ICD-10-PCS Value			Definition
Ø	Atmospheric Control	Definition:	Extracorporeal control of atmospheric pressure and composition
		Examples:	Antigen-free air conditioning, series treatment
1	Decompression	Definition:	Extracorporeal elimination of undissolved gas from body fluids
		Examples:	Hyperbaric decompression treatment, single
2	Electromagnetic Therapy	Definition:	Extracorporeal treatment by electromagnetic rays
		Examples:	TMS (transcranial magnetic stimulation), series treatment
3	Hyperthermia	Definition:	Extracorporeal raising of body temperature
		Examples:	None
4	Hypothermia	Definition:	Extracorporeal lowering of body temperature
		Examples:	Whole body hypothermia treatment for temperature imbalances, series
5	Pheresis	Definition:	Extracorporeal separation of blood products
		Examples:	Therapeutic leukopheresis, single treatment

ICD-10-PCS Root
Operation Definitions

6 Extracorporeal Therapies (continued)

ICD-10-PCS Value			Definition
6	Phototherapy	Definition:	Extracorporeal treatment by light rays
		Examples:	Phototherapy of circulatory system, series treatment
7	Ultrasound Therapy	Definition:	Extracorporeal treatment by ultrasound
		Examples:	Therapeutic ultrasound of peripheral vessels, single treatment
8	Ultraviolet Light Therapy	Definition:	Extracorporeal treatment by ultraviolet light
		Examples:	Ultraviolet light phototherapy, series treatment
9	Shock Wave Therapy	Definition:	Extracorporeal treatment by shock waves
		Examples:	Shockwave therapy of plantar fascia, single treatment
B	Perfusion	Definition:	Extracorporeal treatment by diffusion of therapeutic fluid
		Examples:	Perfusion of donor liver while preparing transplant patient

7 Osteopathic

ICD-10-PCS Value			Definition
Ø	Treatment	Definition:	Manual treatment to eliminate or alleviate somatic dysfunction and related disorders
		Examples:	Fascial release of abdomen, osteopathic treatment

8 Other Procedures

ICD-10-PCS Value			Definition
Ø	Other Procedures	Definition:	Methodologies which attempt to remediate or cure a disorder or disease
		Examples:	Acupuncture, yoga therapy

9 Chiropractic

ICD-10-PCS Value			Definition
B	Manipulation	Definition:	Manual procedure that involves a directed thrust to move a joint past the physiological range of motion, without exceeding the anatomical limit
		Examples:	Chiropractic treatment of cervical spine, short lever specific contact

Note: Sections B-H (Imaging through Substance Abuse Treatment) do not include root operations. The character 3 position represents type of procedure, therefore those definitions are not included in this appendix.

© 2018 Optum360, LLC

Abbreviations, Acronyms, and Symbols

The acronyms, abbreviations, and symbols health care providers use speed communications. The following list includes the most often seen acronyms, abbreviations, and symbols. When abbreviations have more than one meaning, multiple interpretations are separated by a slash (/). Abbreviations of Latin phrases are punctuated.

@	at
"	inch
<	less than
>	greater than
3D	three dimensional
A	assessment/blood type
a (ante)	before
a fib	atrial fibrillation
a flutter	atrial flutter
A&P	auscultation and percussion/anatomy and physiology
a.a.	of each
a.c.	before eating
a.d.	right ear/to, up to
a.m.	morning
a.s.	left ear
a.u.	each ear/both ears
A/G	albumin-globulin ratio
A2	aortic second sound
AAA	abdominal aortic aneurysm
AAC	apical-aortic conduit
AAL	anterior axillary line
AAPC	American Academy of Professional Coders
AAROM	active assistive range of motion
ab	abortion
AB	blood type
abd	abdomen
ABE	acute bacterial endocarditis
ABG	arterial blood gas
abn.	abnormal
ABO	referring to ABO incompatibility
abs. fev.	without fever
ACA	Affordable Care Act
ACD	absolute cardiac dullness
ACE	angiotensin converting enzyme/adrenal cortical extract
ACF	anterior cervical fusion
ACI	autologous chondrocyte implantation
ACL	anterior cruciate ligament
ACLS	advanced cardiac life support
ACP	acid phosphatase
acq.	acquired
ACTH	adrenocorticotropic hormone
ACVD	acute cardiovascular disease
ad lib	as desired, at pleasure
ad. hib.	to be administered
ad. lib.	as desired
ad. us. ext.	for external use
ADEM	acute disseminated encephalomyelitis
ADH	antidiuretic hormone
ADL	activities of daily living
adm	admission, admit
ADM	alcohol, drug or mental disorder
ADP	adenosine diphosphate
ADR	artificial disc replacement
ADS	alternative delivery system
adst. feb.	when fever is present
AE	above the elbow
AEA	anterior ethmoidal artery
AEDs	anti-epileptic drugs
AESOP®	Automated Endoscopic System for Optimal Positioning
AET	ab externo trabeculectomy
AF	atrial fibrillation/amniotic fluid
AFB	acid fast bacilli
AFP	alpha-fetoprotein
ag. feb.	when the fever increases
AGA	appropriate (average) for gestational age
AgNO3	silver nitrate
AHA	American Hospital Association
AHC	alternative health care
AHIMA	American Health Information Management Association
AHTR	acute hemolytic transfusion reaction
AI	aortic insufficiency
AICD	automatic implant cardioverter defibrillator
AID	artificial insemination donor/acute infectious disease
AIDS	acquired immunodeficiency syndrome
AIH	artificial insemination by husband
AIN	anal intraepithelial neoplasia
AIPHI	acute idiopathic pulmonary hemorrhage in infants

© 2018 Optum360, LLC

AIS	androgen insensitivity syndrome
AK	above the knee
AKA	above knee amputation
AKI	acute kidney injury
ALA	aminolevulinic acid
alb. (albus)	white
ALIF	anterior lumbar interbody fusion
alk. phos.	alkaline phosphatase
ALL	acute lymphocytic leukemia
ALOS	average length of stay
ALP	alkaline phosphatase
ALPS	autoimmune lymphoproliferative syndrome
ALS	advanced life support/amyotrophic lateral sclerosis
ALT	alanine aminotransferase/argon laser trabeculoplasty
alt. dieb.	every other day
alt. hor.	every other hour
alt. noc.	every other night
ALTE	apparent life threatening event
ama	against medical advice
AMA	American Medical Association
amb	ambulate
AMI	acute myocardial infarction
AML	acute myelogenous leukemia
AMML	acute myelomonocytic leukemia
AMP	adenosine monophosphate/ampule
ANA	American Nursing Association/ antinuclear antibodies
ANC	absolute neutrophil count
ANS	autonomic nervous system
ant	anterior
AO	aqueous oxygen
AOD	arterial occlusive disease
AODM	adult onset diabetes mellitus
AP	antepartum/anterior-posterior
Ap	apical
A-P	anterior posterior
APC	ambulatory payment classification
APD	automated peritoneal dialysis
APM	arterial pressure monitoring
approx	approximately
appy.	appendectomy
APR	abdominoperineal resection
aq.	water (aqua)
ARC	AIDS-related complex
ARD	acute respiratory disease
ARDS	adult respiratory distress syndrome
ARF	acute respiratory/renal failure

AROM	active range of motion/artificial rupture of membranes
art.	artery, arterial
AS	aortic stenosis/ arteriosclerosis
ASAP	as soon as possible
ASC	ambulatory surgery center
ASC-H	atypical squamous cell cannot exclude high grade squamous intraepithelial lesion
ASC-US	atypical squamous cell of undetermined significance
ASCVD	arteriosclerotic cardiovascular disease
ASD	atrial septal defect
ASHD	arteriosclerotic heart disease
ASO	administrative services only
ASR	age/sex rate
Asst	assistance (min= minimal; mod=moderate)
AST	aspartate aminotransferase
ATP	adenosine triphosphate
ATT	alpha-1 antitrypsin
AUFI	absolute uterine factor infertility
AUS	artificial urinary sphincter
AV	atrioventricular
A-V	arteriovenous
AVF	arteriovenous fistula
AVM	arteriovenous malformation
ax	auxiliary
AxiaLIF	axial lumbar interbody fusion
AZT	azidothymidine
B&B	bowel and bladder
b.i.d.	two times a day
b.i.n.	twice a night
b.i.s.	twice
Ba	barium
BAEP	brainstorm auditory evoked potentials
BAL	bronchoalveolar lavage
bal.	bath
BBB	bundle branch block
BCC	basal cell carcinoma
BCP	birth control pill
BE	barium enema/below the elbow
BI	biopsy
bib.	drink
BiV	biventricular
BK	below the knee
BKA	below knee amputation
BLS	basic life support
BM	bowel movement
BMI	body mass index

© 2018 Optum360, LLC

Abbreviations, Acronyms, and Symbols

BMR	basal metabolic rate		cBMA	concentrated bone marrow stem cell aspirate
BMT	bone marrow transplant		CBR	complete bed rest
BO	body order		cc	chief complaint
BOW	bag of water		CCM	cardiac contractility modulation
BP	blood pressure		C-collar	cervical collar
BPAP	bilevel positive airway pressure		CCPD	continuous cycling peritoneal dialysis
BPC	bare platinum coils		CCS	Certified Coding Specialist
BPD	bronchopulmonary displasia/dysplasia		CCU	coronary care unit
BPH	benign prostatic hyperplasia/benign prostatic hypertrophy		CDC	Centers for Disease Control
Br	breastfeeding		CDG	congenital disorder of glycosylation
BRBPR	bright red blood per rectum		CDGS	carbohydrate-deficient glycoprotein
BrC	breast care		CDH	congenital dislocation of hip
BRM	biological response modifier		CDT	catheter-directed thrombolysis
BRP	bathroom, private/bathroom privileges		CE	cardiac enlargement
BS	Bachelor of Science/breath sounds/bowel sounds		CEA	carcinoembryonic antigen
			CF	cystic fibrosis
BSA	body surface area		Cf-252	Californium 252
BSC	bedside commode		CFC	cardiofasciocutaneous syndrome
BSD	balloon sinus dilation		CGF	congenital generalized fibromatosis
BSO	bilateral salpingo-oophorectomy		CH, Chol	cholesterol
BUN	blood urea nitrogen		CHD	congenital heart disease/congestive heart disease
BUR	back-up rate (ventilator)			
BUS	Bartholin, urethral, Skene's (glands)		CHF	congestive heart failure
bx	biopsy		chgd	changed
C	centigrade/complements/cervical vertebrae		chr.	chronic
			CI	confidence interval/cochlear implant
c̄	with		CIDP	chronic inflammatory demyelinating polyneuropathy
C&S	culture and sensitivity			
c.m.	tomorrow morning		CIED	cardiovascular implantable electronic device(s)
c.n.	tomorrow night			
c/m	counts per minute		CIN	cervical intraepithelial neoplasia
c/o	complaints of		CIS	carcinoma in situ
C/S	cesarean section		CJD	Creutzfeldt-Jakob disease
Ca	calcium/cancer		CKD	chronic kidney disease
CA	cancer		cl liqs	clear liquids
CA 125	cancer antigen 125		Cl	chloride
CABG	coronary artery bypass graft		CLABSI	central line-associated bloodstream infection
CAC	computer assisted coding			
CAD	coronary artery disease		CLC	creative living center
CAL	coracoacromial ligament		CLD	chronic lung disease/chronic liver disease
Cap	capitation		CLL	chronic lymphatic leukemia
CAPD	continuous ambulatory peritoneal dialysis		CLO	clofarabine
			cm	centimeter
caps.	capsule		CM	Chiari malformation
CAR	chimeric antigen receptor		cm2	square centimeters
CAS	computer assisted surgery		CMC	carpometacarpal
CAT	computerized axial tomography		CMG	cystometrogram
cath	catheterize		CML	chronic myelogenous leukemia
CBC	complete blood count		CMRI	cardiac magnetic resonance imaging

© 2018 Optum360, LLC

Abbreviations, Acronyms, and Symbols

CMS	Centers for Medicare and Medicaid Services/ circulation motion sensation		CTA	computed tomographic angiography
CMV	cytomegalovirus/controlled mechanical ventilation		CTLSO	cervical-thoracic-lumbar-sacral-orthosis
			CTZ	chemoreceptor trigger zone
cn	cranial nerves		cu	cubic
CNM	Certified Nurse Midwife		CV	cardiovascular
CNP	continuous negative airway pressure/ Certified Nurse Practitioner		CVA	cerebral vascular accident/ cerebrovascular accident/costovertebral angle
CNS	central nervous system		CVAD	central venous access devices
co	cardiac output		CVD	cardiovascular disease/cerebrovascular disease
CO	carbon monoxide			
CO2	carbon dioxide		CVI	chronic venous insufficiency
COLD	chronic obstructive lung disease		CVL	central venous line
COME	chronic otitis media with effusion		CVMS	clean voided midstream urine
conc.	concentration		CVP	central venous pressure
cont.	continue		CVU	cerebrovascular unit
COPD	chronic obstructive pulmonary disease		CXR	chest x-ray
CP	cerebral palsy		CXy	chest x-ray
CPAP	continuous positive airway pressure		cysto	cystoscopy
CPB	cardiopulmonary bypass		D	day/diopter
CPC	Certified Professional Coder		D&C	dilation and curettage
CPD	cephalopelvic disproportion		D&E	dilation and evacuation
CPK	creatine phosphokinase		D.O.	Doctor of Osteopathic Medicine
CPM	continuous passive motion		D/C	discharge/discontinue
CPR	cardiopulmonary resuscitation/ computer-based patient record		D/R	dayroom
			D/W	dextrose in water
CPT	chest physical therapy		DAW	dispense as written
CPT	Physicians' Current Procedural Terminology		DBE	double balloon enteroscopy
			DBS	deep brain stimulation/deep brain stimulator
CPT 1, CPT 2	carnitine palmitoyltransferase			
CR	creatine/ carrier replacement		DC	Doctor of Chiropractic Medicine/ discontinue
CRBSI	catheter related blood stream infection			
CRF	chronic renal failure		DC'd	discharged/discontinued
CRH	corticotropic releasing hormone		DCES	direct current electrical stimulation
crit.	hematocrit		DCIS	ductal carcinoma in-situ
CROS	contralateral routing of signals		DCR	dacryocystorhinostomy
CRP	C-reactive protein		DCS	direct cortical stimulation
CRPS	chronic regional pain syndrome		DD	down drain
CRRT	continuous renal replacement therapy		DDH	developmental dislocation (dysplasia) of the hip
CRT-D	cardiac resynchronization therapy defibrillator			
			DE	dose equivalent
CRT-P	cardiac resynchronization therapy pacemaker		decem	ten
			decub.	decubitus ulcer/lying down
CS	central service		def.	deficient, deficiency
Cs-137	Cesium 137		del	delivery
C-section	Cesarean section		dep.	dependent
CSF	cerebral spinal fluid/cerebrospinal fluid		DES	drug-eluting stent/diethylstilbestrol
CSM	cortical stimulation mapping		det.	let it be given
CSS	carotid sinus stimulation		DEXA	dual energy x-ray absorptiometry
CT	computerized tomography/corneal thickness/carpal tunnel syndrome		dexter	right

© 2018 Optum360, LLC

dextra	right	DVT	deep vein thrombosis
DHEA	dehydroepiandrosterone	dx	diagnosis
DHT	dihydrotestosterone	DX	diagnosis code
DHTR	delayed hemolytic transfusion reaction	dz	disease
DIC	disseminated intravascular coagulopathy/coagulation	e.g.	exempli gratia (for example)
		e.m.p.	as directed
DIEP	deep inferior epigastric artery perforator	E/M	evaluation and management
DIF	direct immunofluorescence	ead.	the same
dim.	divide in half	EBL	estimated blood loss
DIP	distal interphalangeal (joint)	EBUS	endobronchial ultrasound
disp	disposition	EBV	Epstein-Barr virus
DJD	degenerative joint disease	ECCE	extracapsular cataract extraction
DKA	diabetic ketoacidosis	$ECCO_2R$	extracorporeal carbon dioxide removal
DLIF	direct lateral interbody fusion	ECD	Erdheim-Chester Disease
DM	diabetes mellitus	ECF	extended care facility/extracellular fluid
DMD	Duchenne muscular dystrophy/Doctor of Dental Medicine	ECG	electrocardiogram
		ECHO	enterocytopathogenic human orphan virus/echocardiogram
DME	durable medical equipment		
DNA	deoxyribonucleic acid	EC-IC	extracranial to intracranial
DNP	do not publish	ECMO	extracorporeal membrane oxygenation
DNR	do not resuscitate	ECoG	electrocochleography/ electrocorticogram/ electrocorticography
DNS	do not show		
DO	Doctor of Osteopathy		
DOA	dead on arrival	ECP	extracorporeal photopheresis
DOB	date of birth	ECT	electro-convulsive therapy/emission computerized tomography
doc.	doctor		
DOE	dyspnea on exertion	ECV	external cephalic version
DOS	date of service	ED	effective dose/emergency department/ erectile dysfunction
DPD	dihydropyrimidine dehydrogenase deficiency/ dihydropyrimidine dehydrogenase disease		
		EDC	estimated date of confinement/expected date of confinement
DPR	drug price review	EDI	electronic data interchange
DPT	diphtheria - pertussis – tetanus/days per thousand	EEG	electroencephalogram/ electroencephalography
		EENT	eye, ear, nose, and throat
DR	delivery room	EGA	estimated gestational age
Dr	doctor	EGD	esophagus, stomach and duodenum/ esophagogastroduodenoscopy
DRG	diagnosis-related group		
DS	duodenal switch	EHEC	enterohemorrhagic Escherichia coli
Dsg	dressing	EIN	endometrial intraepithelial neoplasia
DSM-5	Diagnostic and Statistical Manual of Mental Disorders, Fifth Edition	EKG	electrocardiogram
		ELAD	extracorporeal liver assist device
DSS	dioctyl sulfosuccinate	EMG	electromyogram/electromyography
DT	destination therapy	en	clyster/enema
DTRs	deep tendon reflexes	en bloc	in total
DTs	delirium tremens	ENG	electronystagmogram
DUE	drug use evaluation	eng.	engorged
duo	two	ENT	ear, nose, and throat
duodecim.	twelve	EO	elbow orthosis
DUR	drug utilization review	EOG	electrooculography
dur. dolor.	while pain lasts		

© 2018 Optum360, LLC

EOM	end of month/ extraocular motion/ extraocular muscles	F/U	follow-up
EOMI	extraocular motion intact	FAS	fetal alcohol syndrome
EOP	external occipital protuberance	FB	foreign body
EOY	end of year	FBR	foreign body removal
EPAP	expiratory positive airway pressure	FBS	fasting blood sugar
Epis.	episiotomy	FDA	Food and Drug Administration
EPO	epoetin alfa/exclusive provider organization	FDP	fibrin degradation products
		Fe	female/iron
EPS	electrophysiologic stimulation/ electrophysiology study	FEV	forced expiratory volume
		FFI	fatal familial insomnia
EPSDT	early periodic screening, diagnosis and treatment	FFP	fresh frozen plasma
		FFR	fractional flow reserve
ER	emergency room	FFS	fee for service equivalency/fee for service reimbursement
ER-	estrogen receptor negative status		
ER+	estrogen receptor positive status	FH	family history
ERC	endoscopic retrograde cholangiography/ external remote controller	FHR	fetal heart rate
		FHT	fetal heart tone
ERCP	endoscopic retrograde cholangiopancreatography	FHVP	free hepatic venous pressure
		FI	firm one finger down from umbilicus
ERG	electroretinogram	fl	fluid
ERP	endoscopic retrograde pancreatography	f-LITT	focused laser interstitial thermal therapy
ESLD	end-stage liver disease	fluoro	fluoroscopy
ESR	erythrocyte sedimentation rate	FM	face mask
ESRD	end stage renal disease	FME	full-mouth extraction
EST	electroshock therapy	FMG	fine mesh gauze
ESWL	extracorporeal shockwave lithotripsy	FNA	fine needle aspiration
ESWT	extracorporeal shock wave therapy	FNHTR	febrile nonhemolytic transfusion
et	and	FNP	family nurse practitioner
ET	endotracheal	FOD	free of disease
ETD	eustachian tube dysfunction	fort.	strong (fortis)
ETG	episode treatment group	FP	family planning/family practitioner
ETOH	alcohol	FPR	facilitated positional release
ETS	endoscopic thoracic sympathectomy	FR	family relationship/Federal Register
ETV	endoscopic third ventriculostomy	FRAT	free radical assay test
EUS	endoscopic ultrasound	FSE	fetal scalp electrode
EUS-P	endoscopic ultrasound guided paracentesis	FSH	follicle stimulating hormone
		FTND	full term normal delivery
EVA	electric vacuum aspiration	FTSG	full thickness skin graft
EVAR	endovascular aneurysm repair	FTT	failure to thrive
EVD	external ventricular drain	FUO	fever of unknown origin
EVLP	ex vivo lung perfusion	FVC	forced vital capacity
EVR	evoked visual response	fx	fracture
Ex	examination	fxBB	fracture, both bones
exc	excise	G	gram
ext.	extremity	GA	gastric analysis
extr.	extract	GAP	gluteal artery perforator
F	Fahrenheit/female	gav.	gavage
F (on OB)	firm	GAVE	gastric antral vascular ectasia
f.m.	make a mixture	GB	gallbladder

Abbreviations, Acronyms, and Symbols

© 2018 Optum360, LLC

GCA	giant cell arteritis
GDM	gestational diabetes mellitus
GE	gastroesophageal
GEA	global endometrial ablation
GERD	gastroesophageal reflux disease
GFR	glomerular filtration rate
GH	growth hormone
GI	gastrointestinal
GIFT	gamete intrafallopian transfer
GLC	gas liquid chromatography
Gly. supp.	glycerin suppository
GMP	guanosine monophosphate
GNID	gram-negative intracellular diplococci
GnRH	gonadotropin-releasing hormone
GP	general practitioner
gr.	grain
grav	number of pregnancies
GS	general surgeon
GSR	galvanic skin response
GSRA	glycopeptide resistant staphylococcus
GSS	Gerstmann-Straussler-Scheinker
gsw	gunshot wound
gt.	drop
gtt.	drops
GU	genitourinary
Gu	guaiac
GVHD	graft-versus-host disease
gyn	gynecology
H	Hertel measurement
h (hora)	hour
H&P	history and physical
h.d.	at bedtime
H.O.	house officer
h.s.	at bedtime
H_2O	water
H_2O_2	hydrogen peroxide
HA	headache/hearing aide
HAA	hepatitis antigen B
HAAb	hepatitis antibody A
HaAg	hepatitis antigen A
HAI	hemagglutination test/hepatic artery infusion
HAV	hepatitis A virus
HB	headbox/hepatitis B/heart block
HBcAg	hepatitis antigen B
Hbg	hemoglobin
HBO	hyperbaric oxygen
HbO_2	oxyhemoglobin
HBOT	hyperbaric oxygen therapy

HBP	high blood pressure
HBS	hungry bone syndrome
HBsAb	hepatitis surface antibody B
HBsAg	hepatitis antigen B
HBV	hepatitis B vaccine
HCG	human chorionic gonadotropin
HCl	hydrochloric acid
HCM	hypertrophic cardiomyopathy
HCPCS	Healthcare Common Procedural Coding System
Hct	hematocrit
Hctz	hydrochlorothiazide
HCVD	hypertensive cardiovascular disease
HD	hip disarticulation
HDL	high-density lipoproteins
HDR	high dose rate
HEENT	head, eyes, ears, nose, and throat
HeRO	hemodialysis reliable outflow
Hg	hemoglobin
Hgb	hemoglobin
HGH	human growth hormone
HH	hard of hearing
HHA	home health agency
HIAA	hydroxyindoleacetic acid
Hib	Hemophilus influenzae vaccine
HIE	hypoxic-ischemic encephalopathy
HIPAA	Health Insurance Portability and Accountability Act of 1996
HIT	heparin-induced thrombocytopenia
HIV	human immunodeficiency virus
HLHS	hypoplastic left heart syndrome
HLV	herpes-like virus
HMD	hyaline membrane disease
HMO	health maintenance organization
HMS	hepatosplenomegaly
HNAD	hyperosmolar nonacidotic diabetes
HOB	head of bed
HOH	hard of hearing
hor. decub.	at bedtime
HORF	high output renal failure
HPF	high power field
HPG	human pituitary gonadotropin
HPI	history of present illness
HPL	human placental lactogen
HPs	Hanta virus pulmonary syndrome/hot packs
HPV	human papillomavirus
HR	Harrington rod/heart rate/hour
HRT	hormone replacement therapy
hrt.	heart

© 2018 Optum360, LLC

Abbreviations, Acronyms, and Symbols

HS	heelstick/hour of sleep		ID	infective dose
HSBG	heelstick blood gas		Id31	radioactive iodine
HSC	hematopoietic stem cell		IDDM	insulin dependent diabetes mellitus
HSG	hysterosalpingogram		IDH	isocitric dehydrogenase
HSP	health service plan		IDM	infant of diabetic mother
HSV	herpes simplex virus		IEED	involuntary emotional expression
ht.	height		IFIS	intraoperative floppy iris syndrome
HTLV	human T-cell lymphotropic virus		IFVA	intraoperative fluorescence vascular angiography
HTN	hypertension			
HTR	hemolytic transfusion reaction		Ig	immunoglobulin, gamma
HVA	homovanillic acid		IGN	image-guided navigation
HVLA	high velocity low amplitude		IGS	image-guided surgery
HVPG	hepatic venous pressure gradient		IH	infectious hepatitis
Hx	history		IHD	intermittent hemodialysis
hypo	hypodermic injection		IHSS	idiopathic hypertrophic subaortic stenosis
I&D	incision and drainage			
I&O	intake and output		II	icteric index
i.e.	id est (that is)		ILD	interstitial lung disease
I-125	Iodine 125		ILP	interspinous ligamentoplasty
IA	intra-arterial		IM	internal medicine/intramuscular/ infectious mononucleosis/ intramedullary
IAB	intra-aortic balloon			
IABC	intra-aortic balloon counterpulsation		IMC	intermediate care
IABP	intra-aortic balloon pump/intra-arterial blood pressure		IME	independent medical evaluation
			IMO	integrated multiple option
IAEMT	intraoperative anesthetic effect monitoring and titration		IMV	intermittent mandatory ventilation
			In-111	Indium 111
IBM	inclusion body myositis		inc.	incision
IBNR	incurred but not reported		indep	independent
IBS	irritable bowel syndrome		INF	inferior, infusion
IBW	ideal body weight		INH	inhalation solution
IC	infant care		INJ	injection
ICAT	indirect Coombs test		INPH	idiopathic normal pressure hydrocephalus
ICCE	intracapsular cataract extraction			
ICD	implantable cardioverter defibrillator		instill	instillation
ICD-10	International Classification of Diseases, 10th Revision, WHO		IOL	intraocular lens
			IONM	intraoperative neurophysiologic monitoring
ICD-10-CM	International Classification of Diseases, 10th Revision, Clinical Modification, U.S.		IOP	intraocular pressure
ICD-10-PCS	International Classification of Diseases, 10th Revision, Procedure Coding System		IP	intraperitoneal/interphalangeal
			IPA	individual practice association
ICE	intracardiac echocardiography		IPAP	inspiratory positive airway pressure
ICF	International Classification of Functioning, Disability, and Health/ intermediate care facility		IPC	intermittent pneumatic compression
			IPD	interspinous process decompression/ intermittent peritoneal dialysis
IC-Green™	indocyanine green		IPPB	intermittent positive pressure breathing
ICH	intracranial/cerebral hemorrhage			
ICP	intracranial pressure		IPPV	invasive positive pressure ventilation/ intermittent positive-pressure ventilation
ICS	intercostal space			
ICSH	interstitial cell stimulating hormone		IQ	intelligence quotient
ICU	intensive care unit		Ir-192	Iridium 192
			IRDS	idiopathic respiratory distress

Abbreviations, Acronyms, and Symbols

© 2018 Optum360, LLC

ISC	infant servo-control		LBBB	left bundle branch block
ISG	immune serum globulin		LBP	lower back pain
ISN	integrated service network		LCAD	long chain acyl CoA dehydrogenase deficiency
IT	intrathecal administration			
ITP	idiopathic thrombocytopenia purpura		LCHAD	long chain 3-hydroxyacyl CoA dehydrogenase deficiency
IU	international units			
IUD	intrauterine device		LCL	lateral collateral ligament
IV	intravenous		LCLC	lateral collateral ligament complex
IVAD™	implantable ventricular assist device (Thoratec®)		LCP	licensed clinical psychologist
			LCSW	licensed clinical social worker
IVC	inferior vena cava/intravenous cholangiogram		LD	lethal dose
			LDH	lactate dehydrogenase
IVF	in vitro fertilization		LDL	low-density lipoproteins
IVH	intraventricular hemorrhage		LDR	low dose rate
IVIg	intravenous immunoglobulin		LE	lower extremity/lupus erythematosus
IVP	intravenous pyelogram		LED	light-emitting diode
IVUS	intravascular ultrasound		LEEP	loop electrocautery excision procedure/ loop electrosurgical excision procedure
JCAHO	Joint Commission on Accreditation of Healthcare Organizations			
			LFT	liver function test
JODM	juvenile onset diabetes mellitus		LGA	large for gestational age
JVD	jugular venous distention		LGSIL	low grade squamous intraepithelial lesion
JVP	jugular venous pressure		LH	luteinizing hormone
K	potassium		LHC	left heart catheterization
K pouch	Kock pouch		LHF	left heart failure
Kcal	kilocalorie		LHR	leukocyte histamine release
KCL	potassium chloride		Li	lithium
kg	kilogram		lido	lidocaine
KJ	knee jerk		LINAC	linear accelerator
KO	keep open/knee orthosis		liq.	solution (liquor)
Kr-81m	Krypton		LITT	laser interstitial thermal therapy
KUB	kidneys, ureters, bladder		LKS	liver, kidneys, spleen
KVO	keep vein open		LLEC	large loop excision of the cervix
L	left/lumbar vertebrae		LLETZ	large loop excision of transformation zone
L&A	light and accommodation			
L&W	living and well		LLL	left lower lobe
LA	left atrium		LLQ	left lower quadrant
LAA	left atrial appendage		LMD	local medical doctor
LAC	lupus anticoagulant		LML	left medio lateral position
LAD	left anterior descending		LMN	lower motor neuron
LAM	lymphangioleiomyomatosis		LMP	last menstrual period
LAP	leucine aminopeptidase		LMS	left mentum anterior position (chin)
lap.	laparoscopy/laparotomy		LMT	left mentum transverse position
LASH	laparoscopic assisted supracervical hysterectomy		LNS	lymph node sampling
			LNT	lymph node transfer
LAT	lateral		LOA	leave of absence
LAV	lymphadenopathy associated virus		LOC	level of consciousness/loss of consciousness
LAVH	laparoscopic assisted vaginal hysterectomy			
			LOM	limitation of motion
LB	legbag		LOP	left occiput posterior position
LBB	left bundle branch		LOPS	loss of protective sensation

Abbreviations, Acronyms, and Symbols

LOS	length of stay
LOT	left occiput transverse position
LP	lumbar puncture
LPC	licensed professional counselor
LPM	liters per minute
LPT	lymphatic pump treatment
LR	lactated Ringer's/log roll
LS	lumbar sacral
LSA	left sacrum anterior position
LSB	left sternal border
LSF	lumbar spinal fusion
LSH	laparoscopic supracervical hysterectomy
LSO	lumbar sacral orthosis
LT	left
LTC	long term care
LUCL	lateral ulnar collateral ligament
lul	left upper lobe
luq	left upper quadrant
LUTS	lower urinary tract symptoms
LV	left ventriculography/ left ventricle
LVAD	left ventricular assist device
LVAS	left ventricle assist system
LVB	lymphovenous bypass
LVHA	low velocity-high amplitude
lymphs	lymphocytes
lytes	electrolytes
M	manifest refraction/male
M1	mitral first sound
M2	mitral second sound
m^2	meters squared
MA1	volume respirator
MAA	macroaggregated albumin
MAC	maximum allowable cost/monitored anesthesia care
MAD	monoamine oxidase (inhibitor)
MALT	mucosa associated lymphoid tissue
man. prim.	first thing in the morning
MAP	mean arterial pressure
MARS	molecular adsorbent recirculating system
MASER	microwave amplification by stimulated emission of radiation
MBC	minimum bactericidal concentration/ maximum breathing capacity
MBD	minimal brain dysfunction
MBS	modified barium swallow
MCAD	medium chain acyl CoAdehydrogenase deficiency
mcg	microgram
MCGR	magnetically controlled growing rod
MCH	mean corpuscular hemoglobin

MCHC	mean corpuscular hemoglobin concentration
MCI	mild cognitive impairment
MCL	midclavicular line
MCP	metacarpophalangeal
MCT	mediastinal chest tube
MCV	mean corpuscular volume
MD	manic depression/ medical doctor/ muscular dystrophy/myocardial disease
MDC	major diagnostic category
MDD	manic-depressive disorder
MDS	myelodysplastic syndrome
Mec	meconium
MED	minimal effective dose
med/surg	medical, surgical
meds	medications
MELAS	mitochondrial encephalopathy, lactic acidosis and stroke-like episodes
MEN	multiple endocrine neoplasia
MEP	motor evoked potentials
mEq	milliequivalent
mEq/1	milliequivalent per liter
MERRF	myoclonus with epilepsy and with ragged red fibers
MFD	minimum fatal dose
MFR	myofascial release
MFT	muscle function test
Mg	magnesium
mg	milligram
MH/CD	mental health/chemical dependency
MH/SA	mental health/substance abuse
MHC	mental health clinic
MI	myocardial infarction
min	minimum/minimal/minute
MIRPE	minimally invasive repair of pectus excavatum
misce.	miscellaneous
MIVAT	minimally invasive video-assisted thyroidectomy
ML	midline
ml	milliliter
MLC	midline catheter
mm	millimeter
mmHg	millimeters of mercury
MMK	Marshall-Marchetti-Krantz
MMRV	measles, mumps, rubella vaccine
MOD	multiple organ dysfunction
MODS	multiple organ dysfunction syndrome
MOH	medication overuse headache
MOM	milk of magnesia

Abbreviations, Acronyms, and Symbols

© 2018 Optum360, LLC

mono	monocyte/mononucleosis	NIR	near infrared
mor. dict.	in the manner directed	NJ	nasojejunal
MPD	maximum permissible dose	NKA	no known allergies
MPI	myocardial perfusion imaging	NKMA	no known medical allergies
MR	mitral regurgitation	NMDA	N-Methyl-D-aspartate
MRA	magnetic resonance angiography	NNR	new and nonofficial remedies
MRI	magnetic resonance imaging	noc.	night
mRNA	messenger RNA	Non-par	non-participating provider
MRSA	methicillin-resistant staphylococcus aureus	NOS	not otherwise specified
		novem.	nine
MS	morphine sulfate/multiple sclerosis	NP	neuropsychiatry/nurse practitioner
MSLT	multiple sleep latency testing	NPA	national prescription audit/non-par approved
MSSA	methicillin susceptible staphylococcus aureus	NP-CPAP	nasopharyngeal continuous positive airway pressure
MTD	right eardrum	NPN	non-par not approved/nonprotein nitrogen
MTHFR	methylenetetrahydrofolate reductase		
MTP	metatarsophalangeal	Npt	normal pressure and temperature
MTS	left eardrum	NPWT	negative-pressure wound therapy
multip.	multipara - pregnant woman who has more than one child	NS	normal saline/not significant
		NSAID	nonsteroidal anti-inflammatory drug
MVA	manual vacuum aspiration/motor vehicle accident	NSD	nominal standard dose
		NSR	normal sinus rhythm
MVD	microvillous inclusion disease	NST	nonstress test
MVD	microvascular decompression	NSTEMI	non-ST elevation myocardial infarction
MVP	mitral valve prolapse	NSV	no-scalpel vasectomy
N	nitrogen	NSVB	normal spontaneous vaginal bleeding
N&V	nausea and vomiting	NSVD	normal spontaneous vaginal delivery
n.p.o.	nothing by mouth	NT	nasotracheal/nontender
N2O	nitrous oxide	NTE	neutral thermal environment
Na	sodium	NTP	normal temperature and pressure
NaCl	sodium chloride (salt)	nyd	not yet diagnosed
NAD	no appreciable disease	O	blood type/oxygen
NAT	nonaccidental trauma	o	no information
NB	newborn	O&P	ova and parasites
NBICU	newborn intensive care unit	o.d.	right eye
NBT	nitroblue tetrazolium	o.m.	every morning/otitis media
NCA	neurocirculatory asthenia	o.n.	every night
NCPR	no cardiopulmonary resuscitation	o.s.	left eye
NCR	no cardiac resuscitation	o.u.	each eye/both eyes
NCV	nerve conduction velocity	O2	oxygen
NDC	national drug code	OA	open access/osteoarthritis
NDPH	new daily persistent headache	OAG	open angle glaucoma
NEC	necrotizing enterocolitis/not elsewhere classified	OB	obstetrics
		OB-GYN	obstetrics and gynecology
neg.	negative	OC	open crib/oral contraceptive/ office call
NF	National Formulary/neurofibromatosis	OCT	ornithine carbamyl transferase/oxytocin challenge test/optical coherence tomography
NG	nasogastric		
NGU	nongonococcal urethritis		
NIDDM	non-insulin dependent diabetes mellitus		
NIPPV	non-invasive positive pressure ventilation	octo.	eight

Abbreviations, Acronyms, and Symbols

ODS	obstructed defecation syndrome
OFC	occipitofrontal circumference
oint	ointment
OJ	orange juice
OM	otitis media
omn. hor.	every hour
OMS	oromaxillary surgery
OMT	osteopathic manipulative treatment
ONH	optic nerve head
OOA	out-of-area
OOB	out of bed
OPD	outpatient department
OPG	oculoplethysmography
ophth	ophthalmology
OPV	oral polio vaccine
OR	operating room
ORIF	open reduction internal fixation
oris	mouth
ortho.	orthopedics
os	mouth/opening
OSA	obstructive sleep apnea
OST	oxytocin stress test
OT	occupational therapy
OTC	over-the-counter
OTD	organ tolerance dose
OTH	other routes of administration
ov.	ovum/office visit
OW	open ward
oz.	ounce
P	plan/after/pulse/phosphorus
P&A	percussion and auscultation
P&T	pharmacy and therapeutics
p.c.	after eating
p.m.	after noon
p.p.	near point of visual accommodation
p.r.	pulse rate/far point of visual accommodation/through the rectum
p.r.n.	as needed for
p/o	by mouth
P+PD	percussion & postural drainage
P2	pulmonic 2nd sound
PA	physician assistant/posteroanterior/pulmonary artery
PAB	premature atrial beats
PAC	premature atrial contraction/pre-admission certification
PACU	post anesthesia care unit
PAD	peripheral arterial disease/pulmonary artery diastolic
PAH	para-aminohippurate
PAP	Papanicolaou test or smear/pulmonary artery pressure
PAR	parenteral/post anesthesia recovery
para	alongside of/number of pregnancies, e.g., para 1, 2, 3, etc.
PARR	post anesthesia recovery room
part. vic.	in divided doses
PAT	paroxysmal atrial tachycardia
path	pathology
PBA	pseudobulbar affect
PBI	protein-bound iodine
PC	packed cells
PCA	patient controlled analgesia
PCD	polycystic disease
PCF	posterior cervical fusion
PCG	phonocardiogram
PCN	penicillin
PCP	primary care physician
PCPM	per contract per month
PCR	physician contingency reserve/polymerase chain reaction
PCS	ICD-10-PCS (International Classification of Diseases, 10th Revision Procedure Coding System)
PCV	packed cell volume
PCW	pulmonary capillary wedge
PD	postural drainage/Parkinson's disease/peritoneal dialysis/ pilonidal disease
Pd-103	Palladium 103
PDA	patent ductus arteriosus
PDT	percutaneous dilatational tracheostomy
PE	physical examination/pulmonary embolism
PEC	pre-existing condition
Peds	pediatrics
PEEK	polyether-ether-ketone
PEEP	positive end expiratory pressure
PEG	pneumoencephalogram/percutaneous endoscopic gastrostomy
PEGJ	percutaneous endoscopic gastrojejunostomy
PEJ	percutaneous endoscopic jejunostomy
PEMF	pulsed electromagnetic field
PEN	parenteral and enteral nutrition
PENS	percutaneous electrical nerve stimulation
PERRLA	pupils equal, regular, reactive to light and accommodation
PET	positron emission tomography
PFC	persistent fetal circulation
PFO	patent foramen ovale
PFT	pulmonary function test

© 2018 Optum360, LLC

PG	prostaglandin	PRBC	packed red blood cells
PGA	polyglycolic acid	PRCA	pure red cell aplasia
PGLA	polyglycolic-polylactic acid	preg	pregnant
PH	past history	PRES	posterior reversible encephalopathy
pH	potential of hydrogen	previa	placenta previa
PharmD	doctor of pharmacy	primip	primipara—a woman having her first child
PHO	physician-hospital organization		
PI	present illness	PRIND	prolonged reversible ischemic neurologic deficit
PICC	peripherally inserted central catheter		
PID	pelvic inflammatory disease	PROM	premature rupture of membranes
PIP	proximal interphalangeal (joint)	PROMM	proximal myotonic myotonia
PIRRT	prolonged intermittent renal replacement therapy	PSA	prostate specific antigen
		PSP	phenolsulfonphthalein
PK	penetrating keratoplasty	PsyD	Doctor of Psychology
pk.	pack	Pt	patient/prothrombin time
PKU	phenylketonuria	PT	physical therapy/prothrombin time
PLCH	pulmonary Langerhans cell histiocytosis	PTA	prior to admission/percutaneous transluminal angioplasty
PLEVA	pityriasis lichenoides et varioliformis acuta		
		PTB	patellar tendon bearing (cast)
PLF	posterior lumbar fusion	PTCA	percutaneous transluminal coronary angioplasty
PLL	posterior longitudinal ligament		
PMG	primary medical group	PTH	parathyroid hormone
PMHx	past medical history	PTJV	percutaneous transtracheal jet ventilation
PMI	point of maximum intensity	PTLD	posttransplant lymphoproliferative disorder
PMN	polymorphonuclear neutrophil		
PMS	premenstrual syndrome	PTP	posttransfusion purpura
PMT	percutaneous mechanical thrombectomy	PTSD	post-traumatic stress disorder
PNC	premature nodal contraction	PTT	partial thromboplastin time
PND	paroxysmal nocturnal dyspnea/ post nasal drip	PUD	peptic ulcer disease
		pulv.	powder
PNS	peripheral nervous system	PVA	polyvinyl alcohol
PO	(per os) by mouth/postoperative	pVAD	percutaneous ventricular assist device
POAG	primary open-angle glaucoma	PVC	premature ventricular contraction
POD	postoperative day	PVD	premature ventricular depolarization
polys	polymorphonuclear neutrophil	PVL	paraventricular leukomalacia
pos.	positive	Px	prognosis/procedure
post or PM	postmortem exam or autopsy	PZI	protamine zinc insulin
post. clb.	after meals	q.	every
PP	postprandial	q.2h	every two hours
PPD	percussion and postural drainage/ purified protein derivative	q.a.m.	every morning
		q.d.	every day
PPE	palmar plantar erythrodysesthesia	q.h.	every hour
PPH	postpartum hemorrhage	q.h.s.	every night
PPO	preferred provider organization	q.i.d.	four times daily
PPP	protamine paracoagulation	q.n.	every night
PPV	pars plana vitrectomy	q.o.d.	every other day
PPVI	percutaneous pulmonary valve implantation	q.q.h.	every four hours
		QFT	QuantiFERON-TB tuberculosis test
pr	per return	qns	quantity not sufficient
PRB	pressure-regulating balloon	qs	quantity sufficient

© 2018 Optum360, LLC

Abbreviations, Acronyms, and Symbols

quattour	four
quicdecem	fifteen
quinque	five
quotid	daily
R	respiration/right atrium
r	roentgen units (x-rays)
R&C	reasonable and customary
R,R,& E	round, regular, and equal
R/O	rule out
RA	rheumatoid arthritis/refractoryanemia
RAEB-1	refractory anemia w/excess blasts-1
RAEB-2	refractory anemia w/excess blasts-2
RARS	refractory anemia w/ringed sideroblasts
RATx	radiation therapy
RBB	right bundle branch
RBBB	right bundle branch block
RBC	red blood cell
RBOW	ruptured bag of water
RCD	relative cardiac dullness
RCL	radial collateral ligament
RCMD	refractory cytopenia w/multilineage dysplasia
RCMD-RS	refractory cytopenia w/multilineage dysplasia and ringed sideroblasts
RDAVR	rapid deployment aortic valve replacement
RDS	respiratory distress syndrome
REA	resectoscopic endometrial ablation
REM	rapid eye movement
RESA	radial cryosurgical ablation
resp	respiration/respiratory
Retro	retrospective rate derivation
rev.	revise/revision
RF	radiofrequency
RFP	request for proposal
Rh	Rhesus
Rh neg	Rhesus factor negative
RHC	right heart catheterization
RHD	rheumatic heart disease
RHF	right heart failure
RIA	radioimmunoassay
RIND	reversible ischemic neurological deficit
RL	Ringer's lactate
RLE	right lower extremity
RLF	retrolental fibroplasia
RLL	right lower lobe
rlq	right lower quadrant
RLS	restless legs syndrome
RMA	right mentum anterior position
RMC	rating method code

RML	right middle lobe
RMP	right mentum posterior position
RMT	right mentum transverse position
RN	registered nurse
RNA	ribonucleic acid
RNS	responsive neurostimulator system
ROA	right occiput anterior position
ROM	range of motion
ROP	retinopathy of prematurity/right occiput posterior position
ROS	review of systems
RPG	retrograde pyelogram
RR	recovery room
RRR	regular rate and rhythm
RS	reducing substances
RSD	reflex sympathetic dystrophy
RSI	repetitive strain injuries
RSV	respiratory syncytial virus
RT	recreational therapist/respiratory therapist/resting tracing/right
RTC	return to clinic
RUL	right upper lobe
ruq	right upper quadrant
RV	right ventricle
RVAD	right ventricular assist device
RVOT	right ventricular outflow tract
Rx	take (prescription; treatment)
RxN	reaction
s̄	without
S&A	sugar and acetone
s.c.	subcutaneous
s.l.	under the tongue, sublingual
S.O.S.	if necessary (si opus sit)
S/P	status post
SA	sinoatrial
SAH	subarachnoid hemorrhage/ subtotal abdominal hysterectomy
SALT	serum alanine aminotransferase
SAST	serum aspartate aminotransferase
SB	sinus bradycardia
SBFT	small bowel follow through
S-C disease	sickle cell hemoglobin-c disease
SCAD	short chain acyl CoA dehydrogenase deficiency
SCD	sudden cardiac death
SCDs	sequential compression devices
SCI	spinal cord injury
SCID	severe combined immunodeficiency
SCIWORA	spinal cord injury without radiologic (neuroimaging) abnormality

Abbreviations, Acronyms, and Symbols

© 2018 Optum360, LLC

SDAVF	spinal dural arteriovenous fistula	SSNRI	selective serotonin and norepinephrine reuptake inhibitors
sed rate	sedimentation rate of erythrocytes	SSO2	supersaturated oxygen therapy
SEM	systolic ejection murmur	SSRI	selective serotonin reuptake inhibitors
Seno supp	Senokot suppository	ST	sinus tachycardia
SEPS	subdural Evacuating Port System	STA	superficial temporal artery
septem	seven	staph	staphylococcus
sex	six	STARR	stapled transanal rectal resection
SFA	superficial femoral artery	stat	immediately
SG	Swan-Ganz	STD	sexually transmitted disease
SGA	small for gestational age	STEC	shiga toxin-producing Escherichia coli
SGOT	serum glutamic oxaloacetic acid	STEMI	ST elevation myocardial infarction
SH	social history	STEP	serial transverse enteroplasty procedure
SHBG	sex hormone binding globulin	STH	somatotrophic hormone
SHOX	short stature homeobox (gene)	strep	streptococcus
SIADH	syndrome of inappropriate antidiuretic hormone	STS	serology test for syphilis
SIC	standard industry code	STSG	split thickness skin graft
SIDS	sudden infant death syndrome	STU	skin test unit
SIEA	superficial inferior epigastric artery	subcu	subcutaneous
Sig.	write on label (Rx) or let it be labeled	subind.	immediately after
SIRS	systemic inflammatory response syndrome	subq	subcutaneous
SISI	short increment sensitivity index	SUNCT	short lasting unilateral neuralgiform headache with conjunctival injection and tearing
SJS	Stevens-Johnson syndrome	supp	suppository
SLAP	superior labrum anterior and posterior	Sv	scalp vein
SLE	systemic lupus erythematosus	SVC	service
SLNB	sentinel lymph node biopsy	SVCS	superior vena cava syndrome
SLT	selective laser trabeculoplasty	Sx	sign/symptom
SMI	supplementary medical insurance	T	temperature/tender/thoracic vertebrae
SMILE	submucosal minimally invasive lingual excision	T&A	tonsillectomy and adenoidectomy
SMO	slip made out	T&C	type and crossmatch
SNF	skilled nursing facility	t.d.s.	three times a day
SNS	sympathetic nervous system	t.i.d.	three times daily
SOAP	subjective objective assessment plan	T3	triiodothyronine
SOB	shortness of breath	T4	thyroxine
sol.	solution	TAA	tumor-associated antigen
SOP	standard operation procedure	tab.	tablet (tabella)
SPD	semantic pragmatic disorder/summary plan description	TACE	transcatheter arterial chemoembolization/transarterial chemoembolization
SpGr	specific gravity	TACO	transfusion associated circulatory overload
SPIN	standard prescriber identification number	TAH	total abdominal hysterectomy
SPN	solitary pulmonary nodule	TAH-t	Total Artificial Heart
SQ	status quo/subcutaneous	Tap/H_2O/E	tap water enema
SROM	spontaneous rupture of membranes	TAPP	transabdominal preperitoneal
SRS	stereotactic radiosurgery	TAR	thrombocytopenia with absent radii syndrome
SRT	superficial radiation therapy		
ss	half	TAT	tetanus antitoxin/turnaround time
SSE	soap suds enema		
SSEP	somatosensory evoked potential		

Abbreviations, Acronyms, and Symbols

TAVI	transcatheter aortic valve implantation		TPAL	term pregnancies, premature infants, abortions, living children
TAVR	transcatheter aortic valve replacement		TPN	total parenteral nutrition
Tb	tubercle bacillus		TPR	temperature, pulse, respiration
TB	tuberculosis		TPVI	transcatheter pulmonary valve replacement
TBA	to be arranged			
TBG	thyroxine/thyroid binding globulin		TRALI	transfusion-related acute lung injury
TBI	total body irradiation/traumatic brain injury		TRAM	transverse rectus abdominis myocutaneous
TBNA	transbronchial needle aspiration		trans	transverse
TBSA	total body surface area		tres	three
TC&DB	turn, cough, and deep breathe		TRF	thyrotropin releasing factor
Tc-99m	Technetium 99m		TRH	thyrotropin releasing hormone
Td	tetanus		tRNA	transfer ribonucleic acid
TDR	total disc replacement		Ts	tension by Schiotz
TEE	transesophageal echocardiography/ transesophageal echocardiogram temp temperature		TSA	tumor specific antigen
			TSD	Tay-Sachs disease
			TSE	testicular self-exam
TEN	toxic epidermal necrolysis		TSH	thyroid stimulating hormone
TENS	transcutaneous electrical nerve stimulation		TSS	toxic shock syndrome
			TTE	transthoracic echocardiogram
TEP	total extraperitoneal		TTN	transient tachypnea of newborn
TEVAP	transurethral electrovaporization of prostate		TULIP	transurethral ultrasound guided laser induced prostate
TFT	transfer factor test			
TGS	Tactile Guidance System™		TUR	transurethral resection
THA	total hip arthroplasty		TURP	transurethral resection of prostate
Thal	Thalassemia		TVH	total vaginal hysterectomy
THC	tetrahydrocannabinol		TWE	tap water enema
TI	tricuspid insufficiency		Tx	treatment
TIA	transient ischemic attack		U	unit
TIBC	total iron binding capacity		U&C	usual and customary
TIF	transoral incisionless fundoplication		U/A	urinalysis
tinct	tincture		UAC	umbilical artery catheter/catheterization
TIPS	transjugular intrahepatic portosystemic shunt		UAE	uterine artery embolization
			UC	unit clerk
TIVAD	totally implantable subcutaneous central vascular access device		UCHD	usual childhood diseases
			UCR	usual, customary, and reasonable
TKA	total knee arthroplasty		UE	upper extremity
Tl-201	Thallium 201		UFE	uterine fibroid embolization
TLE	temporal lobe epilepsy		UFR	uroflowmetry
TLH	total laparoscopic hysterectomy		UGI	upper gastrointestinal
TLRH	total laparoscopic radical hysterectomy		UMN	upper motor neuron
TM	tympanic membrane		ung.	ointment
TMJ	temporomandibular joint		unus.	one
TNS	transcutaneous nerve stimulator/ stimulation		UPP	urethra pressure profile
			UPPP	uvulopalatopharyngoplasty
TO	telephone order		ur.	urine
TOA	tubo-ovarian abscess		URI	upper respiratory infection
tomo	tomographic		US	unstable spine/ultrasound
TP	total protein		ut dict.	as directed
tPA	tissue plasminogen activator			

Abbreviations, Acronyms, and Symbols

© 2018 Optum360, LLC

UTI	urinary tract infection	VPC	ventricular premature contraction
UV	ultraviolet light	VPRC	volume of packed red cells
UVC	umbilical vein catheter	VPU	video processing unit
V Fib	ventricular fibrillation	VS	vital signs/vesicular sound
V tach	ventricular tachycardia	VSD	ventricular septal defect
Va	visual acuity	VSG	vertical sleeve gastrectomy
VA	ventriculoatrial	VUR	vesicoureteral reflux
VAC	vacuum-assisted closure	vv	veins
VAD	vascular access device/ventricular assist device	w/HSBH	warmed heelstick blood gas
		WAK	wearable artificial kidney
VAIN	vaginal intraepithelial neoplasia	WB	whole blood
VATS	video-assisted thoracoscopic surgery	WBC	white blood count
VBAC	vaginal birth after cesarean	WC	wheelchair
VC	vena cava	WCC	well child care
VCG	vectorcardiogram	WD	well developed
vCJD	variant Creutzfeldt-Jakob disease	W-D	wet to dry (dressings)
VD	venereal disease	WEDI	workgroup for electronic data interchange
VDH	valvular disease of the heart		
VDRL	venereal disease report	WHO	World Health Organization
VE	voluntary effort	WHVP	wedged hepatic venous pressure
VEP	visual evoked potential	WLS	wet lung syndrome
VF	visual field/ventricular fibrillation	WN	well nourished
VFS	videofluoroscopy of swallowing	WNL	within normal limits
VFSS	videofluoroscopic swallowing study	WPW	Wolff-Parkinson-White syndrome
VGD	vein graft disease	Wt	weight
VH-IVUS	virtual histology intravascular ultrasound	x	except
VIN	vulvar intraepithelial neoplasia	Xe-127	Xenon 127
VIP	vasoactive intestinal peptide	Xe-133	Xenon 133
VISC	vitreous infusion suction cutter	XLIF	extreme lateral interbody fusion
Vit	vitamin (followed by specific letter)	XM	cross match
VLCAD	very long chain acyl CoA dehydrogenase deficiency	XVIVO	ex vivo lung perfusion
		Y-O	year-old
VO	verbal order	YTD	year-to-date
VO2	maximum oxygen consumption	ZIFT	zygote intrafallopian transfer
VP	vasopressin/voiding pressure/ ventriculoperitoneal		

© 2018 Optum360, LLC

Procedure Eponyms

Eponym	Description	ICD-10-PCS Table Reference	
Abbe	Vaginal construction — creation of vaginal canal (vaginoplasty) without graft or prosthesis	0UQG	Repair Vagina
Abbe	Vaginal construction — creation of vaginal canal (vaginoplasty) with graft or prosthesis	0UUG	Supplement Vagina
AbioCor®	Implantation of total internal biventricular heart replacement system	02RK 02RL	Replacement Ventricle, Right Replacement Ventricle, Left
Aburel	Intra-amniotic injection of abortifacient for abortion	10A	Abortion Pregnancy
Adams	Excision of palmar fascia for release of Dupuytren's contracture	0JB	Excision Subcutaneous Tissue and Fascia
Adams	Advancement of round ligament(s) of uterus	0US9	Reposition Uterus
Adams	Crushing of nasal septum	09SM	Reposition Nasal Septum
AESOP®	Robotic assisted procedures — Automated Endoscopic System for Optimal Positioning	8E0	Other Procedures Physiological Systems and Anatomical Regions
Albee	Bone peg, femoral neck Graft for slipping patella Sliding inlay graft, tibia	0QU	Supplement Lower Bones
Albert	Arthrodesis, knee	0SG	Fusion Lower Joints
Aldridge (-Studdiford)	Urethral sling	0TSD	Reposition Urethra
Alexander	Shortening of round ligaments of uterus	0US9	Reposition Uterus
Alexander-Adams	Shortening of round ligaments of uterus	0US9	Reposition Uterus
Almoor	Extrapetrosal drainage	099	Drainage Ear, Nose, Sinus
Altemeier	Perineal rectal pull-through operation	0DTP	Resection Rectum
Ammon	Dacryocystotomy incision (for drainage) of a lacrimal sac	089	Drainage Eye
Anderson	Tibial lengthening	0Q8 0QR 0QU	Division Lower Bones Replacement Lower Bones Supplement Lower Bones
Anderson-Hynes	Dismembered Pyeloplasty	0TQ	Repair Urinary System
Anel	Dilation of lacrimal duct	087X 087Y	Dilation Lacrimal Duct, Right Dilation Lacrimal Duct, Left
Arslan	Fenestration of inner ear	09QD 09QE	Repair Inner Ear, Right Repair Inner Ear, Left
Asai	Laryngoplasty	0CQS 0CRS 0CUS	Repair Larynx Replacement Larynx Supplement Larynx
Baffes	Interatrial transposition of venous return	02U5	Supplement Atrial Septum
Baffle	Atrial/interatrial/intra-atrial transposition of venous return	02U5	Supplement Atrial Septum
Baldy-Webster	Uterine suspension	0US9	Reposition Uterus

Procedure Eponyms

Eponym	Description	ICD-10-PCS Table Reference	
Bankhart	Capsular repair into glenoid, for shoulder dislocation	ØRS	Reposition Upper Joints
Bardenheurer	Ligation of innominate artery	Ø3L2	Occlusion Innominate Artery
Barkan	Goniotomy with/without goniopuncture	Ø89	Drainage Eye
Barr	Transfer of tibialis posterior tendon	ØLX	Transfer Tendons
Barsky	Closure of cleft hand	ØXQJ	Repair Hand, Right
		ØXQK	Repair Hand, Left
Bassett	Radical vulvectomy with inguinal lymph node dissection	ØUTM	Resection Vulva
		Ø7B	Excision Lymphatic and Hemic Systems
		Ø7T	Resection Lymphatic and Hemic Systems
Bassini	Inguinal hernia repair (herniorrhaphy)	ØYQ	Repair Anatomical Regions, Lower Extremities
Batch-Spittler-McFaddin	Amputation - knee disarticulation	ØY6	Detachment Anatomical Regions, Lower Extremities
Batista	Partial ventriculectomy, ventricular reduction, ventricular remodeling	Ø2BK	Excision Ventricle, Right
		Ø2BL	Excision Ventricle, Left
		Ø2QK	Repair Ventricle, Right
		Ø2QL	Repair Ventricle, Left
Beck I	Epicardial poudrage/Intrapericardial poudrage	Ø25N	Destruction Pericardium
Beck II	Aorta-coronary sinus shunt	Ø21	Bypass Heart and Great Vessels
Beck-Jianu	Permanent gastrostomy	ØD16	Bypass Stomach
Bell-Beuttner	Subtotal abdominal hysterectomy	ØUT9	Resection Uterus
Belsey	Esophagogastric sphincter	ØDQ	Repair Gastrointestinal System
		ØDU	Supplement Gastrointestinal System
Benenenti	Rotation of bulbous urethra	ØTSD	Reposition Urethra
Berke	Levator resection eyelid	ØKS1	Reposition Facial Muscle
Biesenberger	Bilateral reduction mammoplasty Size reduction of breast, bilateral — cosmetic	ØHØV	Alteration Breast, Bilateral
Biesenberger	Bilateral reduction mammoplasty Size reduction of breast, bilateral — therapeutic	ØHBV	Excision Breast, Bilateral
Bigelow	Litholapaxy	ØTCB	Extirpation Bladder
Billroth I	Partial gastrectomy with anastomosis of the gastric remnant to the duodenum (gastroduodenostomy)	ØDB6	Excision Stomach
Billroth II	Partial gastrectomy with gastrojejunostomy	ØDB6	Excision Stomach
		ØD16	Bypass Stomach
Binnie	Hepatopexy	ØFSØ	Reposition Liver
Bischoff	Ureteroneocystostomy	ØT1	Bypass Urinary System
Bishoff	Spinal myelotomy	ØØ8	Division Central Nervous System and Cranial Nerves
Blalock	Systemic-pulmonary anastomosis	Ø21	Bypass Heart and Great Vessels

Procedure Eponyms

© 2018 Optum360, LLC

Eponym	Description	ICD-10-PCS Table Reference
Blalock-Hanlon shunt	Creation of atrial septal defect	**02B5** Excision Atrial Septum
Blalock-Taussig shunt	Subclavian-pulmonary anastomosis	**021** Bypass Heart and Great Vessels
Blascovic	Resection or advancement of levator palpebrae superioris	**0KS1** Reposition Facial Muscle **0KX1** Transfer Facial Muscle
Blount	Femoral shortening (with blade plate)	**0QB** Excision Lower Bones
Blount	Epiphyseal stapling (temporary epiphysiodesis)	**0QH** Insertion Lower Bones
Boari	Bladder flap ureteroplasty	**0T16** Bypass Ureter, Right **0T17** Bypass Ureter, Left **0T18** Bypass Ureters, Bilateral
Bobb	Cholelithotomy	**0F94** Drainage Gallbladder **0FC4** Extirpation Gallbladder **0FF4** Fragmentation Gallbladder
Bonney	Abdominal hysterectomy	**0UT9** Resection Uterus
Borthen	Iridotasis	**0812** Bypass Anterior Chamber, Right **0813** Bypass Anterior Chamber, Left
Bost	Plantar dissection	**0M8** Division Bursae and Ligaments **0MN** Release Bursae and Ligaments **0SN** Release Lower Joints
Bost	Radiocarpal fusion	**0RG** Fusion Upper Joints
Bosworth	Arthroplasty for acromioclavicular separation	**0MQ** Repair Bursae and Ligaments **0RQ** Repair Upper Joints **0RU** Supplement Upper Joints
Bosworth	Fusion of posterior lumbar spine Fusion of posterior lumbar spine for pseudarthrosis	**0SG0** Fusion Lumbar Vertebral Joint **0SG1** Fusion Lumbar Vertebral Joints, 2 or more
Bosworth	Resection of radial head ligaments (for tennis elbow)	**0MB3** Excision Elbow Bursa and Ligament, Right **0MB4** Excision Elbow Bursa and Ligament, Left
Bosworth	Shelf procedure, hip	**0SQ** Repair Lower Joints
Bottle	Repair of hydrocele of tunica vaginalis	**0VB6** Excision Tunica Vaginalis, Right **0VB7** Excision Tunica Vaginalis, Left
Brauer	Cardiolysis	**02N** Release Heart and Great Vessels
Bricker	Ileoureterostomy	**0DBB** Excision Ileum **0T16** Bypass Ureter, Right **0T17** Bypass Ureter, Left **0T18** Bypass Ureters, Bilateral
Bristow	Repair of recurrent shoulder dislocation	**0RQ** Repair Upper Joints **0RS** Reposition Upper Joints
Brock	Pulmonary valvulotomy	**02NH** Release Pulmonary Valve

Procedure Eponyms

Eponym	Description	ICD-10-PCS Table Reference
Brockman	Soft tissue release for clubfoot	**ØJ8Q** Division Subcutaneous Tissue and Fascia, Right Foot **ØJ8R** Division Subcutaneous Tissue and Fascia, Left Foot **ØLNN** Release Lower Leg Tendon, Right **ØLNP** Release Lower Leg Tendon, Left **ØLNS** Release Ankle Tendon, Right **ØLNT** Release Ankle Tendon, Left **ØLNV** Release Foot Tendon, Right **ØLNW** Release Foot Tendon, Left
Browne (-Denis)	Hypospadias repair	**ØTRD** Replacement Urethra **ØTSD** Reposition Urethra **ØTUD** Supplement Urethra
Brunschwig	Temporary gastrostomy	**ØD16** Bypass Stomach
Bunnell	Tendon transfer	**ØLX7** Transfer Hand Tendon, Right **ØLX8** Transfer Hand Tendon, Left
Burch	Retropubic urethral suspension for urinary stress incontinence	**ØTSD** Reposition Urethra
Burgess	Amputation of ankle	**ØY6** Detachment Anatomical Regions, Lower Extremities
Caldwell	Sulcus extension	**ØCN4** Release Buccal Mucosa
Caldwell-Luc	Maxillary sinusotomy	**Ø99Q** Drainage Maxillary Sinus, Right **Ø99R** Drainage Maxillary Sinus, Left
Caldwell-Luc	Maxillary sinusotomy with removal of membrane lining	**Ø95Q** Destruction Maxillary Sinus, Right **Ø95R** Destruction Maxillary Sinus, Left **Ø99Q** Drainage Maxillary Sinus, Right **Ø99R** Drainage Maxillary Sinus, Left **Ø9BQ** Excision Maxillary Sinus, Right **Ø9BR** Excision Maxillary Sinus, Left **Ø9DQ** Extraction Maxillary Sinus, Right **Ø9DR** Extraction Maxillary Sinus, Left
Callander	Amputation — knee disarticulation	**ØY6** Detachment Anatomical Regions, Lower Extremities
Campbell	Bone block, ankle	**ØSGF** Fusion Ankle Joint, Right **ØSGG** Fusion Ankle Joint, Left
Campbell	Fasciotomy (iliac crest)	**ØJ8C** Division Subcutaneous Tissue and Fascia, Pelvic Region **ØJNC** Release Subcutaneous Tissue and Fascia, Pelvic Region
Campbell	Reconstruction of anterior cruciate ligaments	**ØMQN** Repair Knee Bursa and Ligament, Right **ØMQP** Repair Knee Bursa and Ligament, Left **ØMUN** Supplement Knee Bursa and Ligament, Right **ØMUP** Supplement Knee Bursa and Ligament, Left
Carroll and Taber	Arthroplasty, proximal interphalangeal joint	**ØRQW** Repair Finger Phalangeal Joint, Right **ØRQX** Repair Finger Phalangeal Joint, Left
Cattell	Herniorrhaphy	**ØWQF** Repair Abdominal Wall
Cecil	Urethral reconstruction	**ØTRD** Replacement Urethra **ØTUD** Supplement Urethra

Procedure Eponyms

  © 2018 Optum360, LLC

Eponym	Description	ICD-10-PCS Table Reference	
CentriMag®	Insertion of temporary non-implantable extracorporeal circulatory assist device	02HA	Insertion Heart
		5A02	Assistance Cardiac
Chamberlain	Mediastinotomy	0W9C	Drainage Mediastinum
		0WCC	Extirpation Mediastinum
Chandler	Hip fusion	0SG9	Fusion Hip Joint, Right
		0SGB	Fusion Hip Joint, Left
Charles	Correction of lymphedema	07Q	Repair Lymphatic and Hemic Systems
		07U	Supplement Lymphatic and Hemic Systems
Charnley	Compression arthrodesis	0SG	Fusion Lower Joints
Cheatle-Henry	Repair femoral hernia	0YU7	Supplement Femoral Region, Right
		0YU8	Supplement Femoral Region, Left
Chevalier-Jackson	Partial laryngectomy	0CBS	Excision Larynx
Child	Radical subtotal pancreatectomy	0FBG	Excision Pancreas
Child modification	Radical subtotal pancreatectomy	0FBG	Excision Pancreas
Chopart	Amputation, midtarsal	0Y6M	Detachment Foot, Right
		0Y6N	Detachment Foot, Left
CISH	Classic intrafascial serrated edged macro-morcellator (SEMM) hysterectomy (CISH)	0UT9	Resection Uterus
Clagett	Closure of chest wall following open flap drainage	0WQ8	Repair Chest Wall
Clayton	Resection of metatarsal heads and bases of phalanges	0QBN	Excision Metatarsal, Right
		0QBP	Excision Metatarsal, Left
		0QBQ	Excision Toe Phalanx, Right
		0QBR	Excision Toe Phalanx, Left
Cocked hat	Metacarpal lengthening and transfer of local flap	0PQR	Repair Thumb Phalanx, Right
		0PQS	Repair Thumb Phalanx, Left
		0PRR	Replacement Thumb Phalanx, Right
		0PRS	Replacement Thumb Phalanx, Left
		0PUR	Supplement Thumb Phalanx, Right
		0PUS	Supplement Thumb Phalanx, Left
Cockett	Varicose vein	06D	Extraction Lower Veins
		05D	Extraction Upper Veins
Cody tack	Perforation of footplate	09N9	Release Auditory Ossicle, Right
		09NA	Release Auditory Ossicle, Left
Coffey	Uterine suspension (Meigs' modification)	0US9	Reposition Uterus
Cole	Anterior tarsal wedge osteotomy	0QSL	Reposition Tarsal, Right
		0QSM	Reposition Tarsal, Left
		0QSN	Reposition Metatarsal, Right
		0QSP	Reposition Metatarsal, Left
Collis	Gastroplasty	0DX6	Transfer Stomach
Collis-Nissen	Hiatal hernia repair with esophagogastroplasty	0BQT	Repair Diaphragm
		0DV4	Restriction Esophagogastric Junction
Colonna	Adductor tenotomy (first stage)	0L8	Division Tendons
Colonna	Hip arthroplasty/reconstruction (second stage)	0SQ	Repair Lower Joints

Procedure Eponyms

Eponym	Description	ICD-10-PCS Table Reference		
Commando	Radical glossectomy	**0CT7**	Resection Tongue	
Coventry	Tibial wedge osteotomy	**0QSG** **0QSH**	Reposition Tibia, Right Reposition Tibia, Left	
Cox-maze	Ablation or destruction of heart tissue	**0258**	Destruction Conduction Mechanism	
Crawford	Tarso-frontalis sling of eyelid	**08SN** **08SP** **08UN** **08UP**	Reposition Upper Eyelid, Right Reposition Upper Eyelid, Left Supplement Upper Eyelid, Right Supplement Upper Eyelid, Left	
Culp-Deweerd	Spiral flap pyeloplasty	**0TQ3** **0TQ4** **0TQ6** **0TQ7**	Repair Kidney Pelvis, Right Repair Kidney Pelvis, Left Repair Ureter, Right Repair Ureter, Left	
Culp-Scardino	Ureteral flap pyeloplasty	**0TQ3** **0TQ4** **0TQ6** **0TQ7**	Repair Kidney Pelvis, Right Repair Kidney Pelvis, Left Repair Ureter, Right Repair Ureter, Left	
Curtis	Interphalangeal joint arthroplasty	**0RQW** **0RQX**	Repair Finger Phalangeal Joint, Right Repair Finger Phalangeal Joint, Left	
D'Ombrain	Excision of pterygium with corneal graft	**08R8** **08R9**	Replacement Cornea, Right Replacement Cornea, Left	
Dahlman	Excision of esophageal diverticulum	**0DB1** **0DB2** **0DB3** **0DB4** **0DB5**	Excision Esophagus, Upper Excision Esophagus, Middle Excision Esophagus, Lower Excision Esophagogastric Junction Excision Esophagus	
Dana	Posterior rhizotomy	**0181** **0188** **018B** **018R**	Division Cervical Nerve Division Thoracic Nerve Division Lumbar Nerve Division Sacral Nerve	
Darrach	Ulnar resection	**0PBK** **0PBL**	Excision Ulna, Right Excision Ulna, Left	
Davis	Intubated ureterotomy	**0T96** **0T97** **0T98**	Drainage Ureter, Right Drainage Ureter, Left Drainage Ureters, Bilateral	
de Grandmont	Tarsectomy	**08SN** **08SP**	Reposition Upper Eyelid, Right Reposition Upper Eyelid, Left	
Delorme	Pericardiectomy	**02BN**	Excision Pericardium	
Delorme	Proctopexy - repair of prolapsed rectum	**0DSP**	Reposition Rectum	
Delorme	Thoracoplasty	**0WQ8** **0WU8**	Repair Chest Wall Supplement Chest Wall	
Denker	Radical maxillary antrotomy	**095Q** **095R** **099Q** **099R** **09BQ** **09BR** **09DQ** **09DR**	Destruction Maxillary Sinus, Right Destruction Maxillary Sinus, Left Drainage Maxillary Sinus, Right Drainage Maxillary Sinus, Left Excision Maxillary Sinus, Right Excision Maxillary Sinus, Left Extraction Maxillary Sinus, Right Extraction Maxillary Sinus, Left	

Procedure Eponyms

© 2018 Optum360, LLC

Eponym	Description	ICD-10-PCS Table Reference	
Dennis-Varco	Herniorrhaphy	ØYQ7	Repair Femoral Region, Right
		ØYQ8	Repair Femoral Region, Left
		ØYQE	Repair, Femoral Region, Bilateral
		ØYU7	Supplement Femoral Region, Right
		ØYU8	Supplement Femoral Region, Left
		ØYUE	Supplement, Femoral Region, Bilateral
Denonvillier	Limited rhinoplasty	Ø9ØK	Alteration Nasal Mucosa and Soft Tissue
Derlacki	Tympanoplasty	Ø9Q7	Repair Tympanic Membrane, Right
		Ø9Q8	Repair Tympanic Membrane, Left
		Ø9U7	Supplement Tympanic Membrane, Right
		Ø9U8	Supplement Tympanic Membrane, Left
Dickson	Fascial transplant	ØJX	Transfer Subcutaneous Tissue and Fascia
Dickson-Diveley	Tendon transfer and arthrodesis to correct claw toe	ØSGP	Fusion Toe Phalangeal Joint, Right
		ØSGQ	Fusion Toe Phalangeal Joint, Left
		ØLXV	Transfer Foot Tendon, Right
		ØLXW	Transfer Foot Tendon, Left
Dieffenbach	Hip disarticulation	ØY67	Detachment Femoral Region, Right
		ØY68	Detachment Femoral Region, Left
Doleris	Shortening of round ligaments	ØUS9	Reposition Uterus
D'Ombrain	Excision of pterygium with corneal graft	Ø8R8	Replacement Cornea, Right
		Ø8R9	Replacement Cornea, Left
Dorrance	Push-back for cleft palate	ØCS2	Reposition Hard Palate
		ØCS3	Reposition Soft Palate
Dotter	Transluminal angioplasty	Ø27	Dilation Heart and Great Vessels
		Ø37	Dilation Upper Arteries
		Ø47	Dilation Lower Arteries
Douglas	Suture of tongue to lip for micrognathia	ØCS7	Reposition Tongue
Downstream® System	Aqueous oxygen (AO) therapy	5AØ5	Assistance Circulatory
Doyle	Paracervical uterine denervation	Ø15P	Destruction Sacral Sympathetic Nerve
Duhamel	Abdominoperineal pull-through	ØDTP	Resection Rectum
		ØD1	Bypass Gastrointestinal System
Dührssen	Vaginofixation of uterus	ØUS9	Reposition Uterus
Dunn	Triple arthrodesis	ØSGH	Fusion Tarsal Joint, Right
		ØSGJ	Fusion Tarsal Joint, Left
Dupuytren	Fasciectomy	ØJBJ	Excision Subcutaneous Tissue and Fascia, Right Hand
		ØJBK	Excision Subcutaneous Tissue and Fascia, Left Hand

Procedure Eponyms

Eponym	Description	ICD-10-PCS Table Reference	
Dupuytren	Fasciotomy	ØJ8J	Division Subcutaneous Tissue and Fascia, Right Hand
		ØJ8K	Division Subcutaneous Tissue and Fascia, Left Hand
		ØJNJ	Release Subcutaneous Tissue and Fascia, Right Hand
		ØJNK	Release Subcutaneous Tissue and Fascia, Left Hand
Dupuytren	Shoulder disarticulation	ØX62	Detachment Shoulder Region, Right
		ØX63	Detachment Shoulder Region, Left
Durham (-Caldwell)	Transfer of biceps femoris tendon	ØLXL	Transfer Upper Leg Tendon, Right
		ØLXM	Transfer Upper Leg Tendon, Left
DuToit and Roux	Staple capsulorrhaphy of shoulder	ØRQJ	Repair Shoulder Joint, Right
		ØRQK	Repair Shoulder Joint, Left
DuVries	Tenoplasty	ØLQ	Repair Tendons
Dwyer	Fasciotomy	ØJ8	Division Subcutaneous Tissue and Fascia
		ØJN	Release Subcutaneous Tissue and Fascia
Dwyer	Soft tissue release NEC	ØJ8Q	Division Subcutaneous Tissue and Fascia, Right Foot
		ØJ8R	Division Subcutaneous Tissue and Fascia, Left Foot
		ØLNN	Release Lower Leg Tendon, Right
		ØLNP	Release Lower Leg Tendon, Left
		ØLNS	Release Ankle Tendon, Right
		ØLNT	Release Ankle Tendon, Left
		ØLNV	Release Foot Tendon, Right
		ØLNW	Release Foot Tendon, Left
Dwyer	Wedge osteotomy, calcaneus	ØQBL	Excision Tarsal, Right
		ØQBM	Excision Tarsal, Left
		ØQSL	Reposition Tarsal, Right
		ØQSM	Reposition Tarsal, Left
Eagleton	Extrapetrosal drainage	Ø99B	Drainage Mastoid Sinus, Right
		Ø99C	Drainage Mastoid Sinus, Left
Eden-Hybinette	Glenoid bone block	ØPU7	Supplement Glenoid Cavity, Right
		ØPU8	Supplement Glenoid Cavity, Left
Effler	Heart revascularization by arterial implant	Ø21	Bypass Heart and Great Vessels
Eggers	Tendon release (patellar retinacula)	ØL8Q	Division Knee Tendon, Right
		ØL8R	Division Knee Tendon, Left
		ØLNQ	Release Knee Tendon, Right
		ØLNR	Release Knee Tendon, Left
Eggers	Tendon transfer (biceps femoris tendon) (hamstring tendon)	ØLXL	Transfer Upper Leg Tendon, Right
		ØLXM	Transfer Upper Leg Tendon, Left
Elliot	Scleral trephination with iridectomy	Ø8B6	Excision Sclera, Right
		Ø8B7	Excision Sclera, Left
		Ø8BC	Excision Iris, Right
		Ø8BD	Excision Iris, Left

Procedure Eponyms

© 2018 Optum360, LLC

Eponym	Description	ICD-10-PCS Table Reference	
Ellis Jones	Repair of peroneal tendon	ØLQN	Repair Lower Leg Tendon, Right
		ØLQP	Repair Lower Leg Tendon, Left
		ØLQV	Repair Foot Tendon, Right
		ØLQW	Repair Foot Tendon, Left
Ellison	Reinforcement of collateral ligament	ØMXN	Transfer Knee Bursa and Ligament, Right
		ØMXP	Transfer Knee Bursa and Ligament, Left
Elmslie-Cholmeley	Tarsal wedge osteotomy	ØQBL	Excision Tarsal, Right
		ØQBM	Excision Tarsal, Left
		ØQSL	Reposition Tarsal, Right
		ØQSM	Reposition Tarsal, Left
Eloesser	Thoracoplasty	ØWQ8	Repair Chest Wall
		ØWU8	Supplement Chest Wall
Eloesser	Thoracostomy	ØW99	Drainage Pleural Cavity, Right
		ØW9B	Drainage Pleural Cavity, Left
Emmet	Repair by suture of a laceration of the cervix uteri	ØUQC	Repair Cervix
Estes	Transposition of an ovary to the uterine cavity	ØUSØ	Reposition Ovary, Right
		ØUS1	Reposition Ovary, Left
Estlander	Thoracoplasty	ØWQ8	Repair Chest Wall
ESWL	Extracorporeal shockwave lithotripsy	00F	Fragmentation Central Nervous System and Cranial Nerves
		02F	Fragmentation Heart and Great Vessels
		08F	Fragmentation Eye
		ØBF	Fragmentation Respiratory System
		ØCF	Fragmentation Mouth and Throat
		ØDF	Fragmentation Gastrointestinal System
		ØFF	Fragmentation Hepatobiliary System and Pancreas
		ØTF	Fragmentation Urinary System
		ØUF	Fragmentation Female Reproductive System
		ØWF	Fragmentation Anatomical Regions, General
Evans	Release of clubfoot	ØJ8Q	Division Subcutaneous Tissue and Fascia, Right Foot
		ØJ8R	Division Subcutaneous Tissue and Fascia, Left Foot
		ØLNN	Release Lower Leg Tendon, Right
		ØLNP	Release Lower Leg Tendon, Left
		ØLNS	Release Ankle Tendon, Right
		ØLNT	Release Ankle Tendon, Left
		ØLNV	Release Foot Tendon, Right
		ØLNW	Release Foot Tendon, Left
Farabeuf	Ischiopubiotomy	0Q82	Division Pelvic Bone, Right
		0Q83	Division Pelvic Bone, Left
Fasanella-Servatt	Blepharoptosis repair	08SN	Reposition Upper Eyelid, Right
		08SP	Reposition Upper Eyelid, Left

Eponym	Description	ICD-10-PCS Table Reference
Ferguson	Hernia repair	**0YQ5** Repair Inguinal Region, Right **0YQ6** Repair Inguinal Region, Left **0YQE** Repair, Inguinal Region, Bilateral
Fick	Perforation of footplate	**09N9** Release Auditory Ossicle, Right **09NA** Release Auditory Ossicle, Left
Finney	Pyloroplasty	**0DQ7** Repair Stomach, Pylorus
Foley	Pyeloplasty	**0TQ3** Repair Kidney Pelvis, Right **0TQ4** Repair Kidney Pelvis, Left
Fontan	Creation of conduit between inferior vena cava (IVC) and pulmonary artery or trunk	**0610** Bypass Inferior Vena Cava
Fothergill (-Donald)	Uterine suspension	**0US9** Reposition Uterus
Fowler	Arthroplasty of metacarpophalangeal joint	**0RQU** Repair Metacarpophalangeal Joint, Right **0RQV** Repair Metacarpophalangeal Joint, Left
Fowler	Release mallet finger repair	**0L87** Division Hand Tendon, Right **0L88** Division Hand Tendon, Left
Fowler	Tenodesis (hand)	**0LQ7** Repair Hand Tendon, Right **0LQ8** Repair Hand Tendon, Left
Fowler	Thoracoplasty	**0WQ8** Repair Chest Wall
Fox	Entropion repair with wedge resection	**08BN** Excision Upper Eyelid, Right **08BP** Excision Upper Eyelid, Left **08BQ** Excision Lower Eyelid, Right **08BR** Excision Lower Eyelid, Left
Franco	Suprapubic cystotomy	**0T9B** Drainage Bladder
Frank	Permanent gastrostomy	**0D16** Bypass Stomach
Frazier (-Spiller)	Subtemporal trigeminal rhizotomy	**008K** Division Trigeminal Nerve
Fredet-Ramstedt	Pyloromyotomy	**0D87** Division Stomach, Pylorus
Fredet-Ramstedt	Pyloromyotomy with wedge resection	**0DB7** Excision Stomach, Pylorus
Frenckner	Intrapetrosal drainage	**099B** Drainage Mastoid Sinus, Right **099C** Drainage Mastoid Sinus, Left
Frickman	Abdominal proctopexy	**0DSP** Reposition Rectum
Frommel	Shortening of uterosacral ligaments	**0US9** Reposition Uterus
Gabriel	Abdominoperineal resection of rectum	**0DTP** Resection Rectum **0D1** Bypass Gastrointestinal System
Gant	Wedge osteotomy of trochanter	**0QB6** Excision Upper Femur, Right **0QB7** Excision Upper Femur, Left **0QS6** Reposition Upper Femur, Right **0QS7** Reposition Upper Femur, Left
Garceau	Tibial tendon transfer	**0LXN** Transfer Lower Leg Tendon, Right **0LXP** Transfer Lower Leg Tendon, Left
Gardner	Spinal meningocele repair	**00QT** Repair Spinal Meninges

© 2018 Optum360, LLC

Procedure Eponyms

Eponym	Description	ICD-10-PCS Table Reference	
Gelman	Release of clubfoot	ØJ8Q	Division Subcutaneous Tissue and Fascia, Right Foot
		ØJ8R	Division Subcutaneous Tissue and Fascia, Left Foot
		ØLNN	Release Lower Leg Tendon, Right
		ØLNP	Release Lower Leg Tendon, Left
		ØLNS	Release Ankle Tendon, Right
		ØLNT	Release Ankle Tendon, Left
		ØLNV	Release Foot Tendon, Right
		ØLNW	Release Foot Tendon, Left
Ghormley	Hip fusion	ØSG9	Fusion Hip Joint, Right
		ØSGB	Fusion Hip Joint, Left
Gifford	Destruction of lacrimal sac	Ø85X	Destruction Lacrimal Duct, Right
		Ø85Y	Destruction Lacrimal Duct, Left
Gifford	Keratotomy delimiting	Ø8Q8	Repair Cornea, Right
		Ø8Q9	Repair Cornea, Left
Gifford	Keratotomy radial (refractive)	Ø8Q8	Repair Cornea, Right
		Ø8Q9	Repair Cornea, Left
Gill	Arthrodesis of shoulder	ØRGJ	Fusion Shoulder Joint, Right
		ØRGK	Fusion Shoulder Joint, Left
Gill	Laminectomy	Ø1N1	Release Cervical Nerve
		Ø1N8	Release Thoracic Nerve
		Ø1NB	Release Lumbar Nerve
Gilliam	Uterine suspension	ØUS9	Reposition Uterus
Gill-Stein	Carporadial arthrodesis	ØRGN	Fusion Wrist Joint, Right
		ØRGP	Fusion Wrist Joint, Left
Girdlestone	Laminectomy with spinal fusion	ØRGØ	Fusion Occipital-cervical Joint
		ØRG1	Fusion Cervical Vertebral Joint
		ØRG2	Fusion Cervical Vertebral Joints, 2 or more
		ØRG4	Fusion Cervicothoracic Vertebral Joint
		ØRG6	Fusion Thoracic Vertebral Joint
		ØRG7	Fusion Thoracic Vertebral Joints, 2 to 7
		ØRG8	Fusion Thoracic Vertebral Joints, 8 or more
		ØRGA	Fusion Thoracolumbar Vertebral Joint
		ØSGØ	Fusion Lumbar Vertebral Joint
		ØSG1	Fusion Lumbar Vertebral Joints, 2 or more
		ØSG3	Fusion Lumbosacral Joint
		ØSG5	Fusion Sacrococcygeal Joint
Girdlestone	Tendon transfer for claw toe repair	ØLXV	Transfer Foot Tendon, Right
		ØLXW	Transfer Foot Tendon, Left
Girdlestone	Resection of femoral head and neck without insertion of joint prosthesis	ØQB6	Excision Upper Femur, Right
		ØQB7	Excision Upper Femur, Left
Girdlestone	Resection of femoral head and neck with replacement prosthesis	ØSR9	Replacement Hip Joint, Right
		ØSRB	Replacement Hip Joint, Left
Girdlestone	Resection of hip prosthesis	ØSP9	Removal Hip Joint, Right
		ØSPB	Removal Hip Joint, Left

Procedure Eponyms

Eponym	Description	ICD-10-PCS Table Reference
Girdlestone	Resection of hip prosthesis with replacement prosthesis	ØSP9 Removal Hip Joint, Right ØSPB Removal Hip Joint, Left ØSR9 Replacement Hip Joint, Right ØSRB Replacement Hip Joint, Left ØSRA Replacement Hip Joint, Acetabular Surface, Right ØSRE Replacement Hip Joint, Acetabular Surface, Left
Girdlestone-Taylor	Tendon transfer for claw toe repair	ØLXV Transfer Foot Tendon, Right ØLXW Transfer Foot Tendon, Left
Glenn	Anastomosis of superior vena cava to right pulmonary artery	Ø21V Bypass Superior Vena Cava
Goebel-Frangenheim-Stoeckel	Urethrovesical suspension	ØTSC Reposition Bladder Neck ØTSD Reposition Urethra
Goldner	Clubfoot release	ØM8 Division Bursae and Ligaments ØMN Release Bursae and Ligaments ØSN Release Lower Joints
Goldthwaite	Ankle stabilization	ØSGF Fusion Ankle Joint, Right ØSGG Fusion Ankle Joint, Left
Goldthwaite	Patellar stabilization	ØQSD Reposition Patella, Right ØQSF Reposition Patella, Left
Goldthwaite	Tendon transfer for stabilization of patella	ØLXQ Transfer Knee Tendon, Right ØLXR Transfer Knee Tendon, Left
Goodall-Power	Vaginectomy	ØUTG Resection Vagina
Gordon-Taylor	Hindquarter amputation	ØY62 Detachment Hindquarter, Right ØY63 Detachment Hindquarter, Left ØY64 Detachment Hindquarter, Bilateral
Graber-Duvernay	Drilling femoral head	ØQ9 Drainage Lower Bones ØQB Excision Lower Bones
Green	Scapulopexy	ØPQ5 Repair Scapula, Right ØPQ6 Repair Scapula, Left
Grice	Subtalar arthrodesis	ØSGH Fusion Tarsal Joint, Right ØSGJ Fusion Tarsal Joint, Left
Gritti-Stokes	Knee disarticulation	ØY6F Detachment Knee Region, Right ØY6G Detachment Knee Region, Left
Gross	Umbilical herniorrhaphy	ØWQF Repair Abdominal Wall
Guyon	Amputation of ankle	ØY6M Detachment Foot, Right ØY6N Detachment Foot, Left
Hagner	Epididymotomy	ØV9J Drainage Epididymis, Right ØV9K Drainage Epididymis, Left ØV9L Drainage Epididymis, Bilateral
Halsted	Repair inguinal hernia	ØYQ5 Repair Inguinal Region, Right ØYQ6 Repair Inguinal Region, Left
Hampton	Anastomosis small intestine to rectal stump	ØD1A Bypass Jejunum ØD1B Bypass Ileum ØD1H Bypass Cecum
Hanging hip	Muscle release	ØKNN Release Hip Muscle, Right ØKNP Release Hip Muscle, Left

Procedure Eponyms

© 2018 Optum360, LLC

Eponym	Description	ICD-10-PCS Table Reference	
Harrison-Richardson	Vaginal suspension with graft or prosthesis	**0UUG**	Supplement Vagina
Harrison-Richardson	Vaginal suspension	**0USG**	Reposition Vagina
Hartmann	Resection of the intestine (colectomy) (with pouch)	**0DT**	Resection Gastrointestinal System
Hauser	Achillotenotomy	**0L8N** **0L8P**	Division Lower Leg Tendon, Right Division Lower Leg Tendon, Left
Hauser	Bunionectomy with adductor tendon transfer	**0QBQ** **0QBR** **0LXV** **0LXW**	Excision Toe Phalanx, Right Excision Toe Phalanx, Left Transfer Foot Tendon, Right Transfer Foot Tendon, Left
Hauser	Stabilization of patella	**0QSD** **0QSF**	Reposition Patella, Right Reposition Patella, Left
Heaney	Vaginal hysterectomy	**0UT9** **0UTC**	Resection Uterus Resection Cervix
HeartMate	Implantable heart assist system	**02HA** **5A02**	Insertion Heart Assistance Cardiac
HeartMate II	Left ventricular assist system	**02HL**	Insertion Ventricle, Left
Hegar	Perineorrhaphy	**0WQN**	Repair Perineum, Female
Heine	Cyclodialysis	**0892** **0893**	Drainage Anterior Chamber, Right Drainage Anterior Chamber, Left
Heineke–Mikulicz	Pyloroplasty	**0DQ7**	Repair Stomach, Pylorus
Heller	Esophagomyotomy	**0D84**	Division Esophagogastric Junction
Hellström	Transplantation of aberrant renal vessel	**04S9** **04SA** **06S9** **06SB**	Reposition Renal Artery, Right Reposition Renal Artery, Left Reposition Renal Vein, Right Reposition Renal Vein, Left
Henley	Jejunal transposition	**0D1A** **0DB6**	Bypass Jejunum Excision Stomach
Hey	Amputation of foot	**0Y6M** **0Y6N**	Detachment Foot, Right Detachment Foot, Left
Hey-Groves	Reconstruction of anterior cruciate ligament	**0MUN** **0MUP**	Supplement Knee Bursa and Ligament, Right Supplement Knee Bursa and Ligament, Left
Heyman	Soft tissue release for clubfoot	**0J8Q** **0J8R** **0LNN** **0LNP** **0LNS** **0LNT** **0LNV** **0LNW**	Division Subcutaneous Tissue and Fascia, Right Foot Division Subcutaneous Tissue and Fascia, Left Foot Release Lower Leg Tendon, Right Release Lower Leg Tendon, Left Release Ankle Tendon, Right Release Ankle Tendon, Left Release Foot Tendon, Right Release Foot Tendon, Left

Eponym	Description	ICD-10-PCS Table Reference
Heyman-Herndon (-Strong)	Correction of metatarsus varus	**ØSNK** Release Tarsometatarsal Joint, Right **ØSNL** Release Tarsometatarsal Joint, Left **ØSNM** Release Metatarsal-Phalangeal Joint, Right **ØSNN** Release Metatarsal-Phalangeal Joint, Left
Hibbs	Lumbar spinal fusion (lumbar, lumbosacral)	**ØSGØ** Fusion Lumbar Vertebral Joint **ØSG1** Fusion Lumbar Vertebral Joints, 2 or more **ØSG3** Fusion Lumbosacral Joint
Higgins	Repair femoral hernia	**ØYQ7** Repair Femoral Region, Right **ØYQ8** Repair Femoral Region, Left
Hill-Allison	Hiatal hernia repair, transpleural approach	**ØBQT** Repair Diaphragm
Hitchcock	Anchoring tendon of biceps	**ØLM1** Reattachment Shoulder Tendon, Right **ØLM2** Reattachment Shoulder Tendon, Left **ØLM3** Reattachment Upper Arm Tendon, Right **ØLM4** Reattachment Upper Arm Tendon, Left
Hofmeister	Gastrectomy	**ØDB6** Excision Stomach **ØD16** Bypass Stomach
Hoke	Midtarsal fusion	**ØSGH** Fusion Tarsal Joint, Right **ØSGJ** Fusion Tarsal Joint, Left
Hoke	Triple arthrodesis	**ØSGH** Fusion Tarsal Joint, Right **ØSGJ** Fusion Tarsal Joint, Left
Holth	Iridencleisis	**Ø812** Bypass Anterior Chamber, Right **Ø813** Bypass Anterior Chamber, Left
Holth	Sclerectomy	**Ø812** Bypass Anterior Chamber, Right **Ø813** Bypass Anterior Chamber, Left
Homan	Correction of lymphedema	**Ø7Q** Repair Lymphatic and Hemic Systems **Ø7U** Supplement Lymphatic and Hemic Systems
Hutch	Ureteroneocystostomy	**ØT16** Bypass Ureter, Right **ØT17** Bypass Ureter, Left **ØT18** Bypass Ureters, Bilateral
Hybinette-Eden	Glenoid bone block	**ØPU7** Supplement Glenoid Cavity, Right **ØPU8** Supplement Glenoid Cavity, Left
Impella®	Percutaneous external heart assist device	**Ø2HA** Insertion Heart **5AØ2** Assistance Cardiac
Interleukin-2	Infusion; high-dose, low-dose	**3EØ** Introduction Physiological Systems and Anatomical Regions
Irving	Tubal ligation	**ØUB5** Excision Fallopian Tube, Right **ØUB6** Excision Fallopian Tube, Left **ØUB7** Excision Fallopian Tubes, Bilateral

Procedure Eponyms

© 2018 Optum360, LLC

Eponym	Description	ICD-10-PCS Table Reference	
Irwin	Osteotomy	0QSB	Reposition Lower Femur, Right
		0QSC	Reposition Lower Femur, Left
		0QSG	Reposition Tibia, Right
		0QSH	Reposition Tibia, Left
		0QSJ	Reposition Fibula, Right
		0QSK	Reposition Fibula, Left
IVUS	Ultrasound, intravascular, by site	B24	Ultrasonography Heart
		B34	Ultrasonography Upper Arteries
		B44	Ultrasonography Lower Arteries
		B54	Ultrasonography Veins
Jaboulay	Pyloroplasty by forming a side-to-side gastroduodenal anastomosis (Gastroduodenostomy)	0D1	Bypass Gastrointestinal System
Janeway	Permanent gastrostomy	0D16	Bypass Stomach
Jatene	Arterial switch	02S1	Reposition, Coronary Artery, Two Arteries
		02SP	Reposition Pulmonary Trunk
		02SX	Reposition, Thoracic Aorta, Ascending/Arch
Johanson	Urethral reconstruction	0TRD	Replacement Urethra
		0TUD	Supplement Urethra
Jones	Claw toe repair (transfer of extensor hallucis longus tendon)	0LXV	Transfer Foot Tendon, Right
		0LXW	Transfer Foot Tendon, Left
Jones	Claw toe repair — modified (with arthrodesis)	0SGP	Fusion Toe Phalangeal Joint, Right
		0SGQ	Fusion Toe Phalangeal Joint, Left
Jones	Dacryocystorhinostomy	081X	Bypass Lacrimal Duct, Right
		081Y	Bypass Lacrimal Duct, Left
Jones	Hammer toe repair (interphalangeal fusion)	0SGP	Fusion Toe Phalangeal Joint, Right
		0SGQ	Fusion Toe Phalangeal Joint, Left
Jones	Hammer toe repair — modified (tendon transfer with arthrodesis)	0LXV	Transfer Foot Tendon, Right
		0LXW	Transfer Foot Tendon, Left
		0SGP	Fusion Toe Phalangeal Joint, Right
		0SGQ	Fusion Toe Phalangeal Joint, Left
Jones	Peroneal tendon repair	0LQN	Repair Lower Leg Tendon, Right
		0LQP	Repair Lower Leg Tendon, Left
		0LQV	Repair Foot Tendon, Right
		0LQW	Repair Foot Tendon, Left
Joplin	Exostectomy with tendon transfer	0QBN	Excision Metatarsal, Right
		0QBP	Excision Metatarsal, Left
		0LXV	Transfer Foot Tendon, Right
		0LXW	Transfer Foot Tendon, Left
Kader	Temporary gastrostomy	0D16	Bypass Stomach
Kaufman	For urinary stress incontinence	0TUC	Supplement Bladder Neck
Kazanjiian	Buccal vestibular sulcus extension	0CN4	Release Buccal Mucosa
Kehr	Hepatopexy	0FS0	Reposition Liver
Keller	Bunionectomy	0QBQ	Excision Toe Phalanx, Right
		0QBR	Excision Toe Phalanx, Left
Kelly (-Kennedy)	Urethrovesical plication	0TSC	Reposition Bladder Neck
Kelly-Stoeckel	Urethrovesical plication	0TSC	Reposition Bladder Neck

Procedure Eponyms

Eponym	Description	ICD-10-PCS Table Reference	
Kerr	Low cervical cesarean section	10D0	Extraction Products of Conception
Kessler	Arthroplasty, carpometacarpal joint	0RRS	Replacement Carpometacarpal Joint, Right
		0RRT	Replacement Carpometacarpal Joint, Left
Kidner	Excision of accessory navicular bone (with tendon transfer)	0QBL	Excision Tarsal, Right
		0QBM	Excision Tarsal, Left
		0LXV	Transfer Foot Tendon, Right
		0LXW	Transfer Foot Tendon, Left
Killian	Frontal sinusotomy	099S	Drainage Frontal Sinus, Right
		099T	Drainage Frontal Sinus, Left
King-Steelquist	Hindquarter amputation	0Y62	Detachment Hindquarter, Right
		0Y63	Detachment Hindquarter, Left
		0Y64	Detachment Hindquarter, Bilateral
Kirk	Amputation through thigh	0Y6C	Detachment Upper Leg, Right
		0Y6D	Detachment Upper Leg, Left
Kock pouch	Continent ileostomy	0D1B	Bypass Ileum
Kock pouch	Cutaneous uretero-ileostomy	0T16	Bypass Ureter, Right
		0T17	Bypass Ureter, Left
		0T18	Bypass Ureters, Bilateral
		0DBB	Excision Ileum
Kock pouch	ESWL (electrocorporeal shockwave lithotripsy)	0TF	Fragmentation Urinary System
		0WFR	Fragmentation Genitourinary Tract
Kock pouch	Removal, calculus	0TCB	Extirpation Bladder
		0TCC	Extirpation Bladder Neck
Kock pouch	Revision, cutaneous uretero-ileostomy	0WQF	Repair Abdominal Wall
Kock pouch	Urinary diversion procedure	0T16	Bypass Ureter, Right
		0T17	Bypass Ureter, Left
		0T18	Bypass Ureters, Bilateral
		0DBB	Excision Ileum
Kondoleon	Correction of lymphedema	07Q	Repair Lymphatic and Hemic Systems
		07U	Supplement Lymphatic and Hemic Systems
Krause	Sympathetic denervation	015L	Destruction Thoracic Sympathetic Nerve
		015M	Destruction Abdominal Sympathetic Nerve
Kroener	Partial salpingectomy	0UB5	Excision Fallopian Tube, Right
		0UB6	Excision Fallopian Tube, Left
		0UB7	Excision Fallopian Tubes, Bilateral
Kroenlein	Lateral orbitotomy	0NRP	Replacement Orbit, Right
		0NRQ	Replacement Orbit, Left
Krönig	Low cervical cesarean section	10D0	Extraction Products of Conception

Procedure Eponyms

© 2018 Optum360, LLC

Eponym	Description	ICD-10-PCS Table Reference
Krukenberg	Reconstruction of below-elbow amputation	**ØJQG** Repair Subcutaneous Tissue and Fascia, Right Lower Arm **ØJQH** Repair Subcutaneous Tissue and Fascia, Left Lower Arm **ØJQJ** Repair Subcutaneous Tissue and Fascia, Right Hand **ØJQK** Repair Subcutaneous Tissue and Fascia, Left Hand **ØKQ9** Repair Lower Arm and Wrist Muscle, Right **ØKQB** Repair Lower Arm and Wrist Muscle, Left **ØKQC** Repair Hand Muscle, Right **ØKQD** Repair Hand Muscle, Left
Kuhnt-Szymanowski	Ectropion repair with lid reconstruction	**08RN** Replacement Upper Eyelid, Right **08RP** Replacement Upper Eyelid, Left **08RQ** Replacement Lower Eyelid, Right **08RR** Replacement Lower Eyelid, Left
Labbe	Gastrotomy	**ØD96** Drainage Stomach **ØDC6** Extirpation Stomach
Ladd	Mobilization of intestine	**ØDN** Release Gastrointestinal System
Lagrange	Iridosclerectomy	**0812** Bypass Anterior Chamber, Right **0813** Bypass Anterior Chamber, Left
Lambrinudi	Triple arthrodesis	**ØSGH** Fusion Tarsal Joint, Right **ØSGJ** Fusion Tarsal Joint, Left
Langenbeck	Cleft palate repair	**ØCS2** Reposition Hard Palate **ØCS3** Reposition Soft Palate
Lapidus	Bunionectomy with metatarsal osteotomy	**ØMQS** Repair Foot Bursa and Ligament, Right **ØMQT** Repair Foot Bursa and Ligament, Left **ØQBN** Excision Metatarsal, Right **ØQBP** Excision Metatarsal, Left
Larry	Shoulder disarticulation	**ØX62** Detachment Shoulder Region, Right **ØX63** Detachment Shoulder Region, Left
Lash	Internal cervical os repair	**ØUVC** Restriction Cervix
LASH	Laparoscopically assisted supracervical hysterectomy	**ØUT9** Resection Uterus
Latzko	Cesarean section	**10D0** Extraction Products of Conception
Latzko	Colpocleisis	**ØULG** Occlusion Vagina
Le Fort	Colpocleisis	**ØULG** Occlusion Vagina
Leadbetter	Urethral reconstruction	**ØTRD** Replacement Urethra
Leadbetter-Politano	Ureteroneocystostomy	**ØT16** Bypass Ureter, Right **ØT17** Bypass Ureter, Left **ØT18** Bypass Ureters, Bilateral
LeMesurier	Cleft lip repair	**ØCQ0** Repair Upper Lip **ØCQ1** Repair Lower Lip

© 2018 Optum360, LLC

Procedure Eponyms

Eponym	Description	ICD-10-PCS Table Reference	
Leriche	Periarterial sympathectomy	01BK	Excision Head and Neck Sympathetic Nerve
		01BL	Excision Thoracic Sympathetic Nerve
		01BM	Excision Abdominal Sympathetic Nerve
		01BN	Excision Lumbar Sympathetic Nerve
		01BP	Excision Sacral Sympathetic Nerve
Lindholm	Repair of ruptured tendon	0LQ	Repair Tendons
Linton	Varicose vein	06D	Extraction Lower Veins
Lisfranc	Foot amputation	0Y6M	Detachment Foot, Right
		0Y6N	Detachment Foot, Left
Lisfranc	Shoulder disarticulation	0X62	Detachment Shoulder Region, Right
		0X63	Detachment Shoulder Region, Left
Littlewood	Forequarter amputation	0X60	Detachment Forequarter, Right
		0X61	Detachment Forequarter, Left
Lloyd-Davies	Abdominoperineal resection	0DTP	Resection Rectum
		0D1	Bypass Gastrointestinal System
Longmire	Bile duct anastomosis	0F1	Bypass Hepatobiliary System and Pancreas
Lord	Dilation of anal canal for hemorrhoids	0D7Q	Dilation Anus
Lord	Orchidopexy	0VS9	Reposition Testis, Right
		0VSB	Reposition Testis, Left
		0VSC	Reposition Testes, Bilateral
Lucas and Murray	Knee arthrodesis with plate	0SGC	Fusion Knee Joint, Right
		0SGD	Fusion Knee Joint, Left
Madlener	Tubal ligation	0UL5	Occlusion Fallopian Tube, Right
		0UL6	Occlusion Fallopian Tube, Left
		0UL7	Occlusion Fallopian Tubes, Bilateral
Magnuson (-Stack)	Arthroplasty for recurrent shoulder dislocation	0RSJ	Reposition Shoulder Joint, Right
		0RSK	Reposition Shoulder Joint, Left
Malström's	Vacuum extraction	10D0	Extraction Products of Conception
Malström's	Vacuum extraction with episiotomy	10D0	Extraction Products of Conception
		0W8N	Division Perineum, Female
Manchester (-Donald) (-Fothergill)	Uterine suspension	0US9	Reposition Uterus
Marckwald	Cervical os repair	0UVC	Restriction Cervix
Marshall-Marchetti (-Krantz)	Retropubic urethral suspension	0TSD	Reposition Urethra
Masters'	Stress test (two-step)	4A02	Measurement Cardiac
		4A12	Monitoring Cardiac
Matas	Aneurysmorrhaphy	02V	Restriction Heart and Great Vessels
		03V	Restriction Upper Arteries
		04V	Restriction Lower Arteries
Mayo	Bunionectomy	0STP	Resection Toe Phalangeal Joint, Right
		0STQ	Resection Toe Phalangeal Joint, Left
Mayo	Umbilical herniorrhaphy	0WQF	Repair Abdominal Wall
Mayo	Vaginal hysterectomy	0UT9	Resection Uterus

Procedure Eponyms

© 2018 Optum360, LLC

Eponym	Description	ICD-10-PCS Table Reference
Maze/Cox-Maze	Ablation or destruction of heart tissue	Ø258 Destruction Conduction Mechanism
Mazet	Knee disarticulation	ØY6F Detachment Knee Region, Right ØY6G Detachment Knee Region, Left
McBride	Bunionectomy with soft tissue correction	ØMQS Repair Foot Bursa and Ligament, Right ØMQT Repair Foot Bursa and Ligament, Left ØQBN Excision Metatarsal, Right ØQBP Excision Metatarsal, Left
McBurney	Repair inguinal hernia	ØYQ5 Repair Inguinal Region, Right ØYQ6 Repair Inguinal Region, Left
McCall	Enterocele repair	ØUQF Repair Cul-de-sac ØUUF Supplement Cul-de-sac
McCauley	Release of clubfoot	ØJ8Q Division Subcutaneous Tissue and Fascia, Right Foot ØJ8R Division Subcutaneous Tissue and Fascia, Left Foot ØLNN Release Lower Leg Tendon, Right ØLNP Release Lower Leg Tendon, Left ØLNS Release Ankle Tendon, Right ØLNT Release Ankle Tendon, Left ØLNV Release Foot Tendon, Right ØLNW Release Foot Tendon, Left
McDonald	Encirclement suture, cervix	ØUVC Restriction Cervix
McIndoe	Vaginal construction	ØUQG Repair Vagina ØUUG Supplement Vagina
McKeever	Fusion of first metatarsophalangeal joint for hallux valgus repair	ØSGM Fusion Metatarsal-Phalangeal Joint, Right ØSGN Fusion Metatarsal-Phalangeal Joint, Left
McKissock	Breast reduction	ØHØT Alteration Breast, Right ØHØU Alteration Breast, Left ØHØV Alteration Breast, Bilateral ØHBT Excision Breast, Right ØHBU Excision Breast, Left ØHBV Excision Breast, Bilateral
McReynolds	Transposition of pterygium	Ø8QS Repair Conjunctiva, Right Ø8QT Repair Conjunctiva, Left
McVay	Repair femoral or inguinal hernia	ØYQ5 Repair Inguinal Region, Right ØYQ6 Repair Inguinal Region, Left ØYQ7 Repair Femoral Region, Right ØYQ8 Repair Femoral Region, Left ØYQA Repair Inguinal Region, Bilateral ØYQE Repair, Femoral Region, Bilateral
Mikulicz	Exteriorization of intestine (first stage)	ØD1K Bypass Ascending Colon ØD1L Bypass Transverse Colon ØD1M Bypass Descending Colon ØD1N Bypass Sigmoid Colon

Eponym	Description	ICD-10-PCS Table Reference
Mikulicz	Excision of exteriorized segment of large intestine (second stage)	0DBE Excision Large Intestine 0DBF Excision Large Intestine, Right 0DBG Excision Large Intestine, Left 0DBK Excision Ascending Colon 0DBL Excision Transverse Colon 0DBM Excision Descending Colon 0DBN Excision Sigmoid Colon
Miles	Complete proctectomy	0DTP Resection Rectum
Millard	Cheiloplasty-rotation advancement	0KX1 Transfer facial muscle
Miller	Midtarsal arthrodesis	0SGH Fusion Tarsal Joint, Right 0SGJ Fusion Tarsal Joint, Left
Miller	Urethrovesical suspension	0TSC Reposition Bladder Neck 0TSD Reposition Urethra
Millin-Read	Urethrovesical suspension	0TSC Reposition Bladder Neck 0TSD Reposition Urethra
Mitchell	Hallux valgus repair	0Q8N Division Metatarsal, Right 0Q8P Division Metatarsal, Left 0MQS Repair Foot Bursa and Ligament, Right 0MQT Repair Foot Bursa and Ligament, Left 0QBN Excision Metatarsal, Right 0QBP Excision Metatarsal, Left
Mohs	Chemosurgical excision of skin	0HB Excision Skin and Breast 3E00 Introduction Skin and Mucous Membranes
Moore	Arthroplasty	0SRA Replacement Hip Joint, Acetabular Surface, Right 0SRE Replacement Hip Joint, Acetabular Surface, Left 0SRR Replacement Hip Joint, Femoral Surface, Right 0SRS Replacement Hip Joint, Femoral Surface, Left
Moschowitz	Repair femoral hernia	0YQ7 Repair Femoral Region, Right 0YQ8 Repair Femoral Region, Left 0YQE Repair, Femoral Region, Bilateral
Moschowitz	Enterocele repair	0UQF Repair Cul-de-sac
Moschowitz	Enterocele repair with graft or prosthesis	0UUF Supplement Cul-de-sac
Moschowitz	Sigmoidopexy	0DSN Reposition Sigmoid Colon
Muller	Banding of pulmonary artery	02VQ Restriction Pulmonary Artery, Right 02VR Restriction Pulmonary Artery, Left
Mumford	Partial claviculectomy	0PB9 Excision Clavicle, Right 0PBB Excision Clavicle, Left
Mustard	Interatrial transposition of venous return	02U Supplement Heart and Great Vessels
Nicola	Tenodesis for recurrent dislocation of shoulder	0LS1 Reposition Shoulder Tendon, Right 0LS2 Reposition Shoulder Tendon, Left
Nissen	Fundoplication of stomach	0DV4 Restriction Esophagogastric Junction
Noble	Plication of small intestine	0DS9 Reposition Duodenum 0DSA Reposition Jejunum 0DSB Reposition Ileum

Procedure Eponyms

© 2018 Optum360, LLC

Eponym	Description	ICD-10-PCS Table Reference
Norman Miller	Vaginopexy	**ØUSG** Reposition Vagina
Norton	Cesarean — extraperitoneal	**1ØDØ** Extraction Products of Conception
Norwood	Pulmonary artery homograft patch augmentation of aortic arch	**Ø2UX** Supplement Thoracic Aorta, Ascending/Arch
Ober (-Yount)	Gluteal-iliotibial fasciotomy	**ØJNC** Release Subcutaneous Tissue and Fascia, Pelvic Region **ØJNL** Release Subcutaneous Tissue and Fascia, Right Upper Leg **ØJNM** Release Subcutaneous Tissue and Fascia, Left Upper Leg
O'Donoghue	Triad knee repair	**ØMQN** Repair Knee Bursa and Ligament, Right **ØMQP** Repair Knee Bursa and Ligament, Left **ØSBC** Excision Knee Joint, Right **ØSBD** Excision Knee Joint, Left
Olshausen	Uterine suspension	**ØUS9** Reposition Uterus
Oscar Miller	Midtarsal arthrodesis	**ØSGH** Fusion Tarsal Joint, Right **ØSGJ** Fusion Tarsal Joint, Left
Osmond-Clark	Soft tissue release with peroneus brevis tendon transfer	**ØLXS** Transfer Ankle Tendon, Right **ØLXT** Transfer Ankle Tendon, Left
Oxford	Sling procedure for urinary incontinence	**ØTS** Reposition Urinary System
Panas	Linear proctotomy	**ØD9** Drainage Gastrointestinal System **ØDCP** Extirpation Rectum **ØDNP** Release Rectum
Pancoast	Division of trigeminal nerve at foramen ovale	**ØØ8K** Division Trigeminal Nerve
Pantaloon	Revision of gastric anastomosis	**ØDQ6** Repair Stomach
Paquin	Ureteroneocystostomy	**ØT16** Bypass Ureter, Right **ØT17** Bypass Ureter, Left **ØT18** Bypass Ureters, Bilateral
Partsch	Marsupialization of dental cyst	**ØNBR** Excision Maxilla **ØNBT** Excision Mandible, Right **ØNBV** Excision Mandible, Left
Pattee	Reconstruction of external auditory canal	**09RØ** Replacement External Ear, Right **09R1** Replacement External Ear, Left **09R2** Replacement External Ear, Bilateral **09UØ** Supplement External Ear, Right **09U1** Supplement External Ear, Left **09U2** Supplement External Ear, Bilateral **ØHR2** Replacement Skin, Right Ear **ØHR3** Replacement Skin, Left Ear
Peet	Splanchnic resection	**01BK** Excision Head and Neck Sympathetic Nerve **01BL** Excision Thoracic Sympathetic Nerve **01BM** Excision Abdominal Sympathetic Nerve **01BN** Excision Lumbar Sympathetic Nerve **01BP** Excision Sacral Sympathetic Nerve

Eponym	Description	ICD-10-PCS Table Reference	
Pemberton	Osteotomy of ilium	0Q82	Division Pelvic Bone, Right
		0Q83	Division Pelvic Bone, Left
		0QS2	Reposition Pelvic Bone, Right
		0QS3	Reposition Pelvic Bone, Left
Pemberton	Mobilization and fixation for rectal prolapse repair	0DSP	Reposition Rectum
Pereyra	Paraurethral suspension	0TSC	Reposition Bladder Neck
		0TSD	Reposition Urethra
Pinsker	Obliteration of nasoseptal telangiectasia	09RK	Replacement Nasal Mucosa and Soft Tissue
Piper	Forceps application to aftercoming head	10D	Extraction Pregnancy
Pirogoff	Ankle amputation through malleoli of tibia and fibula	0Y6M	Detachment Foot, Right
		0Y6N	Detachment Foot, Left
Politano-Leadbetter	Ureteroneocystostomy	0T16	Bypass Ureter, Right
		0T17	Bypass Ureter, Left
		0T18	Bypass Ureters, Bilateral
Polya	Gastrectomy	0D16	Bypass Stomach
		0DB6	Excision Stomach
Pomeroy	Ligation and division of fallopian tubes	0UB5	Excision Fallopian Tube, Right
		0UB6	Excision Fallopian Tube, Left
		0UB7	Excision Fallopian Tubes, Bilateral
Poncet	Lengthening of Achilles tendon	0L8N	Division Lower Leg Tendon, Right
		0L8P	Division Lower Leg Tendon, Left
Poncet	Urethrostomy, perineal	0TQD	Repair Urethra
Porro	Cesarean section	10D0	Extraction Products of Conception
Potts-Smith	Descending aorta-left pulmonary artery anastomosis	021W	Bypass Thoracic Aorta, Descending
Printen and Mason	High gastric bypass	0D16	Bypass Stomach
Puestow	Pancreaticojejunostomy	0F1G	Bypass Pancreas
Putti-Platt	Capsulorrhaphy of shoulder for recurrent dislocation	0RQJ	Repair Shoulder Joint, Right
		0RQK	Repair Shoulder Joint, Left
Rabbit ear	Anterior urethropexy (Tudor)	0TSC	Reposition Bladder Neck
		0TSD	Reposition Urethra
Ramadier	Intrapetrosal drainage	099B	Drainage Mastoid Sinus, Right
		099C	Drainage Mastoid Sinus, Left
Ramstedt	Pyloromyotomy (with wedge resection)	0D87	Division Stomach, Pylorus
		0DB7	Excision Stomach, Pylorus
Rankin	Exteriorization of intestine	0D1K	Bypass Ascending Colon
		0D1L	Bypass Transverse Colon
		0D1M	Bypass Descending Colon
		0D1N	Bypass Sigmoid Colon
Rankin	Proctectomy (complete)	0DTP	Resection Rectum
Rashkind	Atrial balloon septostomy	0216	Bypass, Atrium, Right
Rastelli	Creation of conduit between right ventricle and pulmonary artery	021K	Bypass Ventricle, Right
		02LH	Occlusion, Pulmonary Valve
Rastelli	Repair of pulmonary artery atresia	021K	Bypass Ventricle, Right
		02LH	Occlusion, Pulmonary Valve

© 2018 Optum360, LLC

Eponym	Description	ICD-10-PCS Table Reference
Rastelli	Repair of transposition of great vessels	Ø2LH Occlusion, Pulmonary Valve Ø2SP Reposition Pulmonary Trunk Ø2SW Reposition Thoracic Aorta, Descending Ø2SX Reposition, Thoracic Aorta, Ascending/Arch Ø2UP Supplement Pulmonary Trunk Ø2UW Supplement Thoracic Aorta, Descending Ø2UX Supplement Thoracic Aorta, Ascending/Arch
Rastelli	Repair of truncus arteriosus	Ø21K Bypass Ventricle, Right Ø2UM Supplement, ventricular septum Ø24F Creation, aortic valve
Raz-Pereyra	Bladder neck suspension	ØTSC Reposition Bladder Neck
Ripstein	Repair of rectal prolapse	ØDSP Reposition Rectum ØDUP Supplement Rectum
Rodney Smith	Radical subtotal pancreatectomy	ØFBG Excision Pancreas
Rodney Smith modification	Radical subtotal pancreatectomy	ØFBG Excision Pancreas
Roux-en-Y	Bile duct (choledochoenterostomy)	ØF19 Bypass Common Bile Duct
Roux-en-Y	Cholecystojejunostomy (anastomosis of gallbladder to intestine)	ØF14 Bypass Gallbladder
Roux-en-Y	Esophagus (intrathoracic) Intrathoracic esophagoenterostomy — (Anastomosis of esophagus to intestinal segment)	ØD12 Bypass Esophagus, Middle
Roux-en-Y	Gastroenterostomy	ØD16 Bypass Stomach
Roux-en-Y	Gastrojejunostomy	ØD16 Bypass Stomach
Roux-en-Y	Pancreaticojejunostomy — (anastomosis of pancreas (duct) to jejunum)	ØF1D Bypass Pancreatic Duct ØF1F Bypass Pancreatic Duct, Accessory ØF1G Bypass Pancreas
Roux-Goldthwait	Repair of patellar dislocation	ØQSD Reposition Patella, Right ØQSF Reposition Patella, Left
Roux-Herzen-Judine	Jejunal loop interposition	ØD11 Bypass Esophagus, Upper ØD12 Bypass Esophagus, Middle ØD13 Bypass Esophagus, Lower ØD15 Bypass Esophagus ØDB1 Excision Esophagus, Upper ØDB2 Excision Esophagus, Middle ØDB3 Excision Esophagus, Lower ØDB4 Excision Esophagogastric Junction ØDB5 Excision Esophagus ØDT1 Resection Esophagus, Upper ØDT2 Resection Esophagus, Middle ØDT3 Resection Esophagus, Lower ØDT4 Resection Esophagogastric Junction ØDT5 Resection Esophagus ØDX8 Transfer Small Intestine
Ruiz-Mora	Proximal phalangectomy for hammer toe	ØQBQ Excision Toe Phalanx, Right ØQBR Excision Toe Phalanx, Left

© 2018 Optum360, LLC

Procedure Eponyms

Eponym	Description	ICD-10-PCS Table Reference
Russe	Bone graft of scaphoid	ØPUM Supplement Carpal, Right ØPUN Supplement Carpal, Left
S.P. Rogers	Knee disarticulation	ØY6F Detachment Knee Region, Right ØY6G Detachment Knee Region, Left
Saemisch	Corneal section	Ø898 Drainage Cornea, Right Ø899 Drainage Cornea, Left
Salter	Innominate osteotomy	ØQB2 Excision Pelvic Bone, Right ØQB3 Excision Pelvic Bone, Left ØQS4 Reposition Acetabulum, Right ØQS5 Reposition Acetabulum, Left
Sano	Shunt/bypass of right ventricular outflow tract to main pulmonary artery	Ø21K Bypass right ventricle
Sauer-Bacon	Abdominoperineal resection	ØDTP Resection Rectum ØD1 Bypass Gastrointestinal System
Schanz	Femoral osteotomy	ØQS6 Reposition Upper Femur, Right ØQS7 Reposition Upper Femur, Left ØQS8 Reposition Femoral Shaft, Right ØQS9 Reposition Femoral Shaft, Left ØQSB Reposition Lower Femur, Right ØQSC Reposition Lower Femur, Left
Schauta (-Amreich)	Radical vaginal hysterectomy	ØUT4 Resection Uterine Supporting Structure ØUT9 Resection Uterus
Schede	Thoracoplasty	ØWQ8 Repair Chest Wall ØWU8 Supplement Chest Wall
Scheie	Sclerostomy (cautery of sclera)	Ø812 Bypass Anterior Chamber, Right Ø813 Bypass Anterior Chamber, Left
Schlatter	Total gastrectomy	ØDT6 Resection Stomach
Schroeder	Endocervical excision	ØUBC Excision Cervix
Schuchardt	Nonobstetrical episiotomy	ØH89 Division Skin, Perineum
Schwartze	Simple mastoidectomy	Ø9BB Excision Mastoid Sinus, Right Ø9BC Excision Mastoid Sinus, Left
Scott	Intestinal bypass for obesity	ØD1A Bypass Jejunum ØD1B Bypass Ileum ØD1H Bypass Cecum
Scott	Jejunocolostomy (bypass)	ØD1A Bypass Jejunum
Seddon-Brooks	Transfer of pectoralis major tendon	ØLXC Transfer Thorax Tendon, Right ØLXD Transfer Thorax Tendon, Left
Semb	Apicolysis of lung	ØBL4 Occlusion Upper Lobe Bronchus, Right ØBL8 Occlusion Upper Lobe Bronchus, Left
Senning	Correction of transposition of great vessels	Ø2U Supplement Heart and Great Vessels
Sever	Division of soft tissue of arm	ØK87 Division Upper Arm Muscle, Right ØK88 Division Upper Arm Muscle, Left ØK89 Division Lower Arm and Wrist Muscle, Right ØK8B Division Lower Arm and Wrist Muscle, Left

Procedure Eponyms

© 2018 Optum360, LLC

Eponym	Description	ICD-10-PCS Table Reference
Sewell	Indirect heart revascularization	**021** Bypass Heart and Great Vessels
Sharrard	Iliopsoas muscle transfer	**0KXN** Transfer Hip Muscle, Right **0KXP** Transfer Hip Muscle, Left
Shelf	Hip arthroplasty	**0QR4** Replacement Acetabulum, Right **0QR5** Replacement Acetabulum, Left **0QU4** Supplement Acetabulum, Right **0QU5** Supplement Acetabulum, Left
Shirodkar	Encirclement suture, cervix	**0UVC** Restriction Cervix
Silver	Bunionectomy	**0QBN** Excision Metatarsal, Right **0QBP** Excision Metatarsal, Left
Sistrunk	Excision of thyroglossal cyst	**0JB4** Excision Subcutaneous Tissue and Fascia, Right Neck **0JB5** Excision Subcutaneous Tissue and Fascia, Left Neck
SKyphoplasty	Percutaneous vertebral augmentation	**0PS3** Reposition Cervical Vertebra **0PS4** Reposition Thoracic Vertebra **0QS0** Reposition Lumbar Vertebra **0PU3** Supplement Cervical Vertebra **0PU4** Supplement Thoracic Vertebra **0QU0** Supplement Lumbar Vertebra
Slocum	Pes anserinus transfer	**0LXQ** Transfer Knee Tendon, Right **0LXR** Transfer Knee Tendon, Left
Sluder	Tonsillectomy	**0CTP** Resection Tonsils
Smith	Open osteotomy of mandible	**0NQT** Repair Mandible, Right **0NQV** Repair Mandible, Left **0NST** Reposition Mandible, Right **0NSV** Reposition Mandible, Left
Smith-Peterson	Radiocarpal arthrodesis	**0RGN** Fusion Wrist Joint, Right **0RGP** Fusion Wrist Joint, Left
Smithwick	Sympathectomy	**01BK** Excision Head and Neck Sympathetic Nerve **01BL** Excision Thoracic Sympathetic Nerve **01BM** Excision Abdominal Sympathetic Nerve **01BN** Excision Lumbar Sympathetic Nerve **01BP** Excision Sacral Sympathetic Nerve
Soave	Endorectal pull-through	**0DTP** Resection Rectum
Sonneberg	Inferior maxillary neurectomy	**00BK** Excision Trigeminal Nerve
Sorondo-Ferré	Hindquarter amputation	**0Y62** Detachment Hindquarter, Right **0Y63** Detachment Hindquarter, Left **0Y64** Detachment Hindquarter, Bilateral
Soutter	Iliac crest fasciotomy	**0J8C** Division Subcutaneous Tissue and Fascia, Pelvic Region **0JNC** Release Subcutaneous Tissue and Fascia, Pelvic Region
Spalding-Richardson	Uterine suspension	**0US9** Reposition Uterus
Spinelli	Correction of inverted uterus	**0US9** Reposition Uterus
Spivack	Permanent gastrostomy	**0D16** Bypass Stomach
Ssabanejew-Frank	Permanent gastrostomy	**0D16** Bypass Stomach

© 2018 Optum360, LLC

Eponym	Description	ICD-10-PCS Table Reference
Stacke	Simple mastoidectomy	**09BB** Excision Mastoid Sinus, Right **09BC** Excision Mastoid Sinus, Left
Stallard	Conjunctivocystorhinostomy (Conjunctivodacryocystorhinostomy [CDCR])	**081X** Bypass Lacrimal Duct, Right **081Y** Bypass Lacrimal Duct, Left
Stallard	Conjunctivorhinostomy with insertion of tube or stent	**081X** Bypass Lacrimal Duct, Right **081Y** Bypass Lacrimal Duct, Left
Stamm (-Kader)	Temporary gastrostomy	**0D16** Bypass Stomach
Steinberg	Revision of gastric anastomosis	**0DQ6** Repair Stomach
Steindler	Fascia stripping (for cavus deformity)	**0J8Q** Division Subcutaneous Tissue and Fascia, Right Foot **0J8R** Division Subcutaneous Tissue and Fascia, Left Foot **0JDQ** Extraction Subcutaneous Tissue and Fascia, Right Foot **0JDR** Extraction Subcutaneous Tissue and Fascia, Left Foot **0JNQ** Release Subcutaneous Tissue and Fascia, Right Foot **0JNR** Release Subcutaneous Tissue and Fascia, Left Foot
Steindler	Flexorplasty (elbow)	**0KX7** Transfer Upper Arm Muscle, Right **0KX8** Transfer Upper Arm Muscle, Left
Steindler	Muscle transfer	**0KX9** Transfer Lower Arm and Wrist Muscle, Right **0KXB** Transfer Lower Arm and Wrist Muscle, Left
Stewart	Renal plication with pyeloplasty	**0TQ3** Repair Kidney Pelvis, Right **0TQ4** Repair Kidney Pelvis, Left **0TS0** Reposition Kidney, Right **0TS1** Reposition Kidney, Left **0TS2** Reposition Kidneys, Bilateral
Stone	Anoplasty	**0DQR** Repair Anal Sphincter
Strassman	Metroplasty	**0UQ9** Repair Uterus
Strayer	Gastrocnemius recession	**0L8N** Division Lower Leg Tendon, Right **0L8P** Division Lower Leg Tendon, Left **0LSN** Reposition Lower Leg Tendon, Right **0LSP** Reposition Lower Leg Tendon, Left
Stromeyer-Little	Hepatotomy	**0F90** Drainage Liver **0F91** Drainage Liver, Right Lobe **0F92** Drainage Liver, Left Lobe
Strong	Unbridling of celiac artery axis	**04N1** Release Celiac Artery
Sturmdorf	Conization of cervix	**0UBC** Excision Cervix
Summerskill	Dacryocystorhinostomy by intubation	**081X** Bypass Lacrimal Duct, Right **081Y** Bypass Lacrimal Duct, Left
Surmay	Jejunostomy	**0DHA** Insertion Jejunum
Swenson	Bladder reconstruction	**0TUB** Supplement Bladder **0DBB** Excision Ileum **0DBN** Excision Sigmoid Colon
Swenson	Proctectomy	**0DTP** Resection Rectum

Procedure Eponyms

© 2018 Optum360, LLC

Eponym	Description	ICD-10-PCS Table Reference	
Swinney	Urethral reconstruction	**ØTUD**	Supplement Urethra
Syme	Ankle amputation through malleoli of tibia and fibula	**ØY6M** **ØY6N**	Detachment Foot, Right Detachment Foot, Left
Syme	Urethrotomy, external	**ØT7D** **ØT9D** **ØTCD**	Dilation Urethra Drainage Urethra Extirpation Urethra
Taarnhoj	Trigeminal nerve root decompression	**ØØNK**	Release Trigeminal Nerve
Tack	Sacculotomy	**Ø99D** **Ø99E**	Drainage Inner Ear, Right Drainage Inner Ear, Left
Talma-Morison	Omentopexy	**ØDQU**	Repair Omentum
TandemHeart	Insertion of percutaneous external heart assist device	**Ø2HA** **5AØ2**	Insertion Heart Assistance Cardiac
Tanner	Devascularization of stomach	**Ø4L2**	Occlusion Gastric Artery
TAPVC (total anomalous pulmonary venous connection)	One-stage total correction of total anomalous pulmonary venous connection with or without: • Anastomosis between (horizontal) common pulmonary trunk and posterior wall of left atrium (side-to-side) • Enlargement of foramen ovale • Incision (excision) of common wall between posterior left atrium and coronary sinus and roofing of resultant defect with patch graft (synthetic) • Ligation of venous connection (descending anomalous vein) (to left innominate vein) (to superior vena cava) • Repair of atrial septal defect (with prosthesis)	**Ø21** **Ø2L** **Ø2R** **Ø2U**	Bypass Heart and Great Vessels Occlusion Heart and Great Vessels Replacement Heart and Great Vessels Supplement Heart and Great Vessels
Tetralogy of Fallot, total repair (one-stage)	One-stage total correction of tetralogy of Fallot with or without: • Commissurotomy of pulmonary valve • Infundibulectomy • Outflow tract prosthesis • Patch graft of outflow tract • Prosthetic tube for pulmonary artery • Repair of ventricular septal defect (with prosthesis) • Take-down of previous systemic-pulmonary artery anastomosis	**Ø2B** **Ø2N** **Ø2R** **Ø2U**	Excision Heart and Great Vessels Release Heart and Great Vessels Replacement Heart and Great Vessels Supplement Heart and Great Vessels
Thal	Repair of esophageal stricture	**ØDQ3** **ØDQ5** **ØDS6**	Repair Esophagus, Lower Repair Esophagus Reposition Stomach
Thiersch	Rectal prolapse repair	**ØDQR** **ØDUR**	Repair Anal Sphincter Supplement Anal Sphincter
Thiersch	Skin graft	**ØHR**	Replacement Skin and Breast
Thompson	Cleft lip repair	**ØCQØ** **ØCQ1**	Repair Upper Lip Repair Lower Lip

Procedure Eponyms

Eponym	Description	ICD-10-PCS Table Reference	
Thompson	Correction of lymphedema	07Q	Repair Lymphatic and Hemic Systems
		07U	Supplement Lymphatic and Hemic Systems
Thompson	Quadricepsplasty	0KNQ	Release Upper Leg Muscle, Right
		0KNR	Release Upper Leg Muscle, Left
		0KQQ	Repair Upper Leg Muscle, Right
		0KQR	Repair Upper Leg Muscle, Left
Thompson	Thumb apposition with bone graft	0PRR	Replacement Thumb Phalanx, Right
		0PRS	Replacement Thumb Phalanx, Left
		0PUR	Supplement Thumb Phalanx, Right
		0PUS	Supplement Thumb Phalanx, Left
Thoratec	Implantable ventricular assist device (IVAD)	02HA	Insertion Heart
		5A02	Assistance Cardiac
Thoratec	Ventricular assist device (VAD)	02HA	Insertion Heart
		5A02	Assistance Cardiac
Thorek	Partial cholecystectomy	0FB4	Excision Gallbladder
TKP	Thermokeratoplasty	08Q8	Repair Cornea, Right
		08Q9	Repair Cornea, Left
Tomkins	Metroplasty	0UQ9	Repair Uterus
Tommy John surgery	Ulnar collateral ligament reconstruction	0MU3	Supplement Elbow Bursa and Ligament, Right
		0MU4	Supplement Elbow Bursa and Ligament, Left
Torek (-Bevan)	Orchidopexy (first stage) (second stage)	0VS9	Reposition Testis, Right
		0VSB	Reposition Testis, Left
		0VSC	Reposition Testes, Bilateral
Torkildsen	Ventriculocisternal shunt	0016	Bypass Cerebral Ventricle
Torpin	Cul-de-sac resection	0UQF	Repair Cul-de-sac
Toti	Dacryocystorhinostomy (DCR)	081X	Bypass Lacrimal Duct, Right
		081Y	Bypass Lacrimal Duct, Left
Touchas	Size reduction plastic operation	0J0	Alteration Subcutaneous Tissue and Fascia
		0W0	Alteration Anatomical Regions, General
		0X0	Alteration Anatomical Regions, Upper Extremities
		0Y0	Alteration Anatomical Regions, Lower Extremities
Touroff	Ligation of subclavian artery	03L3	Occlusion Subclavian Artery, Right
		03L4	Occlusion Subclavian Artery, Left
Transbronchial needle aspiration (TBNA) biopsy	Transbronchial needle aspiration (TBNA) biopsy of the lung	0B9	Drainage Respiratory System
		0BD	Extraction, Respiratory System
Transbronchial needle aspiration (TBNA) biopsy	Transbronchial needle aspiration (TBNA) biopsy of bronchus	0B9	Drainage Respiratory System
		0BD	Extraction, Respiratory System
Transbronchial needle aspiration (TBNA) biopsy	Transbronchial needle aspiration (TBNA) biopsy of lymph node	07D	Extraction, Lymphatic and Hemic Systems
Trauner	Lingual sulcus extension	0CN4	Release Buccal Mucosa

© 2018 Optum360, LLC

Eponym	Description	ICD-10-PCS Table Reference
Tsuge	Macrodactyly repair	**ØPBR** Excision Thumb Phalanx, Right **ØPBS** Excision Thumb Phalanx, Left **ØPBT** Excision Finger Phalanx, Right **ØPBV** Excision Finger Phalanx, Left **ØQBQ** Excision Toe Phalanx, Right **ØQBR** Excision Toe Phalanx, Left **ØQQQ** Repair Toe Phalanx, Right **ØQQR** Repair Toe Phalanx, Left **ØXQL** Repair Thumb, Right **ØXQM** Repair Thumb, Left **ØXQN** Repair Index Finger, Right **ØXQP** Repair Index Finger, Left **ØXQQ** Repair Middle Finger, Right **ØXQR** Repair Middle Finger, Left **ØXQS** Repair Ring Finger, Right **ØXQT** Repair Ring Finger, Left **ØXQV** Repair Little Finger, Right **ØXQW** Repair Little Finger, Left
Tudor "rabbit ear"	Anterior urethropexy	**ØTSC** Reposition Bladder Neck **ØTSD** Reposition Urethra
Tuffier	Apicolysis of lung	**ØBL** Occlusion Respiratory System **ØBV** Restriction Respiratory System
Tuffier	Vaginal hysterectomy	**ØUT9** Resection Uterus **ØUTC** Resection Cervix
Turco	Release of joint capsules in clubfoot	**ØM8** Division Bursae and Ligaments **ØMN** Release Bursae and Ligaments **ØSN** Release Lower Joints
Uchida	Tubal ligation with or without fimbriectomy	**ØUL5** Occlusion Fallopian Tube, Right **ØUL6** Occlusion Fallopian Tube, Left **ØUL7** Occlusion Fallopian Tubes, Bilateral **ØUB5** Excision Fallopian Tube, Right **ØUB6** Excision Fallopian Tube, Left **ØUB7** Excision Fallopian Tubes, Bilateral
Urban	Mastectomy (unilateral)	**ØHTT** Resection Breast, Right **ØHTU** Resection Breast, Left **Ø7T5** Resection Lymphatic, Right Axillary **Ø7T6** Resection Lymphatic, Left Axillary **Ø7T7** Resection Lymphatic, Thorax **Ø7T8** Resection Lymphatic, Internal Mammary, Right **Ø7T9** Resection Lymphatic, Internal Mammary, Left **ØKTH** Resection Thorax Muscle, Right **ØKTJ** Resection Thorax Muscle, Left
Vectra	Vascular access graft	**ØJH** Insertion Subcutaneous Tissue and Fascia **Ø2H** Insertion Heart and Great Vessels
Vicq D'azyr	Temporary tracheostomy — laryngotracheotomy/cricothyrotomy	**ØB11** Bypass Trachea
Vidal	Varicocele ligation	**Ø6LY** Occlusion Lower Veins
von Kraske	Proctectomy	**ØDBP** Excision Rectum
Voss	Hanging hip operation	**ØK8** Division Muscles **ØKN** Release Muscles

Procedure Eponyms

Eponym	Description	ICD-10-PCS Table Reference	
Vulpius (-Compere)	Lengthening of gastrocnemius muscle	0L8N	Division Lower Leg Tendon, Right
		0L8P	Division Lower Leg Tendon, Left
WANG™ transbronchial needle aspiration biopsy	Transbronchial needle aspiration (TBNA) biopsy of the lung	0B9	Drainage Respiratory System
		0BD	Extraction, Respiratory System
WANG™ transbronchial needle aspiration biopsy	Transbronchial needle aspiration (TBNA) biopsy of bronchus	0B9	Drainage Respiratory System
		0BD	Extraction, Respiratory System
WANG™ transbronchial needle aspiration biopsy	Transbronchial needle aspiration (TBNA) biopsy of lymph node	07D	Extraction, Lymphatic and Hemic Systems
Wardill	Correction of cleft palate by push-back operation	0CS2	Reposition Hard Palate
		0CS3	Reposition Soft Palate
Ward-Mayo	Vaginal hysterectomy	0UT9	Resection Uterus
Waters Cesarean section	Supravesical extraperitoneal cesarean section	10D0	Extraction Products of Conception
Waterston	Aorta to right pulmonary artery anastomosis	021W	Bypass Thoracic Aorta, Descending
		021X	Bypass Thoracic Aorta, Ascending/ Arch
Watkins (-Wertheim)	Interposition operation of uterus	0US9	Reposition Uterus
Watson-Jones	Hip arthrodesis	0SG9	Fusion Hip Joint, Right
		0SGB	Fusion Hip Joint, Left
Watson-Jones	Reconstruction of lateral ligaments, ankle	0MQQ	Repair Ankle Bursa and Ligament, Right
		0MQR	Repair Ankle Bursa and Ligament, Left
Watson-Jones	Shoulder arthrodesis (extra-articular)	0RGJ	Fusion Shoulder Joint, Right
		0RGK	Fusion Shoulder Joint, Left
Watson-Jones	Tenoplasty	0LQ	Repair Tendons
Weir	Appendicostomy	0D9J	Drainage Appendix
Weir	Nostril reduction/correction of nostrils	090K	Alteration Nasal Mucosa and Soft Tissue
Wertheim	Radical hysterectomy	0UT4	Resection Uterine Supporting Structure
		0UT9	Resection Uterus
West	Dacryocystorhinostomy (DCR)	081X	Bypass Lacrimal Duct, Right
		081Y	Bypass Lacrimal Duct, Left
Wheeler	Entropion repair with lid reconstruction	08UN	Supplement Upper Eyelid, Right
		08UP	Supplement Upper Eyelid, Left
		08UQ	Supplement Lower Eyelid, Right
		08UR	Supplement Lower Eyelid, Left
Wheeler	Eyelid halving procedure	08BN	Excision Upper Eyelid, Right
		08BP	Excision Upper Eyelid, Left
		08BQ	Excision Lower Eyelid, Right
		08BR	Excision Lower Eyelid, Left
Whipple	Pancreaticoduodenectomy with or without cholecystectomy (pancreaticoduodenal resection or excision with choledochojejunal anastomosis, pancreaticojejunal anastomosis, and gastrojejunostomy)	0DB7	Excision Stomach Pylorus
		0DT9	Resection Duodenum or
		0DB9	Excision Duodenum
		0FBG	Excision Pancreas
		0DT4	Resection Gallbladder

Procedure Eponyms

© 2018 Optum360, LLC

Eponym	Description	ICD-10-PCS Table Reference
Whipple- Child modification	Radical subtotal (partial) pancreatectomy	ØFBG Excision of Pancreas
Whipple- Rodney Smith modification	Radical subtotal (partial) pancreatectomy	ØFBG Excision of Pancreas
White	Lengthening of tendo calcaneus by incomplete tenotomy	ØL8N Division Lower Leg Tendon, Right ØL8P Division Lower Leg Tendon, Left
Whitehead	Glossectomy, radical	ØCT7 Resection Tongue
Whitehead	Hemorrhoidectomy	Ø6BY Excision Lower Vein ØDBP Excision Rectum
Whitman	Foot stabilization (talectomy)	ØQTL Resection Tarsal, Right ØQTM Resection Tarsal, Left
Whitman	Hip reconstruction	ØSQ9 Repair Hip Joint, Right ØSQB Repair Hip Joint, Left ØQU4 Supplement Acetabulum, Right ØQU5 Supplement Acetabulum, Left
Whitman	Repair of serratus anterior muscle	ØKQH Repair Thorax Muscle, Right ØKQJ Repair Thorax Muscle, Left
Whitman	Talectomy	ØQBL Excision Tarsal, Right ØQBM Excision Tarsal, Left
Whitman	Trochanter wedge osteotomy	ØQS6 Reposition Upper Femur, Right ØQS7 Reposition Upper Femur, Left
Wier	Entropion repair with lid reconstruction	Ø8UN Supplement Upper Eyelid, Right Ø8UP Supplement Upper Eyelid, Left Ø8UQ Supplement Lower Eyelid, Right Ø8UR Supplement Lower Eyelid, Left
Williams-Richardson	Vaginal construction/reconstruction - creation of vaginal canal (vaginoplasty, vulvovaginoplasty) with graft or prosthesis	ØUUG Supplement Vagina
Williams-Richardson	Vaginal construction/reconstruction - creation of vaginal canal (vaginoplasty, vulvovaginoplasty)	ØUQG Repair Vagina
Wilms	Thoracoplasty	ØWQ8 Repair Chest Wall ØWU8 Supplement Chest Wall
Wilson	First metatarsal angulation (oblique) osteotomy for hallux valgus	ØMQ Repair Bursae and Ligaments ØQ8 Division Lower Bones ØQB Excision Lower Bones
Winiwarter	Cholecystoenterostomy	ØF14 Bypass Gallbladder
Witzel	Temporary gastrostomy	ØD16 Bypass Stomach
Woodward	Release of high riding scapula (Sprengel deformity)	ØPQ5 Repair Scapula, Right ØPQ6 Repair Scapula, Left ØPS5 Reposition Scapula, Right ØPS6 Reposition Scapula, Left
Young	Anterior tibialis tendon transfer (repair of flat foot)	ØLXV Transfer Foot Tendon, Right ØLXW Transfer Foot Tendon, Left
Young	Epispadias repair	ØTSD Reposition Urethra

© 2018 Optum360, LLC

Eponym	Description	ICD-10-PCS Table Reference	
Yount	Division of iliotibial band (Z-plasty for tendon lengthening)	0J8L	Division Subcutaneous Tissue and Fascia, Right Upper Leg
		0J8M	Division Subcutaneous Tissue and Fascia, Left Upper Leg
Zancolli	Biceps tendon transfer	0LX3	Transfer Upper Arm Tendon, Right
		0LX4	Transfer Upper Arm Tendon, Left
Zancolli	Capsuloplasty	0RQU	Repair Metacarpophalangeal Joint, Right
		0RQV	Repair Metacarpophalangeal Joint, Left
Zenith Flex® AAA Endovascular Graft	AAA endovascular graft (intraluminal device)	04V0	Restriction Abdominal Aorta
Zenith TX2® TAA Endovascular Graft	TAA endovascular graft (intraluminal device)	02VW	Restriction Thoracic Aorta, Descending
		02VX	Restriction Thoracic Aorta, Ascending/Arch
Zenith® Renu™ AAA Ancillary Graft	AAA ancillary graft (intraluminal device)	04V0	Restriction Abdominal Aorta
Ziegler	Iridectomy	08BC	Excision Iris, Right
		08BD	Excision Iris, Left

Procedure Eponyms

© 2018 Optum360, LLC

Surgical Terms

A special language is spoken in the surgical suite and written in the medical charts documenting procedures. The following list includes many of the medical terms heard most often in the operating room.

ablation. Surgical removal or destruction of a part, using electrocautery, radiofrequency, laser, chemicals, or hot and cold liquids.

abrasion. Removal of layers of skin.

achalasia. Failure of the smooth muscles within the gastrointestinal tract to relax at points of junction; most commonly referring to the esophagogastric sphincter's failure to relax when swallowing.

acromioplasty. Repair of the part of the shoulder blade that connects to the deltoid muscles and clavicle.

advance. To move away from the starting point.

allograft. Transplanted tissue from the same species.

amputation. Removal of a limb or part of a limb.

analysis. Study of a body section or parts.

anastomosis. Surgically created connection between ducts, blood vessels, or bowel segments to allow flow from one to the other.

aneurysm. Circumscribed dilation or outpouching of an artery wall, often containing blood clots connecting directly with the lumen of the artery.

angioplasty. Reconstruction of a blood vessel.

antibody. Immunoglobulin or protective protein encoded within its building block sequence to interact only with its specific antigen.

antigen. Substance inducing sensitivity or triggering an immune response and the production of antibodies.

antrum. Chamber or cavity, typically with a small opening.

appliance. Device providing function to a body part.

arthrocentesis. Aspiration of fluid from a joint with needle.

arthrodesis. Surgical fixation of a joint.

arthroplasty. Restoration of a joint.

arthroscopy. Endoscopic examination of a joint.

arthrotomy. Surgical incision into a joint.

articulate. Comprised of separate segments joined together, allowing for movement of each part on the other.

aspiration. Drawing in or out by suction.

assay. Test of purity.

astragalectomy. Surgical excision of the talus (ankle) bone.

augmentation. Add to or increase the substance of a body site, usually performed as plastic reconstructive measures. Augmentation may involve the use of an implant or prosthesis, especially within soft tissue or grafting procedures, such as bone tissue.

autograft. Any tissue harvested from one anatomical site of a person and grafted to another anatomical site of the same person. Most commonly, blood vessels, skin, tendons, fascia, and bone are used as autografts.

avulse. Tear away from.

benign. Mild or nonmalignant in nature.

bioartificial. Comprising both living tissue or cells and synthetic materials.

biofeedback. Technique allowing the patient to control body function.

biometry. Statistical analysis of biological data.

biopsy. Tissue or fluid removed for diagnostic purposes through analysis of the cells in the biopsy material.

blood type. Classification of blood by group.

bougie. Probe used to dilate or calibrate a body part.

bovine. Of or relating to cattle (cows).

brachytherapy. Radiotherapy proximate to the organ being treated.

bridge. Connection between two parts of an organ.

bronchoscopy. Visual inspection of the airway using a fiberoptic scope.

brush. Tool used to gather cell samples or clean body part.

burr. Drill used to cut and shape bone.

bursa. Cavity or sac containing fluid that occurs between articulating surfaces and serves to reduce friction from moving parts.

bypass. 1) Auxiliary flow. 2) A surgically created pathway altering the route of passage of the contents of a tubular body part.

calculus. Concretion of calcium, cholesterol, salts, or other substances that forms in any part of the body.

cannula. Tube inserted to facilitate passage.

capsulorrhaphy. Suturing or repair of a joint capsule, most frequently done on the glenohumeral joint.

capsulotomy. Incision made into a capsule, such as the lens of the eye, the kidney, or a joint.

c-arm. Portable x-ray machine for surgery.

cast. Rigid encasement for therapeutic purposes.

catheter. Any of a number of tubes inserted in body parts.

cauterize. Heat or chemicals used to burn or cut.

celiotomy. Incision through the abdominal wall into the abdominal cavity, also laparotomy.

cement. Bone cement/polymethyl methacrylate (PMMA), used for orthopedic implant fixation.

centesis. Puncture or perforation.

cephalad. Toward the head.

cerclage. Looping or encircling an organ or tissue with wire or ligature for positional support.

cheiloplasty. Surgery of the lip.

chemodenervation. Chemical destruction of nerves.

chemosurgery. Application of chemical agents to destroy tissue, originally referring to the in situ chemical fixation of premalignant or malignant lesions to facilitate surgical excision.

chemotherapy. Treatment of disease, especially cancerous conditions, using chemical agents.

chisel. Instrument for cutting or planing bone.

chondral. Cartilage.

chromotubation. Medication injection into the uterus and tubes.

cicatricial. Concerning a scar.

ciliary. Pertaining to certain structures in or around the eye and eyelid (ciliary body, ciliary muscle, ciliary process, anterior ciliary vein).

circumcise. Circular cutting around a body part.

clamp. Tool used to grip, compress, join, or fasten body parts.

clipping. Occlusion or completely closing the orifice or lumen.

closure. Suturing of an incision.

clysis. Fluids injected into the body.

coblation. Controlled ablation; shrinking tissue with radiofrequency and saline.

coctolabile. Capable of being destroyed or altered when boiled.

comminuted. Fracture type in which the bone is splintered or crushed.

commissure. Juncture where two corresponding parts come together, especially referring to the union site of adjacent heart valve cusps.

complex. Composite of anatomical parts or surgical procedures.

composite. Made of two or more different parts or elements.

conduit. Channel for passage of fluids or air.

condyle. Rounded end of a bone that forms an articulation.

conization. Excision of a cone-shaped piece of tissue.

constriction. Therapeutic binding of a body part.

contour. Act of shaping along desired lines.

corpectomy. Removal of the body of a bone, such as a vertebra.

correct. Body part modification.

craterization. Formation of a depression in body tissue.

cross match. Test used to match the compatibility of a donor's blood or organ to the recipient.

crus. 1) Any body part resembling a leg. 2) Lower part of the leg.

cryotherapy. Any surgical procedure that uses intense cold for treatment.

culture. Growth of microorganisms in a medium conducive to their development.

curettage. Removal of tissue by scraping.

cutaneous. Relating to the skin.

cystotomy. Incision into the gallbladder or urinary bladder.

debridement. Removal of dead or contaminated tissue and foreign matter from a wound.

decompress. Relieve pressure.

decubitus. 1) Pressure ulcer often spawned by bedrest. 2) Patient's position in bed.

dehiscence. Rupture or bursting open.

deligation. Closure by tying up; sutures, ligatures.

denervation. Destruction or deprivation of nerve connection, by either excision, incision, or injection.

depressor. Tool used to push body tissue out of the way.

dermabrasion. Cosmetic procedure that smooths out flaws and disfigured skin and promotes the growth of a new layer of skin cells by removing the outer layer of skin by mechanical or chemical means such as fine sandpaper, wire brushes, and caustic substances.

© 2018 Optum360, LLC

destruction. Tissue elimination or eradication by the direct use of energy, force, or a destructive agent.

detection. Search for presence of a tissue or material.

diagnostic. Aid in diagnosis.

dialysis. Diffusion of body fluids to restore normal balance.

diaphysis. Central shaft of a long bone.

diathermy. Therapeutic use of heat in a part of the body.

dilation. Expansion or stretching an opening, hollow or tubular structure.

dilution. Concentration reduction of a mixture or solution by adding more fluid.

disarticulation. Amputation through a joint.

discectomy/diskectomy. Removal of an intervertebral disc (disk).

dislocation. Displacement of a body part.

dissection. Cut apart or separate tissues or body structures apart or into pieces.

distension. Stretched or dilated.

diversion. Rechanneling of body fluid through another conduit.

diverticulum. Pouch or sac in the walls of an organ or canal.

division. Separating into two or more parts.

donor. Person from whom tissues or organs are removed for transplantation.

dorsum. Back side or back part of the body or individual anatomical structure.

dosimetry. Component in the administration of radiation oncology therapy in which a radiation dose is calculated to a specific site, including implant or beam orientation and exposure, isodose strengths, tissue inhomogeneities, and volume.

drain. Drawing of fluid or air from a cavity or site.

drill. Making a hole in a bone or hard tissue.

dynamic. Motion in response to forces.

echography. Ultrasonography.

ectopic. Abnormal position.

edentulous. Toothless.

electrocautery. Division or cutting of tissue using high-frequency electrical current to produce heat, which destroys cells.

elevator. Tool for lifting tissues or bone.

elution. 1) Separation of one solid from another, usually by washing. 2) Washing a substance from a material into the fluid in which it is immersed (e.g. drug on a stent in the bloodstream).

embolism. Obstruction of a blood vessel resulting from a clot or foreign substance.

embolization. Natural or artificial formation or development of an embolus.

embolus. An abnormal particle, blood clot or a piece of plaque that travels from the site where it formed to another location in the body.

endobronchial. Within the bronchus.

endoscopy. Visual inspection of the body using a fiberoptic scope.

enteroscopy. Visual inspection of the digestive system using a fiberoptic scope.

enterostomy. Surgical formation of an opening into the intestine through an abdominal wall stoma.

epiphyses. Ends of a long bone.

epithelize. Formation of epithelial cells over a surface. Also epithelialize.

escharotomy. Surgical incision into the scab or crust resulting from a severe burn in order to relieve constriction and allow blood flow to the distal unburned tissue.

esophagoscopy. Internal visual inspection of the esophagus through the use of an endoscope placed down the throat.

evacuation. Removal of material, especially waste material.

evisceration. Removal of contents of a cavity.

examination. Comprehensive visual and tactile screening and specific testing leading to diagnosis or, as appropriate, to a referral to another practitioner.

exchange. Substitution of one thing for another.

excise. Remove or cut out.

exclusion. Closure by any method.

exenteration. Surgical removal of the entire contents of a body cavity, such as the pelvis or orbit.

exfoliate. Skin falling off in layers.

exploration. Examination for diagnostic purposes.

exposure. Displaying, revealing, or making accessible.

expression. Squeezing out of tissue.

exteriorize. 1) Expose an organ temporarily for observation. 2) Transpose an internal organ to the exterior of the body.

external fixation. Rods and pins connected in a lattice to secure bone.

extract. 1) Condensed medication. 2) To draw or pull out with force or effort.

fascia. Fibrous sheet or band of tissue that envelops organs, muscles, and groupings of muscles.

fasciotomy. Cutting through fascia.

fenestrated. Having one or more openings.

fenestration. Openings in tissue or bandage.

fibrosis. Formation of fibrous tissue as part of the restorative process.

filiform. Probe with woven-thread end.

fissure. Deep furrow or groove in tissue structures.

fistula. Tube-like passage between two cavities.

fistulization. Creation of a fistula for therapeutic reasons.

fit. Attack of acute symptoms.

fixate. Hold, secure, or fasten in position.

fixation. Attach tissue or material.

flap. Mass of flesh moved for grafting.

fluoroscopy. Radiology technique that allows real-time visual examination of part of the body or a function of an organ using a device that projects an x-ray image on a fluorescent screen.

follow-up. Visits or treatment following a procedure.

forceps. Tool for grasping or compressing tissue.

fossa. Indentation or shallow depression.

fragment. Division into pieces.

free graft. Unattached tissue moved to another part of the body.

fresh frozen plasma. Fluid, unconcentrated source of all clotting factors without platelets, of a unit of human blood which is centrifuged, separated, and frozen while fresh (within eight hours of collection).

frozen section. Thin slice of frozen tissue removed for microscopic study with a special cutting instrument, often used to confirm the nature of tissue during a procedure.

fulgurate. Destruction by electric current.

full-thickness graft. Skin graft that includes the full thickness of the skin with little or no subcutaneous tissue.

furuncle. Inflamed, painful cyst or nodule on the skin caused by bacteria, often staphylococcus, entering along the hair follicle.

fusion. Union of tissues, especially bone.

Gigli saw. Saw made of thin, flexible wire with teeth along the edge used for cutting bones (e.g., craniotomy).

glomectomy (carotid). Removal of the carotid body framework.

graft. Tissue implant from another part of the body or another person.

guillotine. 1) Surgical instrument with a ring and a handle with a knife blade used for cutting protruding structures such as tonsils. 2) Amputation technique that leaves an open wound at the end of the stump requiring a second stage closure.

halo. Tool for stabilizing the head and spine.

harvest. Removal of cells or tissue from their native site to be used as a graft or transplant to another part of the donor's body or placed into another person.

hematoma. Solidified (clotted or partially clotted) localized tumor-like collection of blood in some part of the body caused by a break in a blood vessel wall, usually as a result of trauma.

hemilaminectomy. Excision of a portion of the vertebral lamina.

hemiphalangectomy. Excision of part of the phalanx.

hemostasis. Interruption of blood flow or the cessation or arrest of bleeding.

hemostat. Tool for clamping vessels and arresting hemorrhaging.

hernia. Protrusion of a body structure through tissue.

hidradenitis. Infection or inflammation of a sweat gland.

homograft. Transplanted tissue from one member of species to another.

hyperthermia. Therapeutic raising of body temperature.

hypertrophic. Description of body part that has grown larger.

hypophysectomy. Destruction of the pituitary gland.

hypothermia. Therapeutic lack of heat.

identification. Recognition of body part or tissue.

imaging. Use of modalities such as X-ray, ultrasound, computerized axial tomography, or magnetic resonance imagery to allow visualization of body tissues.

imbrication. Overlapping of tissues during closure.

immunotherapy. Therapeutic use of antibodies (serum or gamma globulin).

implant. Insertion of a material.

© 2018 Optum360, LLC

impression. Mark made by one organ on another.

in situ. In the normal location or site of origin.

incise. To cut open or into.

incubation. Culture cultivation under controlled conditions.

infusion. Introduction of substance into blood.

inguinal. Groin region.

inject. Introduction into body tissues.

innervate. Supplying a stimulus or energy to nerve fibers connected to a part.

inseminate. Injection of semen.

insert. To put into.

instillation. Administering a liquid slowly over time, drop by drop.

instrumentation. Use of tool or implement for therapeutic reasons.

insufflation. Blowing air or gas into a body cavity.

interpretation. Professional health care provider's review of data with a written or verbal opinion.

interstitial. Within the small spaces or gaps occurring in tissue or organs.

intracavitary. Within a body cavity.

intubate. Insertion of a tube into a body canal or organ.

inversion. Turn inward, inside out, or upside down.

irrigate. Washing out, lavage.

kinetics. Motion or movement.

laminectomy. Removal or excision of the posterior arch of a vertebra to provide additional space for the nerves and widen the spinal canal.

lance. Incision with a lancet.

lancet. Pointed surgical knife.

laparoscopy. Endoscopic examination of the abdomen.

laparotomy. Opening of the abdomen for therapy or diagnosis.

laryngoscopy. Examination of the larynx with an endoscope.

laser. Concentrated light used to cut or seal tissue.

lateral. To the side.

lavage. Washing out of a body cavity.

lesion. Any discontinuity of tissue.

ligation. Tying off a blood vessel or duct with a suture or a soft, thin wire.

limited. Bounded.

lingual. Relating to the tongue.

lithotripsy. Destruction of calcified substance in the gallbladder, urethra, or bladder (also litholapaxy).

localization. Limitation to area.

lysis. 1) Destruction, breakdown, dissolution, or decomposition of cells or substances by a specific catalyzing agent. 2) Surgical mobilization of an organ by division of restraining tissues.

manipulate. Treatment by hand.

manometric. Measurement of pressure or tension in gas or a liquid.

marsupialization. Creation of a pouch in surgical treatment of a cyst in which one wall is resected and the remaining cut edges are sutured to adjacent tissue creating an open pouch of the previously enclosed cyst.

mastectomy. Surgical removal of one or both breasts.

mastotomy. Incision of breast.

measure. 1) Evaluate the level of a physiological or physical function at a point in time. 2) Action intended to achieve a result.

meatus. Opening or passage into the body.

metatarsectomy. Excision of metatarsus.

microdissection. Dissection of tissue using a microscope.

micro repair. Repair of tissue at a level that requires using a microscope.

modification. Changing of tissues.

monitor. Recording of events.

motility. Capability of independent, spontaneous movement.

myotomy. Division of muscle.

necropsy. Autopsy.

necrosis. Death of cells or tissue within a living organ or structure.

nephrotic. Degeneration of renal epithelium.

neurectomy. Excision or resection of a nerve.

neuroplasty. Repair or reconstruction of a nerve.

neurotomy. Dissection of a nerve.

obliterate. Get rid or do away with completely.

observation. Perception of events.

obturate. Occlude an opening.

obturator. Prosthesis used to close an acquired or congenital opening in the palate that aids in speech and chewing.

occlusion. Constriction, closure, or blockage of a passage.

open fracture. Exposed fracture.

orchiectomy. Surgical removal of one or both testicles via a scrotal or groin incision, indicated in cases of cancer, traumatic injury, and sex reassignment surgery. A prosthetic testis may be inserted in the scrotum at the time of surgical removal.

osteomyelitis. Infection and inflammation of bone and bone marrow.

osteophytes. Bony outgrowth.

osteoplasty. Plastic repair of bone.

osteoporotic. Porous condition of bones.

osteotome. Tool used for cutting bone.

osteotomy. Bone incision.

oversewing. Suturing over an edge to form a closure.

packing. Material placed into a cavity or wound, such as gels, gauze, pads, and sponges.

palpate. Examination by feeling with the hand.

paring. Cutting away an edge or a surface.

paronychia. Infection of nail structures.

pedicle. Stem-like, narrow base or stalk attached to a new growth.

pedicle graft. Flap graft that remains attached to the original site by a narrow base of tissue to maintain blood supply during grafting.

peduncle. Connecting structures of the brain.

penetrate. Pierce.

percutaneous. Through the skin.

periosteum. Double-layered connective membrane on the outer surface of bone.

photocoagulation. Application of an intense laser beam of light to disrupt tissue and condense protein material to a residual mass, used especially for treating ocular conditions.

pilonidal. Growth of hair under skin or in cyst.

pinning. Bone fastening.

plethysmography. Measurement of changes in organ volume.

pleurodesis. Injection of a sclerosing agent into the pleural space for creating adhesions between the parietal and the visceral pleura to treat a collapsed

lung caused by air trapped in the pleural cavity, or severe cases of pleural effusion.

plication. Surgical technique involving folding, tucking, or pleating to reduce the size of a hollow structure or organ.

porcine. Of or relating to pigs.

portable. Movable.

probing. Exploration using a slender, often flexible rod.

procedure. Conduct of operation.

process. Anatomical projection or prominence on a bone.

prone. Lying face downward.

prophylaxis. Intervention or protective therapy intended to prevent a disease.

prosthesis. Man-made substitute for a missing body part.

prostrate. Recline on one's front.

pump. Forcing gas or liquid from body part.

puncture. Creating a hole.

pyelotomy. Incision or opening made into the renal pelvis. Pyelotomies are performed to accomplish other procedures such as exploration, drainage, removal of a kidney stone, instill medications, or perform ureteropyelography or renal endoscopy.

radical. Extensive surgery.

radiograph. Image made by an x-ray.

radiopaque dye. Medium injected into the body that is impenetrable by x-rays.

ream. Shape or enlarge a hole.

recess. Small empty cavity in a body part.

reconstruct. Tissue rebuilding.

reduce. Restoration to normal position or alignment.

reduction. Correction of a fracture, dislocation, or hernia to the correct place and alignment, manually or by surgery.

refer. Recommendation to another source.

regulation. Authoritative ruling or law put forth by an executive authority of the law.

reimplant. Reinsert or reattach tissue.

reinforce. Enhancement of strength.

reinnervation. Restoration of nerve function.

release. Disconnection of a tendon or ligament.

reoperation. Repeat performance of operation.

repair. Restore to healthy state or function.

© 2018 Optum360, LLC

replacement. Insertion of new tissue or material in place of old one.

reposition. Return or place in original or normal position.

resect. Cutting out or removing all of a bone, organ, or other structure.

reservoir. Space or body cavity for storage of liquid.

response. Reaction to stimulus.

retraction. Act of holding tissue or a structure back away from its normal position or the field of interest.

revascularize. Restoring blood flow or blood supply to a body part.

revision. 1) Re-ordering of tissue. 2) Replace or correct a failed implant or sequelae of previous surgery.

rod. Straight, slim, cylindrical metal instrument for therapeutics.

rongeur. Sharp-edged instrument with a scoop-tip used to cut through tissue and bone; also a scraping tool.

routine. Normal activity.

sclerose. To become hard or firm.

section. Process of cutting a division or segment out of a part.

selective. Separation.

sequestrectomy. Excision of non-viable bone.

seton. Wire or gauze used to create fistula in tissues.

sever. Separate completely.

shunt. Surgically created passage between blood vessels or other natural passages, such as an arteriovenous anastomosis, to divert or bypass blood flow from the normal channel. Abnormal shunting may occur in the body when fistulas form or congenital anomalies are present that cause blood flow to be rerouted from the normal circulatory path.

sialolith. Salivary calculus.

sigmoidoscopy. Endoscopic examination of the entire rectum and sigmoid colon, often including a portion of the descending colon and usually performed with a flexible fiberoptic scope in conjunction with a surgical procedure.

smear. Specimen for study that is spread out across a glass slide.

snare. Wire used as a loop to excise a polyp or lesion.

sound. Long, slender tool with a type of curved, flat probe at the end for dilating strictures or detecting foreign bodies.

spatulate. Cut the open end of a tubular structure with a lengthwise incision and open the end out further for greater opening size in an anastomosis.

spectroscopy. Endoscopic measurement of emission and absorption of different wavelengths (spectra) of visible and non-visible light. Intravascular spectroscopy characterizes the composition of coronary artery plaques to determine appropriate treatment.

speculum. Tool used to enlarge the opening of any canal or cavity.

spiculum. Small, needle-like body or spike.

split-thickness graft. Skin graft that includes the epidermis and part of the dermis.

steal. Diversion of blood to another channel.

stenosis. Narrowing or constriction of a passage.

stent. Tube to provide support in a body cavity or lumen.

stereotaxis. Three-dimensional method for precisely locating structures in the brain.

stoma. Surgically created opening, usually in the abdominal wall, from an internal organ or structure for diversion of waste elimination, drainage, and access.

strapping. Overlapping strips of plaster.

stricture. Narrowing of a hollow structure, tube, duct, passage or opening.

subluxation. Partial or complete dislocation.

suction. Vacuum evacuation of fluid or tissue.

supine. Lying on the back.

suppression. Holding back, putting in check, or inhibiting an act, function, thought, or desire.

suppurative. Forming pus.

survival. Continued life.

suspension. 1) Fixation of an organ for support. 2) Temporary state of cessation of an activity, process, or experience.

suture. Numerous stitching techniques employed in wound closure.

symphysis. Joint that unifies two opposed bones by a junction of bony surfaces to a plate of fibrocartilage.

synchondrosis. Two bones joined by hyaline cartilage or fibrocartilage.

synovia. Clear fluid lubricant of joints, bursae, and tendon sheaths, secreted by the synovial membrane.

talectomy. Excision of the ankle bone.

tap. Withdraw fluid through a needle or trocar.

Surgical Terms

technique. Manner of performance.

teletherapy. External beam radiotherapy or other treatment applied from a source maintained at a distance away from the body.

tenodesis. Stabilization of a joint by anchoring tendons.

tenolysis. Release of a tendon from adhesions.

therapeutic. Treatment of disease.

thermoplasty. The therapeutic application of a controlled heat source to repair tissue.

thoracentesis. Surgical puncture of the chest cavity with a specialized needle or hollow tubing to aspirate fluid from within the pleural space for diagnostic or therapeutic reasons.

thoracotomy. Incision in the chest wall.

thrombectomy. Removal of venous occlusion (clot).

thromboembolism. Blood clot formed in a blood vessel that has become dislodged and carried through the bloodstream.

thrombus. Blood clot formed of blood platelets, proteins and cells that forms in a vessel and remains there.

tomograph. Method of precise x-ray.

tracheostomy. Creation of an opening into the trachea.

traction. Drawing out or holding tension on an area by applying a direct therapeutic pulling force.

tractor. Instrument for pulling an organ.

transbronchial. Through the bronchus.

transcatheter. Procedure or treatment performed via a catheter.

transection. 1) Transverse dissection. 2) Cut across a long axis.

transfer. Removal or moving body tissue.

transplant. Insertion of an organ or tissue from one person or site into another.

transposition. 1) Removal or exchange from one side to another. 2) Change of position from one place to another.

treatment. Management, care, therapy of patient.

trephine. 1) Specialized round saw for cutting circular holes in bone, especially the skull. 2) Instrument that removes small disc-shaped buttons of corneal tissue for transplanting.

trocar. Sharp pointed device that along with a cannula provides percutaneous access to a body cavity such as the abdominal cavity.

tube. Hollow cylinder or pipe.

ultrasound. Imaging using ultra-high sound frequency.

undiversion. Restoration of continuity, flow, or passage through the normal channel.

unroofing. Incision and removal, by any method, of the surface of lesion that is elevated from the organ below it.

urachus. Embryonic tube connecting the urinary bladder to the umbilicus during development of the fetus that normally closes before birth, generally in the fourth or fifth month of gestation.

ureterostomy. Urinary diversion with connection of the ureter(s) to a stoma on the abdominal skin.

ureterocele. Saccular formation of the lower part of the ureter, protruding into the bladder.

ureteropyelogram. X-ray study of the ureter and bladder.

urostomy. Diversion of urinary flow away from the bladder through an artificial opening (stoma) in the skin.

valve. Prosthesis to replace an existing valve or to shunt body fluids.

valvulotome. Catheter-based device used to cut and destroy venous valves.

varices. Enlarge, dilated, or tortured veins.

vasectomy. Surgical procedure involving the removal of all or part of the vas deferens, usually performed for sterilization or in conjunction with a prostatectomy.

vestigial. Remnant of a structure that functioned in a previous stage of a species or individual development of an embryo or fetus.

vomer. Flat bone that forms the lower, posterior portion of the nasal septum.

xenograft. Graft taken from non-human animal.

© 2018 Optum360, LLC

Medical and Surgical

Abdominoplasty

Body System
Anatomical Regions, General

PCS Root Operation
Alteration

Repair

Supplement

Root Operation Table
ØWØ Anatomical Regions, General, Alteration

ØWQ Anatomical Regions, General, Repair

ØWU Anatomical Regions, General, Supplement

Body Part
Abdominal Wall

Device
Autologous Tissue Substitute (Alteration, Supplement)

Synthetic Substitute (Alteration, Supplement)

Nonautologous Tissue Substitute (Alteration, Supplement)

No Device (Alteration, Repair)

Description
An abdominoplasty is a repair of the abdominal wall, which is classified to the body system "General Anatomical Regions" in PCS. Anatomically, the abdominal wall is subdivided into two general regions: the anterolateral and the posterior abdominal wall. It is composed of three tissue layers: skin, superficial fascia, and muscle. Surgical procedures on the abdominal wall involve all three of these tissue layers. Abdominoplasty may be performed for either cosmetic or medical purposes.

Alteration
Alteration involves modifying an anatomic structure without affecting the function of the body part. The root operation Alteration identifies procedures that are cosmetic in nature. Use of this root operation requires diagnostic confirmation that the abdominoplasty is being performed to improve appearance.

Abdominoplasty performed for cosmetic reasons may also be referred to as a "tummy tuck." The procedure involves removing excess skin and underlying subcutaneous tissue and abdominal fat as well as tightening and restoring abdominal musculature. A cosmetic abdominoplasty may also involve

reinforcement of the abdominal wall with biological or synthetic material, which is reported with the appropriate device value.

> **Focus Point**
> *A cosmetic abdominoplasty (abdominal panniculectomy) that involves only the removal of excess skin, underlying subcutaneous tissue, and fat, without muscle tightening, is assigned a code from table ØJØ.*

Repair
The root operation Repair involves restoring a body part, in this case the abdominal wall, to its normal anatomic structure and function. Repair is primarily used when an injury to the abdominal wall requires layered suture repair. Repair of the abdominal wall may also be required for stoma complications, such as a parastomal hernia. When the repair of the abdominal wall is focused on a stoma, the qualifier Stoma is reported.

> **Focus Point**
> *Do not report the root operation Repair when mesh is used to reinforce a repair of the abdomen. See the root operation Supplement.*

Supplement
When the abdominal wall is repaired and biological or synthetic material is used to reinforce or augment the repair, the correct root operation is Supplement. A common procedure classified to this root operation is the repair of a hernia involving the abdominal wall using mesh to reinforce the repair. Mesh may also be used in the repair of complex abdominal wall anomalies.

> **Focus Point**
> *Do not report the root operation Supplement when biological or synthetic material is used but the objective of the procedure is solely cosmetic in nature. In this case, the correct root operation is Alteration and the biological or synthetic material used to reinforce the abdominal wall is captured using the appropriate device value. All methods, approaches, and devices used to improve appearance are coded as Alteration.*

Coding Guidance
AHA: 2017, 3Q, 8; 2014, 4Q, 38

© 2018 Optum360, LLC

Ablation, Cardiac

Body System
Heart and Great Vessels

PCS Root Operation
Destruction

Division

Root Operation Table
Ø25   Heart and Great Vessels, Destruction

Ø28   Heart and Great Vessels, Division

Body Part
Conduction Mechanism

Approach
Open

Percutaneous

Percutaneous Endoscopic

Description
Electrodes are placed in the heart to measure electrical activity (cardiac mapping). When the source of the arrhythmia is found, the arrhythmogenic focus is destroyed by creating lesions or scars, using either ablation or incision, to permanently interrupt and/or redirect the abnormal electrical conduction to restore normal sinus rhythm. This procedure is performed primarily to treat atrial fibrillation. A cardiac ablation procedure may be performed by one of three different surgical approaches: open, endovascular, or thoracoscopic. The thoracoscopic, or thoracoscopic-assisted, approach is the most recently developed incisional technique. Newer advances now permit therapeutic cardiac ablations using a minimally invasive transcatheter endovascular approach.

Destruction
Cardiac ablation of conduction tissue is reported with the root operation Destruction. In an ablation procedure, anatomically defined triggers are isolated in the left or right atrium and a heat, radiofrequency (microwave), laser, ultrasound, or cold cryoprobe is used to create lesions in the aberrant conduction tissue that will heal into scars. The scar tissue permanently disrupts conduction of electrical impulses through the aberrant conduction tissue. The right and/or left atrial tissue and/or atrial septum may also be treated in this way and additional operative ablation involving the atrioventricular annulus, as well as the atrial tissue around the pulmonary veins, may be performed.

Division
An alternative method of disrupting abnormal electrical conduction is the incision and separation of the aberrant tissue. This surgical technique is reported with the root operation Division, which involves cutting into the abnormal conduction pathways to separate or transect them. The incisions heal forming scar tissue that permanently disrupts conduction along the abnormal pathways. The maze procedure is so named because the treatment creates lines of conduction block in the heart, similar to a maze. The classic maze procedure involves creating the maze lines with sharp scalpel incision, resulting in scar tissue formation and subsequent therapeutic conduction block.

Focus Point
Ablation reported with the root operation Destruction is the preferred technique. The open surgical incision method is a lengthy, demanding, highly invasive procedure. Surgical techniques have evolved from surgical incisions to tissue ablation by energy sources such as radiofrequency, laser, and cryoablation to create the conduction blocks.

Focus Point
Even though the procedure may be performed on various sites within the heart or around the pulmonary veins, the root operation is directed at abnormal conduction pathways and in ICD-10-PCS is always captured by a single body part, Conduction Mechanism. The cardiac conduction system main components are the sinoatrial (SA) node, atrioventricular (AV) node, bundle of His, bundle branches, and Purkinje fibers. The PCS Body Part Key also includes the bundle of Kent in the Conduction Mechanism body part. This is an abnormal extra conduction pathway between atria and ventricles, which causes Wolff-Parkinson-White syndrome (WPW).

Focus Point
A transcatheter endovascular approach does not involve direct visualization of the operative site, so the approach Percutaneous is assigned. Thoracoscopic incisions are classified as Percutaneous Endoscopic approach. Thoracoscopic-assisted via a mini-thoracotomy approach, even though it is minimally invasive, is considered an Open approach. Procedures performed using the open approach with percutaneous endoscopic assistance are coded to the approach Open, according to ICD-10-PCS guidelines.

Coding Guidance
AHA: 2016, 3Q, 43; 2014, 4Q, 47; 2014, 3Q, 20; 2014, 3Q, 19; 2013, 2Q, 38

© 2018 Optum360, LLC

Ablation, Endometrial

Body System
Female Reproductive System

PCS Root Operation
Destruction

Root Operation Table
ØU5   Female Reproductive System, Destruction

Body Part
Endometrium

Approach
Via Natural or Artificial Opening
Via Natural or Artificial Opening Endoscopic

Description
The lining of the uterus (endometrium) proliferates each month in preparation for implantation of an embryo. If no embryo implants, the blood-rich endometrial tissue (menses) sloughs from the uterine wall and is discharged from the uterus as menstrual flow. Endometrial ablation may be performed to reduce abnormally severe menstrual flow (menorrhagia), seen most commonly in premenopausal women.

Endometrial ablation is reported with the root operation Destruction, which is the physical eradication of all or a portion of a body part by the direct use of energy, force, or a destructive agent. None of the body part is physically taken out of the body.

In resectoscopic endometrial ablation (REA), tissue of the endometrium is destroyed using a laser, fulguration, or other heat-related technique during hysteroscopy (device inserted through the vagina for a visual examination). The physician surgically ablates the inner lining of the uterus with the assistance of a fiberoptic resectoscope. The physician advances the hysteroscope through the vagina and into the cervical os to gain entry into the uterine cavity. The physician inspects the uterine cavity with the fiberoptic scope and ablates the endometrium by electrosurgical ablation, roller barrel desiccation, or laser evaporation. Report the approach as Via Natural or Artificial Opening Endoscopic for REA.

In global endometrial ablation (GEA), the entire endometrium is ablated concurrently using a device that is advanced into the vagina, through the cervical os, and into the uterus. Most forms of GEA do not require direct visualization. Heat and/or energy are applied to increase the temperature and destroy the lining.

In GEA balloon technique, a balloon is inserted through the vagina and cervical os into the uterus to destroy tissue using an infusion of heated fluid.

In microwave ablation, microwave energy is emitted from a probe that is inserted through the vagina and cervical os into the uterus. The microwaves destroy the endometrium using heat.

In bipolar energy GEA ablation, a device advanced through the vagina and cervical os into the uterus deploys a metallic mesh. Suction draws uterine tissue into contact with the mesh, and the tissue is ablated with radiofrequency.

When endometrial ablation is performed with a vaginal approach to the uterus without endoscopic (hysteroscopy) guidance, report the approach as Via Natural or Artificial Opening. Hydrothermal ablation is the only GEA technique that requires direct visualization with a hysteroscope. In hydrothermal ablation GEA, hot salt water is circulated in the uterus. This would be reported using the approach Via Natural or Artificial Opening Endoscopic.

In endometrial cryoablation, a cryoprobe destroys surrounding endometrium. The physician inserts a speculum for visualization of the cervix. A numbing block is placed in the cervix. A thin cryoablation device is inserted through the cervix into the uterus. The cryoablation device freezes targeted uterine endometrial tissue. The instrument is withdrawn following completion of the procedure. As the instrumentation is inserted through the vagina into the uterus without endoscopic visualization, report the approach Via Natural or Artificial Opening.

Focus Point
Correct coding of the approach in endometrial ablation requires a careful review of the medical record, as any of the available techniques may be enhanced using hysteroscopy. When use of a scope is documented, report the approach Via Natural or Artificial Opening Endoscopic. All REA techniques use a scope.

Medical and Surgical

Ablation, Vein, Thermal, Endovenous

Body System
Lower Veins

PCS Root Operation
Destruction

Root Operation Table
Ø65 Lower Veins, Destruction

Body Part
Refer to the ICD-10-PCS tabular list for a complete list of body parts.

Approach
Percutaneous

Device
No Device

Qualifier
No Qualifier

Description
Endovenous thermal vein ablation uses a laser or radiofrequency (RF) electrode to create intense local heat in a varicose or incompetent vein in an extremity, thus obliterating and sealing the vein closed. The most common site of treatment is the greater saphenous vein.

A duplex ultrasound is used to map the veins. The extremity is prepped and draped, and a local anesthetic is applied to the puncture site. Using a Percutaneous approach, a needle is inserted into the access site. A guidewire is placed into the vessel using ultrasound guidance. An introducer sheath is placed over the guidewire, after which the guidewire is removed and the ablation catheter system is introduced with the tip advanced to the target venous site under ultrasound guidance. A local anesthetic agent is injected into the tissues surrounding the vein within its fascial sheath along the course of the vein. Ultrasonography is used to position the catheter tip at the level of the terminal valve, and the catheter electrodes are deployed. The electrodes should be just distal to the valve cusps of the terminal valve. Radiofrequency or laser energy is applied until the appropriate temperature is obtained, collapsing and sclerosing the vein to seal it closed. The catheter tip is slowly withdrawn, maintaining the correct temperature, until it reaches the introducer sheath in the distal vein. The vein is again evaluated with ultrasound to confirm successful endovenous obliteration. The ablation catheter and introducer sheath are removed, and hemostasis is obtained with manual pressure applied to the puncture site.

Focus Point
Ablation procedures are reported with root operation Destruction, which is defined as "physical eradication of all or a portion of a body part by the direct use of energy, force, or a destructive agent."

© 2018 Optum360, LLC

Medical and Surgical

Adenoidectomy (without Tonsillectomy)

Body System
Mouth and Throat

PCS Root Operation
Destruction

Excision

Resection

Root Operation Table
ØC5   Mouth and Throat, Destruction

ØCB   Mouth and Throat, Excision

ØCT   Mouth and Throat, Resection

Body Part
Adenoids

Approach
External

Qualifier
Diagnostic (Excision)

No Qualifier

Description
Adenoidectomy is the surgical removal of adenoids. Indications for the removal include recurrent infections and difficulty breathing through the nose. Surgical techniques may vary.

Destruction
Using an External (intraoral) approach, an electrocautery instrument with a suction Bovie removes or reduces the adenoid tissue.

Excision
Using an External (intraoral) approach and a mirror or nasopharyngoscope for visualization, the physician uses an adenotome or a curette and basket punch to excise a portion of the adenoid.

Resection
Using an External (intraoral) approach and a mirror or nasopharyngoscope for visualization, the physician uses an adenotome or a curette and basket punch to excise the entire adenoid.

Focus Point
If adenoid tissue is removed for pathologic or histologic evaluation, the qualifier Diagnostic is used.

Focus Point
The body part Adenoid is reported once whether one or both adenoids are removed.

Focus Point
When the adenoidectomy is done in conjunction with a tonsillectomy, a separate code is needed for the tonsillectomy.

Focus Point
An External approach is used on procedures within an orifice on structures that are visible without the aid of instrumentation. See guideline B5.3a.

Adjustment, Cardiac Pacemaker Lead

Body System
Heart and Great Vessels

PCS Root Operation
Revision

Root Operation Table
Ø2W Heart and Great Vessels, Revision

Body Part
Heart

Approach
Percutaneous

Device
Cardiac Lead

Description
Pacemakers are devices that help regulate abnormal electrical impulses that can cause cardiac arrhythmias, including bradycardia (slow heartbeat), or blocks (disruption of electrical impulses). Pacemakers have two parts: the generator (device that generates the electrical impulse) and the lead(s) (insulated wire[s]) that transmit the impulse to the heart muscle. The pacemaker may have one to three leads.

When a previously placed lead becomes dislodged, the electrical impulse is not being delivered to the correct site within the right atrium or right ventricle. To correct the problem, the physician may perform an adjustment using a Percutaneous or Percutaneous Endoscopic approach.

The patient is brought to the operating room, and a previously placed transvenous right atrial or right ventricular electrode is repositioned. This is done when the system does not function due to improper placement of the electrode wire itself. The incision for the previously placed pacemaker generator is opened, and the generator is removed. The wire is tested to ensure that the wire is not defective but simply in the wrong place. The lead is disconnected and freed from any attachments. Using a guidewire, the lead is guided to the correct position in the heart. It is reattached to the generator in its new position and tested again. The generator is placed back in its pocket, and the pocket is closed.

Focus Point
Do not report an Open approach unless the physician directly visualizes the repositioning of the cardiac portion of the lead. While the generator is removed from the pocket using an Open approach, the actual revision of the lead is via a Percutaneous approach using a guidewire into the heart, which is the site of the procedure. The heart itself is not directly visualized.

Focus Point
The root operation Revision is reported when the objective of the procedure is to reposition a pacemaker lead that has been previously placed but has become dislodged. The lead is not replaced.

Coding Guidance
AHA: 2015, 3Q, 27; 2015, 2Q, 19

© 2018 Optum360, LLC

Medical and Surgical

Adrenalectomy, Unilateral

Body System
Endocrine System

PCS Root Operation
Resection

Root Operation Table
ØGT   Endocrine System, Resection

Body Part
Adrenal Gland, Left
Adrenal Gland, Right

Approach
Open
Percutaneous Endoscopic

Description
The adrenal glands are two small, paired glands, each located above a kidney. The adrenal glands secrete hormones that help regulate many bodily functions, including salt and water balance, the immune system, metabolism, blood sugar levels, blood pressure control, response to stress, and other essential body functions. Unilateral adrenalectomy may be indicated if one of the adrenal glands is producing too much hormone. If one adrenal gland is removed, the other adrenal gland takes over and provides full function.

Adrenalectomy may be performed for disorders such as hyperaldosteronism (Conn syndrome), Cushing syndrome, Addison's disease, pheochromocytoma, large myelolipoma, metastatic tumors, adrenocortical carcinoma, neuroblastoma, and adrenal masses of unknown cause or morphology. The surgical approach depends on the size, location, and the possibility of malignancy.

Using an Open approach, the physician completely removes one adrenal gland. The physician exposes the adrenal gland via an upper anterior midline abdominal or posterior incision. The retroperitoneal space is explored. The capsule of the kidney is incised, and the adrenal capsule is opened. Blood supply to the adrenal gland is ligated, and the gland is removed. The physician closes the incision with sutures.

Alternatively, the physician may perform a laparoscopic unilateral adrenalectomy. Using a Percutaneous Endoscopic approach through the abdomen, the physician places a trocar at the level of the umbilicus, and the abdomen is insufflated. The laparoscope is placed through the umbilical port, and additional trocars are placed into the abdominal cavity as needed. In the back approach, the trocar is placed at the back proximal to the retroperitoneal space, superior to the kidney, and adjacent to the adrenal gland. The physician uses the laparoscope fitted with a fiberoptic camera and an operating tool to remove the entire left or right adrenal gland using a specimen bag inserted through a port. The abdomen is then deflated, the trocars are removed, and the incisions are closed with sutures.

Focus Point
Resection includes all of a body part or any subdivision of the body part that has its own body part value. Removal of all of one or both of the adrenal glands completely is reported as Resection. Removal of a portion of one or both of the adrenal glands is reported as Excision. See ICD-10-PCS guideline B3.8.

Focus Point
ICD-10-PCS code assignment depends on the objective of the procedure. If an adrenal gland Excision for biopsy is performed for diagnostic purposes, followed by a Resection of the affected adrenal gland, both the Excision for biopsy and the more definitive Resection are coded, according to ICD-10-PCS guideline B3.4b.

Alveoloplasty

Medical and Surgical

Body System
Head and Facial Bones

PCS Root Operation
Excision

Replacement

Supplement

Root Operation Table
ØNB   Head and Facial Bones, Excision

ØNR   Head and Facial Bones, Replacement

ØNU   Head and Facial Bones, Supplement

Body Part
Maxilla

Mandible, Right

Mandible, Left

Approach
Open

Device
No Device (Excision)

Autologous Tissue Substitute (Replacement, Supplement)

Synthetic Substitute (Replacement, Supplement)

Nonautologous Tissue Substitute (Replacement, Supplement)

Description
The alveolar process is a bone in either the maxilla (upper jaw) or mandible (lower jaw) that surrounds and supports the teeth. Alveoloplasty is surgical repair or reconstruction of the bone of the alveolar process. An alveoloplasty is performed in areas where teeth have been removed or lost, or where there is a bone irregularity. It can be done to smooth, reconstruct, or recontour the alveolar bone. Alveoloplasty may also be done to repair or to reconstruct defects in the alveolar bone due to surgery or disease.

Excision
Excisional alveoloplasty is a surgical procedure performed to smooth down protruding areas of bone into a more even transition. In ICD-10-PCS, "excisional debridement" is coded using the root operation Excision. The physician alters the contours of the alveolus by selectively performing alveoloplasty to remove lesions, sharp areas, or undercuts of alveolar bone. Using an Open approach, the physician makes incisions in the mucosa overlying the alveolus, exposing the alveolar bone. Drills, osteotomes, or files are used to excise and contour the bone. The mucosa is sutured in place over the contoured bone.

Replacement
The physician removes a portion of the alveolus. Using an Open approach, incisions are made through the mucosa to expose the alveolar bone. Curettes, drills, or osteotomes are used to remove the diseased alveolar bone or sequestrum. If an autograft is used, through a separate incision, the physician harvests the bone graft from the hip or skull and closes the surgically created wound. The bone graft is placed in the alveolar defect created by the removal of the diseased bone, re-establishing normal contours of the maxilla or mandible. The physician closes all incisions in layers and gingival incisions in a single layer. The mucosa may be sutured directly over the surgical wound, or it may be packed and allowed to heal secondarily.

Supplement
Bony reconstruction of the alveolar bone can stabilize the maxillary or mandibular segments and replace bone that was previously excised or was lost due to disease. Using an Open approach, the physician makes an incision in the mucosa adjacent to the alveolar bone. The mucosa is elevated and loosened. If an autograft is used, the physician harvests the bone graft through a separate incision from the hip or skull and closes the surgically created wound. The bone graft is placed in the alveolar defect, re-establishing normal contours of the maxilla or mandible. The physician closes all incisions in layers and gingival incisions in a single layer.

Focus Point
If an autograft is obtained from a different body part, a separate procedure is coded, according to guideline B3.9.

Focus Point
The ICD-10-PCS index also lists Repair under the main term "Alveoloplasty." Repair would be used only when the procedure performed does not meet any other root operation. Review documentation in the operative report carefully to determine the objective of the procedure to assign the appropriate root operation.

© 2018 Optum360, LLC

Alveolotomy

Body System
Head and Facial Bones

PCS Root Operation
Division

Drainage

Root Operation Table
ØN8   Head and Facial Bones, Division

ØN9   Head and Facial Bones, Drainage

Body Part
Maxilla

Mandible, Right

Mandible, Left

Approach
Open

Device
Drainage Device (Drainage)

No Device

Qualifier
Diagnostic (Drainage)

No Qualifier

Description
The alveolar process is a bone in either the maxilla (upper jaw) or mandible (lower jaw) that surrounds and supports the teeth. Alveolotomy may be performed to drain an abscess, cyst, or hematoma on the alveolar process.

Division
In some instances, a bone incision is created or the bone is divided for indications other than drainage of fluid. The physician makes an Open incision into the alveolar bone, separating all or a portion of the bone. The physician then irrigates the area with antibiotic solution, and the soft tissues are sutured closed, or the wound is packed and left open, allowing the area to drain.

Drainage
The physician makes an Open incision into the alveolar bone and drains an abscess, cyst, or hematoma from alveolar structures. The physician then irrigates the area with antibiotic solution, the periosteum is closed over the bone, and the soft tissues are sutured closed; or the wound is packed and left open, allowing the area to drain. An artificial drain may be placed and removed at a later time. If the drain remains in place at the end of the procedure, report the qualifier Drainage Device.

Focus Point
Division should not be confused with the root operation Release. Release involves incising restraining tissue such as scar tissue or adhesions, while Division involves incising and separating a body part.

Amputation, Below Knee

Body System
Anatomical Regions, Lower Extremities

PCS Root Operation
Detachment

Root Operation Table
ØY6 Anatomical Regions, Lower Extremities, Detachment

Body Part
Lower Leg, Right
Lower Leg, Left

Approach
Open

Qualifier
High
Mid
Low

Description
Below-knee amputations (BKA) may be performed for severe injury, peripheral vascular disease, nonhealing ulcers, severe infection, or cancer of the lower leg, foot and/or ankle.

In ICD-10-PCS, amputation is reported with the Detachment root operation using the tables in the body systems Anatomical Regions, Upper Extremities; and Anatomical Regions, Lower Extremities, because amputations are performed only on the extremities, across overlapping body layers. A BKA is an amputation below the knee but above the ankle and is reported using body part Lower Leg.

During a below-knee amputation, the physician makes an incision in the skin of the leg at the level where the amputation is to take place. The incision is carried completely around the leg. The tissue is dissected down to the bones. The large arteries, veins, and nerves are identified and tied off prior to being cut. Tissue is further debrided as needed. The tibia and fibula are identified. The physician surgically cuts the bones, completing the amputation. The wound is thoroughly irrigated and then closed in layers, including the skin. A soft dressing is placed over the stump.

An alternate amputation of the leg through tibia and fibula is a guillotine amputation. The physician places a pneumatic tourniquet on the thigh. The limb is measured for optimal stump length, and marks are made to facilitate skin flap preparation. Progressive incisions are made through soft tissues, and nerves and vessels are ligated. The tibia and fibula are bisected with a circular saw, rounded, and smoothed. The calf muscles are brought forward over the ends of the tibia and fibula and attached to the connective tissue on the front of the stump. The tourniquet is released, and bleeding points are electrocoagulated. A drainage tube is placed deep in the muscle flap, and the skin flaps are closed and sutured. A soft dressing is applied, followed by a rigid dressing in preparation for fabrication of prosthetic devices.

Focus Point
Review the operative report carefully to assign the appropriate level of detachment. BKAs involve amputation of the lower leg through the shaft of the tibia and fibula, reported with the qualifier High, Mid, or Low. Qualifier High represents the portion of the tibia/fibula shaft closest to the knee (proximal), Mid represents the middle portion of the shaft of the tibia and fibula, and Low means the distal or furthest portion of the shaft of the tibia and fibula. The body part Knee Region would be used for disarticulation through the knee joint.

Coding Guidance
AHA: 2017, 2Q, 3

© 2018 Optum360, LLC

Amputation, Foot and Toe Ray

Body System
Anatomical Regions, Lower Extremities

PCS Root Operation
Detachment

Root Operation Table
ØY6 Anatomical Regions, Lower Extremities, Detachment

Body Part
Foot, Right
Foot, Left

Approach
Open

Qualifier
Complete
Complete 1st Ray
Complete 2nd Ray
Complete 3rd Ray
Complete 4th Ray
Complete 5th Ray
Partial 1st Ray
Partial 2nd Ray
Partial 3rd Ray
Partial 4th Ray
Partial 5th Ray

Description
Foot and toe ray amputations, which involve the amputation of the toe and all or part of the corresponding metatarsal bone, may be performed for severe injury, peripheral vascular disease, nonhealing ulcers, severe infection, or cancer of the foot and/or toes.

In ICD-10-PCS, amputation is reported with the Detachment root operation using the tables in the body systems Anatomical Regions, Upper Extremities; and Anatomical Regions, Lower Extremities, because amputations are performed only on the extremities, across overlapping body layers. In ICD-10-PCS, ray amputations are coded using the body part Foot with the qualifier indicating the level of detachment. If the entire foot is removed, qualifier Complete is used.

Ray amputations can involve the partial or complete ray, removal of a single toe and its corresponding metatarsal, or removal of the lateral four toes with the corresponding metatarsals. A Complete ray amputation involves removing the entire metatarsal bone, while a Partial ray amputation occurs anywhere along the shaft or head of the metatarsal bone of the foot.

The physician performs an amputation of a portion of a metatarsal bone and its attached toe. Using an Open approach, an incision is made dorsally over the involved metatarsal and toe. Using a small rongeur, the affected portion of the metatarsal and toe is transected obliquely. Tendons may be retracted, removed, or drained as indicated. The involved metatarsal bone and the toe are completely dissected free from the foot and removed. The wound is irrigated and debrided. It is closed in layers. A dressing and a cast or a brace are applied.

Focus Point
Review the operative report carefully to assign the appropriate level of detachment. The physician may use the words "toe amputation," but if the documentation indicates the amputation is through the midshaft of the fifth metatarsal, this is the foot rather than the toe and is reported with the qualifier Partial 5th Ray.

Focus Point
A code is needed for each individual ray detached, according to guideline B3.2a.

Coding Guidance
AHA: 2017, 2Q, 3; 2015, 1Q, 28

Amputation, Toe

Body System
Anatomical Regions, Lower Extremities

PCS Root Operation
Detachment

Root Operation Table
ØY6 Anatomical Regions, Lower Extremities, Detachment

Body Part
1st Toe, Right
1st Toe, Left
2nd Toe, Right
2nd Toe, Left
3rd Toe, Right
3rd Toe, Left
4th Toe, Right
4th Toe, Left
5th Toe, Right
5th Toe, Left

Approach
Open

Qualifier
Complete
High
Mid
Low

Description
Surgical removal of the toe(s), or amputation, is commonly performed in severe cases of frostbite and gangrene.

In ICD-10-PCS, amputation is reported with the Detachment root operation using the tables in the body systems Anatomical Regions, Upper Extremities;

and Anatomical Regions, Lower Extremities, because amputations are performed only on the extremities, across overlapping body layers. A toe amputation is coded using the body part that specifies the toe being removed, and the qualifier indicates the level at which the amputation is taking place.

The physician performs an amputation of a toe at the metatarsophalangeal joint. Using an Open approach, the physician makes an incision over and around the affected toe where the toe joins the foot. The physician continues the incision deep to the metatarsophalangeal joint. The capsule is identified, and a capsulotomy is performed. The proximal phalanx bone is disarticulated from the metatarsal bone, and the joint is debrided. The tendon and soft tissues are excised for closure and skin coverage. The toe is excised free from the foot. The wound is irrigated and closed in layers. A dressing and firm-soled shoe are applied.

Focus Point
A code is needed for each toe that is removed as per guideline B3.2a.

Focus Point
Review the operative report carefully to assign the appropriate level of detachment. The qualifier Complete is for the detachment at the metatarsal-phalangeal joint, High for amputation along the proximal phalanx, Mid for amputation through the proximal interphalangeal joint or anywhere along the middle phalanx, and Low for amputation through the distal interphalangeal joint or anywhere along the distal phalanx.

Coding Guidance
AHA: 2017, 2Q, 3

© 2018 Optum360, LLC

Medical and Surgical

Amygdalohippocampectomy

Body System
Central Nervous System and Cranial Nerves

PCS Root Operation
Excision

Root Operation Table
00B Central Nervous System and Cranial Nerves, Excision

Body Part
Cerebral Hemisphere

Approach
Open

Description

Amygdalohippocampectomy is the surgical removal of all or a portion of the amygdala, hippocampus, and parahippocampal gyrus, all of which are parts of the temporal lobe of the brain.

Amygdalohippocampectomy is performed to treat medically refractive temporal lobe epilepsy with sparing of unaffected brain tissue and reduced effects of the more conventional anterior temporal lobectomy.

An MRI is done before surgery to map the margins of the involved brain structures. The patient is prepped with a general anesthetic and placement of a lumbar drain. With the patient's head in position, the scalp is incised and the underlying temporalis muscle is dissected to expose the skull. Burr holes are drilled around the periphery of the bone flap area to be raised. Using a craniotome, via Open approach, the bone flap is freed and lifted to expose the dura, which is dissected and retracted out of the operative field. An operating microscope is used. A brain retractor is inserted, and cerebrospinal fluid is carefully suctioned from the ambient cistern. The uncus is elevated with the retractor, and the anatomical positioning of the related structures (fusiform and parahippocampal gyri, uncus, ambient cistern, and tentorium) is examined. Landmarks for cortical incisions, such as the oculomotor nerve, are identified. Cortical incisions are made, and the temporal horn of the lateral ventricle is exposed, using careful suction dissection of the cortex and white matter. The horn is opened, and the amygdala and hippocampus are identified. The parahippocampal gyrus is then incised, exposing the

posterior aspect of the temporal horn and anterior hippocampus. The thin layer of neural tissue connecting the hippocampus and the amygdala is divided with subpial aspiration. The parahippocampal gyrus is removed subpially, the hippocampus is divided transversely, and anterior choroidal and posterior cerebral arteries are coagulated and divided. The hippocampus is completely separated from the arachnoid membrane and removed. The amygdala facing the temporal horn is excised with an ultrasonic aspirator. Closure is done by suturing the dura meticulously and replacing the bone flap into position. Screws or plates are placed to secure the bone flap to surrounding skull bone. The divided muscles are sutured, and the galea and the scalp are closed. The root operation Excision is reported since only a portion of the Cerebral Hemisphere is removed.

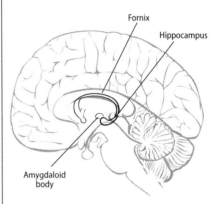

The hippocampus, fornix, and amygdala are part of the limbic system, which governs emotional memory and fear response. Selective removal may be for treatment of intractable temporal lobe epilepsy. The craniotomy may involve stereotactic navigation

Focus Point
Selective amygdalohippocampectomy (SAH) refers to the removal of only those portions of the amygdala and hippocampus that are problematic.

Coding Guidance
AHA: 2016, 2Q, 18

Anastomosis, Billroth I

See also Anastomosis, Billroth II

Body System
Gastrointestinal System

PCS Root Operation
Excision

Resection

Root Operation Table
ØDB   Gastrointestinal System, Excision

ØDT   Gastrointestinal System, Resection

Body Part
Stomach

Stomach, Pylorus

Approach
Open

Percutaneous Endoscopic

Description
A gastrectomy with Billroth I anastomosis is primarily used to treat gastric malignancies and can be performed for gastric ulcer disease. The procedure typically involves removing the stomach pylorus and approximating the proximal stomach to the duodenum. In ICD-10-PCS, Stomach, Pylorus which includes the antrum, is its own distinct body part, and Resection is the root operation reported. If the procedure includes portions of the gastric body, body part Stomach is reported with the root operation Excision since only a portion of the stomach is removed. The Billroth I can be performed with an Open or Percutaneous Endoscopic (laparoscopic) approach.

With the patient under general anesthesia, the physician makes a midline abdominal incision using an Open Approach. The distal stomach (antrum) is dissected free from surrounding structures, and the blood supply to the antrum is divided. Next, the gastroduodenal junction is divided and the stomach is divided in its middle portion, removing the antrum. An anastomosis is made between the proximal stomach and the duodenum with staples or sutures. The incision is closed.

When the procedure involves a Percutaneous Endoscopic approach, the patient is placed in a supine position, and the physician inflates the abdomen with air to visualize the abdominal organs. The physician makes several tiny incisions through which the physician inserts the laparoscope and the surgical instruments to perform the gastrectomy with Billroth I anastomosis.

Focus Point
Anastomosis of the stomach to the duodenum is considered a direct anastomosis since no other tubular body parts are bypassed. Based on guideline B3.1b, this anastomosis is considered inherent in the closure and is NOT coded separately. Only the Excision or Resection is reported in the Billroth I procedure. Conversely, two codes are required for a Billroth II anastomosis. See also Anastomosis, Billroth II.

Coding Guidance
AHA: 2017, 2Q, 17

© 2018 Optum360, LLC

Anastomosis, Billroth II

See also Anastomosis, Billroth I

See also Gastrectomy

Body System
Gastrointestinal System

PCS Root Operation
Bypass

Root Operation Table
ØD1   Gastrointestinal System, Bypass

Body Part
Stomach

Approach
Open
Percutaneous Endoscopic

Qualifier
Jejunum

Description
A Billroth II anastomosis, also referred to as a gastrojejunostomy, is a gastrointestinal reconstruction that may be required after gastrectomy for stomach cancer, pyloric valve dysfunction, gastric outlet obstruction, and peptic ulcers. The procedure typically involves a partial gastrectomy and approximation of the greater curvature of the stomach to the jejunum. Billroth II can be performed with an Open or Percutaneous Endoscopic (laparoscopic) approach.

Using an Open approach through a midline abdominal incision, after removing the distal stomach, the surgeon approximates the proximal stomach (greater curvature) with staples or sutures to the proximal jejunum in an end-to-side fashion for a Billroth II anastomosis. The incision is closed in layers.

Less commonly, a Percutaneous Endoscopic approach may be used. The laparoscope and additional trocars are placed through small portal incisions. After removing the distal stomach, the surgeon approximates the proximal stomach (greater curvature) with stapling devices to the jejunum in an end-to-side fashion for a Billroth II anastomosis. The incisions are closed.

The root operation used for the Billroth II anastomosis is Bypass because contents are being rerouted or bypassed around the duodenum into the jejunum. The body part Stomach represents the site bypassed "from," and the qualifier Jejunum indicates the location it is rerouted "to." The partial gastrectomy is also reported with the root operation Excision.

Focus Point
Since the Billroth II is not a direct gastrojejunostomy anastomosis as in the Billroth I, two codes are required, one for the Bypass and one for the Excision. See also Gastrectomy. See also Anastomosis, Billroth I.

Focus Point
Documentation of bypass procedures must clearly identify the body part bypassed from (body part value) and body part bypassed to (qualifier).

Coding Guidance
AHA: 2017, 2Q, 17

Medical and Surgical

Aneurysmectomy, Abdominal Aortic, with Replacement

Medical and Surgical

Body System
Lower Arteries

PCS Root Operation
Replacement

Root Operation Table
Ø4R   Lower Arteries, Replacement

Body Part
Abdominal Aorta

Approach
Open

Device
Autologous Tissue Substitute
Synthetic Substitute
Nonautologous Tissue Substitute

Description
The aorta is the main blood vessel that supplies blood from the heart to the abdomen, pelvis, and legs. An abdominal aortic aneurysm occurs when an area of the aorta enlarges or becomes weakened and balloons out. Rupture or enlargement of the aneurysm to more than 5.0–5.5 cm in diameter is a life-threatening medical emergency requiring surgical correction.

Using an Open approach, the physician makes an abdominal midline incision. The aorta is clamped. The vessel is opened lengthwise, and any thrombi (blood clots) are removed. The vessel is cut above and below the lesion, and the affected portion of the aorta is excised. A harvested or synthetic replacement graft is inserted into the defect and sutured in place between the two ends. Since vital organs (heart and brain) are not in jeopardy and collaterals provide circulation to the lower abdomen, pelvis, and legs during the lower abdominal aorta aneurysmectomy, circulation may not need to be maintained to the lower portion of the body beyond the aneurysm.

Focus Point

If an Autologous Tissue Substitute is harvested from a different body part, report a code for the excision of the graft tissue in addition to the code for the Replacement procedure.

© 2018 Optum360, LLC

Angioplasty, Percutaneous Transluminal Coronary (PTCA)

Body System
Heart and Great Vessels

PCS Root Operation
Dilation

Root Operation Table
027   Heart and Great Vessels, Dilation

Body Part
Coronary Artery, One Artery
Coronary Artery, Two Arteries
Coronary Artery, Three Arteries
Coronary Artery, Four or More Arteries

Approach
Percutaneous

Device
No Device

Qualifier
Bifurcation
No Qualifier

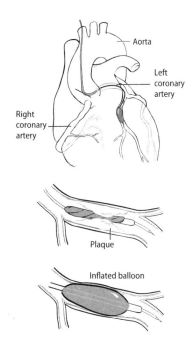

Description
Percutaneous transluminal coronary angioplasty (PTCA), also known as balloon angioplasty, coronary angioplasty, or percutaneous coronary angioplasty, is a minimally invasive procedure using a balloon to expand blocked or narrowed coronary arteries. Coronary artery disease is the narrowing or blockage of the coronary arteries caused by atherosclerosis, which is the buildup of plaque consisting of cholesterol, fatty deposits, calcium, and fibrin on the inner walls of the coronary arteries. This plaque may partially or totally block the blood flow through the coronary artery. This decreased blood flow starves the heart of the oxygen and nutrients it needs to function properly. If the oxygen supply to the heart muscle is reduced, a heart attack may occur.

In the PTCA procedure, the physician makes a small incision in the arm or leg and places two catheters. A catheter is inserted through the femoral, radial, or brachial artery and a second catheter with a balloon tip is threaded up to the heart. The physician inflates the balloon at the tip of the second catheter to flatten plaque obstructing the artery against the walls of the artery. If sufficient results are not obtained after the first inflation, the physician may reinflate the balloon for a longer period of time or at greater pressure. The catheter is removed, and pressure is placed over the incision for 20 to 30 minutes to stem bleeding. The patient is observed for a period afterward.

PTCA is reported with the root operation Dilation, which describes expanding an orifice or the lumen of a tubular body part. No device is reported, as the balloon is removed at the conclusion of the procedure.

The qualifier Bifurcation is reported when the intervention is performed for stenoses (narrowing) located in a main coronary artery and an adjoining side-branch vessel called a bifurcation blockage or bifurcation lesion.

Focus Point
The coronary arteries are classified as a single body part that is further specified by the number of arteries treated. Separate the number of arteries treated in the same manner. Assign the Coronary Artery body part value based on this number. Assign additional code(s) for arteries treated with a different device or qualifier value.

Coding Guidance
AHA: 2016, 4Q, 82; 2015, 4Q, 18; 2015, 3Q, 8; 2015, 2Q, 3; 2014, 2Q, 4

Angioplasty, Percutaneous Transluminal Coronary (PTCA) with Stent(s)

Body System
Heart and Great Vessels

PCS Root Operation
Dilation

Root Operation Table
027   Heart and Great Vessels, Dilation

Body Part
Coronary Artery, One Artery
Coronary Artery, Two Arteries
Coronary Artery, Three Arteries
Coronary Artery, Four or More Arteries

Approach
Percutaneous

Device
Intraluminal Device, Drug-eluting
Intraluminal Device, Drug-eluting, Two
Intraluminal Device, Drug-eluting, Three
Intraluminal Device, Drug-eluting, Four or More
Intraluminal Device
Intraluminal Device, Two
Intraluminal Device, Three
Intraluminal Device, Four or More
Intraluminal Device, Radioactive

Qualifier
Bifurcation
No Qualifier

Description
Percutaneous transluminal coronary angioplasty (PTCA), also known as balloon angioplasty, coronary angioplasty, or percutaneous coronary angioplasty, is a minimally invasive procedure using a balloon to expand blocked or narrowed coronary arteries. Coronary artery disease is the narrowing or blockage of the coronary arteries caused by atherosclerosis, which is the buildup of plaque consisting of cholesterol, fatty deposits, calcium, and fibrin on the inner walls of the coronary arteries. This plaque may partially or totally block the blood flow through the coronary artery. This decreased blood flow starves the heart of the oxygen and nutrients it needs to function properly. If the oxygen supply to the heart muscle is reduced, a heart attack may occur.

In the PTCA with stent(s) procedure, the physician makes a small incision in the arm or leg and places two catheters. A catheter is inserted through the femoral or brachial artery, and a second catheter is threaded up to the heart. Any obstruction is first treated by inflating a balloon at the tip of the second catheter (PTCA) and/or by using a rotary cutter (atherectomy) to flatten or remove the obstruction. Another deflated balloon with a stent mounted on it is introduced through a catheter to the site of the blockage under radiographic guidance. Once the stent is inside the blockage, the balloon is inflated, expanding the stent that surrounds it. This locks the stent in place against the artery wall, forming a scaffold to help keep the artery open. The physician may inflate the balloon multiple times to ensure the stent is firmly pressed against the vessel wall. The balloon catheter, guidewire, and guide catheter are then removed. Pressure is placed over the incision for 20 to 30 minutes to stem bleeding. The patient is observed for a period afterward.

PTCA with stent(s) is reported with the root operation Dilation, which describes expanding an orifice or the lumen of a tubular body part.

The qualifier Bifurcation is reported when the intervention is performed for stenoses (narrowing) located in a main coronary artery and an adjoining side-branch vessel called a bifurcation blockage or bifurcation lesion.

Focus Point
The coronary arteries are classified as a single body part that is further specified by the number of arteries treated. Separate the number of arteries treated in the same manner. Assign the Coronary Artery body part value based on this number. Assign additional code(s) for arteries treated with a different device or qualifier value.

Focus Point
If a procedure is performed on a continuous section of a tubular body part (overlapping lesion), assign the body part value describing the furthest site from the point of entry. See ICD-10-PCS guideline B4.1c.

Coding Guidance
AHA: 2016, 4Q, 84, 87; 2015, 4Q, 18; 2015, 3Q, 8; 2015, 2Q, 3; 2014, 2Q, 4

© 2018 Optum360, LLC

Arterioplasty (Bovine Patch)

Body System
Upper Arteries
Lower Arteries

PCS Root Operation
Supplement

Root Operation Table
03U Upper Arteries, Supplement
04U Lower Arteries, Supplement

Body Part
Refer to the ICD-10-PCS tabular list for a complete list of body parts

Approach
Open

Device
Nonautologous Tissue Substitute

Description
Bovine patch arterioplasty is used to repair an artery during cardiac and vascular and surgery.

After induction of general anesthesia, using an Open approach the physician makes an incision over the site of the affected blood vessel. The vessel is isolated and dissected from adjacent critical structures, and vessel clamps are applied. The physician repairs the injured vessel with a nonautologous tissue substitute. The graft tissue is sutured over the defect. The clamps are removed and the skin incision is repaired with layered closure.

Focus Point
Use the device value Nonautologous Tissue Substitute when the Zooplastic device value is not available.

Focus Point
If a procedure is performed on a continuous section of a tubular body part (overlapping lesion), assign the body part value describing the furthest site from the point of entry. See ICD-10-PCS guideline B4.1c.

Coding Guidance
AHA: 2016, 1Q, 31; 2014, 4Q, 37

Medical and Surgical

Arthrocentesis

Body System
Upper Joints
Lower Joints

PCS Root Operation
Drainage

Root Operation Table
ØR9   Upper Joints, Drainage
ØS9   Lower Joints, Drainage

Body Part
Refer to the ICD-10-PCS tabular list for a complete list of body parts.

Approach
Percutaneous

Device
Drainage Device
No Device

Qualifier
Diagnostic (No Device)
No Qualifier

Description
Arthrocentesis, or drainage (aspiration) of fluid from a joint, is performed either for diagnostic or therapeutic purposes. Arthrocentesis is often performed for diagnostic reasons to identify the etiology of an acute infectious or arthritic process, such as septic bursitis, gout, or rheumatoid arthritis. Therapeutic arthrocentesis is generally performed for drainage of joint effusion causing swelling, or infected joint fluid.

Joint aspiration involves the insertion of a needle to withdraw fluid from a joint. After administering a local anesthetic, using a Percutaneous approach, the physician inserts a sterile needle with a syringe attached through the skin and into the joint. Fluid is withdrawn under suction (aspiration) into the syringe. The needle is withdrawn, and pressure is applied to stop any bleeding.

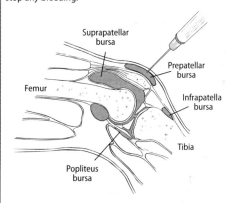

Focus Point
Arthrocentesis performed for diagnostic purposes is reported with the qualifier Diagnostic.

Focus Point
Arthrocentesis performed for therapeutic purposes may require continuous drainage for a period of time after the procedure. In these cases, a drainage catheter may be left in place and removed later. If the drainage catheter remains in place at the end of the procedure, report the device Drainage Device.

© 2018 Optum360, LLC

Banding, Gastric, Laparoscopic Adjustable (LAGB) (Lap-Band® System)

Body System
Gastrointestinal System

PCS Root Operation
Restriction

Root Operation Table
ØDV Gastrointestinal System, Restriction

Body Part
Stomach

Approach
Percutaneous Endoscopic

Device
Extraluminal Device

Description
The physician performs a laparoscopic adjustable gastric banding and port insertion of a gastric restrictive device for treatment of morbid obesity that does not permanently alter the gastrointestinal tract.

Using a Percutaneous Endoscopic approach, the physician places a trocar though an incision, generally above the umbilicus, and insufflates the abdominal cavity. The laparoscope and additional trocars are placed through small portal incisions. The silicone gastric band is introduced into the peritoneal cavity via a trocar and is placed and secured around the upper stomach to form a smaller stomach pouch with a narrowed outlet. A small port, or reservoir, is placed under the skin at the time of surgery and connected to the silicone band by tubing to facilitate postoperative adjustments of the outlet size by the addition or removal of saline via the port. The device may be altered, adjusted, or removed as necessary. The instruments are removed, and the incisions are closed.

The band is not inflated until after surgery. The physician inserts a needle into the access port to add or remove saline to tighten or loosen the band.

Focus Point
Adding saline to tighten the adjustable device is not considered a revision of the device. This procedure refers only to the adjustment of the size of the (adjustable) device, not a revision of the actual device. Report 3EØG3GC Introduction of Other Therapeutic Substance into Upper GI, Percutaneous Approach.

Focus Point
Removal of saline from the adjustable gastric band to correct an obstruction/stenosis due to the device is reported as Revision, with a code from table ØDW. Revision is defined as "correcting, to the extent possible, a portion of a malfunctioning device or the position of a displaced device."

Coding Guidance
AHA: 2018, 1Q, 20

Biopsy, Bone Marrow

Body System
Lymphatic and Hemic Systems

PCS Root Operation
Extraction

Root Operation Table
07D   Lymphatic and Hemic Systems, Extraction

Body Part
Bone Marrow, Sternum
Bone Marrow, Iliac
Bone Marrow, Vertebral

Approach
Open
Percutaneous

Qualifier
Diagnostic

Description
Bone marrow is a fatty substance within bone cavities that helps form blood cells and contains stem cells. Bone marrow biopsy may be performed to evaluate hematologic or lymphoproliferative disorders as well as other nonhematologic conditions when aspiration sampling is insufficient. Bone marrow contains stem cells that produce blood, and stem cells that form a stromal support. Biopsy is performed to evaluate overall cellularity or pathologic infiltration, or to detect focal lesions. Unlike aspirated tissue, tissue extracted via biopsy retains some of its cellular structure for evaluation. Biopsy samples are usually taken from the iliac crest or sternum, but occasionally from the vertebra. Bone marrow biopsies are routinely performed with a needle via a Percutaneous approach but can be accomplished with an Open procedure.

The skin over the bone is first cleaned with an antiseptic solution. A local anesthetic is injected, and the bone biopsy needle is inserted, rotated to the right, to the left, withdrawn, and reinserted at a different angle. This procedure is repeated until a small chip is separated from the bone marrow. The needle is again removed, and a piece of fine wire threaded through its tip transfers the specimen onto gauze. Samples contain bone marrow of which the structure has not been disturbed or destroyed. The bone must be decalcified overnight before it can be properly stained and examined.

During an Open procedure, the provider cuts through the skin and all other body layers, such as fascia and muscle, to expose the site of the procedure and obtains the bone marrow using drills, trephines, or a biopsy needle.

Focus Point
According to ICD-10-PCS guideline B3.4a, biopsy of bone marrow is coded to the root operation Extraction with the qualifier Diagnostic.

Coding Guidance
AHA: 2013, 4Q 111

© 2018 Optum360, LLC

Biopsy, Liver

Body System
Hepatobiliary System and Pancreas

PCS Root Operation
Excision

Extraction

Root Operation Table
ØFB Hepatobiliary System and Pancreas, Excision

ØFD Hepatobiliary System and Pancreas, Extraction

Body Part
Liver

Liver, Right Lobe

Liver, Left Lobe

Approach
Open (Excision)

Percutaneous

Percutaneous Endoscopic

Qualifier
Diagnostic

Description
The liver is a large, multilobed, glandular organ in the upper right abdominal quadrant that is essential to the digestive, metabolic, and hematologic processes of the body because it performs the following functions:

- Secreting digestive enzymes and bile
- Providing metabolism of nutrients from proteins, fats, and carbohydrates
- Storing nutrients such as glycogen for future use
- Filtering and detoxifying substances in the body such as alcohol and medications
- Producing body heat by metabolism
- Producing clotting factors for the blood

If the liver is not functioning properly, a build-up of toxins can occur with a devastating effect on the other organs. Liver biopsy is used to aid in diagnosing, assessing severity, and monitoring the progress of treatment of liver diseases.

Excision
A variety of approaches may be used to obtain liver tissue for biopsy. In one approach, the physician exposes the liver using an Open approach with an upper abdominal incision through the skin, fascia, muscle, and peritoneum. Interrupted mattress sutures are placed on the edge of the liver lobe. A specimen or a wedge- or pie-shaped piece of the liver is excised and sent for pathologic examination. Electrocautery is used to obtain hemostasis of the liver edge. The abdominal incision is closed with layered sutures.

The biopsy may also be obtained using a Percutaneous Endoscopic approach. The physician makes an incision in the umbilicus through which the abdomen is inflated and a fiberoptic laparoscope is inserted. Other incisions are made through which trocars can be passed into the abdominal cavity to deliver instruments, a fiberoptic camera, and light source. The physician manipulates the tools so that the liver can be viewed through the laparoscope and video monitor. Liver biopsy is obtained by using special instruments to excise pieces of liver tissue or lesion. When the specimen is obtained, the abdomen is deflated, instrumentation is removed, and incisions are closed with simple suture. The liver tissue is sent for pathologic diagnostic examination and analysis.

Extraction
The physician may also remove tissue from the liver for examination using ultrasound guidance. Using a Percutaneous approach, the physician inserts a hollow bore needle between the ribs on the patient's right side and extracts tissue from the liver for pathologic diagnostic examination and analysis.

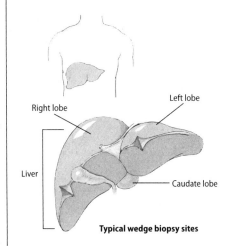

Right lobe

Left lobe

Liver

Caudate lobe

Typical wedge biopsy sites

© 2018 Optum360, LLC

Biopsy, Liver (continued)

Medical and Surgical

Focus Point

Laparotomy performed to reach the site of an open liver biopsy is not coded separately, according to ICD-10-PCS guideline B3.1b.

Focus Point

A needle biopsy of the liver performed during another procedure that is performed via an Open approach is reported as Open rather than Percutaneous. The instrument obtaining the biopsy is a needle, but it is not inserted through the skin or mucous membrane and other body layers to reach the site of the procedure. Although needle biopsies are typically reported with the root operation Extraction, because Open approach is not a valid option in the Hepatobiliary System and Pancreas, Extraction table, open needle biopsy is reported with the root operation Excision.

Focus Point

When liver tissue is removed for biopsy, report either root operation Excision (cutting out or off) or Extraction (pulling or striping out by use of force) with the qualifier Diagnostic. If fluid is removed from the liver for biopsy, use root operation Drainage with the qualifier Diagnostic. If the documentation does not indicate whether the aspiration liver biopsy obtained tissue or fluid, assign root operation Extraction with the qualifier Diagnostic.

Coding Guidance

AHA: 2016, 3Q, 41; 2016, 1Q, 23

© 2018 Optum360, LLC

Biopsy, Lung, Transbronchial

Body System
Respiratory System

PCS Root Operation
Extraction

Root Operation Table
ØBD   Respiratory System, Extraction

Body Part
Upper Lung Lobe, Right
Middle Lung Lobe, Right
Lower Lung Lobe, Right
Upper Lung Lobe, Left
Lung Lingula
Lower Lung Lobe, Left
Lung, Right
Lung, Left
Lungs, Bilateral

Approach
Via Natural or Artificial Opening Endoscopic

Qualifier
Diagnostic

Description
A transbronchial lung biopsy may be performed to diagnose abnormal peripheral lung masses, abnormal findings seen on imaging, hemoptysis, chronic lung or bronchial infections, benign tumors and polyps, as well as cancer, or to assess the stage or cell type of a known malignancy. It is also used in assessing rejection and infectious complications following lung transplantation. Transbronchial biopsy is generally not performed on both lungs in a single operative episode due to the risk of pneumothorax.

The physician views the airway using a Via Natural or Artificial Opening Endoscopic approach with a flexible fiberoptic or rigid bronchoscope (a long, thin tube that has a close-focusing telescope on the end for viewing), which is introduced through the nasal or oral cavity. The airway is anesthetized with a topical anesthetic. The bronchoscope is inserted and advanced through the nasal or oral cavity, past the larynx to inspect the bronchus, including fluoroscopic guidance, if used. The physician uses the views obtained through the bronchoscope to identify abnormal structures in the lung to be biopsied. After diagnostic visualization of the bronchus, fluoroscopy may be used to help navigate the bronchoscope tip to the area to be biopsied. Once the biopsy site is chosen, the distal end of the bronchoscope is directed into the specific segmental or subsegmental bronchus, and the physician passes special closed biopsy forceps through a channel in the bronchoscope. The biopsy forceps is then used to puncture through the bronchial wall (transbronchial) into the lung parenchyma to obtain one or more lung tissue samples from a single lobe. The forceps is closed and is gently retracted. Bleeding is assessed and controlled, and the bronchoscope is removed. Post biopsy chest x-rays may be performed to rule out pneumothorax.

Focus Point
When an imaging service such as fluoroscopic guidance is provided secondary to a principal procedure, the imaging service may be reported separately.

Focus Point
When lung tissue is removed for biopsy, report root operation Extraction with the qualifier Diagnostic. If fluid is removed from the lung for biopsy, use root operation Drainage with the qualifier Diagnostic. If the documentation does not indicate whether the lung biopsy obtained tissue or fluid, assign root operation Extraction with the qualifier Diagnostic.

Coding Guidance
AHA: 2017, 4Q, 41; 2016, 1Q, 26, 27; 2014 1Q, 20-21

Biopsy, Lymph Node

Body System
Lymphatic and Hemic Systems

PCS Root Operation
Excision

Extraction

Root Operation Table
Ø7B   Lymphatic and Hemic Systems, Excision

Ø7D   Lymphatic and Hemic Systems, Extraction

Body Part
Lymphatic, Head

Lymphatic, Right Neck

Lymphatic, Left Neck

Lymphatic, Right Upper Extremity

Lymphatic, Left Upper Extremity

Lymphatic, Right Axillary

Lymphatic, Left Axillary

Lymphatic, Thorax

Lymphatic, Internal Mammary, Right

Lymphatic, Internal Mammary, Left

Lymphatic, Mesenteric

Lymphatic, Pelvis

Lymphatic, Aortic

Lymphatic, Right Lower Extremity

Lymphatic, Left Lower Extremity

Lymphatic, Right Inguinal

Lymphatic, Left Inguinal

Approach
Open (Excision)

Percutaneous

Percutaneous Endoscopic

Via Natural or Artificial Opening Endoscopic (Extraction)

Qualifier
Diagnostic

Description
The lymphatic system picks up clear fluid that naturally leaks from blood vessels in the extremities and carries the fluid toward the chest, where it reenters blood circulation at the subclavian veins. Along the lymphatic channels are lymph nodes, which act as spongy filters to collect potentially dangerous cells to prevent spread of disease. Infectious agents and cancer cells may be captured by the lymph nodes, and biopsy identifies the infectious agent or extent of metastasis. Biopsy of lymph nodes may also be performed to diagnose conditions such as sarcoidosis or lymphoma.

A "sentinel node" is the lymph node immediately downstream, along the lymphatic chain, from a cancer site. In sentinel lymph node biopsy (SLNB) the sentinel node(s) are identified and excised for pathologic examination. In lymph node sampling (LNS), multiple nodes within an anatomical lymphatic chain (body part) are excised for pathologic examination. This is usually performed to stage a malignancy.

Excision
In LNS, the physician removes multiple lymph nodes using an Open or Percutaneous Endoscopic approach. The physician makes a small incision through the skin overlying the lymph node(s) in an Open approach to excise tissue. In a Percutaneous Endoscopic approach, the physician insufflates the targeted site and uses a laparoscope to dissect the nodes. In SLNB, an injection of a radiolabeled colloid or dye may precede surgery. This injection into the lymphatic channel helps the physician identify the lymph node nearest the malignancy. SLNB may also be performed using an Open or Percutaneous Endoscopic approach.

Extraction
In some cases, the sampling site is accessible by needle and a large tissue sample is not needed. When this occurs, fine needle aspiration (FNA) may be performed. In FNA, the physician aspirates a small amount of tissue into a needle. This may require radiologic guidance. Report the root operation Extraction for FNA.

Extraction is also reported for transbronchial needle aspiration (TBNA) lymph node biopsy, for which the approach is reported as Percutaneous Endoscopic. In TBNA, a bronchoscope is inserted and advanced through the nasal or oral cavity past the larynx to inspect the bronchus. The physician uses an FNA needle within the scope device to obtain one or more lymph node samples. The needle is inserted through the bronchial wall and into the lymph node(s). This is usually performed under endobronchial ultrasound (EBUS) guidance. The approach Percutaneous Endoscopic is used as the bronchoscope was used to help access the operative site (lymph node) via puncture through the bronchus (transbronchial).

Focus Point
The purpose of the procedure is to biopsy a sampling of lymphatic tissue rather than remove an entire string of interconnected lymph nodes. Since only a portion of the lymphatic chain (body part) is excised, the sampling procedure is reported as Excision, not Resection. Use Excision when the procedure is documented as a "regional lymph node excision" or "extended regional lymph node excision."

Focus Point
According to ICD-10-PCS guideline B3.4a, lymph node sampling for biopsy is coded to the root operation Excision with the qualifier Diagnostic.

Coding Guidance
AHA: 2017, 4Q, 41;2014, 3Q, 9-10; 2014, 1Q, 26; 2013, 4Q, 111-112

© 2018 Optum360, LLC

Medical and Surgical

Biopsy, Periurethral Tissue

Body System
Urinary System

PCS Root Operation
Excision

Root Operation Table
ØTB   Urinary System, Excision

Body Part
Urethra

Approach
Open
Percutaneous
Via Natural or Artificial Opening
Via Natural or Artificial Opening Endoscopic

Qualifier
Diagnostic

Description
The urethra is the lumen that carries urine from the bladder to the urethral orifice for elimination of urine from the body. The male urethra may be up to 20 cm in length, while the female urethra is usually about 4 cm long. In periurethral biopsy, tissue adjacent to the urethra is sampled for pathological examination.

Using an Open approach, the physician makes an incision in the skin overlying the urethra and removes tissue around the urethra for biopsy. At the site to be analyzed, a portion of the suspect tissue is excised by blunt or sharp dissection. The operative site is closed with sutures.

If a Percutaneous approach is used, the physician passes a needle into the tissue and the sample is removed through the needle. No repair is required.

If the tissue to be sampled lies near the urethral orifice, the approach may be Via Natural or Artificial Opening, meaning the physician can access the site and remove tissue that lies close to the opening of the urethra. This may be done by passing the tip of a biopsy needle into the urethral orifice and through the wall of the urethra to extract a sample of targeted periurethral tissue.

Another possible approach is Via Natural or Artificial Opening Endoscopic, in which the physician uses a urethroscope (cystourethroscope) inserted through the urethra to visualize the site from which the sample is removed through the wall of the urethra. The sample is removed by needle biopsy, through the wall of the urethra and into the targeted periurethral tissue.

Focus Point
The ICD-10-PCS guideline B4.1 directs coders to code the body part that is identified when the prefix "peri" is applied to a body part; for example, periurethral would be reported with the body part Urethra.

Focus Point
The bulbourethral gland (Cowper's) is reported with the body part Urethra, as it is considered a periurethral structure.

Biopsy, Temporal Artery

Body System
Upper Arteries

PCS Root Operation
Excision

Root Operation Table
Ø3B   Upper Arteries, Excision

Body Part
Temporal Artery, Right
Temporal Artery, Left

Approach
Open

Qualifier
Diagnostic

Description
The temporal artery is a branch of the external carotid artery that supplies blood to the head and to the brain. Temporal arteritis, also called giant cell arteritis (GCA), is an inflammatory disorder of the temporal artery. In arteritis, the lining of the artery swells, affecting blood flow. This causes headache or head pain, tenderness surrounding the artery and in the jaw, and varied systemic systems due to the effect of the arteritis on blood flow in the brain and sensory organs.

Under a local anesthetic, through an incision in the skin overlying the artery, the physician isolates and dissects the temporal artery from critical structures and excises a segment of the artery for pathological examination. The artery and skin are repaired in a layered closure.

Blalock-Taussig Shunt Procedure, Modified

See also Conduit, Right Ventricle to Pulmonary Artery (RV-PA) (Sano Shunt)

Body System
Heart and Great Vessels

PCS Root Operation
Bypass

Root Operation Table
Ø21 Heart and Great Vessels, Bypass

Body Part
Pulmonary Trunk
Pulmonary Artery, Right
Pulmonary Artery, Left

Approach
Open

Device
Zooplastic Tissue
Autologous Venous Tissue
Autologous Arterial Tissue
Synthetic Substitute
Nonautologous Tissue Substitute

Qualifier
Innominate Artery
Subclavian Artery
Carotid Artery

Description
Modified Blalock-Taussig shunt procedure is a palliative procedure performed on patients with tetralogy of Fallot and other malformations or defects that affect the flow of blood from the right ventricle, through the pulmonary artery, and to the lungs. These include pulmonary atresia, pulmonary stenosis, and tricuspid atresia. This procedure creates a connection or graft between the innominate, subclavian, or carotid arteries to the pulmonary trunk or right or left pulmonary artery, also known as a systemic-to-pulmonary artery shunt. The procedure

thus increases pulmonary blood flow until a fully corrective procedure can be performed.

In its unmodified form, this operation involves using an Open approach to divide the innominate, subclavian, or carotid artery, tie off the end of the artery, and create a connection between the end of this artery coming from the heart and the side of the pulmonary artery. The difficulty with this operation is making the connection to the pulmonary artery exactly the right size to supply adequate, but not excessive, blood flow to the lungs. Instead, a modified version of the operation is usually performed. Under general anesthesia, using an Open approach, the innominate or subclavian artery is not divided. Instead, one end of a 3 mm to 5 mm diameter graft (usually a Gore-Tex tube) is sewn to the side of the artery, and the other end is sewn to the pulmonary trunk or the side of the pulmonary artery. The size of the tube determines the amount of blood flow to the lungs. Cardiopulmonary bypass is not required. The ductus arteriosus (a connection between the aorta and pulmonary artery that has been supplying blood to the lungs but usually closes at birth) is tied off.

Focus Point
Bypass procedures require clarification of the body part bypassed "from" and body part bypassed "to." Generally, the fourth character for body part specifies the body part bypassed from, and the qualifier specifies the body part bypassed to. However, in this case, the Bypass table reverses the classification of upstream/downstream body parts in this same body system and root operation, similar to coronary artery bypass. Based on the available values in the Heart and Great Vessels, Bypass Table, coding advice from AHA Coding Clinic, 2016, 4Q, pages 102-103, and previous precedence of the guideline B3.6b regarding the reversal of the bypass classification for coronary artery bypass, use the body part value as the "to" and qualifier as the "from."

Coding Guidance
2016, 4Q, 102-103; 2014, 3Q, 3

© 2018 Optum360, LLC

Blepharoplasty

Body System
Eye

PCS Root Operation
Alteration
Repair
Replacement
Reposition
Supplement

Root Operation Table
Ø8Ø   Eye, Alteration
Ø8Q   Eye, Repair
Ø8R   Eye, Replacement
Ø8S   Eye, Reposition
Ø8U   Eye, Supplement

Body Part
Upper Eyelid, Right
Upper Eyelid, Left
Lower Eyelid, Right
Lower Eyelid, Left

Approach
Open
External

Device
Autologous Tissue Substitute (Alteration, Replacement, Supplement)
Synthetic Substitute (Alteration, Replacement, Supplement)
Nonautologous Tissue Substitute (Alteration, Replacement, Supplement)
No Device (Repair, Reposition)

Description
Blepharoplasty is the surgical repair or reconstruction of an eyelid. Blepharoplasty of the upper eyelids is a surgical procedure performed to correct a drooping of the upper eyelid, which is generally caused by excess tissue (ptosis). The most common reason for performing reconstructive functional blepharoplasty is to correct diminished visual fields caused by the weight of excess upper eyelid tissue. Blepharoplasty may also be performed in cases of trauma to the eyelids and orbit, entropion (inversion) or ectropion (eversion) of the edge of the eyelid and trichiasis.

In ICD-10-PCS, the body system Eye contains the body parts Lower and Upper Eyelid with specific values for right and left.

Alteration
Cosmetic blepharoplasty for dermatochalasis with removal of skin and fat is reported with the ICD-10-PCS root operation Alteration because it is performed to modify the natural anatomic structure of a body part without affecting its function. Alteration is coded for all procedures performed solely to improve appearance. All methods, approaches, and devices used for the objective of improving appearance are coded using the root operation Alteration.

Because some surgical procedures can be performed for either medical or cosmetic purposes, coding for Alteration requires diagnostic confirmation that the surgery is in fact performed to improve appearance and is not medically necessary.

Focus Point
The ICD-10-PCS index lists multiple root operation cross-references under the main term "Blepharoplasty." Selection of the appropriate root operation depends on the intent of the procedure being performed. While the ICD-10-PCS index main term "Blepharoplasty" does not include the root operation "Alteration," this may be coded from the Alteration table without consulting the index if the procedure is documented as cosmetic in nature. Blepharoplasty may be performed by other techniques not listed in the index. Review the operative report, and select the appropriate root operation from the ICD-10-PCS tables.

Repair
Blepharoplasty performed to repair trauma to the skin of the eyelid, such as a laceration, would be reported with the root operation Repair. A local anesthetic is injected around the laceration, and the wound is thoroughly cleansed, explored, and often irrigated with a saline solution. For superficial traumas that involve only the skin of the eyelid, the physician performs a simple, one-layer repair with sutures, which is reported as an External approach. For deeper, more complex lacerations, deep subcutaneous or layered suturing techniques are required. The physician may perform a layered closure, which involves suture of tissue layers under the skin with dissolvable sutures before suturing the skin. A repair extending through the skin into the subcutaneous tissue and beyond is considered an Open approach.

Replacement
In some cases, blepharoplasty may be performed to correct a defect, injury, or lesion that requires excision of a portion of the eyelid that must be replaced with a graft. This is reported with the root operation Replacement.

Blepharoplasty (continued)

The physician administers a local anesthetic, and the patient's face and eyelid are draped and prepped for surgery. A section of full-thickness eyelid is excised from the upper or lower eyelid. The section includes the defect and a margin of normal tissue. The edges of the excision site are approximated to reconstitute the eyelid contour. To achieve proper results, a skin graft or flap is performed. When direct wound closure or adjacent tissue transfer is not possible, the physician may take a split-thickness skin autograft from one area of the body and graft it to the area needing repair.

The physician harvests a split-thickness skin graft with a dermatome. The epidermis, or top layer of skin, is taken along with a small portion of the dermis, or bottom layer of the skin. This graft is then sutured or stapled onto the recipient area on the eyelid. Replacement always involves a device, which would be reported as Autologous Tissue Substitute; Synthetic Substitute; or Nonautologous Tissue Substitute. Replacement procedures involving only the eyelid skin are reported with External approach, while procedures that extend beyond the skin into the subcutaneous tissue, fascia, or muscle are reported as Open.

Focus Point

In a Replacement procedure, the excision of the tissue is included in the Replacement procedure and is not reported separately. However, harvest of the autograft, if obtained from a different incision, may be reported in addition to the primary procedure, according to ICD-10-PCS guideline B3.9.

Reposition

The eyelids may be repositioned with various techniques, including skin, muscle, or tendon excision or advancement, and slings.

Ptosis of the eyelid skin can be repaired using an External approach. The eyelid skin region to be resected is identified and marked with a marking pen. With the patient in the supine position, a blade is then used to cut through skin along the fusiform section of the eyelid tissue to be removed. The skin excision performed to reposition the eyelid is integral to the Reposition procedure and is not reported separately.

Alternatively, the physician may perform repositioning of blepharoptosis by resection or advancement of the levator muscle or aponeurosis using an Open approach. During the procedure, the physician administers a local anesthetic, and the patient's face and eyelid are draped and prepped for surgery. An incision line is outlined along the crease of the upper eyelid. A dissection is carried down the normal insertion point of the distal point of the levator tendon. The levator tendon is then isolated. The physician uses sutures to advance the levator tendon onto the tarsal plate in an adjustable fashion.

If the patient is old enough to undergo the procedure under local anesthetic, the patient is placed in a sitting position, and eyelid height and contour are evaluated under the effect of gravity. The amount that the levator tendon is advanced corresponds to the degree of preoperative ptosis. If the patient is not able to undergo the procedure under local anesthetic, general anesthesia is used and a predetermined amount of advancement is performed. In either case, the incision is repaired with sutures once the tendon has been secured in its new location. Any muscle or tendon resected with the intent to reposition the eyelids is integral to the Reposition procedure and not reported separately.

Focus Point

In Reposition procedures, the body part is moved to a new location from an abnormal location or from a normal location where it is not functioning correctly. The body part may or may not be cut out or off to be moved to the new location.

Supplement

Blepharoplasty may be performed to correct a defect in the eyelid by putting in a biologic or synthetic material that reinforces or augments the function of the eyelid. This is reported with the root operation Supplement.

The physician administers a local anesthetic, and the patient's face and eyelid are draped and prepped for surgery. A skin graft or flap is performed in the area in need of repair. The physician may take a split-thickness skin autograft from one area of the body and graft it to the area in need of repair. The physician harvests a split-thickness skin graft with a dermatome. The epidermis, or top layer of skin, is taken along with a small portion of the dermis, or bottom layer of the skin. This graft is then sutured or stapled onto the recipient area on the eyelid. Supplement always involves a device, which would be reported as Autologous Tissue Substitute; Synthetic Substitute; or Nonautologous Tissue Substitute. Supplement procedures involving only the eyelid skin are reported with External approach, while procedures that extend beyond the skin into the subcutaneous tissue, fascia or muscle are reported as Open.

Focus Point

In a Supplement procedure, the body part may have been taken out during a previous procedure but is not taken out as part of the Supplement procedure.

Focus Point

If identical blepharoplasty procedures are performed on both the right and left eyelids, each procedure is coded separately using the appropriate body part value (right, left), according to ICD-10-PCS guideline B4.3.

© 2018 Optum360, LLC

Browpexy

Body System
Anatomical Regions, General

PCS Root Operation
Alteration

Repair

Root Operation Table
ØWØ Anatomical Regions, General, Alteration
ØWQ Anatomical Regions, General, Repair

Body Part
Face

Approach
Open

Description
A browpexy is a procedure with limited applications that is designed to elevate and stabilize the eyebrow. This is commonly done as a cosmetic procedure but can also be performed for cases of facial nerve paralysis or eyebrow ptosis that obstructs the visual field.

Alteration
Browpexy performed for cosmetic purposes is reported using the ICD-10-PCS root operation Alteration because it is performed to modify the natural anatomic structure of a body part without affecting its function. All methods, approaches, and devices used for the sole objective of improving appearance are coded using the root operation Alteration. Because some surgical procedures can be performed for either medical or cosmetic purposes, coding for Alteration requires diagnostic confirmation that the surgery is in fact performed to improve appearance and is not medically necessary.

Repair
A browpexy involves suspending the eyebrow using sutures to the underlying bone. During the procedure, the physician lifts the eyebrow through an upper-eyelid incision or from a small incision above the eyebrow. The brow is raised just above the level of the bone and physically sewn to a higher position on the forehead. Since there is not a more specific code in ICD-10-PCS for reposition of the eyebrow, the default root operation is Repair, which is the most appropriate option, in the Anatomical Regions, General table using the body part Face and Open approach. The root operation Repair is defined as "restoring a body part to its normal structure."

> **Focus Point**
>
> As there is no eyebrow body part in ICD-10-PCS, report the Anatomical Regions, General with Face as the body part. This is consistent with ICD-10-PCS guideline B4.1a, which states: "If a procedure is performed on a portion of a body part that does not have a separate body part value, code the body part value corresponding to the whole body part."

> **Focus Point**
>
> Browpexy is commonly performed in combination with upper lid blepharoplasty. Report the code for browpexy in addition to code(s) for blepharoplasty when performed in combination, according to multiple procedures guideline B3.2c.

Coding Guidance
AHA: 2015, 1Q, 31

Medical and Surgical

Buckling, Scleral (with Implant)

Body System
Eye

PCS Root Operation
Supplement

Root Operation Table
Ø8U Eye, Supplement

Body Part
Eye, Right
Eye, Left

Approach
Percutaneous

Device
Synthetic Substitute

Description
Scleral buckling surgery is performed to treat retinal detachment, when the retina separates from the back wall of the eye. It is a method for closing breaks and flattening the separated retina to the underlying tissue. A scleral buckle is a piece of silicone sponge, rubber, or semi-hard plastic band or sleeve that the physician, usually an ophthalmologist, places on the outside of the eye (the sclera, or the white of the eye) at the site of a retinal tear. The buckle pushes the sclera toward the retinal tear and holds the retina against the sclera until scarring can occur, sealing the retinal tear. The buckle is left permanently in place. In cases of multiple tears, the surgeon may place a silicone band around the entire circumference of the eye.

The patient is placed in the supine position, and after appropriate anesthetic is administered, the eye is prepped and draped in sterile fashion and a lid speculum is placed. The physician explores the sclera to locate the site overlying a retinal detachment, usually with indirect ophthalmoscope. Stay sutures are placed under involved rectus muscles so the eye and the area that will be treated are exposed. The surgeon treats the retinal tear externally, by placing a cold (cryotherapy) or hot (cautery or laser) probe over the sclera and depressing it. The burn seals the choroid to the retina at the site of the tear. The physician cuts a groove in the sclera and mattress sutures are placed across this incision. Any subretinal fluid is drained.

The scleral buckle device is soaked in an antibiotic solution and then laid in the scleral bed underneath the rectus muscle and sutured in place, taking care not to perforate the eye globe with the needle. Sometimes, a silicone sponge is placed under the band. Additional cryotherapy or photocoagulation may be performed at this time. When the retinal detachment has been adequately repaired and supported, the rectus muscle sutures are removed.

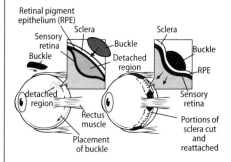

Focus Point
The scleral buckle is considered an implant that physically reinforces and augments the eye externally during healing and is reported as Supplement. While the intent of the procedure is to repair a retinal detachment, the device is not placed on the retina but on the external eye. In conjunction with the formation of chorioretinal adhesions, the implant pressing inward on the wall of the eye enables the attachment of the retina.

Focus Point
ICD-10-PCS does not provide an External approach value for eye Supplement procedures. Report the approach Percutaneous as the closest available equivalent.

© 2018 Optum360, LLC

Bunionectomy

See also Bunionectomy, Double Osteotomy

See also Bunionectomy, Tendon Transfer

Body System
Lower Bones

PCS Root Operation
Excision

Root Operation Table
ØQB   Lower Bones, Excision

Body Part
Metatarsal, Right
Metatarsal, Left

Approach
Open

Description

A bunionectomy is the surgical removal of a bunion. A bunion is an enlargement of the joint at the base of the big toe comprising bone and soft tissue. A bunionette is the same condition but on the outside of the foot at the base of the little toe. A bunionette is also called tailor's bunion. Treatment of bunions is traditionally performed via Open approach using various techniques. The root operation is reported with Excision as only a portion of the metatarsal bone is excised.

Using an Open approach, the physician performs a resection with osteotomy of the first metatarsal head, including imbrication of the capsule, by exposing the joint. The physician makes a lateral incision over the distal third of the first metatarsal bone to expose the metatarsal head. An osteotome is used to remove the medial extension of the bone. The cut is made along the shaft of the bone. The wound is irrigated and the soft tissues are sutured. Soft dressing is applied and weight bearing is allowed as tolerated.

A bunionectomy may be performed using a minimally invasive approach. The patient is given a local or general anesthetic, and the physician makes one or more small incisions close to the metatarsal bone. The bunion is removed. ICD-10-PCS does not offer a minimally invasive approach option. The complete definitions of the approach values must be applied. Although smaller incisions are used, if the site is directly visualized and exposed, Open approach is the appropriate approach value.

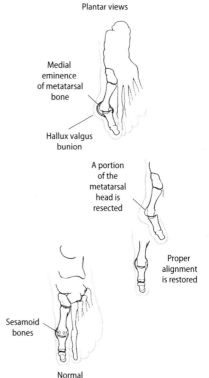

Plantar views

Medial eminence of metatarsal bone

Hallux valgus bunion

A portion of the metatarsal head is resected

Proper alignment is restored

Sesamoid bones

Normal metatarsophalangeal joint

Bunionectomy, Double Osteotomy

See also Bunionectomy

See also Bunionectomy, Tendon Transfer

Body System
Lower Bones

PCS Root Operation
Reposition

Root Operation Table
ØQS   Lower Bones, Reposition

Body Part
Metatarsal, Right
Metatarsal, Left
Toe Phalanx, Right
Toe Phalanx, Left

Approach
Open

Device
Internal Fixation Device

Description
A bunionectomy is the surgical removal of a bunion. A bunion, or bunion deformity, is an enlargement of the joint at the base of the big toe comprising bone and soft tissue that typically causes pain at the first metatarsal head.

The primary purpose of a double osteotomy bunion surgery is to reposition the metatarsal and phalangeal bones that form the first metatarsophalangeal (MTP) joint.

Using an Open approach, a medial incision is made, exposing the proximal phalanx and distal metatarsal. Soft tissues are dissected and the joint capsule is exposed, with incision into the capsule and exposure of the medial eminence. The medial eminence is excised in line with the metatarsal shaft. Medial wedge osteotomy of the proximal phalanx is performed just distally to the phalangeal base, and the phalanx is repositioned. The surgeon then makes a V-shaped cut into the first metatarsal, removing excess bone in the distal aspect near the metatarsal head, allowing the metatarsal bone to be repositioned in the lateral direction. The cut and repositioned phalangeal and metatarsal bones are then fixed in this new position with small screws or suture wires placed though the phalanx and the metatarsal bone. The redundant joint capsule is tightened and closed. The incisions are thoroughly irrigated and closed in layers.

Focus Point
The appropriate root operation for realignment of bones is Reposition. The osteotomies are inherent to the repositioning of the bone and are not reported as additional codes.

Coding Guidance
AHA: 2014, 4Q, 31

© 2018 Optum360, LLC

Bunionectomy, Tendon Transfer

See also Bunionectomy

See also Bunionectomy, Double Osteotomy

Body System
Tendons

PCS Root Operation
Transfer

Root Operation Table
ØLX   Tendons, Transfer

Body Part
Foot Tendon, Right
Foot Tendon, Left

Approach
Open

Description
A bunion, or bunion deformity, is an enlargement of the joint at the base of the big toe comprising bone and soft tissue that typically causes pain at the first metatarsal head. A bunionectomy is the surgical removal of a bunion. In some cases, correction of the bunion deformity requires soft tissue procedures such as tendon transfers.

The physician treats a bunion deformity of the foot with tendon transfers. Using an Open approach, the surgeon makes an incision over the top of the foot between the first and second toes. The incision is carried deep to the metatarsophalangeal joint. The extensor tendon of the big toe is identified and cut and then transferred and reattached at a new position to correct anatomical alignment. Other tendons may also be cut and reattached at new locations until correct anatomical alignment is achieved. Any contracted structures are released as needed. The sesamoid bones are examined and removed as necessary. The bony eminence (exostosis) may be excised in a separately reportable procedure. The incisions are cleansed with sterile saline and closed in layers.

Focus Point
According to ICD-10-PCS multiple procedures guideline B3.2c, multiple procedures with distinct objectives may be reported separately. If the surgeon performs a concomitant metatarsal neck and/or phalangeal osteotomy to reposition the bones, or excision of the bony exostosis at the time of tendon transfer, these procedures may also be reported. See also Bunionectomy, and Bunionectomy, Double Osteotomy.

Bypass Graft, Aorto-bifemoral

Body System
Lower Arteries

PCS Root Operation
Bypass

Root Operation Table
Ø41   Lower Arteries, Bypass

Body Part
Abdominal Aorta

Approach
Open

Device
Autologous Venous Tissue
Autologous Arterial Tissue
Synthetic Substitute
Nonautologous Tissue Substitute
No Device

Qualifier
Femoral Arteries, Bilateral

Description

Aorto-bifemoral bypass surgery is used to bypass diseased large blood vessels in the abdomen and groin in patients with atherosclerosis or peripheral arterial disease.

Under general Anesthesia, using an Open approach, the physician makes an incision in the skin of the abdomen over the lower abdominal aorta into the abdomen, and the aorta is isolated and dissected from adjacent critical structures. Through a separate skin incision in the groin or upper thigh, the femoral artery is isolated and dissected from adjacent critical structures. Once vessel clamps have been affixed above and below the defect, the lower aorta may be cut through or tied off with sutures. The single end of a Y-shaped synthetic or natural autologous or nonautologous graft is sutured to the aorta. One of the two ends, or "limbs," of the Y graft is passed through a tunnel on the inside of the upper thigh and sutured to a point on the femoral artery. The other end of the Y is placed in a similar fashion on the other side. When clamps are removed, the graft forms a new route, bypassing the blocked area. After the graft is complete, the abdominal and groin incisions are repaired with layered closures with sutures and staples.

Focus Point

Documentation of bypass procedures must clearly state the body part bypassed from and body part bypassed to.

Focus Point

If an Autologous Venous or Arterial Tissue is harvested from a different body part, report a code for the Excision of the graft tissue in addition to the code for the Bypass root operation.

© 2018 Optum360, LLC

Medical and Surgical

Bypass Graft, Coronary Artery (CABG)

Body System
Heart and Great Vessels

PCS Root Operation
Bypass

Root Operation Table
Ø21 Heart and Great Vessels, Bypass

Body Part
Coronary Artery, One Artery
Coronary Artery, Two Arteries
Coronary Artery, Three Arteries
Coronary Artery, Four or More Arteries

Approach
Open
Percutaneous Endoscopic

Device
Zooplastic Tissue
Autologous Venous Tissue
Autologous Arterial Tissue
Synthetic Substitute
Nonautologous Tissue Substitute
No Device

Qualifier
Coronary Artery
Internal Mammary, Right
Internal Mammary, Left
Thoracic Artery
Abdominal Artery
Aorta

Description
Under general anesthetic, using an Open approach, the chest is opened via midline sternotomy, and the surgeon examines the heart. Cardiopulmonary bypass is initiated with a single, two-stage venous uptake tube. Saphenous vein is harvested from either leg. Other arterial or vein graft may also be taken from the arm, the back of the leg, or from a cadaver. A clamp is placed on the aorta above the heart. Cold preserving solution is pumped through the coronary arteries to stop the heart. A point is chosen on the diseased coronary arteries beyond the area of disease, and a longitudinal incision is cut in it. The proximal part of the graft is trimmed to the same length as the cut in the coronary artery is cleaned off. One end of each graft is sewn onto the coronary arteries, bypassing the occluded segments, and the other end is attached to the aorta. A 3 mm to 6 mm hole is punched in the ascending aorta, and the other end of the vein graft is sewn to this hole. The clamp on the aorta is released. Cardiopulmonary bypass is discontinued when heart function returns. Because the graft bypasses the blood

flow around the diseased artery, the root operation Bypass is reported.

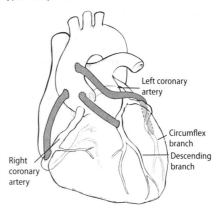

Coronary artery bypass can be performed using limited access or minimally invasive approaches that use smaller incisions with the combinations of robotic instrumentation, laparoscopy and computer-enhanced manipulation systems. These techniques vary with some using minimal sternotomy and may or may not use cardiopulmonary bypass. These still are categorized as Open approach. There are limited cases of CABG being performed with a total endoscopic approach and since ICD-10-PCS does not address minimally invasive procedures, care must be taken to apply the full definitions when determining the correct approach value.

Focus Point
Bypasses are coded differently for coronary artery bypass procedures than other bypasses. In a CABG, the fourth character, body part, identifies the number of coronary arteries bypassed "to" and the seventh character, qualifier, specifies the body part bypassed "from." See guideline B3.6b.

Focus Point
Each coronary artery that uses a different device and/or qualifier is coded separately. See guideline B3.6c.

Focus Point
If an Autologous Venous or Arterial Tissue is harvested from a different body part such as a saphenous vein graft, report a code for the excision of the graft tissue in addition to the code for the Bypass procedure (see guideline B3.9). When the left internal mammary artery graft (LIMA) remains attached or pedicled, it is not considered a device, and no additional code is reported for the harvesting since it was not excised from the patient.

© 2018 Optum360, LLC

Bypass Graft, Coronary Artery (CABG) (continued)

Focus Point

Auxiliary procedures such as transfusion catheters, intra-aortic balloon pumps, and temporary pacing that are routinely done to support the performance of the bypass procedure are not coded separately, with the exception of cardiopulmonary bypass, which is reported as Extracorporeal Performance of Cardiac Output, Continuous, from table 5A1. However, if these procedures are continued after surgery, this is considered more extensive than the temporary support required during the procedure and may be separately reported.

Coding Guidance

AHA: 2016, 4Q, 82; 2016, 1Q, 27; 2014, 3Q, 8; 2014, 3Q, 20; 2014,1Q, 10; 2013, 4Q, 108; 2013, 3Q, 18; 2013, 2Q, 37

© 2018 Optum360, LLC

Bypass, Extracranial-Intracranial

Body System
Upper Arteries

PCS Root Operation
Bypass

Root Operation Table
Ø31   Upper Arteries, Bypass

Body Part
Common Carotid Artery, Right
Common Carotid Artery, Left
Temporal Artery, Right
Temporal Artery, Left

Approach
Open

Device
Autologous Venous Tissue
Autologous Arterial Tissue
No Device

Qualifier
Intracranial Artery

Description
Similar to cardiac bypass surgery in which blocked heart arteries are bypassed, extracranial to intracranial (EC-IC) bypass is done to improve cerebral blood flow. By rerouting blood flow around a blocked artery by connecting a blood vessel from outside the brain (extracranial) to a vessel inside the brain (intracranial), blood supply is restored to the brain, preventing strokes. This bypass can be performed either directly (donor artery) or via a vessel graft.

Donor Artery
The donor artery is a healthy, superficial (extracranial) artery in the scalp or neck that is detached at one end and anastomosed to an intracranial artery, bypassing a diseased portion of another artery and establishing new blood flow. The most common bypass is the superficial temporal to the middle cerebral artery, performed to reroute the blood from a diseased or occluded carotid artery, which normally supplies the blood to the temporal, parietal, and frontal brain lobes.

Using an Open approach, an incision is made in the side of the scalp, and the physician isolates and dissects one end of the superficial temporal artery (STA), separating it from adjacent critical structures. A craniotomy is performed and through the hole in the skull, the physician creates a bypass around the blocked internal carotid artery by connecting the donor artery (STA) to the middle cerebral artery on the surface of the brain (intra- cranial artery). The superficial temporal artery now bypasses the occluded area and supplies blood to the brain.

Vessel Graft
The vessel graft method uses a vein or artery harvested from elsewhere in the body as a conduit around the diseased or occluded artery. The saphenous vein, or radial or ulna arteries are commonly used. Via an Open approach, the physician connects one end of the previously harvested vessel to the carotid artery and tunnels it under the skin up to the scalp. A craniotomy is performed, and the surgeon connects the other end of the graft to an artery in the brain.

Focus Point
The root operation Bypass is used for both types of EC-IC procedures. The body part value identifies the body part bypassed "from," and the qualifier identifies the body part bypassed "to" (see guideline B3.6a). No device is reported for the donor artery method as the artery is still attached to the blood supply and is not a device. The vessel graft device value depends on the type of artery or venous graft harvested.

Focus Point
Harvesting of an autograft from a different site is coded separately, according to guideline B3.9.

Bypass, Femoral to Peroneal with In-Situ Saphenous Vein Graft

Body System
Lower Arteries

PCS Root Operation
Bypass

Root Operation Table
041   Lower Arteries, Bypass

Body Part
Femoral Artery, Right
Femoral Artery, Left

Approach
Open

Device
Autologous Venous Tissue

Qualifier
Peroneal Artery

Description
Arterial bypass procedures may be indicated in patients with occlusive disease with ischemic pain, claudication, nonhealing ulcerations, or gangrene with impending tissue loss.

Using an Open approach, the physician isolates and dissects a section of the femoral artery. Separate incisions are used to expose the greater saphenous vein and to gain access to the peroneal artery. Vessel clamps are affixed above and below the site of anastomosis in the femoral and distal arteries. The physician isolates and dissects the greater saphenous vein from adjacent critical structures. The side branches are clipped and the greater saphenous vein divided and prepared for the femoral anastomosis. An endarterectomy of the femoral artery is performed, and the greater saphenous vein is then anastomosed. After completion of the proximal anastomosis, a valvulotome is passed through the vein to lyse the valves. The distal anastomosis to the peroneal artery is performed under tourniquet control, and the greater saphenous vein is utilized as a vein patch in the distal peroneal arteriotomy. The clamps are removed, and without the vein valves, the blood now flows backward toward the feet, as if the vein were an artery. An angiography is performed to evaluate the anastomoses. The blocked or damaged portion of the artery is not removed. After the graft is complete, the incisions are closed in layers.

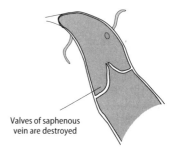

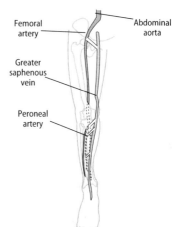

Valves of saphenous vein are destroyed

Femoral artery

Abdominal aorta

Greater saphenous vein

Peroneal artery

Saphenous vein graft is attached to femoral artery at top and the distal peroneal artery at bottom.

Focus Point
Excision of the in situ saphenous vein and lysis of the saphenous vein valves are integral to the bypass procedure and are not reported separately.

Focus Point
If living or biologic autograft or allograft material is mixed with a synthetic material, report qualifier Autologous Tissue Substitute or Nonautologous Tissue Substitute, respectively. If two separate grafts are used, each can be reported separately.

Focus Point
Bypass procedures may be performed using an Open approach with endoscopic assistance. According to ICD-10-PCS guideline B5.2, if a procedure is performed using an Open approach with Percutaneous Endoscopic Assistance, report the approach as Open.

Coding Guidance
AHA: 2016, 3Q, 31; 2014, 2Q, 6

© 2018 Optum360, LLC

Bypass, Lymphovenous (LVB)

Body System
Lymphatic and Hemic Systems

PCS Root Operation
Repair

Root Operation Table
Ø7Q   Lymphatic and Hemic Systems, Repair

Body Part
Lymphatic, Head
Lymphatic, Right Neck
Lymphatic, Left Neck
Lymphatic, Right Upper Extremity
Lymphatic, Left Upper Extremity
Lymphatic, Right Axillary
Lymphatic, Left Axillary
Lymphatic, Thorax
Lymphatic, Internal Mammary, Right
Lymphatic, Internal Mammary, Left
Lymphatic, Mesenteric
Lymphatic, Pelvis
Lymphatic, Aortic
Lymphatic, Right Lower Extremity
Lymphatic, Left Lower Extremity
Lymphatic, Right Inguinal
Lymphatic, Left Inguinal

Approach
Open

Device
No Device

Qualifier
No Qualifier

Description
The lymphatic system is a network of vessels that carry lymphatic fluid throughout the body, draining from the tissues into the blood. Lymphedema is a progressive, painful disorder in which excessive lymph fluid is unable to drain normally and accumulates in the tissues, causing swelling, usually occurring in the arms and legs.

Postmastectomy lymphedema syndrome is a form of lymphedema that occurs after excision of the axillary lymphatic structures during mastectomy. Edema in the arms and hands develops from pooling of interstitial fluids due to reduced lymphatic circulation. Lymphedema can often be treated with nonsurgical interventions, such as medications, compression, massage therapy, and diet modification, to reduce the swelling and discomfort. However, in some cases with advanced lymphedema, or as a preventative measure, surgical intervention may be performed.

With the patient under general anesthesia, the surgeon injects a fluorescent indocyanine green (IC-Green™) dye through a central venous line. The dye lights up, mapping the pathway of the lymphatic system in the affected area using an infrared camera. The identified lymphatic vessels are marked with a pen, and using super resolution microscopic techniques and equipment, an Open approach is used via incisions about an inch long to visualize the lymphatic vessels. Depending on the number of areas affected, the surgeon may make multiple incisions during the procedure. The lymphatic vessels are anastomosed using microscopic suture techniques to veins nearby, bypassing the damaged lymph nodes and shunting the flow of lymphatic fluid directly to the veins. Depending on the size of the recipient vein, either an end-to-end or an end-to-side anastomosis is performed. Patency is confirmed with dye and imaging, and the incisions are closed under the microscope to avoid damaging the anastomoses. Blood loss is minimal.

Focus Point
The intent of a lymphovenous bypass procedure is to bypass or reroute, not drain, the obstructed lymphatic fluid to a new venous location. There is, however, no bypass option in the Lymphatic and Hemic Systems body system in ICD-10-PCS. The root operation Repair is used instead as the closest available alternative.

Coding Guidance
AHA: 2017, 1Q, 34

Cerclage, Cervical

Body System
Female Reproductive System

PCS Root Operation
Restriction

Root Operation Table
ØUV Female Reproductive System, Restriction

Body Part
Cervix

Approach
Open
Percutaneous
Via Natural or Artificial Opening

Device
Extraluminal Device
Intraluminal Device
No Device

Description
Cerclage of the cervix is performed to prevent miscarriage by reinforcing weak cervical muscles in a patient with a history of cervical incompetence, short cervical length, or cervical insufficiency. The cerclage may be performed prior to pregnancy or in early pregnancy, usually between weeks 12 and 16.

Cerclage may be performed transabdominally, but the most common approach is vaginal Via Natural or Artificial Opening. In vaginal cerclage, the physician inserts a speculum into the vagina to view the cervix of a pregnant or nonpregnant patient. A thick, nondissolvable suture or a thin wire is threaded around the cervix and secured to reinforce the cervical muscles and prevent cervical dilation. In McDonald cerclage, the cervix is grasped and a purse-string stitch is placed around the high endo-cervix, near to the internal os (opening) to close it. In the Shirodkar operation, the suture is buried under incisions in the vaginal mucosa and cinched to secure closure of the os. In some cases, a thin piece of fascia or other nondissolvable material may be placed instead of a wire or suture. This would be reported as an Intraluminal Device, as would a device such as a cerclage pessary placed around the cervical os within the vaginal canal (lumen).

An Open abdominal approach for cerclage may be used in instances such as traumatic cervical laceration, congenital shortening of the cervix, previous failed vaginal cerclage, or advanced cervical effacement. In abdominal cervical cerclage, a small abdominal incision just above the pubic hairline gives the physician access to the peritoneal space, and a band is placed around the cervix at the level of the internal os

to prevent spontaneous abortion from an incompetent cervix. The abdominal incision is closed with sutures. In some cases, a thin piece of fascia or other nondissolvable material may be placed instead of a wire or suture. In such cases, report an Extraluminal Device around the external surface of the cervix.

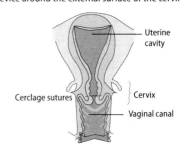

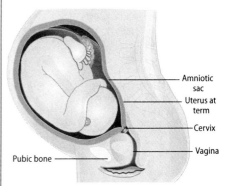

Although it remains in place after the surgery, the suture typically placed during cerclage is considered a surgical supply rather than a device. If material other than a wire or suture is placed, report Extraluminal Device or Intraluminal Device.

Focus Point
Because the cervical os is not completely closed off, restriction is the correct root operation for cervical cerclage. The root operation Restriction describes, "Partially closing an orifice or the lumen of a tubular body part."

Focus Point
Wires and sutures placed in cervical cerclage are considered surgical supplies and are not considered devices. Removal of cervical cerclage in these cases is reported with root operation Extirpation.

Coding Guidance
AHA: 2015, 3Q, 25

© 2018 Optum360, LLC

Chemoembolization, Hepatic Artery

See also Introduction, Antineoplastic Agent, Hepatic Artery, under "Administration" in the Medical and Surgical Related section

Body System
Lower Arteries

PCS Root Operation
Occlusion

Root Operation Table
Ø4L   Lower Arteries, Occlusion

Body Part
Hepatic Artery

Approach
Percutaneous

Device
Intraluminal Device

Description

Chemoembolization delivers chemotherapy drugs combined with embolic material directly to a tumor, which minimizes exposure of healthy tissues to highly toxic chemotherapy drugs. This delivery method minimizes side-effects, like nausea and vomiting, and maximizes the cancer-killing properties of the drugs. The chemotherapy drugs are mixed with particles, called microspheres, that block the flow of blood to the tumor. Without a blood supply, the tumor no longer has the oxygen and nutrients it needs to grow.

This method of chemotherapy is used primarily for the treatment of hepatocellular carcinoma, a type of primary liver cancer, but it may also be used to treat cancers that have spread to the liver from another area of the body (metastasis). It is also known as transcatheter arterial chemoembolization (TACE) of the liver. Unlike other organs, the liver has two blood supplies—the portal vein that feeds most normal liver cells and the hepatic artery that feeds cancer cells in the liver. This unique feature of the liver allows the injection of chemotherapy drugs directly into the hepatic artery branches to kill the cancer cells and block the tumor's blood supply, while sparing the healthy liver tissue.

In ICD-10-PCS, two codes are required to code this method of treatment. A code for the root operation Occlusion is reported for the embolization from the

Medical and Surgical section with a second code for the root operation Introduction from the Administration section to report the infusion of the antineoplastic substance and the embolic material. The Occlusion component of the procedure is described here. Occlusion is defined as completely closing an orifice or the lumen of a tubular body part, which in this procedure involves closing off the hepatic artery branches that feed the tumor.

Before the procedure, diagnostic tests are performed to demonstrate patency of the portal vein to ensure the patient will have an adequate blood supply to the liver after treatment. With the patient under local anesthesia and mild intravenous sedation, a catheter is inserted percutaneously via the femoral artery and threaded into the hepatic artery. Angiography is then performed to identify the branches of the hepatic artery that supply blood to the tumor. Smaller catheters are then threaded into these branches, followed by injection of the embolic chemotherapy mixture. Embolic material may consist of tiny microbeads or microspheres, a viscous collagen agent, gelatin powder or sponges, or polyvinyl alcohol (PVA) particles. Regardless of the type of embolic material, this is reported with the device value Intraluminal Device when used to occlude a tubular body part (blood vessel).

Focus Point

The ICD-10-PCS guideline for Occlusion vs. Restriction for vessel embolization procedures, B3.12, states the following:

"If the objective of an embolization procedure is to completely close a vessel, the root operation Occlusion is coded. If the objective of an embolization procedure is to narrow the lumen of a vessel, the root operation Restriction is coded.

"Examples: Tumor embolization is coded to the root operation Occlusion, because the objective of the procedure is to cut off the blood supply to the vessel. Embolization of a cerebral aneurysm is coded to the root operation Restriction, because the objective of the procedure is not to close off the vessel entirely, but to narrow the lumen of the vessel at the site of the aneurysm where it is abnormally wide."

Coding Guidance
AHA: 2015, 1Q, 38; 2014, 3Q, 26

© 2018 Optum360, LLC

Cholecystectomy

Body System
Hepatobiliary System and Pancreas

PCS Root Operation
Excision

Resection

Root Operation Table
ØFB Hepatobiliary System and Pancreas, Excision

ØFT Hepatobiliary System and Pancreas, Resection

Body Part
Gallbladder

Approach
Open

Percutaneous Endoscopic

Qualifier
Diagnostic (Excision)

No Qualifier

Description
Cholecystectomy is the surgical removal of part or all of the gallbladder, a pear-shaped organ that collects and stores bile produced in the liver. Cholecystectomy is performed to treat stones in both the gallbladder and the bile ducts. A cholecystectomy may also be needed for pancreatic and gallbladder inflammation, gallbladder polyps, or neoplasms.

Excision
Excision is reported for partial removal of the gallbladder or excision of a portion of the gallbladder. A partial removal, reported with root operation Excision, can be performed to prevent bile duct damage when safe dissection of the total gallbladder is difficult.

In an Open approach, the physician removes part of the gallbladder. The physician exposes the liver and gallbladder via a right subcostal incision. The cystic duct and cystic artery are ligated, and a portion of the gallbladder is removed. The incision is closed with layered sutures.

In a Percutaneous Endoscopic approach, the physician performs laparoscopic removal of a portion of the gallbladder. The physician makes a 1 cm infraumbilical incision through which a trocar is inserted. Pneumoperitoneum is achieved by insufflating the abdominal cavity with carbon dioxide. A fiberoptic laparoscope fitted with a camera and light source is inserted through the trocar. Other incisions are made on the right side of the abdomen and in the subxiphoid area to allow other instruments or an additional light source to be passed into the abdomen. The tip of the gallbladder is mobilized and placed in traction. The portion of the gallbladder to be removed

is dissected from the liver bed and removed through a trocar site. The intra-abdominal cavity is irrigated. The trocars are removed, and the incisions are closed.

> **Focus Point**
> A biopsy of the gallbladder may be done for diagnostic purposes and would be reported with the qualifier Diagnostic. Cholecystectomy otherwise would be reported with the qualifier No Qualifier.

Resection
The root operation Resection is reported for a complete removal of the gallbladder.

Using an Open approach, the physician exposes the liver and gallbladder via a right subcostal incision. The cystic duct and cystic artery are ligated, and the gallbladder is totally removed using electrocautery. The incision is closed with layered sutures.

In a Percutaneous Endoscopic approach, the physician performs laparoscopic total removal of the gallbladder. The physician makes a 1 cm infraumbilical incision through which a trocar is inserted. Pneumoperitoneum is achieved by insufflating the abdominal cavity with carbon dioxide. A fiberoptic laparoscope fitted with a camera and light source is inserted through the trocar. Other incisions are made on the right side of the abdomen and in the subxiphoid area to allow other instruments or an additional light source to be passed into the abdomen. The tip of the gallbladder is mobilized and placed in traction. The Hartmann's pouch (junction of the cystic duct and gallbladder neck) is identified.

Tissue is dissected free from around the area to expose Calot's triangle (formed by the cystic artery, and cystic and common bile ducts). Clips are applied to the proximal area of the cystic duct and artery (close to the gallbladder), and the cystic duct and artery are cut. The gallbladder is dissected from the liver bed and removed through a trocar site. Any loose stones that have dropped into the abdominal cavity are retrieved with forceps. The intra-abdominal cavity is irrigated. The trocars are removed, and the incisions are closed.

> **Focus Point**
> If a Percutaneous Endoscopic (laparoscopic) cholecystectomy is converted to an Open procedure, code the Percutaneous Endoscopic Inspection and Open Excision or Resection. See ICD-10-PCS guideline B3.2d.

> **Focus Point**
> An Open cholecystectomy performed with Percutaneous Endoscopic (laparoscopic) assistance is reported as an Open procedure, according to ICD-10-PCS guideline B5.2.

© 2018 Optum360, LLC

Medical and Surgical

Chondroplasty, Knee Abrasion

Body System
Lower Joints

Root Operation Table
Excision

Root Operation Table
ØSB   Lower Joints, Excision

Body Part
Knee Joint, Right
Knee Joint, Left

Approach
Open
Percutaneous Endoscopic

Description
Chondroplasty is a repair or reconstruction of articular (joint) cartilage. Chondroplasty may be performed for patients who have damage to the cartilage of the knee, either from an acute injury or from degenerative wear, commonly referred to as chondromalacia.

An abrasion chondroplasty is a surgical procedure performed to debride, or smooth, the degenerated, worn area. In ICD-10-PCS, excisional debridement is coded using the root operation Excision.

Using a Percutaneous Endoscopic approach, the physician makes 1 cm long portal incisions on either side of the patellar tendon for arthroscopic access into the knee joint. Lesions of the articular cartilage are identified by the arthroscope and the use of a probe. Additional portal incisions may be made to provide better access to the lesions. The unstable or fragmented cartilage is debrided with a motorized suction cutter. The cartilage is smoothed down to the layer of subchondral bone, which promotes bleeding and regeneration of cartilage. Any loose bodies are removed.

The physician may also drill holes into the subchondral bone or create tiny fractures (microfractures) to further promote cartilage regeneration. The joint is then thoroughly flushed. A temporary drain may be applied. Incisions are closed with sutures and Steri-Strips.

In some instances, an Open approach may be indicated. A longitudinal incision is made over the knee to expose the knee joint structures. The unstable or fragmented cartilage is debrided with a motorized suction cutter. The cartilage is smoothed down to the layer of subchondral bone, which promotes bleeding and regeneration of cartilage, and any loose bodies are removed. The physician may also drill holes into the subchondral bone or create tiny fractures (microfractures) to further promote cartilage regeneration. The joint is thoroughly flushed, and a temporary drain may be applied. The incision is closed in layers with sutures and is bandaged.

Focus Point
Chondroplasty that is performed as a component of accomplishing the objective of a main procedure, such as a meniscectomy, is not reported separately, consistent with ICD-10-PCS guideline B3.1b. If the documentation is unclear or there is a question whether the procedure is a component of the main procedure, query the physician for clarification.

Focus Point
To ensure accurate code assignment, it is necessary to review the medical record documentation for information on the approach and surgical technique, and to determine the bones, cartilage, ligaments, tendons, or muscles treated. According to ICD-10-PCS multiple procedures guideline B3.2, multiple procedures may be reported if the same procedure is performed on different body parts with distinct body part characters, or multiple body parts with separate distinct body parts classified to a single body part value. Refer to the ICD-10-PCS Body Part Key and Body Part Definitions for specific body part values.

Coding Guidance
AHA: 2015, 1Q, 34

Circumcision

Body System
Male Reproductive System

PCS Root Operation
Resection

Root Operation Table
ØVT   Male Reproductive System, Resection

Body Part
Prepuce

Approach
External

Description
The physician performs surgical removal of the penile foreskin. Surgical technique may vary. After the administration of a local anesthetic by injection(s), the physician removes the foreskin of the penis by clamping the foreskin in a plastic device and trimming the excess protruding skin. A segment of foreskin on the dorsal or the side of the penis is crushed with forceps. Using a clamp technique, a cut is made through the crushed tissue with scissors, and the divided foreskin is fitted in a plastic bell-shaped clamp. The clamp crushes a ring of the foreskin and holds the skin edges together while the excess skin is trimmed from the top of the device. The clamp is left in place and simply falls off when healing has finished days later. Using a technique without a clamp, a cut is made through the crushed tissue with scissors, and the divided foreskin is pulled down over the head of the penis, while the excess skin is trimmed from around the head of the penis. Bleeding is controlled by chemical cautery or suture ligatures. The skin edges created are sutured together with absorbable suture material.

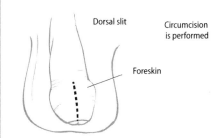

Dorsal slit

Circumcision is performed

Foreskin

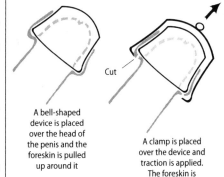

A bell-shaped device is placed over the head of the penis and the foreskin is pulled up around it

Cut

A clamp is placed over the device and traction is applied. The foreskin is then cut

Medical and Surgical

© 2018 Optum360, LLC

Closure, Left Atrial Appendage

Body System
Heart and Great Vessels

PCS Root Operation
Occlusion

Root Operation Table
02L   Heart and Great Vessels, Occlusion

Body Part
Atrium, Left

Approach
Open
Percutaneous
Percutaneous Endoscopic

Device
Extraluminal Device
Intraluminal Device
No Device

Qualifier
Left Atrial Appendage

Description

The left atrial appendage (LAA), also called the left auricle, is a small pouch in the anterior left atrium. It is thought to accept excess blood volume when left atrial pressure is high. The LAA is anatomically insignificant, except for patients who have atrial fibrillation (AF). In AF, the right and left atria beat irregularly, and usually rapidly, although some patients in AF experience bradycardia. The erratic beats disrupt the normal flow of blood in the heart and may cause blood to pool in the LAA, where it may linger and form thrombi. As a result, patients with AF have a fivefold risk of stroke and usually undergo lifelong pharmacological therapy to prevent clot formation. For some patients, anticoagulant therapy is contraindicated, and occlusion of the left atrial appendage provides prophylaxis.

To surgically close the LAA, the surgeon uses a surgical stapler, clip, or suture to pull together the walls of the LAA to permanently close the opening from the left atrium. Occlusion may also be performed by inserting a device that blocks blood from entering the LAA. Cardiovascular surgeons routinely perform closure of the left atrial appendage during major cardiovascular procedures such as coronary artery bypass graft, mitral valve repair, and maze procedures. In patients with atrial fibrillation, prophylactic left atrial appendage removal or exclusion is recommended whenever the chest has been opened for another cardiovascular procedure to prevent future strokes.

Occlusion may be performed using an Open, Percutaneous, or Percutaneous Endoscopic approach.

The Watchman™ is an intraluminal device for percutaneous endovascular, transcatheter closure of the LAA. To implant the Watchman device, the physician places a catheter sheath into the femoral vein and advances it, under fluoroscopic guidance, to the right atrium. The physician then advances a transseptal puncture apparatus through the sheath to the right atrium, punctures the intra-atrial septum, and advances the Watchman device into the opening of the LAA in the left atrium. The device self-expands, sealing off the LAA.

The AtriClip® is an extraluminal device that is clamped on the LAA exterior, sealing the LAA from the rest of the left atrium. It may be placed using an Open approach or by accessing the heart through an incision between the ribs (mini-thoracotomy) using thoracoscopic assistance to view the operative site.

Alternatively, the physician may use sutures or staples to close the LAA, using an Open or Percutaneous Endoscopic approach. Sutures and staples are considered integral to the performance of the procedure and are not coded as devices.

> **Focus Point**
>
> *Medical devices that occlude the LAA are an emerging technology, so watch for changes in status for FDA approval of new and existing devices. Use the ICD-10-PCS Device Key for guidance.*

> **Focus Point**
>
> *A transcatheter endovascular approach does not involve direct visualization of the operative site, so the approach Percutaneous is assigned. Thoracoscopic incisions are classified as Percutaneous Endoscopic approach. Thoracoscopic-assisted via a mini-thoracotomy approach, even though it is minimally invasive, is considered an Open approach. Procedures performed using the open approach with percutaneous endoscopic assistance are coded to the approach Open, according to ICD-10-PCS guidelines.*

Coding Guidance
AHA: 2017, 4Q, 104; 2017, 1Q, 36; 2014, 3Q, 20

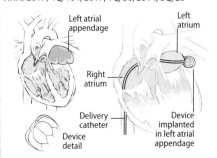

Left atrial appendage

Left atrium

Right atrium

Delivery catheter

Device detail

Device implanted in left atrial appendage

© 2018 Optum360, LLC

Colectomy, Total

Body System
Gastrointestinal System

PCS Root Operation
Resection

Root Operation Table
ØDT   Gastrointestinal System, Resection

Body Part
Large Intestine

Approach
Open

Percutaneous Endoscopic

Description
Total colectomy, or complete removal of the large intestine, is performed for conditions such as late stage malignant neoplasms, diverticulitis, and inflammatory bowel diseases of the intestine, such as Crohn's disease and ulcerative colitis. Total colectomy includes the removal of the large bowel from the cecum to the level of the upper rectum, including the ascending, transverse, and descending colon, the sigmoid colon, and the hepatic and splenic flexures.

In ICD-10-PCS, the entire large intestine (colon) is defined as its own body part of Large Intestine and encompasses all of the previously named individual intestinal body parts. Resection includes all of a body part, or any subdivision of a body part that has its own body part value, while Excision includes only a portion of a body part. If the surgeon removes the entire subdivision of the body part with its own body part value (Large Intestine), the correct root operation is Resection.

For a total colectomy, bowel function is restored either by connecting the small intestine (ileum) to the top of the rectum by anastomosis, or by creating an ileostomy. End-to-side or side-to-side anastomosis can be performed by stapling or suturing. Any anastomosis method is inherent in the resection and is not coded separately. The formation of an ileostomy involves pulling the end of the intestine through a hole or stoma in the abdominal wall for external excretion and requires an additional code from the root operation Bypass table.

For a traditional open total colectomy, reported with ICD-10-PCS approach Open, the physician makes a midline abdominal incision. The large laparotomy incision allows direct visualization and direct access to the abdominal cavity. The colon is mobilized, and the colorectal junction and terminal ileum are divided. The colon is removed. The terminal ileum is either approximated to the rectum with staples or hand-sewn stitches; or is brought out through a separate incision in the abdominal wall onto the skin as an ileostomy. The peritoneum is closed with running Vicryl, fascia with running Vicryl, skin with clips. Sterile dressings are applied.

Laparoscopic total colectomy is reported with the approach Percutaneous Endoscopic. Laparoscopic colon removal involves a 1.5 cm incision near the umbilicus to place the camera (laparoscope) with three to five more small incisions made for other instruments. The Hasson trocar is placed into the abdominal cavity, and gas insufflation is initiated. A laparoscope is inserted to visualize the abdominal cavity, and trocars are placed. The inserted instruments (trocars) are used to mobilize the colon and to divide the colorectal junction and terminal ileum. The colon is extracted through the incisions, and the terminal ileum is either approximated to the rectum with staples or hand-sewn stitches; or is brought out through a separate incision in the abdominal wall onto the skin as an ileostomy. The advantages of laparoscopic colectomy over open colectomy include shorter length of hospital stay and better outcomes for postoperative morbidity and mortality.

> **Focus Point**
>
> According to ICD-10-PCS guideline B3.1b, the anastomosis, regardless of technique, is not reported separately as it is considered a component in the surgery and a procedural step to the closing; only the Resection code is assigned.

> **Focus Point**
>
> A proctocolectomy includes resection of the colon and rectum. An additional code is added for the resection of the rectum.

© 2018 Optum360, LLC

Colporrhaphy (Vaginal Laceration)

Body System
Female Reproductive System

PCS Root Operation
Repair

Root Operation Table
ØUQ   Female Reproductive System, Repair

Body Part
Vagina

Approach
Via Natural or Artificial Opening
Via Natural or Artificial Opening Endoscopic
External

Description
The term colporrhaphy can imply several different types of procedures, from a repair of a simple or complex vaginal laceration to an anterior repair of a cystocele or posterior repair of rectocele. The operative report must be examined carefully to determine the specific objective in order to report the appropriate root operation, body system, and body part value. The following example describes the root operation Repair of a vaginal laceration.

The physician inserts a speculum into the vagina and identifies the extent of the vaginal laceration or wound. Usually a local anesthetic is used; however, some cases may require general anesthesia. The physician then repairs lacerations of the vagina. In a layered closure procedure, a local anesthetic is injected around the laceration, and the wound is thoroughly cleansed, explored, and often irrigated with a saline solution. Due to deeper or more complex lacerations, deep subcutaneous or layered suturing techniques are required. The physician sutures tissue layers under the skin with dissolvable sutures before suturing the skin.

Focus Point
Laxity due to stretching of the pelvic fascia may result in prolapse of the bladder, urethra, or rectum (cystocele, urethrocele, rectocele) into the vagina. The support tissues between the vagina and these structures are tightened to correct the laxity in the pelvic fascia, and the structures are pushed back into their normal position. This would be reported with the root operation Repair, body system Subcutaneous Tissue and Fascia, Pelvic Region.

Coding Guidance
AHA: 2016, 1Q, 15; 2014, 4Q, 44

Medical and Surgical

Component Release, Abdominal Muscle

Body System
Muscles

PCS Root Operation
Release

Root Operation Table
ØKN   Muscles, Release

Body Part
Abdomen Muscle, Right
Abdomen Muscle, Left

Approach
Open

Description
Large or complex abdominal wall defects most commonly result from incisional hernias due to multiple abdominal operations that have failed primary suture closure or mesh repair. They may also result from trauma, surgical resection of the abdominal wall due to neoplasm or necrotizing abdominal wall infections, or therapeutic open abdomen that cannot be closed primarily.

The anterior abdominal wall consists of three flat muscles and a pair of vertical muscles. The flat muscles are the right and left external and internal oblique, and the right and left transversus abdominis muscles. The right and left vertical rectus abdominus muscles are covered by a sheath divided into two regions.

Abdominal component separation enlarges the circumference of the abdomen by incising and moving muscle layers on each side to bridge the abdominal wall defect. In component separation of the abdominal wall, the surgeon elevates skin flaps over the rectus abdominis muscle and the internal and external oblique or transversus abdominis muscles are incised lateral to the abdominal wall defect. This separation enables mobilization of the vertical rectus muscles toward the midline to reduce the size of the defect and facilitate primary musculofascial wound closure. This may be reinforced with synthetic or bioprosthetic mesh in a separately reportable procedure. In larger defects, mesh is used to bridge the musculofascial edges, which is also reported separately.

Release
As the flat muscles are being incised to allow the mobilization of the vertical rectus abdominis muscles, the appropriate root operation is Release. Release is defined as "freeing a body part from an abnormal physical constraint by cutting or by the use of force." In the root operation Release, the body part value coded is the body part being freed (rectus abdominis muscle) rather than the tissue being cut (internal and external oblique or transversus abdominis muscles) to free the body part. If the sole objective of the procedure is freeing a body part without cutting the body part, the root operation is Release.

Focus Point
If mesh is used to reinforce the abdominal wall, use the appropriate root operation Supplement for placement of the mesh in addition to the Release procedure.

Coding Guidance
AHA: 2014, 4Q, 39

© 2018 Optum360, LLC

Medical and Surgical

Conduit, Right Ventricle to Pulmonary Artery (RV-PA) (Sano Shunt)

See also Fontan Stage I (Norwood Procedure)

See also Fontan Stage II (Glenn Procedure) (Caval-pulmonary Artery Anastomosis)

See also Fontan Stage III, Completion

See also Blalock-Taussig Shunt Procedure, Modified

Body System
Heart and Great Vessels

PCS Root Operation
Bypass

Root Operation Table
Ø21   Heart and Great Vessels, Bypass

Body Part
Ventricle, Right

Approach
Open

Device
Zooplastic Tissue
Autologous Venous Tissue
Autologous Arterial Tissue
Synthetic Substitute
Nonautologous Tissue Substitute

Qualifier
Pulmonary Trunk

Description
A three-staged surgical approach is performed for children born with a functional single ventricle, known as hypoplastic left heart syndrome (HLHS). Stage I is performed within several days of birth. The purpose of this procedure is to enlarge the hypoplastic aorta to provide blood flow to the body. *See also* Fontan Stage I (Norwood Procedure). An additional connection must be made to provide blood flow to the lungs via a shunt placed between the right ventricle and pulmonary artery. This portion of the procedure ensures that blood-flow is controlled enough to prevent damage to the heart and lungs while ensuring adequate oxygen delivery to the lungs.

The patient is placed under general anesthesia and on cardiopulmonary bypass. Using an Open approach, a median sternotomy incision through the middle of the chest is performed. After the Norwood procedure enlarging the aorta is performed, incisions are made on the main pulmonary artery and right ventricle. An appropriate sized RV-PA conduit is selected. One end of the conduit is sewn onto the incision on the main pulmonary artery, and the other end is sewn onto the incision on the right ventricle. A delayed sternal closure may be necessary with skin closed in layers. A chest tube(s) may be used to provide drainage for the chest cavity.

Focus Point
Many different types of materials may be used for the conduit. Synthetic Substitute conduits made of Gore-Tex, Nonautologous Tissue Substitutes using valved tissue from a cadaver, Zooplastic Tissue grafts using a valved bovine (cow) jugular vein, or composite Dacron tube graft containing a porcine (pig) valve can be used. Composite graft material using a mixture of biologic and synthetic material is always coded as a Nonautologous Tissue Substitute.

Focus Point
Multiple surgical procedures may be performed concomitantly to correct congenital heart disorders. ICD-10-PCS guidelines on multiple procedures should be followed when assigning codes for these procedures.

Coding Guidance
AHA: 2017, 1Q, 19; 2014, 3Q, 30

Conization, Cervix, LEEP

Body System
Female Reproductive System

PCS Root Operation
Excision

Root Operation Table
ØUB   Female Reproductive System, Excision

Body Part
Cervix

Approach
Via Natural or Artificial Opening

Qualifier
Diagnostic
No Qualifier

Description
A loop electrosurgical excision procedure (LEEP) is the surgical excision and simultaneous cautery of the wound site of the cervix using a thin wire through which an electrical current is delivered. It may also be documented as a large loop excision of the transformation zone (LLETZ), large loop excision of the cervix (LLEC) or loop cone biopsy of the cervix. The procedure is performed to remove neoplasia or otherwise aberrant tissue from the cervix. LLETZ has a more specific goal than does LEEP. LLETZ removes through the loop excision process the entire transformation zone, while LEEP's goal is to remove the lesion and a margin of healthy tissue surrounding it. The transformation zone (squamocolumnar junction) is an area of the cervix with normally evolving cells, found on the outer surface of an immature cervix or higher in the cervical canal in an older cervix. The transformation zone is more susceptible to the risk of intraepithelial neoplasia resulting from HPV infection than are other parts of the cervix, vagina, or vulva.

Using a vaginal, Via Natural or Artificial Opening approach, the physician views the cervix—including the upper/adjacent portion of the vagina—through a colposcope, a binocular microscope used for enhanced visualization of the vagina, ectocervix, and endocervix. The physician inserts a weighted speculum into the vagina to fully expose the cervix. Cervical tissue is removed by LEEP using a hot cautery wire containing a high frequency, low voltage electrical cutting current as a cutting instrument. Due to the electrical current, a grounding pad is attached to the patient's leg during the procedure. Usually, if the lesions are not too deep, the tissue is excised in one pass of the cutting wire to excise the entire transformation zone. The LEEP procedure can be both diagnostic and therapeutic for the excision of abnormal cervical tissue, e.g., tissue positive for CIN I, II or III. The cone of cervical tissue usually undergoes pathological examination. It is generally standard surgical protocol that specimens removed during surgery must be submitted for pathologic gross and/or microscopic examination. The documentation must state the objective of the procedure is diagnostic to report the qualifier Diagnostic.

Focus Point

By definition, to report the approach Via Natural or Artificial Opening Endoscopic, the scope instrumentation must enter through the natural or artificial opening. A colposcope remains outside the body and does not enter the vaginal vestibule. Therefore, LEEP using colposcopy is reported with the approach Via Natural or Artificial Opening.

Focus Point

Although some tissue is destroyed by the electrocautery in LEEP, the goal of the procedure is excision of abnormal cervical tissue, so Excision is the root operation reported.

Medical and Surgical

© 2018 Optum360, LLC

Control, Epistaxis, Ligation Anterior Ethmoidal Arteries

Body System
Upper Arteries

PCS Root Operation
Occlusion

Root Operation Table
Ø3L   Upper Arteries, Occlusion

Body Part
Internal Carotid Artery, Right
Internal Carotid Artery, Left

Approach
Open

Device
Extraluminal Device
No Device

Description
Clinically, epistaxis (bleeding from the nostril, nasal cavity, or nasopharynx) can be divided into two categories—anterior bleeds and posterior bleeds—based on the site of the hemorrhage. Epistaxis often occurs when the nasal mucosa becomes eroded, causing the vessel walls to become weakened and break. Approximately 90 percent of nosebleeds occur in the anterior nose at a network of vessels called the Kiesselbach plexus, near the nasal septum. This vascular plexus contains a convergence of the internal and external carotid and maxillary venous and arterial branches. Posterior epistaxis occurs in the posterior nasal cavity and is often of arterial origin. Posterior nasal hemorrhages are often more complex or difficult to control than anterior epistaxis and present a greater risk of airway difficulty and aspiration of blood into the respiratory tract.

When site of bleeding is determined to be the anterior ethmoidal artery (AEA), the physician may administer a local anesthetic and control the epistaxis by ligation of the ethmoidal vessels. The physician administers a local anesthetic and makes an Open incision along the side of the nose near the inner canthus of the right or left eye to expose the ethmoid arteries. The periosteum (periorbitum) is elevated. The anterior ethmoidal artery is identified in the suture line between the frontal and ethmoid bones. The posterior ethmoid artery is located upon entering the posterior medial wall near the orbital apex. A clip or suture completes the ligation of the anterior ethmoidal artery. The incision is repaired with layered closure.

Focus Point
The anterior ethmoidal artery extends from the ophthalmic artery, which is a branch of the extracranial portion of the internal carotid artery. According to the ICD-10-PCS Body Part Key, only the intracranial portion of the internal carotid artery is reported with Intracranial Artery. ICD-10-PCS guideline B4.2 states that where a specific branch of a body part does not have its own body part value in PCS, the body part is typically coded to the closest proximal branch that has a specific body part value.

Focus Point
A clip across the outside lumen of the artery is considered an Extraluminal Device; sutures are coded as No Device per guideline B6.1b.

Focus Point
When documentation specifies only "control of acute epistaxis" with no further description of a more definitive root operation being performed, use root operation Control of body part Nasal Mucosa and Soft Tissue from the Ear, Nose and Sinus body system (table 093).

Medical and Surgical

Conversion, Gastrostomy to Jejunostomy (PEG-PEJ)

Body System
Gastrointestinal System

PCS Root Operation
Insertion

Root Operation Table
ØDH   Gastrointestinal System, Insertion

Body Part
Jejunum

Approach
Via Natural or Artificial Opening Endoscopic

Device
Feeding Device

Description
A conversion of gastrostomy to jejunostomy is the endoscopic advancement of a jejunostomy tube through an existing gastrostomy tube into the proximal jejunum.

An endoscopy of the proximal small bowel is performed. The physician inserts an endoscope through the previously made gastrostomy tube. The jejunostomy tube is grasped with forceps placed through the endoscope and advanced using the endoscope into the proximal jejunum. The endoscope is withdrawn.

Since no device is removed, only a code for the root operation Insertion is reported for the placement of the jejunostomy tube (Feeding Device) through the gastrostomy tube. The gastrostomy tube becomes a part of the jejunostomy and is not removed. The approach value is Via Natural or Artificial Opening Endoscopic since the Feeding Device is advanced through the previously placed tube or ostomy (artificial opening) using the endoscope.

Focus Point
If a previously placed gastrostomy tube is exchanged for a new gastrostomy tube, the root operation reported would be Change.

© 2018 Optum360, LLC

Medical and Surgical

Cordotomy, Spinal (Chordotomy)

Body System
Central Nervous System and Cranial Nerves

PCS Root Operation
Destruction

Division

Root Operation Table
005 Central Nervous System and Cranial Nerves, Destruction

008 Central Nervous System and Cranial Nerves, Division

Body Part
Cervical Spinal Cord

Thoracic Spinal Cord

Lumbar Spinal Cord

Approach
Open

Percutaneous

Percutaneous Endoscopic

Description
Cordotomy (also chordotomy) is the surgical cutting or ablation of the anterolateral sensory tracts in the spinal cord in an attempt to relieve severe and otherwise uncontrollable pain.

Destruction
Cordotomy may also be done using radiofrequency or electrical stimulation to ablate or destroy the pain signal pathway. This is reported with the root operation Destruction, since the intent of this procedure is to physically eradicate the body part by the direct use of energy, force, or a destructive agent.

Using image guidance via a Percutaneous approach, the cordotomy needle is inserted. The needle used is part of a radiofrequency system that uses specially designed needles and electrodes that can cause electrical stimulation or create lesions. Electrical stimulation is used to determine the correct area to place the needle. The patient is continuously monitored, and motor functions are regularly tested. The surgeon uses the patient's sensory feedback to determine the precise area to perform the cordotomy. Using the needle-electrode system, lesions are created to block the pathway pain signals used to reach the brain.

In some instances, a cordotomy may be performed using a Percutaneous Endoscopic approach. A lateral puncture of the spinal canal is performed, guided by fluoroscopy. A guide cannula is inserted percutaneously. As soon as the guide cannula reaches the cerebrospinal fluid (CSF), the endoscope is inserted to visualize the spinal cord and surrounding structures. After the target for electrode insertion into the spinal

cord is determined, cordotomy is performed by radiofrequency.

Focus Point
The ICD-10-PCS index lists only Division under the main terms "Cordotomy" and "Chordotomy." Selection of the appropriate root operation depends on the intent of the procedure being performed. In ICD-10-PCS, a valid code may be chosen directly from the tables without consulting the index. For example, while the index main terms do not include the root operation Destruction, the procedure may be coded from the Destruction table without consulting the index if the intent of the procedure is documented as Destruction of the spinal sensory tract. Review the operative report and select the appropriate root operation from the ICD-10-PCS tables.

Division
Cordotomy or tractotomy of the spinal cord involves the surgical incision or severing of a sensory tract of the spinal cord. Transection of spinal cord tracts involves the use of a transverse incision using an Open approach. The patient is placed prone, and the physician makes a midline incision overlying the affected vertebrae, the fascia is incised, and the paravertebral muscles are retracted. A laminectomy is performed. The physician identifies the anterolateral tracts in the appropriate level on the side opposite the pain. The dentate ligament is divided at the level of the cordotomy and is drawn posteriorly toward the midline to expose the anterolateral part of the cord. A cordotomy knife is introduced into the spinal cord anterior to the dentate ligament and directed toward the anterior spinal artery. The tissue in front of this artery is divided with the knife. The incision is closed with layered sutures.

In a Percutaneous cordotomy, also known as a stereotactic cordotomy, the physician performs a neurosurgical procedure to relieve pain by cutting the tracts of the spinal cord that transmit pain impulses through the nerve pathways. Percutaneous cordotomy is usually done with fluoroscopic or CT guidance under local anesthesia.

Focus Point
In ICD-10-PCS, cordotomy by surgical incision or severing of the nerve tract is coded to the root operation Division. In Division, all or a portion of the body part is separated into two or more portions. Coders should not confuse the root operation Division with Release. If the sole objective of the procedure is to free a body part, the root operation is Release. If the sole purpose is separating or transecting a body part, the root operation is Division.

Cordotomy, Spinal (Chordotomy) (continued)

Focus Point

The laminectomy in these cases is performed as the approach for adequate visualization during the division procedure and is not reported. See ICD-10-PCS guideline B3.1b.

Correction, Syndactyly

Body System
Skin and Breast

PCS Root Operation
Division

Root Operation Table
0H8   Skin and Breast, Division

Body Part
Skin, Right Hand
Skin, Left Hand

Approach
External

Description

Syndactyly is a genetically linked disorder and may appear in conjunction with other syndromes. Syndactyly involves fusion or webbing of the digits and is one of the more common musculoskeletal malformations. Fusion involves the bones of the digits as well as the soft tissues, while webbing involves only the soft tissues. When the webbing occurs in the fingers and is confined to the skin, surgery is generally performed early in childhood to allow normal digit development. The corrective operation for a simple syndactyly involves splitting the webbing and at times applying skin grafts. When the bones are fused, the situation is more complex and surgery may not be able to provide optimal function, particularly when all five bones are involved.

The physician repairs a simple syndactyly (web finger) using skin flaps. Using an External approach, the physician incises the skin of the web for digital release, and the underlying tissues are freed. The repair is accomplished with skin flaps from the incision area.

Focus Point

When skin grafts are needed to accomplish the repair of a simple syndactyly, review the operative report to select the correct root operation(s) to use.

© 2018 Optum360, LLC

Medical and Surgical

Creation, Colostomy

Body System
Gastrointestinal System

PCS Root Operation
Bypass

Root Operation Table
ØD1   Gastrointestinal System, Bypass

Body Part
Cecum
Ascending Colon
Transverse Colon
Descending Colon
Sigmoid Colon

Approach
Open
Percutaneous Endoscopic

Device
Autologous Tissue Substitute
Synthetic Substitute
Nonautologous Tissue Substitute
No Device

Qualifier
Cutaneous

Description
A colostomy is an artificial opening, or stoma, from the large intestine through the abdominal wall, to the exterior of the body. It may be performed to provide a temporary opening to facilitate postsurgical bowel healing or be a permanent opening that allows for the elimination of waste products in a dysfunctional or absent bowel and/or rectum/anus. Conditions that may require a colostomy include malignancies, ulcerative colitis, Crohn's disease, volvulus, obstruction, or trauma.

A colostomy can be formed from any part of the large intestine. The colostomy is permanent if resection includes the distal rectum and anorectal sphincter. A temporary colostomy may be performed in an emergency to relieve a perforated or obstructed colon or as a planned procedure to provide postoperative or post-infectious bowel rest. The preferred method for a temporary colostomy is a diverting loop colostomy. Although an end colostomy is often permanent, it can also be used temporarily.

There are several types of temporary diverting colostomies. For a loop colostomy, after the resection or excision of large intestine or rectum, the remaining colon ends are anastomosed. A loop of colon proximal to the anastomosis is brought out through the abdominal wall onto the skin as a stoma with one ostomy for fecal excretion and one for venting of the bowel.

Other temporary or permanent colostomy procedures can be referred to as end-loop, double barrel, or Hartmann's procedures. The objective for all of these procedures is the same and is coded with the root operation Bypass. The body part reflects the part of the bowel being bypassed "from," and the qualifier reported is Cutaneous to indicate the site bypassed "to." These procedures can be performed using either an Open or Percutaneous Endoscopic (laparoscopic) approach.

Focus Point
Code separately any synchronous bowel resection performed in the same encounter with either root operation Excision or Resection.

Focus Point
For a reversal or takedown (closure) of a colostomy, typically the transected ends of the bowel are excised to facilitate a clean anastomosis. The root operation Excision is coded for this excision of the bowel ends. If no excisions are performed, the root operation reported is Repair.

Coding Guidance
AHA: 2016, 3Q, 3; 2014, 4Q, 41

Medical and Surgical

Creation, Ileostomy

Body System
Gastrointestinal System

PCS Root Operation
Bypass

Root Operation Table
0D1 Gastrointestinal System, Bypass

Body Part
Ileum

Approach
Open
Percutaneous Endoscopic

Device
Autologous Tissue Substitute
Synthetic Substitute
Nonautologous Tissue Substitute
No Device

Qualifier
Cutaneous

Description
An ileostomy involves creating an artificial opening (stoma) from the intestine to the exterior of the body. It may be performed to provide a temporary opening to facilitate postsurgical bowel healing or be a permanent opening that allows for the elimination of waste products in a dysfunctional or absent bowel. Conditions that may require an ileostomy include malignancies, ulcerative colitis, Crohn's disease, volvulus, obstruction, or trauma.

An ileostomy is formed from the small intestine, body part Ileum. There are two main types of ileostomy: a loop ileostomy is typically for temporary use, and the end ileostomy is often permanent but can also be for temporary use.

For a loop ileostomy, after the resection or excision of large intestine, the ileus and remaining colon are anastomosed. A loop of ileum proximal to the anastomosis is brought out through the abdominal wall onto the skin as a stoma. This section is opened up and stitched to the skin. The bowel can be folded upon

itself and approximated to form a loop or pouch in which to divert the stool while the large bowel heals. This type of ileostomy is easier to reverse and mainly for temporary use until the large intestine is functional. An end ileostomy is necessary when the entire large intestine, including rectum, is resected because there is no large intestine to anastomose with the ileum. The distal segment of ileum that was divided from the large intestine is brought out through the abdominal wall onto the skin. A common method, called Brooke's technique, rolls back the edges of the bowel to expose the mucosa with suturing of the mucosa to the skin edges to create an end stoma. It protrudes slightly above the level of the skin to help with better fit of the external appliance, which eases drainage and prevents spillage.

A permanent ileostomy or continent ileostomy is less common and uses an internal pouch or reservoir referred to as a Kock pouch (K pouch). The internal pouch is fashioned from the terminal ileum and uses a valve mechanism that is controlled by the patient via catheterization to excrete the fecal waste.

The root operation for all of the ileostomy procedures is Bypass with the body part Ileum as the site bypassing "from" and the qualifier Cutaneous as the site bypassed "to." These procedures can be performed using either an Open or Percutaneous Endoscopic (laparoscopic) approach.

Focus Point

Code separately any synchronous bowel resection performed in the same encounter with root operation Excision or Resection.

Focus Point

For a reversal or takedown (closure) of an ileostomy, typically the transected ends of the bowel are excised to facilitate a clean anastomosis. The root operation Excision is coded for this excision of the bowel ends. If no excisions are performed, the root operation reported is Repair.

Coding Guidance
AHA: 2016, 3Q, 3; 2014, 4Q, 41

© 2018 Optum360, LLC

Cystectomy (Bladder)

Body System
Urinary System

PCS Root Operation
Excision

Resection

Root Operation Table
ØTB Urinary System, Excision

ØTT Urinary System, Resection

Body Part
Bladder

Approach
Open

Percutaneous Endoscopic

Via Natural or Artificial Opening

Via Natural or Artificial Opening Endoscopic

Qualifier
Diagnostic (Excision)

No Qualifier

Description
A cystectomy is a surgical procedure commonly used to treat bladder cancer. This procedure may involve removing all or part of the bladder.

Excision
The removal of a portion of diseased or damaged bladder tissue is reported with the root operation Excision. Using an Open approach, the physician makes an incision in the skin above the pubic bone and cuts the corresponding muscles, fat, and fibrous membranes (fascia) to access the bladder. The bladder and the major vesical blood vessels are mobilized, and the physician incises the bladder wall to access the diseased or damaged bladder tissue. After removing the tissue, the physician inserts catheters into the bladder and urethra and sutures the bladder tissues. The physician performs layered closure and inserts a drain tube, bringing it out through a separate stab

incision in the skin. The cystectomy procedure may be complicated because of prior administration of radiation, a previous surgery, or difficult access to the diseased or damaged bladder tissue.

The approach may also be Via Natural or Artificial Opening Endoscopic. The physician examines the urinary collecting system with a cystourethroscope passed through the urethra into the bladder and excises a tumor, lesion, or other tissue of the bladder. The physician removes the instruments and cystourethroscope.

Resection
The root operation Resection is reported when a total cystectomy is performed. Using an Open approach to access the bladder, the physician makes an incision in the skin of the lower abdomen and cuts the corresponding muscles, fat, and fibrous membranes (fascia). In some cases, the physician dissects and ties (ligates) the hypogastric and vesical vessels and severs the bladder from the urethra, rectum, surrounding peritoneum, vas deferens, and prostate (if applicable). After removing the bladder and controlling bleeding, the physician inserts drain tubes and performs layered closure. In other cases, the physician bilaterally removes the pelvic lymph nodes.

In a Percutaneous Endoscopic approach, several small incisions along with laparoscope are used to access the bladder. The Percutaneous Endoscopic approach employs the same principles as the Open approach.

Focus Point
In a radical cystectomy, the surgery may involve removal of the bilateral pelvic lymph nodes, bladder, and, in some cases, the urethra. In men, the prostate gland and seminal vesicles may also be removed and in women, the uterus and ovaries, if present. Code separately any organs or structures that are actually removed and for which there is a distinctly defined body part.

Cystostomy, Suprapubic (Suprapubic Catheter)

Body System
Urinary System

PCS Root Operation
Drainage

Root Operation Table
ØT9   Urinary System, Drainage

Body Part
Bladder

Approach
Open

Percutaneous

Device
Drainage Device

Description
Urine is collected in the bladder and released by the urinary sphincters into the urethra during urination. A cystostomy is an opening from the skin into the bladder for the drainage of urine. If a patient is unable to void normally and urethral catheterization is contraindicated, a suprapubic cystostomy may be performed. In suprapubic cystostomy, a tube is placed through the patient's skin overlying and into the bladder for the drainage of urine.

A suprapubic cystostomy may be accomplished using an Open approach during which the physician makes an incision in the skin over the lower abdomen and above the pubic symphysis (suprapubic) and cuts the corresponding muscles, fat, and fascia. The Open approach may be performed because the patient's bladder is empty, making a percutaneous approach difficult.

If the patient's bladder is full of urine, the physician may perform the cystostomy using a Percutaneous approach, in which a needle is inserted through the abdomen into the bladder. Urine is aspirated to ensure the needle is correctly positioned. Using guidewires and sheaths, the physician establishes a route through which a catheter is introduced into the bladder. In some cases, the physician may use a flexible cystoscope to help visualize catheter placement. In either approach, once the catheter is in place, a balloon is inflated at the end of the catheter in the bladder to prevent the catheter from dislodging.

A cystostomy may also be documented as a vesicostomy or epicystotomy.

Insertion of a cystostomy tube or catheter is reported with the root operation Drainage and the device Drainage Device.

Focus Point
If an Open or Percutaneous approach is assisted by cystoscopy, report the Open or Percutaneous approach. Percutaneous Endoscopic approach is limited to those cases in which the scope is inserted through the skin. Inspection of a body part(s) performed to achieve the objective of a procedure is not coded separately. See ICD-10-PCS guideline B3.11a.

© 2018 Optum360, LLC

Cystourethroscopy, with Inspection, Bladder and Ureters

Body System
Urinary System

PCS Root Operation
Inspection

Root Operation Table
ØTJ   Urinary System, Inspection

Body Part
Ureter

Approach
Via Natural or Artificial Opening Endoscopic

Description
Waste fluid (urine) is extracted from the blood in the bilateral kidneys and transported from the kidneys to the bladder through the ureters. The bladder acts as a urinary collection device, pooling urine from both ureters and releasing urine into the urethra and out of the body. Urethral sphincters control the release of urine. To examine the ureters, an endoscope can be threaded into the urethral orifice and into the bladder and ureters.

The physician inserts the cystourethroscope into the urethra and threads it into the bladder. From there, the physician identifies a ureter and advances the scope into it. The physician slowly withdraws the scope from the ureter while examining the lumen on a projected video display screen. From the bladder, the scope is advanced into the contralateral ureter, and the examination is repeated in the second ureter. The physician examines the bladder, and then examines the urethra as the scope is withdrawn.

The intent of the procedure is to examine the body part(s) and does not include any treatment. The root operation Inspection is reported when the physician visually or manually explores a body part without performing any procedures on the body part.

Focus Point

According to ICD-10-PCS guideline B3.11b, if multiple tubular body parts (e.g. urethra, bladder, ureters) are inspected, only the most distal (farthest point reached) is reported. For example, in cystourethroscopy of the bladder and ureter, the ureter is the farthest point reached. Therefore, inspection of the bladder and urethra are bundled into inspection of the ureter.

Focus Point

If cystourethroscopy is performed during a therapeutic operation that is performed on the same body part from an approach other than Via Natural or Artificial Opening Endoscopic, the Inspection code may be reported in addition to the therapeutic operation. This is consistent with advice in ICD-10-PCS guideline B3.11c.

Debridement (Excisional)

Body System
Skin and Breast
Subcutaneous Tissue and Fascia
Muscles
Tendons
Bursae and Ligaments
Head and Facial Bones
Upper Bones
Lower Bones

PCS Root Operation
Excision

Root Operation Table
ØHB Skin and Breast, Excision
ØJB Subcutaneous Tissue and Fascia, Excision
ØKB Muscles, Excision
ØLB Tendons, Excision
ØMB Bursae and Ligaments, Excision
ØNB Head and Facial Bones, Excision
ØPB Upper Bones, Excision
ØQB Lower Bones, Excision

Body Part
Refer to the ICD-10-PCS tabular list for a complete list of body parts.

Approach
External
Open

Description
The physician surgically removes devitalized or necrotic tissue by a sharp cutting instrument to promote healing of the wound. The extent of the debridement depends on the tissue affected, in some cases requiring all layers of the wound, including the bony layer, to be debrided.

Debridement by excision is the definite cutting away of or excising of tissue in a wound/ulcer that is damaged, necrotic, devitalized, dead, infected, abscessed, burned, ischemic, has gross contamination, slough, or eschar, with delayed or no healing or foreign material. Debridement is carried down to viable, bleeding tissue when vascularization is not impaired. The procedure can be performed in the operating room, emergency department, or at bedside by physician, nurse, physical therapist, or physician assistant. The tissue does not require a pathological exam.

The physician uses a scalpel to excise the affected skin until viable, bleeding tissue is encountered. A topical antibiotic is placed on the wound. A gauze dressing or an occlusive dressing may be placed over the surgical site.

The root operation Excision describes a single, precise surgical objective, defined as "cutting out or off, without replacement, a portion of a body part."

Debridement is coded to the root operation that best describes the specific objective of the procedure performed and the body part of the deepest level of tissue removed. The correct approach for excisional debridement of the skin is External, defined as "procedures performed directly on the skin or mucous membrane." Excisional debridement that extends deeper than the skin into the subcutaneous tissue and beyond is considered an Open approach.

Focus Point
The use of a sharp instrument or vague terms such as knife dissection do not necessarily indicate an excisional debridement. The person performing the procedure must document that excisional debridement was carried out by describing in detail the surgical removal, including the tissue depth, technique, and all instrumentation used. A code is assigned for excisional debridement when the provider documents "excisional debridement" and/or the documentation meets the root operation definition of Excision.

Focus Point
Documentation of excisional debridement should include the level of tissue removed. Report excision of the specific body system/part rather than Anatomical Regions, Body Systems.

Focus Point
According to ICD-10-PCS guideline B3.5, if the root operation Excision is performed on overlapping layers of the musculoskeletal system, the body part specifying the deepest layer is coded. For example, excisional debridement that includes skin, subcutaneous tissue, and muscle is coded to the Muscle body part.

Focus Point
Some debridement procedures are integral components of a more definitive procedure and are not coded separately. According to ICD-10-PCS Multiple Procedures guideline B3.2, multiple procedures with distinct objectives may be reported separately.

Debridement performed in preparation for another procedure is not reported separately, according to guideline B3.1b, which states: "Procedural steps necessary to reach the operative site and close the operative site are not coded separately."

If the documentation is unclear or if there is any question about the procedures performed, the provider should be queried for clarification.

© 2018 Optum360, LLC

Debridement (Excisional) (continued)

Coding Guidance
AHA: 2016, 3Q, 20; 2016, 1Q, 40; 2015, 3Q, 3-7; 2015, 1Q, 29; 2015, 1Q, 34; 2014, 4Q, 32; 2014, 3Q, 14-15; 2014, 3Q, 18

Debridement (Nonexcisional)

Body System
Skin and Breast
Subcutaneous Tissue and Fascia
Muscles
Tendons
Bursae and Ligaments
Head and Facial Bones
Upper Bones
Lower Bones

PCS Root Operation
Extraction

Root Operation Table
ØHD Skin and Breast, Extraction
ØJD Subcutaneous Tissue and Fascia, Extraction
ØKD Muscles, Extraction
ØLD Tendons, Extraction
ØMD Bursae and Ligaments, Extraction
ØND Head and Facial Bones, Extraction
ØPD Upper Bones, Extraction
ØQD Lower Bones, Extraction

Body Part
Refer to the ICD-10-PCS tabular list for a complete list of body parts.

Approach
External
Open

Description
The physician removes damaged skin, subcutaneous tissue, fascia, muscles, tendons, bursae and ligaments, and/or bone by methods other than excision.

Debridement by extraction is the removal of tissue by instrumentation via nonexcisional methods such as pulling, stripping, scraping, pressurized irrigation, brushing, water scalpel, or scrubbing to promote healing of the wound. This may be performed on wounds, ulcers, or any tissue contaminated by bacteria or that is damaged, necrotic, devitalized, dead,

infected, abscessed, burned, ischemic, has gross contamination with foreign material, slough, eschar, or granulation, or with delayed or no healing. Debridement is carried down to viable, bleeding tissue when vascularization is not impaired. The wound is cleansed, and a dressing is applied. It can be performed in the operating room, emergency department, or at bedside by physician, nurse, physical therapist, or physician assistant. The tissue does not require pathological exam.

Extraction is coded when the method employed to take out the body part is pulling or stripping (scraping). Minor cutting (such as trimming of loose fragments) is included in the root operation Extraction if the objective of the procedure is met by pulling or stripping.

Debridement is coded to the root operation that best describes the specific objective of the procedure performed and the deepest level of tissue removed.

The correct approach for nonexcisional debridement (extraction) of the skin is External, defined as "procedures performed directly on the skin or mucous membrane." Nonexcisional debridement that extends deeper than the skin into the subcutaneous tissue and beyond is considered an Open approach.

Focus Point
Examples of procedures coded as extraction include forceps removal of devitalized tissue, scraping with a scalpel or other sharp instrument, trimming of loose tissue fragments, and scrubbing. VersaJet, Pulsavac, pulsed lavage digressive debridement, mechanical lavage, pulsatile lavage, mechanical irrigation, and high-pressure irrigation involve more than simple irrigation and are reported as Extraction, rather than Irrigation.

Focus Point
Documentation of nonexcisional debridement should include the level of tissue removed. Report extraction of the specific body system rather than the anatomical regions body systems.

Debridement (Nonexcisional) (continued)

Focus Point

Some debridement procedures are integral components of a more definitive procedure and are not separately coded. According to ICD-10-PCS Multiple Procedures guideline B3.2, multiple procedures with distinct objectives may be reported separately.

Debridement performed in preparation for another procedure is not reported separately, according to guideline B3.1b, which states: "Procedural steps necessary to reach the operative site and close the operative site are not coded separately."

If the documentation is unclear or if there is any question about the procedures performed, the provider should be queried for clarification.

Coding Guidance

AHA: 2016, 3Q, 20-22; 2016, 1Q, 40; 2015, 3Q, 3-7; 2015, 3Q, 12; 2015, 2Q, 22; 2015, 1Q, 23; 2015, 1Q, 29; 2015, 1Q, 34; 2014, 4Q, 32; 2014, 3Q, 14; 2014, 3Q, 18

Decompression, Posterior Fossa (Chiari Malformation)

See also Graft, Dura Mater, Intracranial

Body System
Central Nervous System and Cranial Nerves

PCS Root Operation
Release

Root Operation Table
ØØN Central Nervous System and Cranial Nerves, Release

Body Part
Cerebellum

Approach
Open

Device
No Device

Qualifier
No Qualifier

Description

A Chiari malformation (CM) is a structural abnormality in the cerebellum that is usually considered a congenital condition, although it can be acquired later in life due to traumatic injury, disease, or infection. It is characterized by displacement of the cerebellar tonsils through the foramen magnum and into the upper spinal canal, sometimes causing noncommunicating hydrocephalus due to obstruction of cerebrospinal fluid (CSF) outflow.

A posterior fossa decompression is a surgical procedure performed to remove the bone at the back of the skull and spine to relieve compression of the brainstem and spinal cord, and to restore the normal flow of CSF.

Under general anesthesia, the patient is placed in the prone position on the operating table, and the head is held in position for surgery with a 3-pin skull-fixation device. A strip of hair is shaved along the planned incision site, and the scalp is prepped. Using an Open approach, the physician makes an incision in the midline extending from the posterior mid-scalp to the midcervical region down the middle of the neck. The skin and muscles are gently spread apart and retracted to allow the surgeon access to the skull and the top of the spine. Dissection is continued to the skull, and a small section of the skull in the occipital bone is removed to enter the posterior fossa. In some cases, a C1 vertebral laminectomy may be required to access the procedure site. The removal of the occipital bone may provide enough decompression to restore normal CSF flow, or the stretched and damaged cerebellar tonsils may be shrunk with electrocautery to correct any blockage of CSF flow out of the fourth ventricle. In other cases, an enlargement of the dura is required to decompress. The dura covering the brain and spinal cord is exposed and opened to view the cerebellar tonsils and the cisterna magna. If a larger dural opening is required, in a separately reportable procedure, a patch of synthetic or biologic material or pericranial autograft tissue from the patient's scalp tissue just outside the skull is sutured into place. This patch graft enlarges the dural opening to provide more space around the cerebellar tonsils. The dural patch is sutured and covered with a sealant to prevent CSF leakage. The incision site is sutured closed in layers and covered with a dressing.

Focus Point

The occipital craniectomy and C1 laminectomy (if performed) are procedural steps performed only to the reach the decompression site and should not be coded separately. See guideline B3.1b.

© 2018 Optum360, LLC

Decompression, Posterior Fossa (Chiari Malformation) (continued)

Focus Point

Autograft pericranial tissue harvested from the operative site is not reported separately, according to ICD-10-PCS guideline B3.9.

Focus Point

An additional procedure from table 00U Central Nervous System and Cranial Nerves, Supplement, is reported for a dural graft, if performed. According to ICD-10-PCS guideline B3.2c, multiple procedures with distinct objectives may be reported separately.

Coding Guidance
AHA: 2017, 3Q, 10; 2014, 3Q, 24

Decompression, Subacromial, Rotator Cuff Tendon

See also Release, Coracoacromial Ligament

See also Repair, Rotator Cuff (Shoulder)

Body System
Tendons

PCS Root Operation
Release

Root Operation Table
ØLN   Tendons, Release

Body Part
Shoulder Tendon, Right
Shoulder Tendon, Left

Approach
Open
Percutaneous Endoscopic

Description
Subacromial decompression is commonly performed to treat subacromial impingement syndrome, caused by pinching of the rotator cuff tendon between the humeral head and the undersurface of the acromion.

Subacromial decompression of the rotator cuff tendon can be performed with an Open or Percutaneous Endoscopic approach. In an Open approach, the technique is similar, with a larger incision and direct visualization of the shoulder structures. The Percutaneous Endoscopic approach is the most commonly performed due to the smaller incisions and shorter recovery period.

Under appropriate anesthesia, the patient is placed in the lateral decubitus position. Using a Percutaneous Endoscopic (arthroscopic) approach, the physician makes two or three small portal incisions, through which the arthroscope with attached camera and surgical instruments are inserted. A sterile solution is pumped into the shoulder joint, expanding it to allow better visualization of the joint structures.

Bone spurs from the acromion are removed, as well as any inflamed bursal tissue, and in some cases a portion of the clavicle, until enough tissues are removed to allow the rotator cuff tendons to move freely between the humeral head and the acromion without pinching or catching on the bone. The incisions are closed with sutures; dressings and a sling are applied.

Focus Point

Review the operative report carefully to determine the true objective of the procedure(s) performed in order to report the appropriate root operation. In the root operation Release, report the body part being freed rather than the tissue that is cut or excised. See ICD-10-PCS guideline B3.13.

Focus Point

Subacromial decompression of the rotator cuff tendon is frequently performed in conjunction with additional procedures such as rotator cuff repair, tenodesis, superior labrum anterior and posterior repair, and coracoacromial ligament release. ICD-10-PCS guidelines on multiple procedures should be followed when assigning codes for these procedures.

Decortication, Pulmonary

Body System
Respiratory System

PCS Root Operation
Release

Root Operation Table
ØBN   Respiratory System, Release

Body Part
Upper Lung Lobe, Right
Middle Lung Lobe, Right
Lower Lung Lobe, Right
Upper Lung Lobe, Left
Lung Lingula
Lower Lung Lobe, Left
Lung, Right
Lung, Left
Lungs, Bilateral

Approach
Open
Percutaneous Endoscopic

Description
Decortication of the lung is the removal of thickened serous membrane for lung expansion. This procedure is typically performed for trapped lungs due to fibrothorax, or fibrosis in the pleural space, caused by inflammatory response to conditions such as hemothorax, empyema, tuberculosis, and other forms of pleuritis.

In an Open pulmonary decortication, the physician removes a constricting membrane or layer of tissue from the surface of the lung (decortication) to permit the lung to fully expand. The physician opens the chest cavity wide. Using a scalpel, the surgeon makes a long incision around the side of the chest between two of the ribs.

The incision is carried through all the tissue layers into the chest cavity. Rib spreaders are inserted into the wound, and the ribs are spread apart to expose the lung. The constricting membrane is then stripped off the entire surface of the lung; other times, only a portion of the lung surface is removed. The chest wall incision is then sutured closed in layers. A chest tube(s) may be used to provide drainage for the chest cavity. Alternatively, the chest cavity can be opened by a vertical incision in the front of the chest through the sternum. The skin incision is carried down to the sternum bone, and then a saw is used to split the sternum. With the sternum split in half, the chest is entered by spreading the sternum apart with a set of rib spreaders. When the procedure is complete, the wound is closed by using wires to bring the two halves of the sternum together, and the skin is closed by suturing.

Using a Percutaneous Endoscopic approach, the physician removes a constricting membrane or layer of tissue from the surface of the lung (decortication) to permit the lung to fully expand using thoracoscopy. The surgeon makes a small incision between two ribs and by blunt dissection and the use of a trocar enters the thoracic cavity. The endoscope is passed through the trocar and into the chest cavity. The constricting membrane is then stripped off the entire surface of the lung; at other times, only a portion of the lung surface is removed using a device through the endoscope or the insertion of an instrument through a second incision in the chest. At the conclusion of the procedure, the endoscope and the trocar are removed. A chest tube for drainage and re-expansion of the lung is usually inserted through the wound used for the thoracoscopy.

Focus Point
The term decortication has two unique definitions, each of which is reported with a different root operation. One meaning of decortication is removing the cortex (outer layer) of a structure or organ such as the pleura of the lung. This is represented with the root operation Extraction, which is the stripping off all or a portion of that cortex. The other definition of decortication is removal of the fibrous bands or tissues that prevent lung expansion, which is best represented by the root operation Release.

© 2018 Optum360, LLC

Medical and Surgical

Denervation, Facet (Percutaneous)

Body System
Peripheral Nervous System

PCS Root Operation
Destruction

Root Operation Table
Ø15   Peripheral Nervous System, Destruction

Body Part
Cervical Nerve
Thoracic Nerve
Lumbar Nerve
Sacral Nerve

Approach
Percutaneous

Description
Percutaneous facet denervation is also referred to as radiofrequency facet ablation, facet rhizotomy, radiofrequency facet denervation, and facet thermocoagulation. This procedure is used to treat back pain transmitted through the sensory nerves within the facet joint of spinal vertebrae. Radiofrequency delivers heat and destroys selected nerve fibers, blocking pain transmission.

Using a Percutaneous approach, a needle is inserted into the nerve that connects to the damaged joint facet. Local anesthetic is applied to numb the nerve. The needle is heated to damage the affected nerve, which no longer allows the nerve to send pain signals.

Medical and Surgical

Dilation and Curettage (D&C)

Body System
Female Reproductive System

PCS Root Operation
Extraction

Root Operation Table
ØUD   Female Reproductive System, Extraction

Body Part
Endometrium

Approach
Via Natural or Artificial Opening
Via Natural or Artificial Opening Endoscopic

Qualifier
Diagnostic
No Qualifier

Description
The lining of the uterus (endometrium) proliferates each month in preparation for implantation of an embryo. Dilation and curettage (D&C) may be performed to diagnose abnormalities in the lining of the uterus, or to treat abnormal uterine bleeding.

The physician may remove the endometrial lining of the uterus by suction D&C using a sharp instrument to remove tissue from inside the uterus. The physician inserts a speculum into the vagina to view the cervix and uses a tenaculum to grasp the cervix, pull it down, and exert traction. After dilating the cervical canal with a small probe, the physician passes a curette into the uterus. The curette is used to scrape the lining of the uterus and the endometrial tissue is aspirated from the uterus via the vagina for diagnostic or therapeutic purposes. When there is no visualization during this

procedure, report the approach as Via Natural or Artificial Opening. The qualifier Diagnostic is assigned when the documented purpose of the D&C is diagnostic.

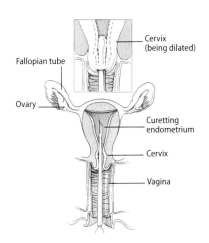

Cervix
(being dilated)

Fallopian tube

Ovary

Curetting
endometrium

Cervix

Vagina

The physician may advance a hysteroscopy into the vagina and uterus to provide visualization of the D&C, which is performed for diagnostic or therapeutic reasons. When a hysteroscope is used during the D&C, the approach is Via Natural or Artificial Opening, Endoscopic.

> **Focus Point**
> *A code from the Obstetrics section would be reported if the D&C is performed subsequent to an abortion or delivery.*

Dilation, Esophagus

Medical and Surgical

Body System
Gastrointestinal System

PCS Root Operation
Dilation

Root Operation Table
ØD7   Gastrointestinal System, Dilation

Body Part
Esophagus, Upper
Esophagus, Middle
Esophagus, Lower
Esophagogastric Junction
Esophagus

Approach
Via Natural or Artificial Opening, Endoscopic

Device
No Device

Description
Dilation of the esophagus is performed by the passage of balloon or hydrostatic dilators through the esophagus to enlarge the esophagus and relieve obstruction. A stricture, a decrease in the esophagus opening as a result of a scar or a deposit of abnormal tissue, is often the cause of obstruction. The technique and approach may vary, including the following.

Dilation by Balloon or Dilator Device
Using flexible endoscopy, the physician can directly view the stricture and pass a dilator through the endoscope into the patient's throat down into the esophagus and across the stricture. The dilating balloon or plastic dilator stretches and breaks the stricture, and the dilator is withdrawn. This may be repeated several times to dilate the esophagus to an acceptable size.

Dilation by Guidewire
The physician dilates the esophagus by passing dilators over a guidewire. The physician uses an endoscope to place a guidewire into the patient's throat, down the esophagus, and into the stomach. If the endoscope cannot traverse the stricture, fluoroscopy is used to confirm placement of the guidewire. A series of dilators are passed over the guidewire and withdrawn. The process is repeated until the esophagus is dilated to an acceptable size.

Retrograde Dilation
The physician dilates the esophagus using a dilator that passes from the stomach through the esophagus. The physician uses an endoscope to place a guidewire into the patient's throat, down the esophagus, and into the stomach. If the endoscope cannot traverse the stricture, fluoroscopy is used to confirm placement of the guidewire. A dilator is inserted through a gastrostomy tube and attached to the guidewire. Tension on the oral end of the wire pulls the dilator into the distal esophagus. The process is repeated until the esophagus is dilated to an acceptable size.

> **Focus Point**
> *All of the described techniques are reported with the root operation Dilation. No Device value is reported since there is no device left in the body after the procedure is completed. See guideline B6.1a.*

> **Focus Point**
> *If an endoscopic inspection is performed in conjunction with the Dilation procedure, it is considered inherent to the procedure and is not coded separately. See guideline B3.11a.*

© 2018 Optum360, LLC

Discectomy

See also Laminectomy, Decompressive (Hemilaminectomy)

See also Replacement, Intervertebral Disc, Artificial

Body System
Upper Joints

Lower Joints

PCS Root Operation
Excision

Resection

Root Operation Table
ØRB   Upper Joints, Excision

ØRT   Upper Joints, Resection

ØSB   Lower Joints, Excision

ØST   Lower Joints, Resection

Body Part
Cervical Vertebral Disc

Cervicothoracic Vertebral Disc

Thoracic Vertebral Disc

Thoracolumbar Vertebral Disc

Lumbar Vertebral Disc

Lumbosacral Disc

Approach
Open

Description
Intervertebral discs, which are contained between each of the spinal joints, are made up of a stronger, outer fibrous ring called the annulus fibrosus, which protects and absorbs compression, and the softer, inner center, called the nucleus pulposus, which acts as a shock absorber. ICD-10-PCS includes the intervertebral disc body part values in the Upper Joints and Lower Joints body systems.

Discectomy is generally performed with a spinal fusion and often with a decompressive laminectomy. It is performed with the fusion to access the site and make way for the grafting material. During a decompression, it is typically performed to ensure that there are no stray pieces of material compressing the nerve root or spinal canal. If the documentation says only part of the disc material was removed, Excision is the appropriate root operation. If the documentation specifies total discectomy, Resection is the root operation reported.

In a microdiscectomy performed to remove a portion of a herniated disc that is irritating a lumbar nerve root, a small incision is made in the low back, and the back muscles are moved gently out of the way. The spine is entered by removing the ligamentum flavum (membrane) over the nerve roots. A portion of the inside facet joint is removed to release the pressure over the nerve (*see also* Laminectomy, Decompressive [Hemilaminectomy]). Only the herniated portion of the disc is removed, reported with the root operation Excision. The microdiscectomy is reported as an Open procedure since the surgeon is using the incision to directly visualize the site of the procedure.

Focus Point
If an entire disc is removed and immediately replaced with an artificial disc, Replacement is reported, which by definition includes the removal of the body part. See also Replacement, Intervertebral Disc, Artificial.

Focus Point
Certain discectomies may be documented as minimally invasive procedures. There is no specific approach value for minimally invasive surgery, and no current guidelines addressing them. Each operative report must be carefully reviewed and the ICD-10-PCS approach definitions applied to determine the correct approach value.

Coding Guidance
AHA: 2016, 2Q, 16; 2014, 2Q, 6, 7; 2013, 4Q, 108

Diversion, Urinary, Ileal Conduit

Body System
Urinary System

PCS Root Operation
Bypass

Root Operation Table
ØT1   Urinary System, Bypass

Body Part
Ureter, Right
Ureter, Left
Ureters, Bilateral

Approach
Open
Percutaneous Endoscopic

Qualifier
Ileocutaneous

Description
Ileal conduit urinary diversion is a surgical technique for creating a new urinary passage by attaching the ureters to a portion of the ileum, which is brought out through the abdominal wall for direct emptying of urine through a stoma. Bypass is used as the root operation; urine bypasses the bladder by going directly from the ureters to the stoma via the ileal conduit. Also known as a Bricker procedure, it is often performed in conjunction with the removal of the bladder (radial cystectomy).

Ileal conduit urinary diversion may be performed using an Open or Percutaneous Endoscopic (laparoscopic) approach. The surgeon performs the ileoureteral anastomosis by removing a small section of the ileum, which serves as a conduit. The ureters are sutured to one end of the conduit, and the other end is brought through an incision in the abdominal wall, creating a stoma to empty urine. A urostomy pouch is used to collect the urine.

Focus Point
Code separately any synchronous bladder resection performed during the same encounter.

Focus Point
Bypass procedures require clarification of the body part bypassed "from" and body part bypassed "to," according to guideline B3.6a.

Focus Point
If robotic assistance is used, an additional code from table 8EØ should be appended.

© 2018 Optum360, LLC

Drainage, Floor of Mouth

Body System
Anatomical Regions, General

PCS Root Operation
Drainage

Root Operation Table
ØW9   Anatomical Regions, General, Drainage

Body Part
Oral Cavity and Throat

Approach
Open

Percutaneous

Device
Drainage Device

No Device

Qualifier
Diagnostic

No Qualifier

Description

A soft tissue enlargement in the floor of the mouth may be caused by a liquefied hematoma, cyst, or infection. These swellings are often painful and may be drained to reduce the symptoms or remove the defect. Approach to the infection may be intraoral or, for deeper defects, extraoral.

In an extraoral Open approach, the physician drains an abscess, a cyst, or liquefied hematoma from the floor of the mouth by making an incision in the skin below the inferior border of the mandible and dissecting through the tissue to reach the affected space. The physician may dissect through the supra mylohyoid muscle and submental space into the sublingual space below the tongue to drain the abscess. The dissection may be taken to the supra mylohyoid muscle to drain an abscess in the submental space. The physician makes an incision under the angle of the mandible, or between the angle and the chin, and below the inferior border of the mandible. Dissection may be limited to the submandibular space. An incision is made just below the angle of the ramus of the mandible, the posterior part of the mandible, and into the masticator space containing the masticator muscles to drain the abscess, cyst, or liquefied hematoma. A drain may be placed for continued drainage or to facilitate healing, which is later removed.

Using an intraoral Open approach, the physician makes an intraoral incision, opening the mucosa of the tongue or floor of the mouth overlying an abscess, cyst, or liquefied hematoma and drains the fluid.

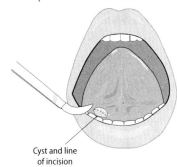

A small incision is made in the floor of the mouth; the cyst is opened and the fluid is drained

Cyst and line
of incision

The physician may use an Open approach to dissect through the anterior floor of the mouth into the supra mylohyoid muscle to drain an abscess in the submental space. The physician may incise through the mucosa of the floor of the mouth to the supra mylohyoid muscle or carry the dissection deeper into the tissue to reach the submandibular space. The physician may dissect down through the mucosa in the posterior floor of the mouth and into the masticator space, containing the ramus, the posterior part of the mandible, and the masticator muscles, to drain a deep abscess or other lesion.

In some cases, a needle with an attached syringe may be inserted extraorally or intraorally to draw fluid from the area to be drained using a Percutaneous approach.

Focus Point
When therapeutic drainage is the focus of the procedure, No Qualifier is reported even when the extracted material is sent to pathology for examination. If the purpose of the procedure is diagnostic, report the qualifier Diagnostic.

Focus Point
A temporary postoperative wound drain placed to facilitate healing is not reported; use qualifier No Device. When a drainage tube or catheter is placed and remains in place at the end of the procedure for continued drainage of an abscess, cyst, or liquefied hematoma, report the qualifier Drainage Device.

The root operation Drainage with the qualifier Drainage Device is reported when a separate procedure is performed to put in a drainage device. See ICD-10-PCS guidelines B6.1a, B6.1b and B6.2.

Coding Guidance
AHA: 2017, 2Q, 16

Elevation, Skull Fracture

See also Debridement (Excisional)

Body System
Head and Facial Bones

PCS Root Operation
Reposition

Root Operation Table
ØNS   Head and Facial Bones, Reposition

Body Part
Skull

Approach
Open

Device
Internal Fixation
External Fixation
No Device

Description
This procedure involves elevating the depressed skull fracture to restore anatomical position. Reposition is the appropriate root operation, as it is defined as moving to its normal location, or other suitable location, all or a portion of a body part.

Using an Open approach, the scalp is incised and retracted to expose the skull depression. The physician may drill a burr hole and pull up on the skull to elevate the bone. If there are multiple fracture lines, the bony pieces are approximated and stabilized in anatomic position. The scalp is reapproximated and closed in sutured layers.

If internal fixation is used, a more specific body part value may be reported as well as a device value of Internal Fixation Device. Refer to the ICD-10-PCS tabular list, table ØNS, for complete list of body parts.

> **Focus Point**
> *If the fracture has damaged tissue beyond the skull, such as the dura and brain, any debridement of the brain and dura are performed in a separately reportable open procedure. See also* Debridement (Excisional).

Coding Guidance
AHA: 2013, 3Q, 25

Medical and Surgical

© 2018 Optum360, LLC

Embolization, Uterine Artery, Percutaneous

Body System
Lower Arteries

PCS Root Operation
Occlusion

Root Operation Table
Ø4L   Lower Arteries, Occlusion

Body Part
Internal Iliac Artery, Right
Internal Iliac Artery, Left

Approach
Percutaneous

Device
Intraluminal Device

Qualifier
Uterine Artery, Right
Uterine Artery, Left

Description
Percutaneous uterine artery embolization (UAE) is a minimally invasive procedure that is used to occlude the blood supply to a focused area of the uterus without disrupting collateral uterine circulation. UAE is most commonly used to treat uterine fibroids as an alternative to hysterectomy or other surgical intervention (e.g., myomectomy). However, UAE may also be used to treat other conditions that result in pelvic pain, pressure, and excessive vaginal bleeding.

Using a Percutaneous approach, under local anesthesia and radiological guidance, a catheter is introduced into the femoral artery at the groin and advanced over a guidewire into the uterine artery. Small metal coils, biospheres, or Gelfoam are deployed into the vessel through the catheter. If necessary, multiple areas of the uterus can be treated. Contrast imaging may be performed to confirm filling of the uterine artery. As the blood supply is eliminated, the fibroid tissue withers, relieving the associated symptoms. Fibroid recurrence or the development of new fibroids may require re-embolization or hysterectomy. Complications include migration of the coils, which can result in organ damage, infection (e.g.,

endometritis, septicemia), infertility, uterine adhesions, and iatrogenic menopause.

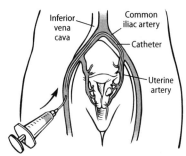
The catheter is inserted in the femoral artery at the groin, and advanced to branches of the uterine artery

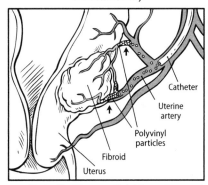
Uterine fibroid tumors will shrink over time after granules injected into arterial branches stop the blood flow to the fibroids

Focus Point

In the ICD-10-PCS Body Part Key, the uterine arteries are defined as Internal Iliac Artery, Right or Internal Iliac Artery, Left. Qualifiers Uterine Artery, Right and Uterine Artery, Left are reported to specify the type of artery and laterality.

Coding Guidance
AHA: 2015, 2Q, 27

Endarterectomy, Carotid

Medical and Surgical

Body System
Upper Arteries

PCS Root Operation
Extirpation

Root Operation Table
Ø3C   Upper Arteries, Extirpation

Body Part
Common Carotid Artery, Right
Common Carotid Artery, Left
Internal Carotid Artery, Right
Internal Carotid Artery, Left
External Carotid Artery, Right
External Carotid Artery, Left

Approach
Open

Description
Carotid endarterectomy is a procedure that treats carotid artery disease, the build-up of plaques in one or both of the carotid arteries, which supply oxygenated blood to the brain. This build-up of plaques (atherosclerosis) may restrict blood flow to the brain. Removing the plaques causing the narrowing in the artery can improve the blood flow in the carotid artery, reducing the risk of stroke.

Endarterectomy procedures involve removing the tunica intima (the innermost membrane of the vessel) that is clogged by disease or other obstruction. The surgical technique may vary depending on the nature of the obstruction or disease. In ICD-10-PCS, the removal of plaque is coded to the root operation Extirpation, which is defined as taking or cutting out solid matter from a body part.

With the patient under general anesthesia and using an Open approach, the physician makes an incision in the skin over the site of a blood clot, plaque, or abnormal lining of the affected vessel. The vessels are isolated and dissected from adjacent critical structures, and vessel clamps are applied. The vessels are incised. Using a blunt, spatula-like tool, the plaque and the vessel lining are separated from the arteries and removed. The edge of the normal artery linings may be sutured to the artery walls to prevent separation when blood flow resumes. After the plaque and lining are removed, patch grafts taken from another portion of the patient's body, a cadaver, or a synthetic source may be applied and sutured to the vessels. This enlarges the diameter of the arteries. The vessel clamps are removed, and the skin incision is repaired with layered closure.

Alternatively, surgeons may use another technique called eversion carotid endarterectomy, in which the carotid artery is cut and turned inside out (everted) and the plaque removed. The surgeon then reattaches the artery. The vessel clamps are removed, and the skin incision is repaired with layered closure.

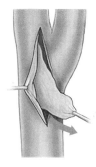

Plaque is removed

Focus Point
If a plaque lesion extends as a continuous lesion of one vessel into another—for example starting at the bifurcation of the common carotid artery but ending at the internal carotid artery—code the internal carotid artery body part value as it corresponds to the furthest anatomical site from the point of entry. See ICD-10-PCS guideline B4.1c.

Focus Point
The reinforcement of the vessel using a patch graft is coded separately in ICD-10 PCS using the root operation Supplement, according to ICD-10-PCS multiple procedures guideline B3.2. If a separate procedure is performed to harvest autograft tissue from another incision, it is coded to the appropriate root operation in addition to the primary procedure, according to ICD-10 PCS coding guideline B3.9.

Focus Point
Reattachment of the artery in eversion carotid endarterectomy is integral to the extirpation procedure and is not reported separately, according to ICD-10-PCS guideline B3.1b.

Coding Guidance
AHA: 2016, 2Q, 11; 2015, 1Q, 29

© 2018 Optum360, LLC

Enteroscopy, Double Balloon (DBE)

Body System
Gastrointestinal System

PCS Root Operation
Destruction

Excision

Extirpation

Root Operation Table
ØD5 Gastrointestinal System, Destruction

ØDB Gastrointestinal System, Excision

ØDC Gastrointestinal System, Extirpation

Body Part
Small Intestine

Approach
Via Natural or Artificial Opening Endoscopic

Qualifier
No Qualifier

Diagnostic (Excision)

Description
Double balloon enteroscopy (DBE), also known as "push-pull enteroscopy," is a new endoscopic technique that allows for extensive examination and endoscopic treatment of abnormalities found in the small intestine (small bowel), located between the stomach and colon (large intestine). DBE is frequently performed to help diagnose and treat abnormalities found during previous diagnostic studies of the small intestine, such as capsule endoscopy or radiology imaging, when therapeutic intervention is needed and/or diagnostic biopsies are required in areas beyond the reach of conventional endoscopes. DBE is used to evaluate and manage gastrointestinal bleeding, abdominal pain, chronic diarrhea, neoplasms, and other small intestinal disorders. In some cases after capsule endoscopy, the capsule is retained in the small bowel and can be retrieved using DBE, preventing more extensive surgical retrieval.

The system consists of a specifically designed, lighted, flexible video endoscope with two latex balloons. One balloon is attached to the tip of the enteroscope and the other at the distal end of an overtube. Using a balloon-pump controller, the overtube balloon is inflated to grip the intestinal wall, using alternating balloon inflation and deflation using a push-and-pull technique to move the inner endoscope within the tube step by step forward within the small intestine. Electrocautery or biopsy instruments are guided through the endoscope to the tip. The DBE scope can be inserted either via an oral or rectal approach depending on the location of the abnormality.

Under appropriate anesthesia, the patient is placed on the left side and the double balloon endoscope is passed down the throat, through the stomach, and into the small intestine. The endoscope may also be passed through the rectum, the entire colon, and into the small intestine in a rectal approach. Both of these approaches are reported as Via Natural or Artificial Opening Endoscopic. In both approaches, the endoscope is advanced using a push-pull technique, inflating and deflating the balloon to progress the endoscope to the area of interest in the small intestine. The small intestine is carefully examined, and the physician may take biopsies or remove polyps, cauterize bleeding sites, retrieve a capsule, or perform other therapeutic interventions.

Destruction
The endoscope is advanced using a push-pull technique, inflating and deflating the balloon to progress the endoscope to the area of interest in the small intestine. Once the bleeding sites are located, they are cauterized using endoscopic lasers or bipolar cautery. The endoscope is removed.

Excision
The endoscope is advanced using a push-pull technique, inflating and deflating the balloon to progress the endoscope to the area of interest in the small intestine. The physician may take a biopsy of a random location or specific lesion of the small intestine. The base of the lesion may be electrocoagulated and severed using biopsy forceps or bipolar cautery. A snare loop may be placed around the base of the lesion and closed (the tissue is electrocoagulated and severed as the loop is closed). The severed tissue is withdrawn through the endoscope. The endoscope is removed.

Extirpation
The endoscope is advanced using a push-pull technique, inflating and deflating the balloon to progress the endoscope into the small intestine. Once the retained capsule or other foreign body is located, it is grasped with forceps and retracted using the endoscope.

Focus Point
According to ICD-10-PCS multiple procedures guideline B3.2c, multiple procedures with distinct objectives may be reported separately. Review the operative report carefully, and select all appropriate root operations with distinct objectives from the ICD-10-PCS tables.

Focus Point
In a double balloon endoscopy, the balloon is part of the surgical instrumentation used to access the procedure site. It is not the objective of the balloon to dilate the intestine in these cases.

Enucleation, Eyeball, with Synchronous Implant

Medical and Surgical

Body System
Eye

PCS Root Operation
Replacement

Root Operation Table
Ø8R   Eye, Replacement

Body Part
Eye, Right
Eye, Left

Approach
Open

Device
Synthetic Substitute

Description
Eyeball enucleation is the surgical removal of the entire globe of the eye. An ocular prosthesis is an artificial eye that is placed in the eye socket after the enucleation procedure. The most common indications for an eyeball enucleation procedure are intraocular malignancy and trauma.

Under general anesthesia, the patient is prepped and draped. After an ocular speculum has been inserted, using an Open approach, the physician dissects the conjunctiva free at the corneal-scleral juncture (the limbus). The physician cuts each extraocular muscle at its juncture to the eyeball and severs the optic nerve. The eyeball is removed, but the extraocular muscles remain attached at the back of the eye socket. A spherical implant that has been washed with an antibiotic solution is placed deep into the eye socket. The extraocular muscles are attached to the permanent implant to allow normal movement of the prosthesis. The orbital implant is covered surgically with conjunctiva. A temporary eye patch is placed.

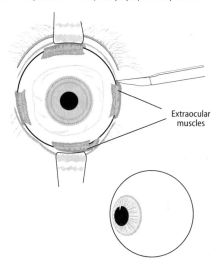

Extraocular muscles

Permanent prosthesis

© 2018 Optum360, LLC

Epiglottopexy, Transoral Endoscopic

See also Excision, Lingual, Submucosal Minimally Invasive (SMILE)

See also Tonsillectomy, Lingual

Body System
Mouth and Throat

PCS Root Operation
Reposition

Root Operation Table
ØCS   Mouth and Throat, Reposition

Body Part
Epiglottis

Approach
Via Natural or Artificial Opening Endoscopic

Description
Laryngomalacia is a congenital laryngeal anomaly defined as collapse of supraglottic structures during inspiration. It frequently causes stridor in infants, as well as feeding problems, failure to thrive, and apnea. Severe laryngomalacia with life-threatening stridor and apnea may require surgical correction to prevent resulting cardiopulmonary diseases. Epiglottopexy is performed to treat laryngomalacia by repositioning the epiglottis to improve airway conditions.

Surgical treatment of laryngomalacia is performed under general anesthesia, using the approach Via Natural or Artificial Opening Endoscopic with direct laryngoscopy. Local anesthesia of the glottic and supraglottic regions is administered. The laryngoscope is advanced into the laryngeal lumen, and laser-surgical vaporization of the corresponding mucosal areas of the epiglottis and the base of the tongue is performed to create a raw surface. Suspension of the epiglottis to the base of the tongue is then performed with resorbable suture material. Bleeding is assessed and controlled. Photographs of the epiglottic suspension may be taken at the conclusion of the procedure.

Focus Point
Epiglottopexy is frequently performed with other procedures such as lingual tonsillectomy and excision of the base of the tongue. When performed, these procedures are coded in addition to the epiglottopexy with a code from table ØCBM Excision of Pharynx. See also Tonsillectomy, Lingual.

Coding Guidance
AHA: 2016, 3Q, 28

Episiotomy

Medical and Surgical

Body System
Anatomical Regions, General

PCS Root Operation
Division

Root Operation Table
0W8   Anatomical Regions, General, Division

Body Part
Perineum, Female

Approach
External

Description

An episiotomy is the surgical incision of the perineum to widen the outlet of the vagina to facilitate delivery of the infant (childbirth). During childbirth, the emergence of the infant head through the vaginal canal may stretch the perineal tissue to the point that it tears. To prevent this trauma, the physician attending the delivery may incise under local anesthesia the perineum with scissors or a scalpel to accommodate the crowning head. The incision (episiotomy) may be midline (median or midline episiotomy) or lateral, beginning at the vaginal orifice and is continued to the right or left, away from the rectum (mediolateral). Episiotomy may also be performed to extend a perineal tear with a smooth incision, making the laceration easier to repair. Following delivery, the episiotomy incision is repaired.

An episiotomy is reported with root operation Division, as it involves cutting into the body part (perineum), without draining fluids and/or gases, and separating it.

The approach is External as the incision is directly on the skin and mucous membrane. This is currently the only approach value available in the Division, Anatomical Regions, General table for the body part Perineum, Female.

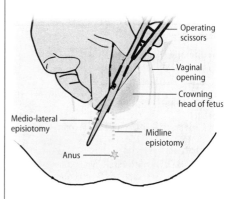

Focus Point

In ICD-10-PCS, the episiotomy and delivery are reported with separate codes. Repair of the episiotomy is not separately reported.

Focus Point

If the physician extends a laceration, it remains an episiotomy and is coded as such. If an episiotomy extends spontaneously, it becomes a laceration and is classified as to degree.

© 2018 Optum360, LLC

Esophagectomy, Partial

Body System
Gastrointestinal System

PCS Root Operation
Excision

Resection

Root Operation Table
ØDB   Gastrointestinal System, Excision

ØDT   Gastrointestinal System, Resection

Body Part
Esophagus, Upper

Esophagus, Middle

Esophagus, Lower

Esophagogastric Junction

Esophagus (Excision)

Approach
Open

Percutaneous Endoscopic

Description
During a partial esophagectomy, the physician surgically removes part of the esophagus. Indications for partial removal of the esophagus include injury, gastroesophageal reflux disease, and the presence of esophageal cancer. The surgical approach and technique may vary, depending on the nature and anatomic site of the esophageal resection. ICD-10-PCS contains body part values for segments of the esophagus (Upper, Middle, Lower, Esophagogastric Junction) as well as a body part for the entire esophagus.

Partial esophagectomies may be performed via an Open or Percutaneous Endoscopic (laparoscopic) approach. Using an Open approach, the physician gains access to the esophagus through a cervical, thoracic, thoracoabdominal, or abdominal incision. Access during a Percutaneous Endoscopic approach is made with several small incisions in the abdomen in order to manipulate the laparoscopic instruments. With the exception of the lower esophagus, the physician resects the affected portion of the esophagus and reconnects (anastomoses) the remaining esophagus.

If the physician resects the most distal part of the esophagus, the stomach is dissected free of surrounding structures, and the esophagus is mobilized as it passes through the diaphragm to the stomach. The esophagus is divided at its connection to the stomach. Part of the esophagus is excised and removed, without synchronous resection of gastric tissue. Next, a right chest incision is made between the ribs to expose the esophagus. The distal esophagus is mobilized under direct vision and divided above its diseased segment. The distal esophagus, attached proximal stomach, and the esophageal segment are removed. The remaining stomach is pulled into the chest and connected to the stump of the proximal esophagus. Drains are placed into the chest near the new anastomosis, and the incisions are closed.

Focus Point
The anastomosis is not coded separately, according to guideline B3.1b.

Focus Point
The root operation Resection is used for a partial esophagectomy if the entire body part Upper, Lower, Middle, or Esophagogastric Junction is removed but the remainder of the esophagus is intact, according to guideline B3.8.

Esophagectomy, Total

Body System
Gastrointestinal System

PCS Root Operation
Resection

Root Operation Table
0DT   Gastrointestinal System, Resection

Body Part
Esophagus

Approach
Open
Percutaneous Endoscopic

Description

The most common indication for an esophagectomy is a malignancy such as adenocarcinoma or squamous cell carcinoma. Other reasons include narrowing or damage from severe acid reflux disease, achalasia, or injury.

The physician surgically removes the entire esophagus. Surgical technique may vary depending on whether or not a thoracotomy approach is used.

Resection and Anastomosis
The physician removes the esophagus and attaches the stump to the stomach and the pharynx. The physician gains access to the esophagus through two incisions when using an Open approach: an oblique cervical incision and a horizontal upper midline abdominal incision. The physician divides the esophagus at the cervical level (for an esophagogastrostomy) or at its origin at the pharynx (for a pharyngogastrostomy). The esophagus is removed through the abdominal incision and divided from the stomach. The stomach is pulled through the posterior mediastinum and anastomosed to the pharynx or the remaining cervical esophagus. The incisions are repaired in sutured layers.

Resection with Thoracotomy and Anastomosis
The physician removes the esophagus through abdominal, chest, and neck incisions and replaces esophagus with stomach. Using an Open approach, the physician makes a midline abdominal incision. Next, the stomach is dissected free of surrounding structures, and the esophagus is mobilized as it passes through the diaphragm to the stomach. The physician makes an incision in the right chest between the ribs and exposes the esophagus. The esophagus is mobilized under direct vision in the chest from diaphragm to the neck. The surgeon makes a longitudinal incision in the left or right neck and identifies and mobilizes the esophagus in the neck. The esophagus is divided at its junction with the stomach and in the neck, and the esophagus is removed. The stomach is pulled through the middle of the chest into the neck, and the stomach is connected to the stump of the esophagus. The incisions are closed.

Both techniques can be performed using a Percutaneous Endoscopic approach in which several small incisions are made in the abdomen in order to manipulate the laparoscopic instruments.

Focus Point
The anastomosis is not coded separately, according to guideline B3.1b.

© 2018 Optum360, LLC

Medical and Surgical

Esophagogastroduodenoscopy with Biopsy

Body System
Gastrointestinal System

PCS Root Operation
Excision

Extraction

Root Operation Table
ØDB   Gastrointestinal System, Excision

ØDD   Gastrointestinal System, Extraction

Body Part
Esophagus, Upper

Esophagus, Middle

Esophagus, Lower

Esophagogastric Junction

Esophagus

Stomach

Stomach, Pylorus

Duodenum

Approach
Via Natural or Artificial Opening Endoscopic

Qualifier
Diagnostic

Description
In esophagogastroduodenoscopy (EGD) with biopsy, the physician passes an endoscope through the sedated patient's mouth into the esophagus. The esophagus, stomach, duodenum, and sometimes the jejunum are viewed to determine if bleeding, tumors, erosions, ulcers, or other abnormalities are present.

Excision
The physician examines the upper gastrointestinal tract for diagnostic purposes. The physician passes an endoscope through the patient's mouth into the esophagus. The esophagus, stomach, and duodenum are viewed and inspected to determine if bleeding, tumors, erosions, ulcers, or other abnormalities are present. Single or multiple tissue samples from the upper gastrointestinal tract in the esophagus, stomach, and/or duodenum are obtained for biopsy using forceps through the endoscope. The endoscope is withdrawn at the completion of the procedure.

Extraction
The physician examines the upper gastrointestinal tract for diagnostic purposes. The physician passes an endoscope through the patient's mouth into the esophagus. The esophagus, stomach, and duodenum are viewed and inspected to determine if bleeding, tumors, erosions, ulcers, or other abnormalities are present. Single or multiple tissue specimens are obtained from the esophagus, stomach, and/or duodenum by brushing. The endoscope is withdrawn at the completion of the procedure.

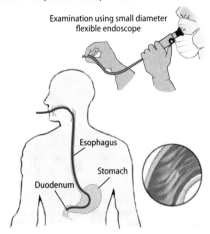

Examination using small diameter flexible endoscope

Esophagus

Stomach

Duodenum

Focus Point
Because the objective of the EGD with biopsy is to remove tissue for diagnostic purposes, the root operations are Excision and Extraction with the qualifier Diagnostic. The endoscope is used only as the approach to view the site of the biopsy and is included in the approach value Via Natural or Artificial Opening Endoscopic. Inspection performed using the same approach is not reported separately as it is considered intrinsic to the biopsy procedure.

Focus Point
Biopsies may be taken from multiple areas of the upper gastrointestinal system during an EGD. Consistent with ICD-10-PCS Multiple Procedures guidelines, report each code separately if the biopsies are done in areas that have a specific named body part.

Coding Guidance
AHA: 2016, 1Q, 24; 2015, 3Q, 21

Evacuation, Acute Subdural Hematoma

Body System
Central Nervous System and Cranial Nerves

PCS Root Operation
Extirpation

Root Operation Table
00C   Central Nervous System and Cranial Nerves, Extirpation

Body Part
Subdural Space, Intracranial

Approach
Open
Percutaneous
Percutaneous Endoscopic

Description
An acute subdural hematoma usually occurs due to trauma. Blood collects in the subdural space between the dura and the arachnoid. In some instances the hemorrhage organizes or becomes solid, resulting in pressure on the brain, and must be removed.

The physician evacuates a solid subdural hematoma by craniectomy or craniotomy by drilling a burr hole in the cranium. In an Open approach, a flap of skull is cut open and the site of the hematoma is directly visualized after removing the bone. In a Percutaneous approach, the instrumentation is inserted through a small burr hole to reach the site of the procedure. In some instances, an endoscope might be needed to visualize the site of the procedure and evacuate the hematoma. This is reported with the approach Percutaneous Endoscopic.

The hematoma is identified using imaging. First, the patient's head is stabilized, and the area is shaved, prepped, and draped. The physician incises the scalp and peels it away from the area to be drilled. A drill is used to drill or cut through the cranium to the dura mater, which is opened with an incision. The hematoma is then removed. The area is irrigated and suctioned. The dura mater is sutured closed, and the scalp is repositioned and sutured into place.

Focus Point
Evacuation of a liquefied hematoma, removing only liquid or fluid, is reported with root operation Drainage. If both liquid and solid matter are removed, report only Extirpation. If the documentation does not specify, use Extirpation as the default for evacuation of hematoma.

Focus Point
Removal of bone flaps that are cryopreserved and stored to be reinserted into the skull defect during a subsequent operative episode are integral to the evacuation procedure and are not reported separately.

Coding Guidance
AHA: 2016, 2Q, 29; 2015, 3Q, 9, 10, 11

© 2018 Optum360, LLC

Excision, Lingual, Submucosal Minimally Invasive (SMILE)

See also Epiglottopexy, Transoral Endoscopic

See also Tonsillectomy, Lingual

Body System
Mouth and Throat

PCS Root Operation
Excision

Root Operation Table
ØCB   Mouth and Throat, Excision

Body Part
Pharynx

Approach
Via Natural or Artificial Opening Endoscopic

Qualifier
Diagnostic
No Qualifier

Description
Airway obstruction and sleep apnea can be the result of many conditions, including hypertrophy of the tongue. Submucosal minimally invasive lingual excision (SMILE) is a surgical procedure that removes base of tongue tissue to reduce the size of the tongue.

Submucosal minimally invasive lingual excision is performed under general anesthesia, using the approach Via Natural or Artificial Opening Endoscopic with direct laryngoscopy. The physician makes a small incision in the tongue through which the coblation wand is inserted. Radiofrequency from the coblation wand is used to remove tissue at the base of the tongue. A coblation wand excises tissue with precision while minimizing the heat to surrounding tissue. At the conclusion of the procedure, the wand is removed and a stitch is placed over the incision.

Focus Point
The base of the tongue is anatomically considered part of the oropharynx and, according to the ICD-10-PCS Body Part Key, is included in the body part Pharynx.

Focus Point
If the base of tongue is removed for pathologic or histologic evaluation for diagnostic purposes (e.g., neoplasm), the qualifier Diagnostic is used.

Focus Point
Submucosal minimally invasive lingual excision is frequently performed with epiglottopexy. An additional code for the epiglottopexy is coded. See also Epiglottopexy, Transoral Endoscopic. For removal of the lingual tonsils, see Tonsillectomy, Lingual.

Coding Guidance
AHA: 2016, 3Q, 28; 2016, 2Q, 19

Excision, Radical, Skin Lesion

Body System
Skin and Breast
Subcutaneous Tissue and Fascia

PCS Root Operation
Excision

Root Operation Table
ØHB Skin and Breast, Excision

ØJB Subcutaneous Tissue and Fascia, Excision

Body Part
Refer to the ICD-10-PCS tabular list for a complete list of body parts.

Approach
Open
External

Qualifier
Diagnostic
No Qualifier

Description
Radical excision of a skin lesion is the removal of diseased and/or inflamed tissue that may include removal of a portion of surrounding normal tissue.

After administering the anesthetic, the physician uses an External approach to make a skin incision with a scalpel, usually in an elliptical shape around and under the lesion to remove it. Wide and radical excision may include dissection and removal of adjacent soft tissue of other structures and requires an Open approach. Closure is usually complex and may require a skin graft.

Focus Point
The operative report stating the depth of the removal determines the body system to report when coding a radical excision of skin lesion. Code the deepest layer as instructed by guideline B3.5.

Focus Point
The harvesting of the graft for the closure needs to be coded separately if the graft is taken from a different body part, according to coding guideline B3.9.

Focus Point
Assignment of the qualifiers Diagnostic and No Qualifier depends on the objective of the procedure (therapeutic or diagnostic). However, surgical specimens are routinely sent to pathology for study without necessarily being considered diagnostic. If the documentation is unclear, query the physician.

Medical and Surgical

© 2018 Optum360, LLC

Excision, Thoracic Spinal Dural Arteriovenous Fistula

Body System
Upper Arteries
Upper Veins

PCS Root Operation
Excision

Root Operation Table
Ø3B   Upper Arteries, Excision
Ø5B   Upper Veins, Excision

Body Part
Vertebral Artery, Right
Vertebral Artery, Left
Vertebral Vein, Right
Vertebral Vein, Left

Approach
Open

Description
Dural arteriovenous fistulas are the most common variety of spinal cord arteriovenous malformations (AVMs). A spinal dural arteriovenous fistula (SDAVF) is an abnormal direct connection between the arteries and veins in the dura (outer lining of the spinal cord). The capillaries that normally handle the transition of blood from an artery under high pressure to the veins under lower pressure are missing. This abnormal circulation causes increased high-pressure flow of arterial blood into the lower pressure veins, resulting in swelling and pressure on the spinal cord. The lack of capillaries can result in insufficient nutrient delivery to the tissues, causing neurologic injury and dysfunction. If the SDAVF cannot be occluded with endovascular embolization due to blood flow and vessel anatomy, it may require surgical removal.

Under general anesthesia, the patient is placed in prone (face down) position. Using an Open approach, the physician makes an incision overlying the thoracic vertebra in the area of the SDAVF. The fascia and paraspinal muscles are retracted, and a laminectomy is performed to access the spinal cord at the appropriate location. Using a surgical operating microscope and microsurgical techniques, the surgeon excises the malformation and restores normal blood flow to the spinal cord. The muscles, fascia, and ligaments are repaired, and the incision is closed in layers.

Focus Point
The spinal cord is supplied by three longitudinal arteries; one anterior spinal artery, which supplies the anterior two-thirds of the spinal cord; and paired posterior spinal arteries, which supply the posterior one-third of the spinal cord. The spinal veins are the anterior and posterior spinal veins and anterior and posterior radicular veins. The veins of the spinal cord and vertebral column are valveless.

Exploration, Common Bile Duct

Medical and Surgical

Body System
Hepatobiliary System and Pancreas

PCS Root Operation
Inspection

Root Operation Table
ØFJ Hepatobiliary System and Pancreas, Inspection

Body Part
Hepatobiliary Duct

Approach
Open
Percutaneous Endoscopic

Description
Common bile duct exploration is performed to verify the presence of an obstruction (such as a stone). An obstruction may result in insufficient flow of bile from the liver and gallbladder to the intestine.

Using a Percutaneous Endoscopic approach, a trocar is placed at the umbilicus, and the abdominal cavity is insufflated. The laparoscope is placed through the umbilical port, and additional trocars are placed into the abdominal cavity. The physician locates the bile duct and injects dye into the duct. A contrast study of the bile ducts is usually obtained through the cystic duct. The common duct is visualized with a choledochoscope. The trocars are removed, and the incisions are closed.

An Open approach may be used for common bile duct exploration when done concurrently with another open procedure.

Focus Point
If a common bile duct exploration results in another procedure such as removal of calculi, or stent or drainage tube placement using the same approach as the inspection, the inspection is not coded separately.

Focus Point
In percutaneous cholangiography, a radiographic medium is injected into the common bile duct and fluoroscopy is used to obtain images for diagnostic purposes. This is reported with a code from the Ancillary Section, Imaging, table BF1.

Exploratory Laparotomy/Laparoscopy

Body System
Anatomical Regions, General

PCS Root Operation
Inspection

Root Operation Table
ØWJ Anatomical Regions, General, Inspection

Body Part
Peritoneal Cavity
Gastrointestinal Tract

Approach
Open
Percutaneous Endoscopic

Description
The word "explore" in ICD-10-PCS is defined with the root operation Inspection. This exploratory procedure may also be referred to as a diagnostic laparotomy or laparoscopy. A laparotomy is an Open approach, while laparoscopy is a Percutaneous Endoscopic approach. If a physician uses one of these approaches for an Inspection, all the structures are viewed in the area of the Inspection, which is captured in the Anatomical Regions, General, body system. If the Inspection is performed on the entire abdominal contents, the ICD-10-PCS index instructs the coder to use the Peritoneal Cavity body part value, although Gastrointestinal Tract is an option for reporting more focused inspection.

To explore the intra-abdominal organs and structures, the physician performs an exploratory laparotomy. Using an Open approach, the physician makes a large incision extending from just above the pubic hairline to the rib cage. The abdominal cavity is opened for a systematic examination of all organs. The incision is closed with sutures.

Using a Percutaneous Endoscopic approach for a laparoscopy, small incisions are made and the abdomen insufflated with CO_2. A scope with a light and a camera is inserted. Additional tools for grasping, cutting, and other manipulation are inserted. The physician performs a detailed examination. The incisions are closed with sutures.

Focus Point
According to ICD-10-PCS guideline B3.11c, an Inspection procedure is coded separately if the Inspection procedure and another procedure are performed on the same body part during the same episode and the Inspection procedure is performed using a different approach from the approach used to perform the other procedure.

© 2018 Optum360, LLC

Extraction, Extracapsular Cataract with Intraocular Lens Implantation

Body System
Eye

PCS Root Operation
Replacement

Root Operation Table
Ø8R   Eye, Replacement

Body Part
Lens, Right
Lens, Left

Approach
Percutaneous

Device
Synthetic Substitute

Description

A cataract is a common condition of aging, causing clouding of the lens of the eye, which, left untreated, will cause blurry vision or eventually loss of vision.

Extracapsular cataract extraction with intraocular lens implantation is a one-stage procedure in which a cataract is removed and intraocular prosthesis inserted during the same operative episode.

A local anesthetic is injected into the periorbital area. A small horizontal incision is made where the cornea and sclera meet and, upon entering the eye through the incision, the physician opens the front of the capsule and removes the hard center, or nucleus, of the lens. Using a microscope, the ophthalmologist suctions out the soft lens cortex, leaving the capsule in place. The area is irrigated and aspirated, and an intraocular lens (IOL) (plastic disc that replaces the natural lens) is inserted. The haptics (securing attachments) lodge into the ciliary sulcus or the lens capsule, occupying the exact position of the native lens. The incision may be sutured, antibiotic ointment administered, and eye patch applied.

Another method used is standard phacoemulsification in which the cataract nucleus is shattered with an ultrasonic oscillating probe. After this fragmentation, the phaco probe is inserted into the eye and the cataract is suctioned out through an irrigation-aspiration probe. An intraocular lens (IOL) is inserted once all of the material is removed. The haptics (securing attachments) lodge into the ciliary sulcus or the lens capsule, occupying the exact position of the native lens. The incision may be sutured, antibiotic ointment administered, and eye patch applied.

Focus Point
The removal of the lens is included in the Replacement code.

Fasciectomy, Plantar

Body System
Subcutaneous Tissue and Fascia

PCS Root Operation
Excision

Root Operation Table
ØJB   Subcutaneous Tissue and Fascia, Excision

Body Part
Subcutaneous Tissue and Fascia, Right Foot
Subcutaneous Tissue and Fascia, Left Foot

Approach
Open

Qualifier
Diagnostic
No Qualifier

Description
When the foot's connective tissue, called the fascia, becomes irritated or inflamed, pain can result. Known as plantar fasciitis, it is a common cause of heel pain. There are a number of treatment options available, surgery being one of them. During a plantar fasciectomy the inflamed or scarred tissue is removed. Before surgery, a tourniquet is applied to the ankle. Using an Open approach, the physician makes a longitudinal incision inside the heel, and the fat that has filled the wound is separated with a key elevator. The plantar fascia is identified using right-angle retractors under direct vision. The affected connective tissue of the plantar fascia is incised and a segment removed. The tourniquet is released and the skin closed with nonabsorbable sutures. A dressing and a removable walking boot are applied. The sutures are removed in about three weeks and weight-bearing is increased, though the radical procedure increases the postoperative recovery period.

Focus Point
If the less extensive procedure, plantar fasciotomy, is performed, a code from table ØM8 Division of Bursae and Ligaments, is reported. This procedure can be performed via Open or Percutaneous Endoscopic approach and consists of making an incision through approximately a third of the plantar fascia ligament to release the tension of that ligament. Function is preserved by leaving the remaining two-thirds of the ligament in place.

© 2018 Optum360, LLC

Fasciotomy, Palmar (Dupuytren's Contracture)

Body System
Subcutaneous Tissue and Fascia

PCS Root Operation
Division

Root Operation Table
ØJ8   Subcutaneous Tissue and Fascia, Division

Body Part
Subcutaneous Tissue and Fascia, Right Hand
Subcutaneous Tissue and Fascia, Left Hand

Approach
Open
Percutaneous

Description
A Dupuytren's contracture is a progressive shortening and thickening of the palmar fascia, resulting in flexion contracture deformity of a finger.

In an Open approach, under appropriate anesthesia, the subcutaneous tissue is incised and retracted to expose and visualize the contracted palmar fascia. The palmar fascia cord is incised to relieve tension and allow the finger to extend correctly. The operative wound is closed in layers with sutures.

Under local anesthetic, the physician uses a Percutaneous approach, making a puncture wound with a needle through the subcutaneous tissue to the palmar fascia. During this needling technique, the cord of tissue causing the tension is divided by stabbing it with the needle.

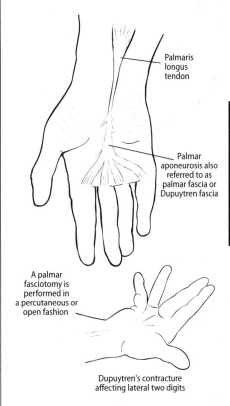

Palmaris longus tendon

Palmar aponeurosis also referred to as palmar fascia or Dupuytren fascia

A palmar fasciotomy is performed in a percutaneous or open fashion

Dupuytren's contracture affecting lateral two digits

Dupuytren's contracture is an increase in the fibrous tissues of the palmar aponeurosis, which results in a shortening of the bands that extend from this fascial tissue to the base of the fingers. The result is fixed flexion of digits

Focus Point
The root operation Division is used since the body part (fascia) is being cut and separated to accomplish the procedure. Root operation Release is not appropriate since the cutting does not involve an abnormal constraint or attachment around the body part.

© 2018 Optum360, LLC

Fistula, Arteriovenous (AV)

Medical and Surgical

Body System
Upper Arteries

PCS Root Operation
Bypass

Root Operation Table
Ø31   Upper Arteries, Bypass

Body Part
Brachial Artery, Right
Brachial Artery, Left
Radial Artery, Right
Radial Artery, Left

Approach
Open

Qualifier
Upper Arm Vein
Lower Arm Vein

Description

This procedure describes formation of an internal arteriovenous fistula (shunt) for dialysis. Surgical technique may vary depending on the site selected for dialysis access and associated factors. The fistula can be created with several different combinations of veins and arteries. Commonly used in the arm are the radial and brachial arteries to the cephalic, basilica, or median vein.

Through an incision, usually in the skin over an artery in the nondominant wrist or antecubital fossa, the physician isolates a desired section of artery and neighboring vein. Vessel clamps are placed on the vein and adjacent artery. The vein is dissected free, divided, and the downstream portion of the vein is sutured to an opening created in the adjacent artery, usually in an end-to-side fashion, allowing blood to flow both down the artery and into the vein. Large branches of the vein may be tied off to cause flow down a single vein. The skin incision is repaired with layered closure. This arteriovenous anastomosis allows an increased blood flow through the vein, usually for hemodialysis. The fistula is allowed to mature for three to six months or more before it is used for hemodialysis.

This type of AV fistula is a simple direct fistula and is reported with the root operation Bypass, which includes as part of its definition, the rerouting of the contents (blood) of a body part (artery) to a downstream area (vein) of the normal route. The upper stream—or "from"—is the artery, which is represented by the body part Radial or Brachial, and the downstream—or "to"—is the vein, reported with the appropriate Upper Arm Vein or Lower Arm Vein qualifier value.

Focus Point

Sometimes, a second stage procedure called a vein transposition is required two to four weeks later. It involves repositioning the vein to a more superficial location to ensure the vein is conducive for safe cannulation. The root operation for the transposition procedure is Reposition.

Coding Guidance
AHA: 2013, 4Q, 125; 2013, 1Q, 27

© 2018 Optum360, LLC

Fistulectomy, Anal

Body System
Gastrointestinal System
Skin and Breast
Subcutaneous Tissue and Fascia

PCS Root Operation
Excision

Root Operation Table
ØDB   Gastrointestinal System, Excision
ØHB   Skin and Breast, Excision
ØJB   Subcutaneous Tissue and Fascia, Excision

Body Part
Anus
Anal Sphincter
Skin, Buttock
Skin, Perineum
Subcutaneous Tissue and Fascia, Buttock
Subcutaneous Tissue and Fascia, Perineum

Approach
Open
External

Description
An anal fistula is an abnormal opening on the skin surface near or around the anus with a tract that connects with the anal canal, which can be the source of both painful bleeding and discharge when passing stools. In some cases, an anal fistula may also occur after surgery performed to drain an anal abscess.

Anal fistulectomy is the surgical removal of the fistula tract that may be needed in cases of recurrent abscesses or chronic drainage from the fistula site. Treatment of anal fistulas depends on the location of the fistula.

The physician explores the anal canal and identifies the location of the fistula in relation to the sphincter muscles. The skin and subcutaneous and connective tissues overlying the fistula are incised, and the fistula tract is dissected free and removed. The incision may be left open to allow continued drainage or closed in layered sutures. In ICD-10-PCS, an anal fistulectomy procedure is coded to the root operation Excision.

Focus Point
Review the operative report carefully, as the body part values and approaches can vary depending upon the location of the fistulous tissue excised. If the anal fistulectomy involves only excision of the anal or perianal skin, report the approach as External. If the excision extends through the skin into the subcutaneous tissue and beyond, report an Open approach.

Focus Point
According to ICD-10-PCS guideline B3.5, if the root operation Excision is performed on overlapping layers of the musculoskeletal system, the body part specifying the deepest layer is coded. For example, fistulectomy that includes perineal skin, subcutaneous tissue, and fascia is coded to the Subcutaneous Tissue and Fascia, Perineum body part.

Coding Guidance
AHA: 2015, 1Q, 29

Fistulectomy, Vesicovaginal

Body System
Urinary System
Female Reproductive System

PCS Root Operation
Repair

Root Operation Table
ØTQ   Urinary System, Repair
ØUQ   Female Reproductive System, Repair

Body Part
Bladder
Vagina

Approach
Open
Percutaneous Endoscopic (Bladder)
Via Natural or Artificial Opening (Vagina)

Description
The primary cause of vesicovaginal fistula, an abnormal opening between the bladder and vagina, is a complication of female pelvic surgery such as a hysterectomy. The symptoms are urinary incontinence and possible hematuria.

With the patient under general anesthesia, using an Open approach, the physician makes a vertical abdominal incision from just above the umbilicus to the pubic symphysis. The anterior bladder wall is opened and the bladder interior explored. The fistula is excised along with the surrounding tissue to ensure preservation of only healthy tissue. The resulting defect is closed with layered sutures starting with the vaginal wall, then the bladder walls, and finally the abdominal incision. A catheter is left in the bladder to prevent distension of the bladder and tension to the sutured areas.

The root operation Repair is reported for suturing of the bladder portion, which can be performed using either an Open or a Percutaneous Endoscopic approach. Repair of the vagina can be performed using an Open approach, as well as Via Natural or Artificial Opening.

Focus Point
Repair of a fistula with a flap or graft is reported with root operation Supplement, along with the appropriate device value. In ICD-10-PCS, Supplement is reported for repairs with a device.

Focus Point
Repair of a vesicovaginal fistula requires reporting two codes, one for Repair of the bladder wall and one for Repair of the vaginal wall. This is consistent with multiple procedures guideline B3.2.a, as the same root operation is being repeated on different body parts with distinct body part values.

Coding Guidance
AHA: 2015, 1Q, 28

© 2018 Optum360, LLC

Fistulotomy, Anal

Body System
Gastrointestinal System
Skin and Breast
Subcutaneous Tissue and Fascia

PCS Root Operation
Division
Drainage

Root Operation Table
ØD8   Gastrointestinal System, Division
ØD9   Gastrointestinal System, Drainage
ØH8   Skin and Breast, Division
ØH9   Skin and Breast, Drainage
ØJ8   Subcutaneous Tissue and Fascia, Division
ØJ9   Subcutaneous Tissue and Fascia, Drainage

Body Part
Anus (Drainage)
Anal Sphincter
Skin, Buttock
Skin, Perineum
Subcutaneous Tissue and Fascia, Buttock
Subcutaneous Tissue and Fascia, Perineum

Approach
Open
External

Device
Drainage Device (Drainage)
No Device

Description
An anal fistula is an abnormal opening on the skin surface near the anus that may connect with a tract that connects with the anal canal, which can be the source of both painful bleeding and discharge when passing stools. In some cases, an anal fistula may also occur after surgery is performed to drain an anal abscess.

Anal fistulotomy is a surgical procedure that may be needed in cases of acute or recurrent abscesses or chronic drainage from the fistula site. Treatment of anal fistulas depends on the location of the fistula.

Division
The physician identifies the location of the internal and external openings of the anal fistula in relation to the sphincter muscles. An incision is made in the perianal skin, and the fistula tract is opened. The mucosa, skin, and internal sphincter muscle overlying the fistula are incised, and the fistula is spread open and laid flat to heal. If the fistula goes beneath the external sphincter muscle, a stitch (Seton) may be placed through the fistula tract to allow future drainage and preserve continence. The incision may be left open to allow drainage.

Drainage
The physician identifies the location of the internal and external openings of the anal fistula in relation to the sphincter muscles. An incision is made in the perianal skin, and the fistula tract may be opened and drained. The mucosa, skin, and internal sphincter muscle overlying the fistula may be incised, and the fistula is spread open and laid flat to heal. If the fistula goes beneath the external sphincter muscle, a stitch (Seton) may be placed through the fistula tract to allow drainage and preserve continence. The incision may be left open to drain.

> **Focus Point**
> Review the operative report carefully, as the body part values and approaches can vary depending upon the location of the fistulous tissue incised. If the anal fistulotomy involves only incision of the anal or perineal skin, report the approach as External. If the incision extends through the skin into the subcutaneous tissue and beyond, report an Open approach.

> **Focus Point**
> Temporary postoperative wound drains are considered integral to the performance of a procedure and are not coded as devices. See guideline B6.1.b.

© 2018 Optum360, LLC

Fontan Stage I (Norwood Procedure)

See also Fontan Stage II (Glenn Procedure) (Caval-pulmonary Artery Anastomosis)

See also Fontan Stage III, Completion

See also Blalock-Taussig Shunt Procedure, Modified

See also Conduit, Right Ventricle to Pulmonary Artery (RV-PA) (Sano Shunt)

Body System
Heart and Great Vessels

PCS Root Operation
Supplement

Root Operation Table
Ø2U   Heart and Great Vessels, Supplement

Body Part
Thoracic Aorta, Ascending/Arch

Approach
Open

Device
Nonautologous Tissue Substitute

Qualifier
No Qualifier

Description
A three-staged surgical approach is performed for children born with a functional single ventricle, known as hypoplastic left heart syndrome (HLHS). Stage I is performed within several days of birth. The purpose of the Norwood procedure is to enlarge the hypoplastic aorta to provide blood flow to the body. It is generally performed in conjunction with a procedure to make an additional connection or shunt to provide blood flow to the lungs, with either a right-ventricle-to-pulmonary-artery shunt, or an innominate/subclavian artery shunt to the pulmonary artery or pulmonary trunk. *See also* Conduit, Right Ventricle to Pulmonary Artery (RV-PA) (Sano Shunt) or Blalock-Taussig Shunt Procedure, Modified.

The patient is placed under general anesthesia and on cardiopulmonary bypass. Using an Open approach, the physician makes a median sternotomy incision through the middle of the chest. The aorta is cross-clamped. The original hypoplastic Thoracic Aorta, Ascending/Arch is made larger, providing blood flow to the body by augmenting/reconstructing it, usually with homograft tissue (Nonautologous Tissue Substitute). Pulmonary blood flow is provided by placing a Sano or modified Blalock-Taussig shunt.

A delayed sternal closure may be necessary with skin closed in layers. A chest tube or tubes may be used to provide drainage for the chest cavity.

Focus Point
Multiple surgical procedures may be performed concomitantly to correct congenital heart disorders. ICD-10-PCS guidelines on multiple procedures should be followed when assigning codes for these procedures.

Coding Guidance
AHA: 2017, 1Q, 19

 © 2018 Optum360, LLC

Fontan Stage II (Glenn Procedure) (Caval-pulmonary Artery Anastomosis)

See also Fontan Stage I (Norwood Procedure)

See also Fontan Stage III, Completion

See also Blalock-Taussig Shunt Procedure, Modified

Body System
Heart and Great Vessels

PCS Root Operation
Bypass

Root Operation Table
Ø21   Heart and Great Vessels, Bypass

Body Part
Superior Vena Cava

Approach
Open

Device
No Device

Qualifier
Pulmonary Artery, Right

Description

A three-staged surgical approach is performed for children born with a functional single ventricle, known as hypoplastic left heart syndrome (HLHS). Stage II of the Fontan procedure, also known as the bidirectional Glenn procedure, is usually performed within six months of birth. The superior vena cava (large vein that carries deoxygenated blood from the upper body into the heart) is disconnected from the heart and attached to the right pulmonary artery, diverting the deoxygenated blood through the lungs, bypassing the right side of the heart.

The patient is placed under general anesthesia and on cardiopulmonary bypass. Circulatory arrest and deep cooling of the body are usually employed. Using an Open approach through the chest, the right (or the persistent left) superior caval vein is occluded and its connection with the heart is divided. The heart end of the superior caval vein is closed. The free end of the superior caval vein is sewn to the right pulmonary

artery. It is assumed that the pulmonary artery is isolated from the opposite lung congenitally or surgically. The goal is to permit blood to flow directly from the superior caval vein to the lungs, thereby bypassing the right side of the heart.

Alternatively, the main pulmonary artery may be tied-off. The superior caval vein is detached from its connection to the right atrium. The hole left in the right atrium is closed with sutures. The free end of the superior caval vein is sewn to a hole in the side of the pulmonary artery. In this way, blood can flow to the lungs without passing through the right side of the heart.

Focus Point
Cardiopulmonary bypass is an exception to the usual practice of not reporting supporting procedures that are components of a larger operation. When a surgical procedure is performed with cardiopulmonary bypass, it is coded as an additional procedure and reported as 5A1221Z Performance of Cardiac Output, Continuous.

Focus Point
Documentation of bypass procedures must clearly state the body part bypassed from and body part bypassed to.

Focus Point
Device value No Device is reported since the free end of the superior caval vein is sewn directly to the side of the corresponding pulmonary artery without a graft.

Focus Point
The Glenn procedure may be referred to as the modified or bidirectional Glenn shunt or a cavo-pulmonary shunt. The bidirectional procedure in this description, which is performed currently, supplies blood to both lungs. It is a modified form of the original operation, which supplied blood only to the right lung.

Coding Guidance
AHA: 2017, 4Q, 36

Fontan Stage III, Completion

See also Fontan Stage I (Norwood Procedure)

See also Fontan Stage II (Glenn Procedure)
(Caval-pulmonary Artery Anastomosis)

Body System
Lower Veins

PCS Root Operation
Bypass

Root Operation Table
041   Lower Veins, Bypass

Body Part
Inferior Vena Cava

Approach
Open

Device
Synthetic Substitute

Qualifier
Pulmonary Trunk
Pulmonary Artery, Right
Pulmonary Artery, Left

Description
The treatment of congenital heart defects such as hypoplastic left heart syndrome usually requires a three-stage surgical procedure. The Fontan completion stage III procedure is the last stage.

The right pulmonary artery (or left in situs inversus) is exposed from the main pulmonary trunk to the hilum of the lung using an Open approach. The superior vena cava is detached from the right atrium. The atrial hole is closed. A hole is made in the top part of the pulmonary artery, and the cut end of the superior vena cava is connected to the hole in the pulmonary artery. Pulmonary blood flow comes directly from the venous system and bypasses the heart. Cardiopulmonary bypass with or without circulatory arrest is required. Blood flow is directed from the inferior caval vein, through a tunnel created inside the right atrium to the pulmonary artery. This tunneled connection may be completed using a synthetic tube graft. All systemic venous return is diverted away from the heart and directly into the pulmonary circulation. The right atrium is widely opened. A large patch of pericardium or Dacron is used for one wall of the tunnel. The lateral wall of the right atrium forms the other half of the tunnel. The tunnel leads from the inferior caval vein, where it joins the right atrium, to the undersurface of the pulmonary artery. The mouth of the tunnel is connected to a hole on the undersurface of the pulmonary artery.

Focus Point
Cardiopulmonary bypass is an exception to the usual practice of not reporting supporting procedures that are components of a larger operation. When a surgical procedure is performed with cardiopulmonary bypass, it is coded as an additional procedure and reported as 5A1221Z Performance of Cardiac Output, Continuous.

Coding Guidance
AHA: 2017, 4Q, 36; 2014, 3Q, 29

© 2018 Optum360, LLC

Medical and Surgical

Frenectomy, Labial

Body System
Mouth and Throat

Root Operation Table
ØCB   Mouth and Throat, Excision

Body Part
Upper Lip
Lower Lip

Approach
Open

Description
A labial frenectomy is the removal of a mucosal band of tissue (labial frenum) that connects the mucosa of

the inner lip to the alveolar (dental) ridge in the oral vestibule. The frenum effectively joins the lip to the gums at the inside mid-center of the upper and lower jaw. When the labial frenum is too bulky or is attached too close to the crest of the alveolar ridge, it can interfere with eating and speaking, disrupt dentures, or cause pain.

The physician removes or excises the labial frenum. Using an Open approach, the physician makes incisions around the frenum and through the mucosa and submucosa. The underlying muscle is removed as well. The excision may extend to the interincisal papilla. The mucosa is closed simply, or the physician may rearrange the tissue as in a Z-plasty technique.

Medical and Surgical

Frenotomy, Labial

Body System
Mouth and Throat

PCS Root Operation
Release

Root Operation Table
ØCN   Mouth and Throat, Release

Body Part
Upper Lip
Lower Lip

Approach
External

Description
A labial frenotomy is the release of a mucosal band of tissue (labial frenum) that connects the mucosa of the

inner lip to the alveolar (dental) ridge in the oral vestibule. The frenum effectively joins the lip to the gums at the inside mid-center of the upper and lower jaw. When the labial frenum is attached too close to the crest of the alveolar ridge, it can interfere with eating and speaking, disrupt dentures, or cause pain.

The physician performs a frenotomy by incising the labial frenum with an External approach. This procedure is often performed to release tension on the frenum and surrounding tissues. The labial frenum is simply incised and not removed.

Focus Point
In the root operation Release, report the body part being freed rather than the tissue that is cut or excised. See ICD-10-PCS guideline B3.13.

Fundoplication, Gastroesophageal

Body System
Gastrointestinal System

PCS Root Operation
Restriction

Root Operation Table
ØDV   Gastrointestinal System, Restriction

Body Part
Esophagogastric Junction

Approach
Open
Percutaneous Endoscopic

Description
Gastroesophageal fundoplication is performed to treat severe gastroesophageal reflux disease (GERD) resulting from mechanical dysfunction of the lower esophageal sphincter, which may occur with or without a paraesophageal (hiatal) hernia. The fundoplication procedure is performed to reduce the size of the gastroesophageal opening. When the objective of the procedure is to partially close the orifice or lumen of a tubular body part, Restriction is the root operation being performed.

Gastroesophageal fundoplication can be performed by a number of techniques, but one of the more common is a Nissen (360-degree wrap) fundoplication or a variation on this procedure. Nissen fundoplication is most commonly performed laparoscopically but may be performed with an open surgical technique if necessary. The procedure involves mobilizing both the lower esophagus and fundus of the stomach. A bougie (dilating instrument) is placed in the distal esophagus to maintain the desired size of the esophageal opening. The hiatus, which is the opening in the diaphragm through which the esophagus and other structures pass, is repaired with sutures, and the hiatal opening is narrowed to a diameter of no more than 2.5 cm. The gastric fundus is then wrapped around and sutured to the distal esophagus to narrow the lumen of the gastroesophageal junction.

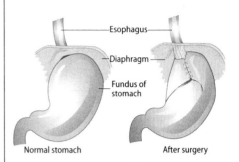

Esophagus

Diaphragm

Fundus of stomach

Normal stomach   After surgery

Focus Point
Endoscopic "transoral incisionless fundoplication (TIF)" is a new procedure that may be performed using an endoscope. The TIF creates a 240-degree partial wrap from the inside of the stomach. Because it is performed from the inside of the stomach, this approach does not require incisions. It is performed only for patients who have either very small or no hiatal hernias. This would be reported with the approach Via Natural or Artificial Opening Endoscopic.

Coding Guidance
AHA: 2016, 2Q, 22; 2014, 3Q, 28

© 2018 Optum360, LLC

Medical and Surgical

Fusion, Ankle (Arthrodesis)

Body System
Lower Joints

PCS Root Operation
Fusion

Root Operation Table
ØSG   Lower Joints, Fusion

Body Part
Ankle Joint, Right
Ankle Joint, Left

Approach
Open
Percutaneous
Percutaneous Endoscopic

Device
Internal Fixation Device
External Fixation Device
Autologous Tissue Substitute
Synthetic Substitute
Nonautologous Tissue Substitute

Description
The ankle joint (or talocrural or tibiotalar joint) is a hinge-type synovial joint located in the lower limb formed by the distal tibia, distal fibula, and talus that permits plantarflexion and dorsiflexion of the foot. An ankle fusion, also known as arthrodesis, is accomplished using various surgical techniques and is usually performed on patients with degenerative arthritis. The fusion reduces range of motion of the ankle joint.

Using an Open approach, the physician reaches the ankle joint through an incision on the outside or the front of the ankle. After accessing the ankle joint,, the physician uses a surgical saw to remove the articulating cartilage on both sides and any bone spurs to prepare the joint surface for fusion. Screws and/or plates may be used to hold the ankle in the correct position for fusion. A bone graft may be used, either a Synthetic, Nonautologous, or Autologous graft, which may be taken from the pelvis, heel bone, or just below the knee. The hardware will remain in place unless it starts to cause pain or becomes displaced. X-rays are used during the procedure to check the placement of hardware and alignment of the joint. The incisions are closed with staples or sutures. The patient may be placed in a splint or plastic boot during healing.

In a Percutaneous approach, the fusion hardware may be inserted into the operative site through small puncture sites. In some cases, external fixators using pins and bars may be inserted through the punctures and connected to metal rods and bolts outside the skin to hold the joint in position. The external fixator is removed after the fusion has healed.

The Percutaneous Endoscopic approach is not significantly different from the Open procedure. An arthroscope and surgical instruments inserted into the ankle joint through small incisions are used to perform osteotomies and place fixation devices.

Focus Point
In some cases, a subtalar (talocalcaneal) joint fusion is performed at the same time as ankle fusion. This is reported with an additional code using Tarsal Joint, Left, or Tarsal Joint, Right, according to the ICD-10-PCS Body Part Key.

Focus Point
Bone graft harvested from the local incision is not reported separately. However, if a separate incision is required to harvest the graft, such as from the pelvis or iliac crest, this may be reported in addition to the primary procedure (fusion). This is consistent with ICD-10-PCS guideline B3.9.

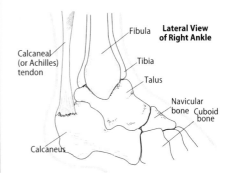

Lateral View of Right Ankle

Fusion, Cervical Spine, Anterior (ACF)

See also Fusion, Cervical Spine, Posterior (PCF)

See also Fusion, Spinal, Interbody Fusion Device, Radiolucent Porous, in the New Technology section

Body System
Upper Joints

PCS Root Operation
Fusion

Root Operation Table
ØRG   Upper Joints, Fusion

Body Part
Occipital-Cervical Joint
Cervical Vertebral Joint
Cervical Vertebral Joints, 2 or more
Cervicothoracic Vertebral Joint

Approach
Open

Device
Autologous Tissue Substitute
Interbody Fusion Device
Synthetic Substitute
Nonautologous Tissue Substitute

Qualifier
Anterior Approach, Anterior Column

Description

Spinal fusion, also known as spinal arthrodesis, fuses together one or more vertebral joints with bone graft, allograft implants or dowels, graft-filled titanium cages, spacers, and in some cases is supplemented by screws, plates, and rods. Spinal arthrodesis may be performed to treat conditions such as herniated discs or degenerative, traumatic, or congenital lesions; or to stabilize fractures or dislocations of the spine. Codes identify the specific body parts for a single vertebral joint or multiple vertebral joints at each spine level where the procedure is performed (cervical, thoracic, or lumbar), the approach, and the spinal column fused (anterior, posterior) as well as devices.

Anterior cervical fusion may be performed in conjunction with posterior cervical spinal fusion, usually when multiple levels are involved.

Under general anesthesia, the patient is placed in a supine (lying on the back, with the face upward)

position. Using an Open approach, an incision is made in the front of the neck beside the trachea. The underlying musculature of the neck is dissected carefully, exposing the anterior (front) of the cervical spine by retracting the esophagus and trachea toward the midline and the carotid artery and associated structures to one side. The muscles overlying the anterior cervical spine are dissected and retractors placed. Bone and degenerated or herniated intervertebral disc material are removed at the levels to be decompressed, down to the level of the posterior longitudinal ligament (PLL), which overlies the dura. The PLL may also be removed if it is compressing the spinal cord or as an approach to the herniated disc material. After the spinal cord and nerve roots have been decompressed at the appropriate levels, distractor instruments are used to restore the normal height of the disc space and to determine the appropriate size for the spacer to be placed. A bone graft, (Autologous, Synthetic, or Nonautologous Tissue Substitute) with or without an interbody device, also called a spacer or cage, is inserted into the disc space. If a spacer or cage is inserted, the bone graft is placed into and sometimes in front of the cage. If the patient's own bone graft is used (Autologous Tissue Substitute), it is harvested from the iliac crest through a separate incision. Fluoroscopic x-rays are used to confirm that the spacer is in the correct position. Additional fixation of the cage may be performed by inserting screws through the cage, or by the surgeon securing a titanium plate and screw device to the remaining vertebral bodies to provide extra stability, prevent dislodgement of the bone graft, and promote adequate fusion.

After the spine is stabilized, the wound area is irrigated with sterile water containing antibiotics. The retractors are removed, restoring the retracted tissues to normal anatomic position, and the incision is closed in layers with sutures. The skin is closed with sutures or staples. Temporary drains may be inserted in the surgical wound to prevent fluid buildup. A sterile bandage is applied.

Focus Point
Discectomy is usually performed with spinal fusion surgery. Report an additional code for the discectomy procedure, using root operation Excision for a partial discectomy and Resection for a total discectomy.

© 2018 Optum360, LLC

Fusion, Cervical Spine, Anterior (ACF) (continued)

Focus Point

Additional corpectomy (excision of vertebral body) and excision of thickened ligaments performed to decompress the cervical spinal cord and/or spinal nerves in conjunction with anterior cervical spinal fusion are reported separately as Release, Cervical Spinal Cord and/or Release, Cervical Nerve, based on which structures (spinal cord or nerve roots) are decompressed. The root operation Release meets the objective of removing the bone or ligaments to complete the decompression. Excision of the posterior longitudinal ligament as an approach to the discectomy procedure is integral to the discectomy and is not reported separately.

Report only one code for any procedures done to Release a single body part. If both spinal cord and spinal nerves are decompressed, two codes can be reported using Release, Cervical Spinal Cord and Release, Cervical Nerve. Multiple procedures guideline B3.2b applies only when the procedure is performed on separate and distinct body parts.

Focus Point

Bone graft harvested from the local incision is not reported separately. However, if a separate incision is required to harvest the graft, such as from the iliac crest, this may be reported in addition to the primary procedure (fusion). This is consistent with ICD-10-PCS guideline B3.9.

Focus Point

When multiple devices are used, code to the highest value listed highest to lowest (with the same approach, body part, and qualifier):

- Interbody Fusion Device (alone or with any other material)
- Autologous Tissue Substitute (alone or with nonautologous and/or with synthetic material)
- Nonautologous Tissue Substitute (alone or with synthetic)
- Synthetic Tissue Substitute

When multiple vertebral joints are fused, each vertebral joint that uses a different device and/or a different qualifier is coded separately. See guidelines B3.10b and B3.10c.

Focus Point

When the spinal fusion procedure is performed through two separate approaches—both anterior and posterior—requiring that the patient be repositioned, two codes are reported: one for the anterior approach through the front of the neck and one for the posterior approach through the back of the neck.

Focus Point

Reporting placement of bone morphogenic protein (BMP) placed during a spinal fusion is optional and at the discretion of the facility. It is reported with a code from the Administration section (3E0).

Focus Point

To code an anterior spinal fusion using an interbody fusion device documented as nanotextured surface or radiolucent porous, use New Technology table XRG. See also Fusion, Spinal, Interbody Fusion Device, Radiolucent Porous, in the New Technology section.

Coding Guidance

AHA: 2018, 1Q, 8; 2018, 1Q, 22; 2017, 2Q, 23; 2016, 2Q, 17; 2015, 2Q, 21; 2014, 3Q, 9, 30; 2014, 2Q, 6-8; 2013, 3Q, 25; 2013, 1Q, 21, 29

Fusion, Cervical Spine, Posterior (PCF)

See also Fusion, Cervical Spine, Anterior (ACF)

Body System
Upper Joints

PCS Root Operation
Fusion

Root Operation Table
ØRG   Upper Joints, Fusion

Body Part
Occipital-Cervical Joint
Cervical Vertebral Joint
Cervical Vertebral Joints, 2 or more
Cervicothoracic Vertebral Joint

Approach
Open

Device
Autologous Tissue Substitute
Synthetic Substitute
Nonautologous Tissue Substitute

Qualifier
Posterior Approach, Posterior Column

Description

Spinal fusion, also known as spinal arthrodesis, fuses together one or more vertebral joints with bone graft, allograft implants or dowels, graft-filled titanium cages, and spacers, and in some cases is supplemented by screws, plates, and rods. Graft-filled titanium cages or spacers, referred to as Interbody Fusion devices in ICD-10-PCS, are specifically used for fusions of the anterior spinal column and are not an option for posterior column fusions. Spinal arthrodesis may be performed to treat conditions such as herniated discs or degenerative, traumatic, or congenital lesions; or to stabilize fractures or dislocations of the spine. Codes identify the specific body parts for a single vertebral joint or multiple vertebral joints at each spine level where the procedure is performed (cervical, thoracic, or lumbar), the approach, and the spinal column fused (anterior, posterior) as well as devices.

The goal of posterior cervical fusion is to stabilize the spine, reducing pain and deformity. Posterior cervical fusion may also be performed in conjunction with anterior cervical spinal fusion, usually when multiple levels are involved. It may be performed with or without a posterior laminectomy for decompression, and with or without instrumentation such as metal screws and rods. Screws and rods are usually used to add stability and increase fusion success rates.

The patient is placed under general anesthesia and positioned in the prone (lying on the stomach)

position. Using an Open approach, a small incision is made in the midline of the back of the neck, the muscles are dissected and retracted off the lamina, and the vertebrae and facet joints are exposed. The surgeon uses a high-speed burr to perform a laminectomy, cutting a trough of bone, and thickened ligaments and/or bone spurs may be removed, decompressing the spinal cord and/or nerve roots. Herniated or degenerated disc material may also be removed. The soft tissue and cartilage of the facet joints are removed, and the surfaces are prepared for the bone graft by burring, allowing surface area for growth of bone.

Autologous Tissue Substitute bone graft may be obtained from the iliac crest, or Synthetic Substitute bone graft or Nonautologous Tissue donor graft may be used. The bone graft material is packed into the facet joints. The back muscles are then released over the bone graft, using tension to hold the bone graft in place. Instrumentation such as wires, screws, and plates, or screws and rods may be added to hold the vertebrae together in a natural position, preventing facet motion and increasing the success of the fusion. After the spine is stabilized, the wound area is irrigated with sterile water containing antibiotics. The deep fascial layer and subcutaneous layers are closed with sutures, and the skin is closed with sutures or staples. Temporary drains may be inserted in the surgical wound to prevent fluid buildup. A sterile bandage is applied.

Focus Point

Discectomy is usually performed with spinal fusion surgery. Report an additional code for the discectomy procedure, using root operation Excision for a partial discectomy and Resection for a total discectomy.

Focus Point

Additional procedures such as laminectomy, foraminotomy, and excision of thickened ligaments performed to decompress the cervical spinal cord and/ or spinal nerves in conjunction with posterior cervical spinal fusion are reported separately as Release, Cervical Spinal Cord and/or Release, Cervical Nerve, based on which structures (spinal cord or nerve roots) are decompressed. The root operation Release meets the objective of removing the lamina, bone spurs (foramina), or ligaments to complete the decompression.

Report only one code for any procedures done to Release a single body part. If both spinal cord and spinal nerves are decompressed, two codes can be reported using Release, Cervical Spinal Cord and Release, Cervical Nerve. Multiple procedures guideline B3.2b applies only when the procedure is performed on separate and distinct body parts.

© 2018 Optum360, LLC

Medical and Surgical

Fusion, Cervical Spine, Posterior (PCF) (continued)

Focus Point

Bone graft harvested from the local incision is not reported separately. However, if a separate incision is required to harvest the graft, such as from the iliac crest, this may be reported in addition to the primary procedure (fusion). This is consistent with ICD-10-PCS guideline B3.9.

Focus Point

When multiple devices are used, code to the highest value listed highest to lowest (with the same approach, body part, and qualifier):

• Interbody Fusion Device (alone or with any other material)

• Autologous Tissue Substitute (alone or with nonautologous and/or with synthetic material)

• Nonautologous Tissue Substitute (alone or with synthetic)

• Synthetic Tissue Substitute

When multiple vertebral joints are fused, each vertebral joint that uses a different device and/or a different qualifier is coded separately. See guidelines B3.10b and B3.10c.

Focus Point

When the spinal fusion procedure is performed through two separate approaches—both anterior and posterior—requiring that the patient be repositioned, two codes are reported: one for the anterior approach through the front of the neck and one for the posterior approach through the back of the neck.

Focus Point

Reporting placement of bone morphogenic protein (BMP) placed during a spinal fusion is optional and at the discretion of the facility. It is reported with a code from the Administration section (3E0).

Coding Guidance

AHA: 2018, 1Q, 8; 2018, 1Q, 22; 2017, 2Q, 23; 2016, 2Q, 17; 2015, 2Q, 21; 2014, 3Q, 9, 30; 2014, 2Q, 6-8; 2013, 3Q, 25; 2013, 1Q, 21, 29

Medical and Surgical

Fusion, Lumbar, Anterior Interbody (ALIF) (Anterior Lumbar Vertebral Arthrodesis)

See also Fusion, Lumbar Posterior (PLF)

See also Fusion, Spinal, Interbody Fusion Device, Radiolucent Porous, in the New Technology section

Body System
Lower Joints

PCS Root Operation
Fusion

Root Operation Table
ØSG Lower Joints, Fusion

Body Part
Lumbar Vertebral Joint
Lumbar Vertebral Joints, 2 or more
Lumbosacral Joint

Approach
Open

Device
Interbody Fusion Device

Qualifier
Anterior Approach, Anterior Column

Description

Spinal fusion, also known as spinal arthrodesis, fuses together one or more vertebral joints with bone graft, allograft implants or dowels, graft-filled titanium cages, spacers, and in some cases is supplemented by screws, plates, and rods. Spinal arthrodesis may be performed to treat conditions such as degenerative, traumatic, or congenital lesions; herniated discs; or to stabilize fractures or dislocations of the spine. Codes identify the specific body parts for a single vertebral joint or multiple vertebral joints at each spinal level where the procedure is performed (cervical, thoracic, or lumbar); the approach; and the spinal column fused (anterior, posterior) as well as devices.

The spine can be fused using various surgical techniques, including:

- Open, Percutaneous, or Percutaneous Endoscopic approaches
- Anterior approach, anterior column: Approaching the anterior spinal column through the front of the body to perform a procedure on the vertebral body or the disc
- Posterior approach, posterior column: Approaching the posterior spinal column (vertebral foramen, spinous process, facets and/or lamina) through the back (posterior) of the body
- Posterior approach, anterior column: Approaching the anterior spinal column through the back (posterior) of the body to perform a procedure on the vertebral body or the disc
- Devices: Autologous tissue substitute, interbody fusion device, nonautologous tissue substitute (allograft)

An anterior lumbar interbody fusion (ALIF) is performed to fuse two (or more) lumbar vertebral bones together at the anterior portion of the spinal column using an interbody fusion device that is typically filled with autologous (autograft) or nonautologous (allograft) bone tissue.

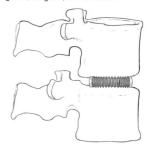

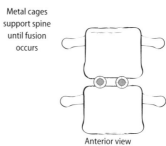

Metal cages support spine until fusion occurs

Anterior view

Spinal fusion with metal cages

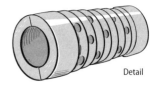

Detail

Under general anesthesia, the patient is placed in supine position, prepped, and draped. Using an Open approach, a 3 inch to 5 inch transverse or oblique incision is made on the left side of the abdomen, and the abdominal muscles are not cut but are retracted to the side. The abdominal contents inside the peritoneal sac are also retracted without cutting, allowing the physician to access the front of the spine without actually entering the peritoneal cavity of the abdomen.

© 2018 Optum360, LLC

Medical and Surgical

Fusion, Lumbar, Anterior Interbody (ALIF) (Anterior Lumbar Vertebral Arthrodesis) (continued)

The aorta and vena cava are located on top of the spine and may require surgical assistance from a vascular surgeon to safely mobilize these vessels. After the aorta and vena cava have been moved away from the spine, special retractors are used to allow the surgeon to visualize the anterior aspect of the intervertebral discs. The intervertebral disc is removed using rongeurs or curettes.

Distractor instruments are used to restore the normal height of the disc space and to determine the appropriate size spacer to be placed. An interbody device, also called a spacer or cage, is inserted into the disc space. A bone graft (Autologous, Synthetic, or Nonautologous Tissue Substitute) is placed into and sometimes in front of the cage. Fluoroscopic x-rays are used to confirm that the spacer is in the correct position.

Additional fixation of the cage may be performed by inserting screws through the cage. If the patient's own bone graft is used, it is harvested from the iliac crest through a separate incision. An ALIF may be combined with a separately reportable posterior or posterolateral lumbar fusion (PLF) from another incision in the back of the spine. The wound is irrigated with sterile solution with antibiotics. The retractors are removed, returning the abdominal contents to normal anatomic position, and the incision is closed in layers with sutures.

Focus Point
Spinal fixation devices such as rods, plates, and screws are included in the fusion and are not coded separately.

Focus Point
If a physician performs a partial or total discectomy with spinal fusion, the discectomy would be coded separately.

Focus Point
Bone graft harvested from the local incision is not reported separately. However, if a separate incision is required to harvest the graft, such as from the iliac crest, this may be reported in addition to the primary procedure (fusion). This is consistent with ICD-10-PCS guideline B3.9.

Focus Point
When multiple devices are used, code to the highest value listed highest to lowest (with the same approach, body part, and qualifier):
- *Interbody Fusion Device (alone or with any other material)*
- *Autologous Tissue Substitute (alone or with nonautologous and/or with synthetic material)*
- *Nonautologous Tissue Substitute (alone or with synthetic)*
- *Synthetic Tissue Substitute*

When multiple vertebral joints are fused, each vertebral joint that uses a different device and/or a different qualifier is coded separately. See guidelines B3.10b and B3.10c.

Focus Point
When the spinal fusion procedure is performed through two separate approaches—both anterior and posterior—requiring that the patient be repositioned, two codes are reported: one for the anterior approach through the abdomen and one for the posterior approach through the back.

Focus Point
Reporting placement of bone morphogenic protein (BMP) placed during a spinal fusion is optional and at the discretion of the facility. It is reported with a code from the Administration section (3E0).

Focus Point
To code an anterior spinal fusion using an interbody fusion device documented as nanotextured surface or radiolucent porous, use New Technology table (XRG). See also Fusion, Spinal, Interbody Fusion Device, Radiolucent Porous, in the New Technology section.

Coding Guidance
AHA: 2018, 1Q, 8; 2018, 1Q, 22; 2017, 2Q, 23; 2014, 3Q, 30; 2014, 3Q, 36; 2014, 2Q, 6-8; 2013, 3Q, 25; 2013, 1Q, 21, 29

Medical and Surgical

Fusion, Lumbar, Posterior (PLF)

See also Fusion, Lumbar Anterior Interbody (ALIF) (Anterior Lumbar Vertebral Arthrodesis)

Body System
Lower Joints

PCS Root Operation
Fusion

Root Operation Table
ØSG   Lower Joints, Fusion

Body Part
Lumbar Vertebral Joint
Lumbar Vertebral Joints, 2 or more
Lumbosacral Joint

Approach
Open

Device
Autologous Tissue Substitute
Synthetic Substitute
Nonautologous Tissue Substitute

Qualifier
Posterior Approach, Posterior Column

Description
Spinal fusion, also known as spinal arthrodesis, fuses together one or more vertebral joints with bone graft, allograft implants or dowels, graft-filled titanium cages, spacers, and in some cases, supplemented by screws, plates, and rods. Spinal arthrodesis may be performed to treat conditions such as degenerative, traumatic, or congenital lesions, herniated discs, or to stabilize fractures or dislocations of the spine. Codes identify the specific body parts for a single vertebral joint or multiple vertebral joints at each spinal level where the procedure is performed (cervical, thoracic, or lumbar), the approach and spinal column fused (anterior, posterior), as well as devices.

The spine is fused using various surgical techniques, including:

- Open, Percutaneous, or Percutaneous Endoscopic approach
- Anterior approach, anterior column: Approaching the anterior spinal column through the front of the body to perform a procedure on the vertebral body or the disc
- Posterior approach, posterior column: Approaching the posterior spinal column (vertebral foramen, spinous process, facets and/or lamina) through the back (posterior) of the body
- Posterior approach, anterior column: Approaching the anterior spinal column through the back

(posterior) of the body to perform a procedure on the vertebral body or the disc

- Devices: Autologous tissue substitute, interbody fusion device, nonautologous tissue substitute (allograft)

Posterior lumbar fusion (PLF) is performed to fuse two (or more) lumbar spine bones together along the sides of the bone. PLF is performed for various spinal conditions, including spondylolisthesis, spinal fractures, tumors, infections, and scoliosis.

Under general anesthesia, with the patient in prone (lying on the stomach) position, the back is prepped and draped. A longitudinal incision is made in the midline of the back directly over the levels to be fused. The fascia and muscle are divided and retractors used to visualize the vertebral arches. An x-ray is used to confirm the appropriate spinal level(s). The lamina, facet joints, and transverse processes are exposed on both sides of the spinous processes. At the levels to be fused, the facet joints and transverse processes are decorticated, and a bone graft is placed alongside of the vertebrae. Pedicle screws connected by titanium rods are placed at each spinal level being fused.

A complete or partial laminectomy and foraminotomy may also be performed if necessary, taking care to protect the nerve roots and neurologic structures. A laminectomy/foraminotomy performed to better access the site is considered inherent to the procedure and not coded separately. If is it done with the specific objective of decompressing a nerve root, an additional code is reported. The wound is irrigated with sterile water containing antibiotics. The deep fascial layer and subcutaneous layers are closed with sutures, and the skin is closed with stitches or surgical staples. A sterile bandage is applied.

> **Focus Point**
> Spinal fixation devices such as rods, plates, and screws are included in the fusion and are not coded separately.

> **Focus Point**
> If a physician performs a partial or total discectomy with spinal fusion, the discectomy would be coded separately.

> **Focus Point**
> Bone graft harvested from the local incision is not reported separately. However, if a separate incision is required to harvest the graft, such as from the iliac crest, this may be reported in addition to the primary procedure (fusion). This is consistent with ICD-10-PCS guideline B3.9.

© 2018 Optum360, LLC

Fusion, Lumbar, Posterior (PLF) (continued)

Focus Point

When multiple devices are used, code to the highest value, listed highest to lowest (with the same approach, body part, and qualifier):

- *Interbody Fusion Device (alone or with any other material)*
- *Autologous Tissue Substitute (alone or with nonautologous and/or with synthetic material)*
- *Nonautologous Tissue Substitute (alone or with synthetic)*
- *Synthetic Tissue Substitute*

When multiple vertebral joints are fused, each vertebral joint that uses a different device and/or a different qualifier is coded separately. See guidelines B3.10b and B3.10c.

Focus Point

When the spinal fusion procedure is performed through two separate approaches, both anterior and posterior, requiring that the patient be repositioned, two codes are reported: one for the anterior approach through the abdomen and one for the posterior approach through the back.

Focus Point

Reporting placement of bone morphogenic protein (BMP) placed during a spinal fusion is optional and at the discretion of the facility. It is reported with a code from the Administration section (3E0).

Coding Guidance

AHA: 2018, 1Q, 8; 2018, 1Q, 22; 2017, 2Q, 23; 2014, 3Q, 30; 2014, 3Q, 36; 2014, 2Q, 6-8; 2013, 3Q, 25; 2013, 1Q, 21, 29

Medical and Surgical

Gastrectomy

See also Gastrectomy, Vertical Sleeve (VSG)

See also Anastomosis, Billroth II

Body System
Gastrointestinal System

PCS Root Operation
Excision

Resection

Root Operation Table
ØDB   Gastrointestinal System, Excision

ØDT   Gastrointestinal System, Resection

Body Part
Esophagogastric Junction

Stomach

Stomach, Pylorus

Approach
Open

Percutaneous Endoscopic

Description

Gastrectomy is the surgical removal of all or part of the stomach to treat conditions such as malignancies, polyps, ulcers, or other diseases/disorders affecting the function of the stomach. Removal of a large portion of the left side of the stomach to treat obesity is referred to as a sleeve gastrectomy (*see also* Gastrectomy, Vertical Sleeve [VSG]).

What is commonly referred to as the stomach is represented by different body parts in ICD-10-PCS, with different body part values. For instance, the proximal stomach or cardia is captured in Esophagogastric Junction, the distal stomach or antrum is described with Stomach, Pylorus, and the body or fundus, captured with body part Stomach. If only a portion of one of these body parts is removed, the root operation Excision is used. If one of these body parts is removed entirely, the root operation Resection is used. If a complete, total, or radical Resection is performed, the body part Stomach captures the entire stomach and all body part values. See guideline B3.8.

Open Excision
The physician performs a partial excision of the stomach fundus using an Open approach. The physician makes a midline abdominal incision, dissects the stomach free from surrounding structures, and identifies and excises the diseased area. The defect created in the stomach is closed with sutures or a stapling device, and the incision is closed. Since only a portion of the stomach fundus was removed, Excision is reported as the root operation.

Open Resection
The physician makes a midline abdominal incision, dissects the distal stomach (pyloric antrum) free from surrounding structures, and divides the blood supply to the antrum. Next, the gastroduodenal junction is divided, and the stomach is divided in its middle portion, removing the antrum. An anastomosis is made between the stomach and the duodenum with staples or sutures. The incision is closed. The entire pyloric antrum is removed, which is reported with root operation Resection.

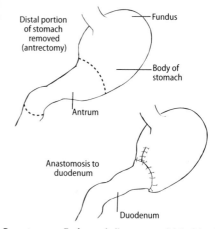

Percutaneous Endoscopic (Laparoscopic) Excision/Resection
A partial or total gastrectomy, considered a minimally invasive procedure, is commonly performed using a Percutaneous Endoscopic (laparoscopic) approach. The physician makes a 1 cm incision in the umbilicus through which the abdomen is inflated and a fiberoptic laparoscope is inserted. Other incisions are made through which trocars can be passed into the abdominal cavity to deliver instruments, a video camera, and when needed an additional light source. The physician manipulates the tools so that the stomach can be viewed through the laparoscope and/or video monitor. The rest of the procedure follows that of an Open approach.

> **Focus Point**
>
> *The anastomosis of the proximal stomach to the esophagus or the distal stomach to the duodenum is considered inherent to the procedure and not coded separately (see guideline B3.1b). If the distal stomach is removed and anastomosed to the jejunum, it is referred to as a Billroth II procedure. See also Anastomosis, Billroth II.*

Coding Guidance
AHA: 2017, 2Q, 17

© 2018 Optum360, LLC

Medical and Surgical

Gastrectomy, Vertical Sleeve (VSG)

See also Gastrectomy

See also Switch, Duodenal (Biliopancreatic Diversion)

Body System
Gastrointestinal System

PCS Root Operation
Excision

Root Operation Table
ØDB   Gastrointestinal System, Excision

Body Part
Stomach

Approach
Open
Percutaneous Endoscopic

Qualifier
Vertical

Description

Sleeve gastrectomy is used to treat morbid obesity by restricting the volume of the stomach by excising a large portion of it. The procedure can be performed as a one-stage, primary procedure or as the initial procedure in a two-stage surgery for patients with severe morbid obesity. In the two-stage procedure, the patient is required to lose a significant amount of weight after the first surgery. Months later, the patient undergoes a gastric bypass or duodenal switch procedure.

A vertical sleeve gastrectomy (VSG) can be performed using an Open or Percutaneous Endoscopic (laparoscopic) approach. The laparoscopic technique is preferred because it involves only small incisions, just large enough for trocars and instrumentation to fit that enable the physician to visualize the site and perform the procedure. The left side of the stomach (greater curvature) is removed, and the remaining portion of the stomach is greatly reduced to approximately the size and shape of a banana.

VSG is a purely restrictive procedure intended to reduce the volume of the stomach, resulting in weight loss. The nerves of the stomach and pyloric valve remain intact, thus preserving the function of the stomach. As a one-stage procedure, VSG does not require reanastomosis of the intestine, and is therefore less complex than gastric bypass or duodenal switch. The absence of bypass greatly reduces the risk of postoperative malabsorption, ulcerations, and obstruction. Additionally, no artificial device implantation is required as in laparoscopic banding, greatly reducing the risk of device complications, including erosion, migration, stricture, and infection. Some surgeons suggest prophylactic removal of the gallbladder to prevent postoperative gallstone complications associated with the procedure.

The root operation Excision is reported for this procedure, as only a portion of the stomach is removed. The qualifier value of Vertical distinguishes this procedure from other types of stomach excisions.

Focus Point
Vertical sleeve gastrectomy may also be documented as sleeve gastrectomy, vertical gastrectomy, greater curvature gastrectomy, gastric reduction, longitudinal gastrectomy, or vertical gastroplasty. Review the operative report carefully to determine the appropriate procedure code. If the documentation is incomplete or inconclusive, query the physician for clarification.

Focus Point
The duodenal switch may be done at the same time or in a staged procedure. See also Switch, Duodenal (Biliopancreatic Diversion).

Coding Guidance
AHA: 2016, 2Q, 31

Medical and Surgical

Gastrojejunostomy, Roux-en-Y (Gastric Bypass for Morbid Obesity)

Body System
Gastrointestinal System

PCS Root Operation
Bypass

Root Operation Table
0D1   Gastrointestinal System, Bypass

Body Part
Stomach

Approach
Open
Percutaneous Endoscopic

Qualifier
Jejunum

Description
Weight-loss surgery is generally performed for people who are morbidly obese with a body mass index (BMI) of 40 or higher, who have not been able to lose weight with traditional methods such as diet, exercise, and medication. It may also be performed for people with obesity with a BMI of 35 or higher who also have a weight-related risk factor such as type 2 diabetes that is difficult to control with diet, exercise, and medication.

Roux-en-Y gastric bypass (gastrojejunostomy) procedure is accomplished by creating a small stomach pouch to restrict food intake. Next, a Y-shaped section of the small intestine is attached to the pouch to allow food to bypass the lower stomach, the duodenum (the first segment of the small intestine), and the first portion of the jejunum (the second segment of the small intestine). This type of bypass reduces the amount of calories and nutrients the body absorbs. The small pouch serves as the stomach and holds only 2 to 6 ounces per serving. Initially, patients experience rapid weight loss, leveling off in 8 to 24 months at 20 percent to 40 percent above the ideal body weight.

The physician performs a gastric bypass for morbid obesity by partitioning the stomach and performing a small bowel division and anastomosis to the proximal stomach (Roux-en-Y gastrojejunostomy). This bypasses the majority of the stomach. Using an Open approach, the physician makes a midline abdominal incision. The stomach is mobilized, and the proximal stomach is divided with a stapling device along the lesser curvature, leaving only a small proximal pouch in continuity with the esophagus. A short limb of the

proximal small bowel (150 cm or less) is divided, and the distal end of the short intestinal limb is brought up and anastomosed to the proximal gastric pouch. The other end of the divided bowel is connected back into the small bowel distal to the short limb's gastric anastomosis to restore intestinal continuity. The incision is closed.

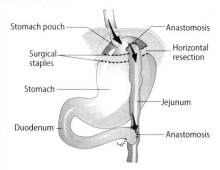

Using a Percutaneous Endoscopic approach, the physician performs a laparoscopic gastric bypass (gastrojejunostomy) for morbid obesity by partitioning the stomach and performing a small bowel division with anastomosis to the proximal stomach (Roux-en-Y gastrojejunostomy). This bypasses the majority of the stomach. The physician places a trocar though an incision above the umbilicus and insufflates the abdominal cavity. The laparoscope and additional trocars are placed through small portal incisions. The stomach is mobilized, and the proximal stomach is divided with a stapling device along the lesser curvature, leaving only a small proximal pouch in continuity with the esophagus. A short limb of the proximal small bowel (150 cm or less) is divided, and the distal end of the short intestinal limb is brought up and anastomosed to the proximal gastric pouch. The other end of the divided bowel is connected back into the small bowel distal to the short limb's gastric anastomosis to restore intestinal continuity. The instruments are removed.

Focus Point
Documentation for bypass procedures must identify the body part bypassed from and body part bypassed to. The fourth character body part specifies the body part bypassed from, and the qualifier specifies the body part bypassed to.

© 2018 Optum360, LLC

Gastroplasty, Collis

See also Fundoplication, Gastroesophageal

Body System
Gastrointestinal System

PCS Root Operation
Transfer

Root Operation Table
ØDX   Gastrointestinal System, Transfer

Body Part
Stomach

Approach
Open
Percutaneous Endoscopic

Qualifier
Esophagus

Description
A Collis gastroplasty is performed as an esophageal lengthening procedure (also called a wedge gastroplasty). It is often performed in conjunction with a separate reportable fundoplasty procedure in order to extend a short esophagus. *See also* Fundoplication, Gastroesophageal.

Collis gastroplasty may be performed using a laparoscopic (Percutaneous Endoscopic) or Open approach. Laparoscopic Collis gastroplasty is similar to other minimally invasive laparoscopic procedures. The physician makes a small incision in or just below the navel and inflates the abdomen with air to visualize the abdominal organs. The laparoscope is inserted through the incision, and the instruments to perform the Collis gastroplasty are inserted through other small incisions in the lower abdomen. A bougie (dilating instrument) is passed through the esophagus into the stomach so that the bougie spans the gastroesophageal junction. The stomach is divided along the bougie with a gastric stapler, forming a gastric tube that effectively lengthens the esophagus. The bougie is removed, and the staple line is sutured.

An Open approach is used in both transthoracic (incision in the chest) and transabdominal (incision in the abdomen) techniques. Following incision, a bougie (dilating instrument) is passed through the esophagus into the stomach so that the bougie spans the gastroesophageal junction. The stomach is divided along the bougie with a gastric stapler, forming a gastric tube that effectively lengthens the esophagus. The bougie is removed and the staple line is sutured.

Focus Point
The root operation Transfer is used since the stomach, while still maintaining its original vasculature, is modified to function as the distal esophagus.

Coding Guidance
AHA: 2016, 2Q, 22

Medical and Surgical

Gastrostomy, Percutaneous Endoscopic (PEG)

Body System
Gastrointestinal System

PCS Root Operation
Drainage

Insertion

Root Operation Table
ØD9   Gastrointestinal System, Drainage

ØDH   Gastrointestinal System, Insertion

Body Part
Stomach

Approach
Percutaneous

Device
Drainage Device (Drainage)

Feeding Device (Insertion)

Description
The gastrointestinal tract is essentially one long lumen that begins at the mouth and continues to the anus. At times, portions of the tract may be blocked or malfunctioning. During these times, the dysfunctioning site can be bypassed so that normal nutritional uptake may continue.

A percutaneous endoscopic gastrostomy (PEG) tube can help patients continue to absorb nutrients through their stomachs without requiring the use of the mouth and esophagus. This is useful in patients who are debilitated by brain injury or disease, in whom the swallowing function is impaired. Other candidates for PEG tubes are patients in whom malignancies are blocking the esophagus, or patients for whom the bypass allows the esophagus to recover following esophageal reconstruction.

In some cases, a PEG tube may be placed for decompression, when malignancy causes an obstruction preventing the natural release of gases from the intestinal tract.

The physician uses an endoscope to examine the upper gastrointestinal tract to guide placement of a PEG tube. The physician passes an endoscope through the patient's mouth into the esophagus to view the esophagus, stomach, duodenum, and sometimes the jejunum. The endoscope is used to guide the placement of a PEG tube from inside the stomach. Externally, the tube is inserted through an incision of the abdomen. The two views allow for a coordinated and accurate PEG tube placement. When in place, the tube connects the gastric lumen with the exterior abdominal wall. A PEG tube inserted percutaneously from the outside into the stomach using endoscopic guidance is reported with the approach Percutaneous. The endoscopic guidance is performed to meet the objective of the procedure and is not reported separately.

Drainage
If the PEG tube is placed for decompression, the root operation is Drainage and the device is Drainage Device.

Insertion
If the tube is placed to provide nutrition, (nutritional substances are directed through the tube directly into the stomach for digestion) the root operation is Insertion and the device is Feeding Device.

> **Focus Point**
> Review documentation carefully to determine whether the PEG tube is being placed for feeding or for decompression, as the coding is different in each circumstance.

> **Focus Point**
> Inspection of a body part(s) performed to achieve the objective of a procedure is not coded separately. Therefore, guidance using esophagogastroduodenoscopy may be required for PEG placement, but this endoscopic guidance is not reported separately. See ICD-10-PCS guideline B3.11a.

> **Focus Point**
> In some cases, a PEG tube is inserted into the stomach and an extension to the PEG tube is guided into the jejunum. This may be documented as PEG/J tube placement. In this case, report the body part Jejunum, since the jejunum is the terminal point of the tube.

Coding Guidance
AHA: 2013, 4Q, 117

© 2018 Optum360, LLC

Gender Reassignment Surgery

Body System
Anatomical Regions, General

PCS Root Operation
Creation

Root Operation Table
ØW4 Anatomical Regions, General, Creation

Body Part
Perineum, Male
Perineum, Female

Approach
Open

Device
Autologous Tissue Substitute
Synthetic Substitute
Nonautologous Tissue Substitute

Qualifier
Vagina
Penis

Description
The process of gender transformation from one sex to another occurs over a period of time in a series of staged procedures and supplemental medical treatment.

Male to female: In a series of staged procedures, the physician removes portions of the male genitalia and forms female external genitals. The penis is dissected, and portions are removed with care to preserve vital nerves and vessels to fashion a clitoris-like structure. The urethral opening is moved to a position similar to that of a normal female. A vagina is made by dissecting and opening the perineum. This opening is lined using pedicle or split-thickness grafts. Labia are created out of skin from the scrotum and adjacent tissue. A stent or obturator is usually left in place in the newly created vagina for three weeks or longer.

Female to male: In a series of staged procedures, the physician forms a penis and scrotum using pedicle flap grafts and free skin grafts. Portions of the clitoris are used as well as the adjacent skin. Prostheses are often placed in the penis to make it sexually functional. Prosthetic testicles are fixed in the scrotum. The vagina is closed or removed.

Focus Point
The coding of sex change operations requires that the body part value identify the current sex of the patient—either body part Perineum, Male or body part Perineum, Female, while the qualifier value identifies the body part being created as either a Vagina or a Penis.

If a separate procedure is performed to harvest autogenous tissue, it is coded to the appropriate root operation in addition to the primary creation operation.

Genioplasty, Augmentation

Body System
Anatomical Regions, General

PCS Root Operation
Alteration

Root Operation Table
ØWØ   Anatomical Regions, General, Alteration

Body Part
Lower Jaw

Approach
Open

Device
Autologous Tissue Substitute
Synthetic Substitute
Nonautologous Tissue Substitute

Description
Augmentation genioplasty is plastic surgery on the chin that involves the addition of bone or other tissue by graft or implant to increase size, symmetry, or otherwise improve the appearance of the chin.

The physician places an Autologous Tissue Substitute, Synthetic Substitute or Nonautologous Tissue Substitute implant or a graft onto the chin to augment or enlarge it. Various materials can be used, including tissue grafted from the patient's own body or a tissue bank, or synthetic prosthetic devices such as silicone may also be used. This procedure is most commonly performed from an intraoral approach. The physician makes an Open incision in the mandibular labial vestibule inside the lower lip. The mucosa is then reflected from the chin and the implanted material placed between the mucosa and the bone. An Open skin incision may also be made under the chin. The implant may be secured to the bone using wires or screws or may simply be held in place by the surrounding tissue. The incisions are then sutured closed.

Focus Point
Augmentation genioplasty for cosmetic purposes, performed solely to improve the patient's appearance, is assigned to the ICD-10-PCS root operation Alteration because it is performed to modify the natural anatomic structure of a body part without affecting its function.

Alteration is coded for all procedures performed solely to improve appearance and includes all methods, approaches, and devices used for the objective of improving appearance. Because chin augmentation with a chin implant is usually a cosmetic procedure, reporting with root operation Supplement rather than Alteration requires diagnostic confirmation that the surgery is in fact being performed for a medically necessary reason, rather than to improve appearance.

© 2018 Optum360, LLC

Medical and Surgical

Graft, Arteriovenous (AV)

Body System
Upper Arteries

PCS Root Operation
Bypass

Root Operation Table
Ø31   Upper Arteries, Bypass

Body Part
Brachial Artery, Right
Brachial Artery, Left
Radial Artery, Right
Radial Artery, Left

Approach
Open

Device
Synthetic Substitute

Qualifier
Upper Arm Vein
Lower Arm Vein

Description
Although an arteriovenous (AV) fistula is the preferred method of vascular access for hemodialysis, an arteriovenous graft can be used for patients who are not good candidates for AV fistula, such as older patients or those with inadequate or smaller veins.

Surgical technique for an arteriovenous graft for dialysis may vary depending on the site selected for dialysis access and associated factors. Using an Open approach through an incision, usually in the skin over an artery in the nondominant wrist or antecubital fossa, the physician isolates a desired section of artery and neighboring vein. Vessel clamps are placed on the vein and adjacent artery. The vein is dissected free and divided, and synthetic tubing made of Teflon or fabric is attached on one end to the artery and the other to the vein, allowing blood to flow both down the artery and into the vein. The skin incision is repaired with layered closure. The tube is then punctured during the performance of the dialysis. This graft takes only about two to three weeks to mature but it is more prone to infection and clots than the AV fistula.

The arteriovenous graft is reported with the root operation Bypass, which includes as part of its definition the rerouting of the contents (blood) of a body part (artery) to a downstream area (vein) of the normal route. The upper stream—or "from"—is the artery, which is represented by the body part Radial or Brachial, and the downstream—or "to"—is the vein, reported with the appropriate Upper Arm Vein or Lower Arm Vein qualifier value. The device value differentiates the AV graft from the AV fistula with the use of Synthetic Substitute for the graft as compared with No Device for the fistula.

Focus Point
A possible complication of an AV graft is clotting with thrombus. When declotting or thrombectomy of the graft is performed without the removal or replacement of the existing graft, the root operation Revision is reported.

Coding Guidance
AHA: 2016, 3Q, 37, 39; 2013, 1Q, 27

Graft, Dura Mater, Intracranial

See also Decompression, Posterior Fossa (Chiari Malformation)

Body System
Central Nervous System and Cranial Nerves

PCS Root Operation
Supplement

Root Operation Table
ØØU   Central Nervous System and Cranial Nerves, Supplement

Body Part
Dura Mater

Approach
Open

Device
Autologous Tissue Substitute
Synthetic Substitute
Nonautologous Tissue Substitute

Qualifier
No Qualifier

Description
During a separately reportable procedure performed via an Open craniotomy, it is sometimes necessary to graft or Supplement the intracranial dura mater to expand the space or to correct a dural/cerebrospinal fluid leak or pseudomeningocele.

At the end of an Open procedure during which the dura mater has been incised, the physician prepares a graft. Suction is used to keep the incision free of cerebral spinal fluid. Single dural stitches may be used to close the dura mater. A patch of synthetic or biologic material or pericranial autograft tissue from the patient's scalp tissue just outside the skull is sutured into place using a needle passed through the graft, which is tied down outside of the area of dura repaired to achieve watertight closure. If the dural defect is small and difficult to access, the graft may be placed inside the dura. The dural patch is sutured and covered with a sealant to prevent cerebrospinal fluid (CSF) leakage. After verifying that the repair is watertight, the surgeon sutures the incision site closed in layers and covers it with a dressing.

Focus Point
Graft material may include material from the patient's own body (autologous), a synthetic implant such as silicone, or material from another living or biologic source (nonautologous).

Focus Point
Autograft pericranial tissue harvested from the operative site is not reported separately, but an additional code can be assigned for Autologous Tissue Substitute (graft) harvested from a separate incision site, according to ICD-10-PCS guideline B3.9.

Focus Point
If a composite graft consisting of a mixture of biologic cellular or acellular material and synthetic material is used for the graft, assign the qualifier Nonautologous Tissue Substitute. Composite material always has a biologic component and therefore is always coded as a nonautologous tissue substitute.

Coding Guidance
AHA: 2017, 3Q, 10; 2015, 4Q, 39; 2014, 3Q, 24; 2014, 2Q, 6

© 2018 Optum360, LLC

Graft, Skin, Split-Thickness (STSG)

Body System
Skin and Breast

PCS Root Operation
Replacement

Root Operation Table
ØHR   Skin and Breast, Replacement

Body Part
Refer to the ICD-10-PCS tabular list for a complete list of body parts.

Approach
External

Device
Autologous Tissue Substitute
Nonautologous Tissue Substitute

Qualifier
Partial Thickness

Description
The skin consists of two layers, the epidermis and dermis. A split-thickness skin graft (STSG) includes the epidermis and part of the dermis. The thickness of the graft depends on the donor site and the needs of the patient. Depending on how much of the dermis is included, an STSG may be thin, intermediate (medium), or thick. STSG is used to cover a large skin defect or injury, often in cases of deep or extensive burns, to provide coverage and promote healing. It may be placed as a meshed (with slits or cuts) or a sheet (whole) graft. Skin harvested from one location and grafted to another on the same individual is termed an Autologous Tissue Substitute. Tissue bank grafts and skin substitute products are reported as Nonautologous Tissue Substitute.

Under appropriate anesthesia, the physician takes a dermal autograft from one area of the body and grafts it to an area in need of repair. This procedure is performed when direct wound closure or adjacent tissue transfer is not possible. A dermal skin graft is harvested by first raising a split-thickness skin graft 0.010 to 0.015 inches in depth with a dermatome, but not removing it. The dermatome is adjusted to remove the desired graft, and a second pass is made over the newly created donor site at that depth to remove a dermal layer autograft.

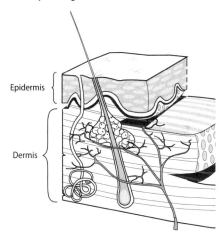

The graft may then be used for grafting with or without meshing by passing it through a meshing device. Meshing the graft allows the graft surface area to be expanded up to nine times the donor site surface area. This may be indicated in large wounds such as major burns. The recipient wound bed is prepared for grafting using saline irrigation and debridement of any nonviable tissue and contaminants. Once the recipient site has been prepared, the graft is placed over the wound bed, dermal side down. The graft is then secured in place by suturing the graft to the surrounding wound bed with absorbable sutures. A nonadherent dressing is applied. Negative-pressure wound therapy (NPWT) with a vacuum-assisted closure (VAC) device may be applied to enhance healing.

Focus Point
Debridement done as preparation of the wound bed for the graft is not reported separately unless the debridement includes layers deeper than skin level.

Focus Point
The harvesting of an autograft from a different procedure site is coded separately, according to guideline B3.9.

Coding Guidance
AHA: 2014, 3Q, 14

Harvest, Graft, Autologous Bone Marrow

See also Biopsy, Bone Marrow

See also Therapy, Bone Marrow Cell, Autologous, Intramuscular in the New Technology section

See also Transplant, Bone Marrow (BMT) in the Medical and Surgical related section, Administration

Body System
Lymphatic and Hemic Systems

PCS Root Operation
Extraction

Root Operation Table
Ø7D   Lymphatic and Hemic Systems, Extraction

Body Part
Bone Marrow, Sternum
Bone Marrow, Iliac
Bone Marrow, Vertebral

Approach
Open
Percutaneous

Device
No Device

Qualifier
No Qualifier

Description

Bone marrow is a fatty substance within bone cavities that helps form blood cells and contains stem cells. Bone marrow may be harvested for transplantation into the bloodstream, to be used in combination with other graft materials for bone grafts or for injection into the muscles. An autologous transplant uses the patient's own bone marrow for the transplant. The harvested bone marrow is usually obtained from a large bone such as the iliac crest or sternum.

Once harvested, the bone marrow is processed with a centrifuge to remove blood and bone fragments and may be used immediately or cryopreserved for later transplantation. If cryopreserved, at the time of transplantation the bone marrow is thawed and infused into the bloodstream of the recipient through an intravenous catheter.

Bone marrow graft harvest procedures are routinely performed with a needle via a Percutaneous approach but can be performed using an Open approach.

With the patient under the appropriate anesthesia, the skin over the bone is first cleaned with an antiseptic solution. A local anesthetic is injected at the site, and the bone extraction needle is inserted into the marrow in the center of the bone using a Percutaneous approach. The needle is rotated to the right, to the left, withdrawn, and reinserted at a different angle. This procedure is repeated in an alternating clockwise/counterclockwise motion until the holes in the needle contain sufficient bone marrow. Once the needle is in place, the stylet is removed by pulling it straight out, and a syringe is connected. The bone marrow is extracted through the needle with the syringe. Several bone punctures may be required to extract sufficient bone marrow for transplant. A bandage is applied to the collection sites. The specimen contains bone marrow whose structure has not been disturbed or destroyed.

During an Open procedure, the provider cuts through the skin and all other body layers such as fascia and muscle to expose the site of the procedure and obtains the bone marrow using drills, trephines, or a biopsy needle.

Focus Point
According to ICD-10-PCS guideline B3.4a, biopsy of bone marrow is coded to the root operation Extraction with the qualifier Diagnostic.

Focus Point
Bone marrow graft harvested from the local incision or operative site is not reported separately. However, if a separate incision in a different body part/location is required to harvest the graft, such as from the pelvis or iliac crest, this may be reported in addition to the primary procedure, according to ICD-10-PCS guideline B3.9.

Coding Guidance
AHA: 2017, 4Q, 74; 2015, 1Q, 30; 2013, Q4, 111

© 2018 Optum360, LLC

Harvesting, Knee Chondrocytes

See also Implantation, Autologous Chondrocyte (ACI), Knee

Body System
Lower Joints

PCS Root Operation
Excision

Root Operation Table
ØSB   Lower Joints, Excision

Body Part
Knee Joint, Right
Knee Joint, Left

Approach
Percutaneous Endoscopic

Description

Autologous chondrocyte implantation (ACI) is performed to treat knee defects caused by damage to the hyaline cartilage in acute or repetitive trauma, or due to a prior surgical procedure. This is a two-stage procedure in which some of the patient's own cartilage is collected from a minor load-bearing area within the knee during an arthroscopic procedure during the first stage. The harvested chondrocytes are sent to a special laboratory where they are isolated from the cartilage matrix and cultured for three to four weeks to increase the number of viable cells. The cells are returned in suspension for surgical implantation during the second stage.

The chondrocytes are harvested during the first stage. After administration of a local anesthetic, the physician removes a small amount of articular cartilage from a healthy, non-weight-bearing section of the knee joint using a Percutaneous Endoscopic approach. The harvested cartilage is transferred to a laboratory, which isolates the chondrocytes. The arthroscopic harvesting of cartilage typically takes less than 30 minutes to perform.

Focus Point
For the implantation of the harvested chondrocytes, see Implantation, Autologous Chondrocyte (ACI), Knee.

Hemicolectomy

Medical and Surgical

Body System
Gastrointestinal System

PCS Root Operation
Resection

Root Operation Table
ØDT   Gastrointestinal System, Resection

Body Part
Large Intestine, Right
Large Intestine, Left

Approach
Open
Percutaneous Endoscopic

Description
Right or left hemicolectomy procedures are performed for conditions such as malignant neoplasms, diverticulitis, inflammatory bowel diseases, volvulus, ischemia, infection, or trauma.

Right hemicolectomy involves removing the cecum, ascending colon, hepatic flexure, the proximal to mid portion of the transverse colon, and a distal portion of the ileum. When a right hemicolectomy is performed, the root operation reported is Resection with the body part value Large Intestine, Right.

Left hemicolectomy refers to the removal of a distal portion of the transverse colon, the descending colon, and sigmoid colon to the level of the upper rectum. When a left hemicolectomy is performed, the root operation is Resection with the body part value Large Intestine, Left.

In ICD-10-PCS, the right or left large intestine (colon) is defined as its own body part. Resection includes all of a body part, or any subdivision of a body part that has its own body part value in ICD-10-PCS, while Excision includes only a portion of a body part. If the surgeon removes the entire subdivision of the body part with its own body part value (the right or left half of the large intestine), the correct root operation is Resection.

For both left and right hemicolectomies, bowel function is restored either by connecting the remaining bowel ends (called anastomosis) or by creating a colostomy. End-to-side or side-to-side anastomosis can by performed by stapling or suturing. Any anastomosis method is inherent in the resection and is not coded separately. The formation of a colostomy involves pulling the end of the intestine

through a hole or stoma in the abdominal wall for external excretion and requires an additional code from the root operation Bypass table.

Open Hemicolectomy
For a traditional open hemicolectomy, reported with ICD-10-PCS approach value Open, the physician makes a midline abdominal incision. The large laparotomy incision allows direct visualization and direct access to the abdominal cavity. The colon is mobilized, and the selected segments of bowel are isolated and divided proximally and distally to the remaining bowel and removed. The remaining bowel ends are reapproximated using staples or sutures, or a colostomy is formed. The peritoneum is closed with running Vicryl, fascia with running Vicryl, skin with clips. Sterile dressings are applied.

Laparoscopic Hemicolectomy
Laparoscopic hemicolectomy is reported with the ICD-10-PCS approach value of Percutaneous Endoscopic. Laparoscopic colon removal involves a 1.5 cm incision near the umbilicus to place the camera (laparoscope) with two or more small incisions made for other instruments. The Hasson trocar is placed into the abdominal cavity, and gas insufflation is initiated. A laparoscope is inserted to visualize the abdominal cavity, and trocars are placed. The inserted instruments (trocars) are used to mobilize and divide the colon. The colon is extracted through the incisions, and the remaining ends of the colon are reattached. The advantages of laparoscopic colectomy over open colectomy are shorter length of hospital stay and better outcomes for postoperative morbidity and mortality.

Focus Point
According to ICD-10-PCS guideline B3.1b, the anastomosis, regardless of technique, is not reported separately as it is considered a component in the surgery and a procedural step to the closing; only the resection code is assigned.

Focus Point
If the sigmoid colon alone is resected, the sigmoidectomy is coded using the body part value Sigmoid Colon. The root operation depends on whether partial (Excision) or total (Resection) sigmoidectomy is performed.

Coding Guidance
AHA: 2014, 4Q, 42; 2014, 3Q, 6

© 2018 Optum360, LLC

Hemorrhoidectomy

Body System
Lower Veins

PCS Root Operation
Excision

Root Operation Table
Ø6B   Lower Veins, Excision

Body Part
Lower Vein

Approach
Open

Qualifier
Hemorrhoidal Plexus

Description
Hemorrhoids are swollen, painful veins in the rectum and anus that are caused by increased pressure that causes the veins to bulge. Patients who suffer from hemorrhoids often have difficulty sitting due to the swelling of the veins, itching, and swelling of the anus. The most common causes of hemorrhoids include prolonged sitting, constipation, or straining during bowel movements. Hemorrhoids are also a common complication of pregnancy and childbirth, or may manifest secondary to the effects of other chronic diseases.

Hemorrhoids are classified as internal or external, meaning that external hemorrhoids are those around the outside under the skin of the anus, and internal hemorrhoids are inside the anus or rectum. Treatment of hemorrhoids usually consists of topical methods intended to decrease discomfort, unless complications develop that require further intervention. Complications of hemorrhoids include bleeding from the varicosities, or thrombus (clot) formations. These complications are treated with a variety of relatively minor surgical procedures that remove the clot, coagulate the area of hemorrhage, or excise, ligate (i.e., tie-off), and inject the offending vein.

If conservative measures to treat hemorrhoids are unsuccessful, a surgical excision of the hemorrhoidal veins (qualifier Hemorrhoidal Plexus) may be required.

The physician performs the root operation Excision of internal and external hemorrhoids using an Open approach. The physician explores the anal canal and identifies the hemorrhoid column. An incision is made in the rectal mucosa around the hemorrhoids, and the lesions are dissected from the underlying sphincter muscles and removed. The incisions are closed with sutures.

Medical and Surgical

Herniorrhaphy, Femoral

Body System
Anatomical Regions, Lower Extremities

PCS Root Operation
Repair

Supplement

Root Operation Table
ØYQ Anatomical Regions, Lower Extremities, Repair

ØYU Anatomical Regions, Lower Extremities,
        Supplement

Body Part
Femoral Region, Right

Femoral Region, Left

Femoral Region, Bilateral

Approach
Open

Percutaneous Endoscopic

Description
A hernia occurs when part of an organ or other tissue protrudes through a weak point or a tear in the overlying muscular wall and fascia. A femoral hernia is protrusion of a loop of intestine or other tissue into the femoral canal. The femoral canal is tubular passage in the groin just below the inguinal ligament through which the femoral artery, other blood vessels, and nerves pass. In ICD-10-PCS the body system Anatomical Regions, Lower Extremity contains the body part Femoral Region with specific values for right, left, and bilateral.

Femoral hernias are more common in women and may be caused by congenital (defects at birth), childbirth-related, or age-related weaknesses in the abdominal walls.

Femoral hernias can be repaired using a laparoscopic or open approach. Laparoscopic hernia repair is similar to other minimally invasive laparoscopic procedures. The physician makes a small incision in or just below the navel and inflates the abdomen with air to visualize the abdominal organs. The laparoscope is inserted through the incision, and the instruments to repair the hernia are inserted through other small incisions in the lower abdomen.

Most laparoscopic herniorrhaphies are performed using either the transabdominal preperitoneal (TAPP) approach or the total extraperitoneal (TEP) approach. The TAPP approach involves placing laparoscopic trocars in the abdominal cavity and entering the peritoneal space for dissection, allowing the mesh to be placed and covered with peritoneum. In the TEP procedure, an inflatable balloon is insufflated in the extraperitoneal space, pushing the peritoneum posteriorly, creating a working space for the laparoscope. This is similar to the TAPP approach, except that the peritoneum is never entered. The mesh can be held in place using staples or by the pressure of the peritoneum after removing the balloon.

Using an Open approach, the physician makes an incision over the femoral canal. Dissection is continued through scar tissue, and the hernia sac is identified and dissected from surrounding structures. The hernia contents may be reduced or the hernia sac opened and the contents examined. The hernia sac may be ligated and resected. The physician may implant a graft or prosthesis of mesh or other material to strengthen and reinforce the hernia repair.

Repair
The root operation Repair involves restoring the body part—in this case, the femoral canal and surrounding structures—to their normal anatomic structure and function. Use the root operation Repair when the femoral hernia repair does not use a tissue graft or synthetic substitute such as mesh.

Supplement
The root operation Supplement involves repair of the tear or weakness in the femoral canal with the use of biological or synthetic material, such as a tissue graft or mesh. The tissue graft or synthetic material is used to reinforce or augment the muscles and fascia in the femoral region.

© 2018 Optum360, LLC

Herniorrhaphy, Inguinal

Body System
Anatomical Regions, Lower Extremities

PCS Root Operation
Repair

Supplement

Root Operation Table
ØYQ Anatomical Regions, Lower Extremities, Repair

ØYU Anatomical Regions, Lower Extremities, Supplement

Body Part
Inguinal Region, Right

Inguinal Region, Left

Inguinal Region, Bilateral

Approach
Open

Percutaneous Endoscopic

Description
A hernia occurs when part of an organ or other tissue protrudes through a weak point or tear in the overlying muscular wall and fascia. An inguinal hernia is protrusion of a loop of intestine or, less commonly, the urinary bladder into the inguinal canal. The inguinal canal is tubular passage through the lower layers of the abdominal wall. In ICD-10-PCS the body system Anatomical Regions, Lower Extremity contains the body part Inguinal Region with specific values for Right, Left, and Bilateral.

Hernias may be caused by congenital (defects at birth) or age-related weaknesses in the abdominal walls. In males, they are often congenital and caused by an improper closure of the abdominal cavity. They can also be caused by an increase in pressure within the abdominal cavity due to heavy lifting, straining, violent coughing, obesity, or pregnancy.

Inguinal hernias can be repaired using a laparoscopic or open approach. Laparoscopic hernia repair is similar to other minimally invasive laparoscopic procedures. The physician makes a small incision in or just below the navel and inflates the abdomen with air to visualize the abdominal organs. The laparoscope is inserted through the incision and the instruments to repair the hernia are inserted through other small incisions in the lower abdomen.

Most laparoscopic herniorrhaphies are performed using either the transabdominal preperitoneal (TAPP) or the total extraperitoneal (TEP) approach. The TAPP approach involves placing laparoscopic trocars in the abdominal cavity and entering the peritoneal space for dissection, allowing the mesh to be placed and covered with peritoneum. In the TEP procedure, an inflatable balloon is insufflated in the extraperitoneal space, pushing the peritoneum posteriorly and creating a working space for the laparoscope. This is similar to the TAPP approach, except that the peritoneum is never entered. The mesh can be held in place using staples or by the pressure of the peritoneum after removing the balloon.

Using an open approach, the physician makes a groin incision. Dissection is continued through scar tissue, and the spermatic cord and hernia sac are identified and dissected from surrounding structures. The hernia contents may be reduced or the hernia sac opened and the contents examined. The hernia sac may be ligated and resected. The physician may implant a graft or prosthesis of mesh or other material to strengthen and reinforce the hernia repair.

Repair
The root operation Repair involves restoring the body part, in this case the inguinal region, inguinal canal, or inguinal triangle, to its normal anatomic structure and function. Use the root operation Repair when the inguinal hernia repair does not use a tissue graft or synthetic substitute such as mesh.

Supplement
The root operation Supplement involves repair of the inguinal hernia with the use of biological or synthetic material, such as a tissue graft or mesh. The tissue graft or synthetic material is used to reinforce or augment the muscles and fascia in the inguinal region.

© 2018 Optum360, LLC

Herniorrhaphy, Paraesophageal (Diaphragmatic)

Body System
Respiratory System

PCS Root Operation
Repair
Supplement

Root Operation Table
ØBQ   Respiratory System, Repair
ØBU   Respiratory System, Supplement

Body Part
Diaphragm

Approach
Open
Percutaneous Endoscopic

Device
No Device (Repair)
Autologous Tissue Substitute (Supplement)
Synthetic Substitute (Supplement)
Nonautologous Tissue Substitute (Supplement)

Description
A paraesophageal herniorrhaphy is performed on patients with a paraesophageal hiatal hernia, which occurs when the gastroesophageal (GE) junction remains in its normal anatomic position but the upper part of the stomach pushes through an opening in the diaphragm, called the esophageal or diaphragmatic hiatus, and up into the chest next to the esophagus. The stomach cannot return to its normal anatomic position. This is different from a "sliding" hiatal hernia, in which the stomach may slide back into its normal place.

Repair
Under general anesthesia, using an Open abdominal approach, the physician makes an incision across the abdomen. The herniated stomach is returned to its appropriate position in the abdomen, and the hernia sac is cut away and removed. The enlarged opening in the diaphragm through which the esophagus passes is narrowed by placing sutures in the two pillars connecting the spinal column and the diaphragm. The physician may reform the stomach, cut the vagus nerve, or alter the size of the stomach-intestinal opening, as well. Drains are placed and the wound is sutured closed.

Alternatively, the Open approach may be thoracic or thoracoabdominal. The physician makes an incision across the chest, which may be extended into the upper abdomen. Tissues are dissected and the esophagus, diaphragm, and upper part of the stomach are exposed. The connective tissue is used to stitch folds or tucks into the diaphragm to restore it to its original position. Drains are placed, and the incision is closed with sutures or staples.

In a Percutaneous Endoscopic repair, the physician makes several tiny incisions through which the laparoscope and surgical instruments are inserted, which are used to reposition the herniated stomach and repair the hernia defect with direct sutures.

Supplement
Under general anesthesia, using an Open abdominal approach, the physician makes an incision across the abdomen. The herniated stomach is returned to its appropriate position in the abdomen, and the hernia sac is cut away and removed. The enlarged opening in the diaphragm through which the esophagus passes is narrowed by placing biologic or synthetic mesh in the defect. The physician may reform the stomach, cut the vagus nerve, or alter the size of the stomach-intestinal opening, as well. Drains are placed and the wound is sutured closed.

Alternatively, the Open approach may be thoracic or thoracoabdominal. The physician makes an incision across the chest, which may be extended into the upper abdomen. Tissues are dissected and the esophagus, diaphragm, and upper part of the stomach are exposed. The enlarged opening in the diaphragm through which the esophagus passes is narrowed by placing biologic or synthetic mesh in the defect. Drains are placed and the incision is closed with sutures or staples.

In a Percutaneous Endoscopic approach, the physician makes several tiny incisions through which the laparoscope and the surgical instruments are inserted, which are used to reposition the herniated stomach and repair the hernia defect with mesh.

Focus Point
The diaphragm is classified to the Respiratory body system in ICD-10-PCS.

Focus Point
Report concomitant Nissen fundoplication for gastroesophageal reflux as a separate procedure, using root operation Restriction.

Coding Guidance
AHA: 2014, 3Q, 28

© 2018 Optum360, LLC

Herniorrhaphy, Ventral, Incisional (Hernia Repair)

Body System
Anatomical Regions, General

PCS Root Operation
Repair

Supplement

Root Operation Table
ØWQ Anatomical Regions, General, Repair

ØWU Anatomical Regions, General, Supplement

Body Part
Abdominal Wall

Approach
Open

Percutaneous Endoscopic

Device
No Device (Repair)

Synthetic Substitute (Supplement)

Description
A ventral, incisional herniorrhaphy is the repair of a tear or bulge through an opening in the abdominal muscles usually occurring at a previous surgical site.

Repair
Under general anesthesia, the physician makes an incision over the hernia using an Open approach. Dissection is continued through scar tissue, and the hernia sac is identified and dissected from surrounding structures. The fascial defect is identified circumferentially. The hernia is reduced, and the hernia sac may be resected. The hernia defect is closed with sutures. The incision is closed.

In a Percutaneous Endoscopic repair, the physician makes several small abdominal incisions and inflates the abdomen with air to visualize the abdominal organs. The laparoscope is inserted through the incision, and the surgical instruments to repair the hernia are inserted through other small incisions in the lower abdomen.

Supplement
The physician repairs an incisional, ventral, or other anterior abdominal wall hernia. Under general anesthesia, the physician makes an incision over the hernia using an Open approach. Dissection is continued through scar tissue, and the hernia sac is identified and dissected from surrounding structures. The fascial defect is identified circumferentially. The hernia is reduced, and the hernia sac may be resected. The hernia defect is closed with mesh or some other prosthetic material. The incision is closed.

In contrast, a Percutaneous Endoscopic approach may also be used. The laparoscopic repair of incisional, or ventral, hernias involves the placement of a synthetic patch into the abdomen through small trocar incisions.

Coding Guidance
AHA: 2014, 4Q, 38; 2014, 1Q, 4-5

© 2018 Optum360, LLC

Hysterectomy

Body System
Female Reproductive System

PCS Root Operation
Resection

Root Operation Table
0UT   Female Reproductive System, Resection

Body Part
Uterus

Approach
Open

Percutaneous Endoscopic

Via Natural or Artificial Opening

Via Natural or Artificial Opening Endoscopic

Via Natural or Artificial Opening With Percutaneous Endoscopic Assistance (Uterus)

Qualifier
Supracervical

No Qualifier

Description

Hysterectomy is surgery to remove the uterus with or without the cervix. A total hysterectomy includes the resection of the uterus and cervix. When performed abdominally, this is documented as TAH, or total abdominal hysterectomy. A total hysterectomy may be performed via an Open abdominal approach, laparoscopically via a Percutaneous Endoscopic approach, or by accessing the uterus through the vagina, with or without laparoscopic assistance. Percutaneous endoscopic assistance in a vaginal hysterectomy is documented as an LAVH, or laparoscopically assisted vaginal hysterectomy. In LAVH, the uterus and cervix are resected. Without laparoscopic assistance, a vaginal hysterectomy may be documented as TVH (total vaginal hysterectomy).

In some cases, the ovaries and fallopian tubes are removed during a hysterectomy. This is separately reported and documented as a BSO, or bilateral salpingo-oophorectomy. Documentation may read TVH/BSO to indicate all organs resected.

A "partial" or "subtotal" hysterectomy removes the uterus but does not remove the cervix. This is reported with qualifier "Supracervical." If the uterine Resection is performed through the vagina with laparoscopic assistance, it may be documented as a LASH or LSH, for laparoscopically-assisted supracervical hysterectomy. For an abdominal approach, documentation may state SAH, for subtotal abdominal hysterectomy.

In a radical hysterectomy, the uterus and cervix are resected as well as structures surrounding the uterus. This procedure is usually limited to diagnoses of

malignancy and is sometimes called a Schauta operation.

In an Open, or abdominal, hysterectomy the surgeon makes either a vertical midline incision or a horizontal incision just within the pubic hairline through which the physician removes the uterus and may elect to remove the cervix. The supporting pedicles containing the tubes, ligaments, and arteries are clamped and cut free. The abdominal incision is closed by suturing.

In a laparoscopic, or Percutaneous Endoscopic hysterectomy, the patient is placed in the dorsal lithotomy position. After inserting a speculum in the vagina, the physician grasps the cervix with an instrument to manipulate the uterus during the surgery. A trocar is inserted periumbilically, and the abdomen is insufflated with gas. Additional trocars are placed in the right and left lower quadrants. The uterus is dissected free from the bladder and surrounding tissue. Coagulation is achieved with the aid of electrocautery instruments. Alternatively, some vessels may be ligated. The uterus is morcellized and removed using endoscopic tools. The uterus and one or both ovaries and/or one or both fallopian tubes are removed in similar fashion. Once the excisions are complete, the abdominal cavity is deflated and instruments and trocars removed. The fascia and skin are closed with sutures.

In a vaginal hysterectomy, reported with the approach Via Natural or Artificial Opening, an incision is made around the cervix through the full thickness of the vaginal membrane. The cut vaginal edge is pulled toward the lower cervix, and vaginal dissection is continued with countertraction. The posterior peritoneum is opened to admit a finger examination of the pelvis. The uterosacral ligaments are clamped and possibly shortened, cut from the uterus, and secured to the vagina. The vesicovaginal space is entered. The connective tissue fusing the bladder and vagina is dissected, and the bladder is separated from the cervix. The bladder pillars are clamped, cut, and ligated near their cervical attachments, as well as the cardinal ligament tissue on each side of the cervix and the left and right uterine vessels. The physician clamps, cuts, and ligates the upper cardinal and lower broad ligament complex. Traction applied to the cervix moves the uterus down until the fundus is low in the pelvis. Hemostats are applied to the angle of the uterus on each side, and the physician removes the uterus above the cervix. The peritoneum is closed with purse-string sutures that incorporate the proximal part of the uterosacral ligaments. In some cases, the physician inserts a laparoscope into the patient's abdomen to enhance visualization of the surgical field. This is a laparoscopically assisted vaginal hysterectomy, reported with the approach Via Natural

© 2018 Optum360, LLC

Hysterectomy (continued)

or Artificial Opening With Percutaneous Endoscopic Assistance.

Focus Point

If, in the performance of a laparoscopic or vaginal hysterectomy, the procedure is converted to an Open (abdominal) procedure, report the appropriate Inspection code to identify the aborted approach. For example, in the case of an attempted laparoscopic total hysterectomy converted to Open procedure, report Inspection of Uterus and Cervix, Percutaneous Endoscopic approach, in addition to the code for open resection of the uterus.

Focus Point

When coding radical hysterectomy procedures in ICD-10-PCS, code separately the organs or structures that are actually removed for which there is a distinctly defined body part, using either root operation Excision or Resection depending on the extent of the structures removed. Use the ICD-10-PCS Body Part Key to help define body parts.

Focus Point

In a robotic-assisted laparoscopic hysterectomy, the robotic assistance may be coded in addition to the primary procedure.

Coding Guidance

AHA: 2017, 4Q, 68; 2015, 1Q 33; 2014, 4Q, 34; 2013, 3Q, 28

Implant, Cochlear (CI)

Body System
Ear, Nose, Sinus

PCS Root Operation
Insertion

Root Operation Table
Ø9H   Ear, Nose, Sinus, Insertion

Body Part
Inner Ear, Right
Inner Ear, Left

Approach
Open

Device
Hearing Device, Single Channel Cochlear Prosthesis
Hearing Device, Multiple Channel Cochlear Prosthesis

Description
A cochlear implant is a surgically implanted electronic device that stimulates the nerve endings within the inner ear, providing a sense of sound to a person who is profoundly deaf or severely hard of hearing. The implants are equipped with software that allows for different programming specific to the patient's daily activities. Threshold levels, volume, pulse widths, live-voice speech adjustments, input dynamic range, and frequency shaping templates can be evaluated and set according to individual needs.

A cochlear implant consists of one or more external microphones that pick up sound from the environment; an external speech processor that filters sound, splits it into channels (Single or Multiple), and sends the sound signals through a thin cable to a transmitter; and a transmitter, which may be a coil held in place by a magnet placed behind the external ear.

The transmitter sends the power and sound to the internal receiver and stimulator that are surgically implanted in the skull bone. The receiver and stimulator convert the signals into electric impulses and send them through an internal cable to an electrode array that winds through the cochlea. The cochlea transmits the electric impulses through the auditory nerve system to the brain, which recognizes them as sound. The external system may be worn entirely behind the ear or its parts may be worn in a pocket, belt pouch, or harness.

Using an Open approach, which allows direct visualization of the operative site, the physician makes a U-shaped incision, creating a skin flap well behind the mastoid, and drills a circular depression in the squamous portion of the temporal bone in which the internal coil will be housed. The mastoid air cells are removed with a drill, and a facial recess approach is used. The bony ear canal is preserved. The internal coil is secured in the depressed area of the temporal bone, and the electrode is introduced through the facial recess and the round window into the cochlea. The ground wire attached to the internal coil is introduced into the temporalis muscle. The incision is sutured.

Focus Point
This procedure is reported with the root operation Insertion, which represents procedures with the sole objective of putting in a nonbiological appliance (device) that assists or performs a physiological function without physically taking the place of the body part and doing nothing else to the body part.

Focus Point
A single procedure code is used to report the implantation of the receiver (within skull) and insertion of electrode(s) in the cochlea.

© 2018 Optum360, LLC

Implantation, Artificial Urinary Sphincter (AUS)

Body System
Urinary System

PCS Root Operation
Insertion

Root Operation Table
ØTH   Urinary System, Insertion

Body Part
Bladder Neck
Urethra

Approach
Open

Device
Artificial Sphincter

Description
An artificial urinary sphincter is a device that mimics the function of a biological urinary sphincter. The artificial urinary sphincter system is filled with saline, using the fluid in a pressure-regulating balloon reservoir to open and close a cuff surrounding the urethra or the bladder neck. When the patient needs to urinate, a pump in the scrotum or labia is squeezed and released several times to remove fluid from the cuff, allowing urine to flow out of the bladder. The cuff automatically refills with saline in a few minutes, squeezing the urethra closed to restore bladder control.

The most common use is to treat men with post prostatectomy urinary incontinence. In men, the cuff is usually implanted around the bulbous urethra. Bladder neck placement is most often used in young men and in patients who need frequent catheterization, and is always used for females and small children. The pressure-regulating balloon (PRB) is usually implanted next to the bladder in the retropubic space, and the pump-control assembly is implanted in a pouch in the scrotum in males. In females, the plane between the bladder neck and vagina is dissected to serve the same purpose as the scrotum.

Under general anesthesia, the patient is placed in the dorsal lithotomy (on the back with the hips and knees flexed and the thighs apart) position, prepped and draped for both perineal and abdominal incisions. Using an Open approach, a midline or transverse suprapubic incision is made. The space of Retzius (between the bladder and the pubis) is opened. Using blunt dissection, a space is made for the balloon, which is filled with saline. A perineal incision is made below the scrotum, a space is created, and the control pump is passed into this position. The Colles fascia and bulbocavernosus muscle are dissected off, exposing the bulbar urethra. A measuring tape is passed around the bulbar urethra to measure for the appropriate size of the cuff for implantation. The artificial urinary sphincter cuff is passed around the urethra and snapped into place. The tubing from the cuff is passed to the suprapubic wound and connected to the control pump. The balloon reservoir has been placed into the subrectus space, and the control pump has been inserted into one side of the scrotum, on the patient's hand-dominant side. The cuff, pump, and reservoir tubing are all connected. The incisions are closed in layers. A Foley catheter may be inserted for the postoperative period.

The device is left deactivated at the time of implantation to allow for healing and is unlocked and activated in the physician's office approximately six to eight weeks after surgery.

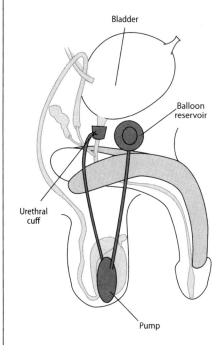

Bladder

Balloon reservoir

Urethral cuff

Pump

Medical and Surgical

Implantation, Autologous Chondrocyte (ACI), Knee

See also Harvesting, Knee Chondrocytes

Body System
Lower Joints

PCS Root Operation
Supplement

Root Operation Table
ØSU   Lower Joints, Supplement

Body Part
Knee Joint, Right
Knee Joint, Left

Approach
Open

Device
Autologous Tissue Substitute

Description

Autologous chondrocyte implantation (ACI) is performed to treat knee defects caused by damage to the hyaline cartilage in acute or repetitive trauma, or due to a prior surgical procedure. This is a two-stage procedure. Some of the patient's own cartilage is collected from a minor load-bearing area within the knee in an arthroscopic procedure in the first stage.

The harvested chondrocytes are sent to a special laboratory where they are isolated from the cartilage matrix and cultured for three to four weeks to increase the number of viable cells. The cells are returned in suspension for surgical implantation in the second stage.

The cultivated chondrocyte cells are implanted during the second stage. Using an Open approach, a knee arthrotomy incision is made into the knee joint. Any necessary debridement is done, and a periosteal flap graft is removed from the proximal medial tibia and sutured around the periphery of the defect to a rim of normal cartilage. A gel-like medium containing the cultured chondrocytes is injected into the defect area under the periosteal graft, which functions as a cover for the chondrocytes while they grow and mature. The incision is closed in layers.

Focus Point
In ICD-10-PCS, root operation Supplement can function as a Repair with device option when a more specific code is not available.

Focus Point
Autograft periosteal tissue harvested from the operative site is not reported separately, according to ICD-10-PCS guideline B3.9.

© 2018 Optum360, LLC

Medical and Surgical

Implantation, Biventricular Heart Replacement System (Artificial Heart)

See also Insertion, Ventricular Assist Device

Body System
Heart and Great Vessels

PCS Root Operation
Replacement

Root Operation Table
Ø2R   Heart and Great Vessels, Replacement

Body Part
Ventricle, Right
Ventricle, Left

Approach
Open

Device
Synthetic Substitute

Description

An implantable heart assist system (artificial heart), also known as an internal biventricular heart replacement system, is indicated in patients with end-stage, irreversible left and right ventricular heart failure for whom surgery or medical therapy is inadequate. To qualify for the device, patients must have end-stage heart failure, a life expectancy of less than 30 days, be ineligible for a natural heart transplant, and have no other treatment options available.

An artificial heart differs from a ventricular assist device. The artificial heart requires resection of the ventricles so the native heart is no longer intact; however, a ventricular assist device is attached to the heart at the ventricle, leaving the heart intact. An example of an artificial heart currently in use is the SynCardia temporary Total Artificial Heart (TAH-t), which is used as a bridge in cardiac transplant-eligible candidates at risk of death from biventricular failure.

This replacement heart system (artificial heart) consists of two artificial polyurethane ventricular chambers with disc valves that are implanted into the chest, replacing the native heart ventricles. These ventricles are pneumatically driven by a line connected to an external driver pump component. The battery-operated pneumatic pump and controller are housed either in a larger, hospital-based, rolling console or in a smaller, portable backpack or shoulder pack container. The artificial ventricles fill and push out the blood when compressed by air from the external pump.

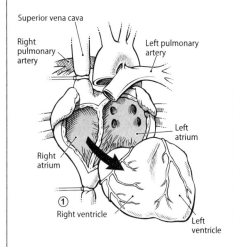

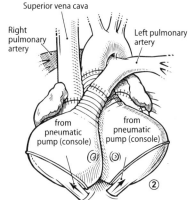

With the patient under general anesthesia, submuscular upper abdominal peritoneal pockets are created for the pneumatic drivelines and tunneled through the rectus fascia. The patient is placed on cardiopulmonary bypass, and using an Open approach, the physician exposes the heart by median sternotomy. The aorta is cross-clamped, and the aortic root and pulmonary artery are divided. A ventriculectomy is performed, after which the artificial ventricles are attached to the left atrium, right atrium, pulmonary artery, and aorta. The drivelines are passed through the previously made tunnels and connected to the ventricles. The device is tested and the sternotomy wired closed.

© 2018 Optum360, LLC

Implantation, Biventricular Heart Replacement System (Artificial Heart) (continued)

Focus Point
This procedure includes ventriculectomy and a substantial removal of part or all of the biological heart. Both ventricles are resected, and the native heart is no longer intact. Do not report a separate code for the ventriculectomy portion of the procedure.

Focus Point
Insertion of this type of device is reported as Replacement, because it involves replacing the resected ventricles with a Synthetic Substitute that physically takes the place and/or function of the resected body part.

Focus Point
Cardiopulmonary bypass is an exception to the usual practice of not reporting supporting procedures that are components of a larger operation. A surgical procedure performed with cardiopulmonary bypass is coded as an additional procedure.

Coding Guidance
AHA: 2017, 1Q, 13

Implantation, Epiretinal Visual Prosthesis

See also Buckling, Scleral (with Implant)

See also Vitrectomy

Body System
Eye

PCS Root Operation
Insertion

Root Operation Table
Ø8H   Eye, Insertion

Body Part
Eye, Right
Eye, Left

Approach
Open

Device
Epiretinal Visual Prosthesis

Description
An epiretinal visual prosthesis is used for treating blindness due to severe to profound or advanced retinitis pigmentosa. The prosthesis is placed on the inner retinal layer and induces artificial electrical stimulation to the remaining functioning retinal cells, thus providing the brain with light perception via the optic nerve. The external equipment includes glasses with a built-in miniature video camera, a video processing unit (VPU) with a rechargeable battery, and a cable. The retinal implant consists of a receiving unit for the transmissions from the external data and power source and the electronics to stimulate the retina to induce visual perception.

Epiretinal implant surgery is performed under general anesthesia using an Open approach and is reported with the root operation Insertion. Phacoemulsification of the lens is followed by a vitrectomy via the pars plana followed by dissection of any epiretinal membrane in the area where the electrode array will be placed. A posterior capsulotomy is created, and the receiving unit is inserted into the capsular bag through an 11-mm corneal incision, which is partially closed using sutures. The electrode array is inserted through a temporal sclerotomy and secured onto the retina using titanium retinal tacks. The electrode array is connected to the receiver unit by a flexible transscleral cable. At the end of the surgery, the eye is filled with balanced salt solution.

Postoperatively, when the implant is activated and functional, the miniature video camera built into the glasses records images in real-time and sends them to the VPU, which converts the images into data wirelessly communicated to the receiver unit. The receiver unit transmits the data to the electrode array, which produces electrical impulses that stimulate the retina's remaining functional cells. The optic nerve transmits visual information to the brain.

Focus Point
Implantation of an epiretinal visual prosthesis includes the implant and the external equipment. Lens removal if present, scleral buckling, vitrectomy, capsulotomy, and epiretinal membrane peeling are integral to the procedure and are not reported separately.

© 2018 Optum360, LLC

Incision and Loop Drainage, Suprapubic Subcutaneous Abscess

Body System
Subcutaneous Tissue and Fascia

PCS Root Operation
Drainage

Root Operation Table
ØJ9   Subcutaneous Tissue and Fascia, Drainage

Body Part
Subcutaneous Tissue and Fascia, Pelvic Region

Approach
Open

Device
Drainage Device
No Device

Qualifier
Diagnostic
No Qualifier

Description
Incision and drainage by loop technique is a minimally invasive technique for treating cutaneous abscesses. It allows for continuous drainage while eliminating the need for repeated packing or wicking changes, making the wound easier for the patient to care for.

Under local anesthesia, the physician makes a small incision through the skin and subcutaneous tissue overlying an abscess. The abscess cavity is opened with a surgical instrument, allowing the contents to drain. The abscess cavity may be curetted and irrigated. A second incision into the abscess cavity is made on the other side of the abscess, and a hemostat is used to extend a tunnel from one incision to the other, looping a sterile drain, either a Penrose drain or a vessel loop, into the tunnel between the two incisions. The drain is tied together to form a loop, which is left in the abscess cavity to facilitate continued drainage. After the infection resolves, the tube is snipped with scissors and removed.

Focus Point
When therapeutic drainage is the focus of the procedure, the Diagnostic qualifier is not reported even when a specimen is sent for pathologic examination. If the purpose of the procedure is diagnostic, the drainage is reported with qualifier Diagnostic.

Focus Point
A drain placed to facilitate healing is not reported. Drains such as Penrose or vessel loops are not classified as drainage devices in ICD-10-PCS. Drainage Device is reported only when the procedure's objective is placement of the device.

Focus Point
The body part for the suprapubic space is Pelvic Region. The retropubic space (space of Retzius) lies behind the symphysis pubis and is reported with Pelvic Cavity.

Coding Guidance
AHA: 2015, 3Q, 20

Insertion, Baclofen Pump

Body System
Subcutaneous Tissue and Fascia

Central Nervous System and Cranial Nerves

PCS Root Operation
Insertion

Root Operation Table
ØJH   Subcutaneous Tissue and Fascia, Insertion

ØØH   Central Nervous System and Cranial Nerves, Insertion

Body Part
Subcutaneous Tissue and Fascia, Abdomen

Subcutaneous Tissue and Fascia, Trunk

Spinal Canal

Approach
Open

Percutaneous

Device
Infusion Device, Pump

Infusion Device

Description
An intrathecal Baclofen pump system is used to treat moderate to severe muscle stiffness and spasticity from conditions such as multiple sclerosis, cerebral palsy, stroke, and spinal cord injuries by restoring normal signals from the nerves to the muscles. Baclofen can be taken orally or with the use of an intrathecal pump. The pump system consists of a pump that is a small metal disk that delivers the Baclofen directly into the spinal canal via a catheter connected to the pump. The Baclofen is stored in the disk and is pushed into the catheter by a tiny motor. An external computer can control the pump, making adjustments to dose, rate, and timing, or the pump can be set to a consistent release.

Reported with the root operation Insertion, the 1" x 3" metal disc or pump is implanted under general anesthesia with an incision, which is an Open approach, into the subcutaneous tissue and fascia of the abdomen or lateral side of the trunk near the waistline. The device value for the pump is Infusion Device, Pump.

A second code reports the Insertion of a small catheter that is inserted through a needle intrathecally, reported as Percutaneous approach, and is threaded upwards, staying within the spinal canal. This is considered a central line catheter with a device value of Infusion Device. The other end of the catheter is then tunneled subcutaneously to the pump and connected. The incision is closed with sutures.

Focus Point
The battery in the Baclofen pump lasts generally from five to seven years. At the end of the battery life, the pump must be replaced. Two codes must be reported reflecting root operations Removal and Insertion, Infusion Device, Pump, using an Open approach into the Subcutaneous Tissue and Fascia, Abdomen.

Focus Point
It is not always necessary to replace the catheter when the battery is replaced; however, if the catheter is also replaced, two additional codes are reported, one for Removal and one for Insertion of the percutaneously placed Infusion Device into the Spinal Canal.

Coding Guidance
AHA: 2014, 3Q, 19

© 2018 Optum360, LLC

Medical and Surgical

Insertion, Bone Growth Stimulator

Body System
Upper Bones

Lower Bones

PCS Root Operation
Insertion

Root Operation Table
ØPH   Upper Bones, Insertion

ØQH   Lower Bones, Insertion

Body Part
Refer to the ICD-10-PCS tabular list for a complete list of body parts.

Approach
Open

Percutaneous

Percutaneous Endoscopic

Device
Bone Growth Stimulator

Description
Electrical bone growth stimulation involves the use of a device that uses an electric current to stimulate the growth of bone tissue. These devices are used to treat many orthopaedic conditions such as fracture nonunions, bone fusion procedures, and other conditions where bone growth is abnormal.

The device is implanted surgically into the bone at the area requiring treatment. One type of implanted device uses a wire coil that is wrapped around the bone site.

Not all treatments using bone stimulation require implantation of devices. Current treatment includes invasive, semi-invasive, and noninvasive electrical bone growth stimulation devices. The different types of implantable electrical bone growth stimulation devices include:

- Direct current electrical stimulation (DCES), which applies an electrical current directly to the treatment area via one or two implanted leads
- Pulsed electromagnetic fields (PEMF), which create an electrical field to stimulate bone growth; these devices may be implanted or worn externally

Focus Point
The root operation Insertion is not assigned to report noninvasive (transcutaneous) (surface) bone stimulators. Use Introduction in the Administration section for these types of bone stimulators. Report root operation Insertion only when the power source, implant cathodes, leads, or electrodes are implanted.

Insertion, Cardiac Defibrillator Generator (ICD)

See also Insertion, Cardiac Lead(s)

See also Insertion, Cardiac Resynchronization Therapy Defibrillator (CRT-D) Pulse Generator

See also Insertion, Cardiac Resynchronization Therapy Pacemaker (CRT-P) Pulse Generator

Body System
Subcutaneous Tissue and Fascia

PCS Root Operation
Insertion

Root Operation Table
ØJH   Subcutaneous Tissue and Fascia, Insertion

Body Part
Subcutaneous Tissue and Fascia, Chest
Subcutaneous Tissue and Fascia, Abdomen

Approach
Open

Device
Defibrillator Generator

Description
An implantable cardioverter defibrillator (ICD) is a device designed to administer an electric shock to control cardiac arrhythmias and restore a normal heartbeat. An ICD consists of a generator, which is placed under the skin, and two leads, which connect the generator to the heart. The device keeps a record of the heart's activity that the provider can retrieve to adjust the programming. Many also offer antitachycardia pacing, which delivers five to 10 paced beats to correct arrhythmia. Most modern ICDs also can function as pacemakers.

The root operation Insertion describes the implantation of the defibrillator generator. An Open approach is used to make an incision into the subcutaneous tissue, creating a pocket either below the clavicle (chest), often referred to as prepectoral, or less commonly in an upper abdominal location. The generator is inserted into the pocket. Once the leads are placed either transvenously into the right atrium and right ventricle or subcutaneously for totally subcutaneous ICD, they are tested and connected to the generator, and the pocket incision is closed. Insertion of the leads is not included and must be coded additionally. *See also* Insertion, Cardiac Lead(s), for the description of the lead placement.

> **Focus Point**
> *Adjustments and revisions to the defibrillator generator are reported with the root operation Revision.*

> **Focus Point**
> *When a generator that has reached the end of its battery life, generally within five to 10 years, is replaced with the same or similar type of generator, it is reported with Removal and Insertion.*

> **Focus Point**
> *Device Cardiac Resynchronization Defibrillation Pulse Generator is used when a third lead is inserted in the left ventricle.*

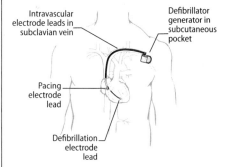

Intravascular electrode leads in subclavian vein

Defibrillator generator in subcutaneous pocket

Pacing electrode lead

Defibrillation electrode lead

Coding Guidance
AHA: 2012, 4Q, 104

© 2018 Optum360, LLC

Medical and Surgical

Insertion, Cardiac Lead(s)

See also Insertion, Cardiac Defibrillator Generator (ICD)

See also Insertion, Cardiac Pacemaker Generator

See also Insertion, Cardiac Resynchronization Therapy Defibrillator (CRT-D) Pulse Generator

See also Insertion, Cardiac Resynchronization Therapy Pacemaker (CRT-P) Pulse Generator

See also Adjustment, Cardiac Pacemaker Lead

Body System
Heart and Great Vessels

PCS Root Operation
Insertion

Root Operation Table
Ø2H   Heart and Great Vessels, Insertion

Body Part
Coronary Vein
Atrium, Right
Ventricle, Right
Ventricle, Left

Approach
Percutaneous

Device
Cardiac Lead, Pacemaker
Cardiac Lead, Defibrillator

Description
Pacemakers and defibrillators are devices that help regulate abnormal electrical impulses that can cause cardiac arrhythmias, including bradycardia (slow heartbeat), tachycardia (rapid heartbeat), atrial fibrillation, or blocks (disruption of electrical impulses). Pacemakers and defibrillators have two parts: the generator (device that generates the electrical impulse) and the lead(s) (insulated wire(s)) that transmits the impulse to the heart muscle. There may be one to three leads.

Cardiac Lead, Pacemaker
Placement of a Cardiac Lead, Pacemaker into the heart chamber is reported with the root operation Insertion for lead(s) used with single- and dual-chamber pacemakers and cardiac resynchronization therapy pacemaker (CRT-P) pulse generators.

The central caval veins are accessed through the subclavian or jugular vein. Using a Percutaneous approach, the vein is penetrated with a large needle, and a wire is passed transvenously. Fluoroscopy is used to guide the thin, flexible wire into the right atrium or right ventricle for a single-chamber device or both for a dual-chamber or CRT-P device. For the CRT-P, since biventricular pacing is required, a third lead is placed in the left ventricle. Fluoroscopy is used for guidance, and a pacing wire (lead) is inserted in the left ventricular chamber of the heart, through the coronary sinus tributary. Depending on the patient's anatomy and difficulty with insertion, it is also common to see the lead tip end in the coronary vein rather than advanced all the way into the left ventricular chamber. When this occurs, the body part value Coronary Vein is reported rather than Ventricle, Left. Once all leads are placed, they are tested and connected to the generator, which is placed in the previously prepared pocket. The creation of the pocket with generator insertion is reported separately. *See also* Insertion, Cardiac Pacemaker Generator and Insertion, Cardiac Resynchronization Therapy Pacemaker (CRT-P) Pulse Generator.

Cardiac Lead, Defibrillator
Placement of a Cardiac Lead, Pacemaker into the heart chamber is reported with the root operation Insertion for lead(s) used with implantable cardioverter defibrillator (ICD) and cardiac resynchronization therapy, defibrillator (CRT-D) pulse generators.

The central caval veins are accessed through the subclavian or jugular vein. Using a Percutaneous approach, the vein is penetrated with a large needle, and a wire is passed transvenously. Fluoroscopy is used to guide the thin, flexible wire into the right atrium and right ventricle for a defibrillator (ICD). For the CRT-D, since biventricular pacing is required, a third lead is placed in the left ventricle. Fluoroscopy is used for guidance, and a pacing wire (lead) is inserted in the left ventricular chamber of the heart, through the coronary sinus tributary. Depending on the patient's anatomy and difficulty with insertion, it is also common to see the lead tip end in the coronary vein rather than advanced all the way into the left ventricular chamber. When this occurs, the body part value reported is Coronary Vein rather than Ventricle, Left. Once all leads are placed, they are tested and connected to the generator, which is placed in the previously prepared pocket. The creation of the pocket with generator insertion is reported separately. *See also* Insertion, Cardiac Defibrillator Generator (ICD) and Insertion, Cardiac Resynchronization Therapy Defibrillator (CRT-D) Pulse Generator.

> **Focus Point**
> *The wires leading from the pacemaker to the electrode are referred to as the leads. The end of a lead includes an electrode. Since the two cannot be separated, they are referred to as a lead in the ICD-10-PCS device values.*

Insertion, Cardiac Lead(s) (continued)

Focus Point

If a lead is displaced and needs only repositioning, the root operation Revision is reported with the body part Heart and the device value Cardiac Lead. See also Adjustment, Cardiac Pacemaker Lead(s).

Focus Point

Report the ICD-10-PCS device value according to the type of cardiac generator device the lead is attached to, rather than the manufacturer's designation as pacing or defibrillator. Some devices combine a pacemaker and ICD in one unit for patients who may require both. After the shock is delivered by the defibrillator lead, a pacing mode is available if needed intermittently.

Focus Point

Two codes are necessary if a lead is replaced. Use a code with the root operation Removal, Cardiac Lead, Heart and one with the root operation, Insertion, Cardiac Lead Pacemaker or Defibrillator, with the appropriate body part value.

Coding Guidance

AHA: 2018, 2Q, 19; 2015, 3Q, 32, 33; 2012, 4Q, 104

Insertion, Cardiac Pacemaker Generator

See also Insertion, Cardiac Lead(s)

Body System
Subcutaneous Tissue and Fascia

PCS Root Operation
Insertion

Root Operation Table
ØJH   Subcutaneous Tissue and Fascia, Insertion

Body Part
Subcutaneous Tissue and Fascia, Chest
Subcutaneous Tissue and Fascia, Abdomen

Approach
Open

Device
Pacemaker, Single Chamber
Pacemaker, Single Chamber Rate Responsive
Pacemaker, Dual Chamber

Description

A pacemaker is an implantable cardiac device that controls the heart's rhythm and maintains regular beats using artificial electric discharges. This device consists of the generator with a battery and the electrodes, or leads. A single-chamber pacemaker has one lead in the right atrium or ventricle. A dual-chamber pacemaker has one lead in the right atrium and one in the right ventricle. Most modern pacemakers have rate responsive capability in which a sensor detects differences in activity or respiratory rates and adjusts accordingly.

The root operation Insertion describes the implantation of the generator. An Open approach is used to make an incision into the subcutaneous tissue, creating a pocket either below the clavicle (chest), often referred to as prepectoral, or less commonly in an upper abdominal location. The generator is inserted into the pocket. Once the lead(s) are placed, they are tested and connected to the generator, and the pocket incision is closed. Insertion of the lead(s) is not included and must be coded additionally. *See also* Insertion, Cardiac Lead(s), for the description of the lead placement.

Focus Point

A single-chamber system may be converted to a dual-chamber system. The existing pacemaker generator pocket is opened and the single-chamber generator removed. The dual-chamber generator is then placed into the existing pocket. The existing pacer wire is tested and connected to the generator. A second lead is placed and tested. The pocket is closed. The root operation Removal, Cardiac Rhythm Related Device, Subcutaneous Tissue and Fascia of Trunk is used for the removal of the single-chamber generator along with Insertion, Pacemaker, Dual Chamber and Insertion, Cardiac Lead, Pacemaker into the appropriate location.

© 2018 Optum360, LLC

Insertion, Cardiac Resynchronization Therapy Defibrillator (CRT-D) Pulse Generator

See also Insertion, Cardiac Lead(s)

See also Insertion, Cardiac Defibrillator Generator (ICD)

Body System
Subcutaneous Tissue and Fascia

PCS Root Operation
Insertion

Root Operation Table
ØJH   Subcutaneous Tissue and Fascia, Insertion

Body Part
Subcutaneous Tissue and Fascia, Chest
Subcutaneous Tissue and Fascia, Abdomen

Approach
Open

Device
Cardiac Resynchronization Defibrillator Pulse Generator

Description
CRT-D uses a resynchronization pulse generator with defibrillation capable of delivering an electrical shock and three transvenous leads to monitor and provide electrical stimulation to the right atrium, right ventricle, and left ventricle. Unlike a standard defibrillator with two leads, the CRT-D includes a third lead implanted within the coronary venous system of the left ventricle to synchronize ventricular contractions. Indications for CRT-D include the treatment of congestive heart failure, cardiomyopathy, and ventricular dysfunction.

The root operation Insertion describes the implantation of the CRT-D pulse generator. An Open approach is used to make an incision into the subcutaneous tissue, creating a pocket either below the clavicle (chest), often referred to as prepectoral, or less commonly in an upper abdominal location. Once all leads are placed, they are tested and connected to the pulse generator. The generator is inserted into the pocket, and the incisions are closed. Insertion of the leads is not included and must be coded additionally. *See also* Insertion, Cardiac Lead(s), for the description of the lead placement.

> **Focus Point**
> *A standard two-lead defibrillation system may be converted to a CRT-D system. The existing defibrillator generator pocket is opened and the defibrillator generator removed. The CRT-D generator is placed into the existing pocket. The existing leads are tested and connected to the generator. A third lead is placed through the coronary sinus tributary, tested, and connected to the generator, and the pocket is closed. The root operation Removal, Cardiac Rhythm Related Device, Subcutaneous Tissue and Fascia of Trunk is used for the removal of the standard defibrillator generator along with Insertion, Cardiac Resynchronization Defibrillator Pulse Generator and Insertion, Cardiac Lead, Defibrillator into the appropriate location.*

> **Focus Point**
> *Also known as BiV ICD, BiV pacing with defibrillation, or biventricular pacing with internal cardiac defibrillator.*

> **Focus Point**
> *The wires leading from the pacemaker to the electrode are referred to as the lead. The end of a lead includes an electrode. Since the two cannot be separated, they are referred to as a lead in the ICD-10-PCS device values.*

© 2018 Optum360, LLC

Insertion, Cardiac Resynchronization Therapy Pacemaker (CRT-P) Pulse Generator

See also Insertion, Cardiac Lead(s)

See also Insertion, Cardiac Defibrillator Generator (ICD)

See also Insertion, Cardiac Pacemaker Generator

Body System
Subcutaneous Tissue and Fascia

PCS Root Operation
Insertion

Root Operation Table
ØJH   Subcutaneous Tissue and Fascia, Insertion

Body Part
Subcutaneous Tissue and Fascia, Chest
Subcutaneous Tissue and Fascia, Abdomen

Approach
Open

Device
Cardiac Resynchronization Pacemaker Pulse Generator

Description

Used to provide electrical stimulation therapy to patients with ventricular dysfunction, the cardiac resynchronization therapy pacemaker (CRT-P) is indicated for those patients who do not require an implantable cardioverter defibrillator (ICD). A standard pacemaker can be single- or dual-chamber, but the CRT-P is a triple-chamber device as the electrodes (leads) are inserted not only into the right atrium and ventricle, but also into the coronary vein behind the heart to pace the left ventricle. This synchronizes the contractions of the left heart with the right heart for better function and can be used to alleviate symptoms for heart failure patients.

The root operation Insertion describes the implantation of the CRT-P pulse generator. An Open approach is used to make an incision into the subcutaneous tissue, creating a pocket either below the clavicle (chest), often referred to as prepectoral, or less commonly in an upper abdominal location. Once the three leads are placed, they are tested and connected to the generator. The generator is inserted into the pocket, and the pocket incision is closed. Insertion of the leads is not included and must be coded additionally. *See also* Insertion, Cardiac Lead(s), for the description of the lead placement.

Focus Point
A single- or dual-chamber system may be converted to a CRT-P system. The existing pacemaker generator pocket is opened and the single-/dual-chamber generator removed. The CRT-P generator is placed into the existing pocket. The existing lead or leads are tested and connected to the generator. A third lead is placed through the coronary sinus tributary, tested, and connected to the generator, and the pocket is closed. The root operation Removal, Cardiac Rhythm Related Device, Subcutaneous Tissue and Fascia of Trunk describes the removal of the single-/dual-chamber generator along with Insertion, Cardiac Resynchronization Pacemaker Pulse Generator and Insertion, Cardiac Lead, Pacemaker, into the appropriate location.

Focus Point
CRT-P is also known as biventricular or BiV pacemaker, or biventricular pacing without internal cardiac defibrillator.

Focus Point
The wires leading from the pacemaker to the electrode are referred to as the lead. The end of a lead includes an electrode. Since the two cannot be separated, they are referred to as a lead in the ICD-10-PCS device values.

© 2018 Optum360, LLC

Insertion, Central Line

See also Insertion, Infusion Pump into Subcutaneous Tissue and Fascia

See also Insertion, Vascular Access Device (VAD, TIVAD, Port-A-Cath)

Body System
Heart and Great Vessels

PCS Root Operation
Insertion

Root Operation Table
Ø2H   Heart and Great Vessels, Insertion

Body Part
Superior Vena Cava

Approach
Percutaneous

Device
Infusion Device

Description
Central venous lines, also known as central venous catheters, are inserted for long-term medication treatment for infections, pain, and cancer.

Venous catheterization techniques may vary depending on the purpose for the catheterization and anatomic site. The physician places a needle or a catheter through a puncture in the skin and into a peripheral vein. For insertion of a nontunneled catheter, the site over the access vein (e.g., subclavian, jugular) is injected with local anesthesia and punctured with a needle. A guide wire is inserted. The central venous catheter is placed over the guide wire. Ultrasound guidance may be used to gain venous access and/or fluoroscopy to check the positioning of the catheter tip in the superior vena cava. The catheter is secured into position and dressed.

A tunneled catheter has an entrance site at a distance from its entrance into the vascular system; it is "tunneled" through the skin and subcutaneous tissue to a great vein. The site over the access vein (e.g., subclavian, jugular) is injected with local anesthesia and punctured with a needle or accessed by cutdown

approach. A guide wire is inserted. A subcutaneous tunnel is created using a blunt pair of forceps or sharp tunneling tools, often over the clavicle from the anterior chest wall to the venotomy site, which is dilated to the right size. The catheter is passed through this tunnel over the guide wire and into the target vein. Ultrasound guidance may be used to gain venous access and/or fluoroscopy to check the positioning of the catheter tip in the superior vena cava. The catheter is secured into position, and any incisions are sutured.

Focus Point
Imaging guidance such as fluoroscopy or ultrasound done to assist in the catheter placement can be coded separately using a code from the Imaging section with the qualifier Guidance.

Focus Point
When coding the placement of a central venous catheter, report the body part for the site where the tip of the catheter ends up rather than the percutaneous entry point. If imaging confirmation of the end placement of a central line catheter inserted via the femoral vein is not performed or the end placement is otherwise unknown or unavailable, assign as the default the code for Insertion, Infusion Device into Lower vein, Percutaneous approach.

Focus Point
Central catheters may also be connected to a subcutaneously inserted pump, port, or reservoir, which may be coded as an additional procedure. Refer to ICD-10-PCS table ØJH Insertion, Subcutaneous Tissue and Fascia.

Focus Point
The tunneled vascular access portion of the central venous catheter is captured using Insertion, Vascular Access Device with the device Vascular Access Device, Tunneled.

Coding Guidance
AHA: 2017, 2Q, 24, 26; 2017, 1Q, 31; 2015, 4Q, 26; 2014, 3Q, 5; 2013, 3Q, 18

Insertion, Deep Brain Stimulator (DBS)

See also Insertion, Intracranial Responsive Neurostimulator (RNS)

See also Insertion, Intracranial Responsive Neurostimulator or Deep Brain Stimulator Lead(s)

Body System
Subcutaneous Tissue and Fascia

PCS Root Operation
Insertion

Root Operation Table
ØJH   Subcutaneous Tissue and Fascia, Insertion

Body Part
Subcutaneous Tissue and Fascia, Chest

Approach
Open

Device
Stimulator Generator, Single Array
Stimulator Generator, Single Array, Rechargeable
Stimulator Generator, Multiple Array
Stimulator Generator, Multiple Array, Rechargeable
Stimulator Generator

Description

Deep brain stimulators (DBS) are used to control tremors in patients diagnosed with essential tremor, epilepsy, Parkinson's disease, or certain psychiatric diseases such as obsessive-compulsive disorder. These intracranial neurostimulator devices consist of a battery-operated generator inserted into a subcutaneous pocket connected to an electrode (lead) implanted into the brain, often the thalamus, for DBS. Electrical impulses from the generator are sent through the lead, interrupting the thalamic signals that play a role in causing the tremor.

Thalamic stimulator implantation for the control of tremor consists of implanting a lead or leads in the thalamus connected to an indwelling battery pack inserted subcutaneously, typically in the chest. The generator and leads may be inserted during the same procedure or may be inserted in a staged process. The leads are considered permanent unless there is a complication. Generators, on the other hand, are battery-operated, and the batteries must be replaced periodically.

Using blunt dissection, a pocket is created for the generator or receiver by incising the skin with an Open approach. Reported with the root operation Insertion, a single- or multiple-array device is placed into the subcutaneous pocket under the clavicle. The unit is connected to an electrode array. After ensuring that the device is functioning, the generator is sutured into place within its subcutaneous pocket.

Focus Point
Insertion of the leads is not included and must be coded additionally. See also Insertion, Intracranial Responsive Neurostimulator or Deep Brain Stimulator Lead(s).

Focus Point
A Single Array is a unilateral device that can connect to only one lead. If a bilateral electrode (lead) is placed, the Multiple Array value is reported as it is a device that can connect to two or more leads. To find out if the device is rechargeable, query the surgeon to see which brand the facility uses.

Focus Point
Deep brain stimulator is not the same as responsive neurostimulator (RNS) and is reported with different PCS values. See also Insertion, Intracranial Responsive Neurostimulator (RNS).

© 2018 Optum360, LLC

Medical and Surgical

Insertion, Endobronchial Valve, Endoscopic

Body System
Respiratory System

PCS Root Operation
Insertion

Root Operation Table
ØBH   Respiratory System, Insertion

Body Part
Main Bronchus, Right
Upper Lobe Bronchus, Right
Middle Lobe Bronchus, Right
Lower Lobe Bronchus, Right
Main Bronchus, Left
Upper Lobe Bronchus, Left
Lingula Bronchus
Lower Lobe Bronchus, Left

Approach
Via Natural or Artificial Opening Endoscopic

Device
Intraluminal Device, Endobronchial Valve

Description
Endobronchial endoscopic valve insertion is typically performed to treat severe emphysema or to manage prolonged air leaks. Emphysema is a chronic, progressive disease characterized by the destruction of lung tissue in multiple lobes, which can lead to the lungs becoming over inflated. Air leaks can have traumatic, iatrogenic, or spontaneous causes, but air leaks most commonly occur following surgery (e.g., lobectomy, segmentectomy, or lung volume reduction surgery) as a result of lung tissue that has not completely closed and sealed. Endoscopic bronchial valve insertion is a minimally invasive procedure because the valves are placed via a bronchoscopic procedure that does not require a surgical incision.

The physician uses a CT scan to determine the location and number of valves to be placed based on the extent of the disease in each lobe. The procedure is performed Via Natural or Artificial Opening Endoscopic, with a bronchoscope with a small flexible camera. Using an airway sizing kit, a balloon is inflated with saline at the target implantation site or sites to determine the appropriate valve sizes for each location. A catheter is passed through the bronchoscope, and the small one-way, umbrella-shaped valves are deployed into the segmental and subsegmental bronchi, blocking the airflow to the diseased area. The valve allows air to flow through the valve on expiration but closes on inspiration, blocking the air from entering that segment of lung, which then collapses.

Focus Point
According to ICD-10-PCS multiple procedures guideline B3.2, multiple procedures may be reported if the same procedure is performed on different body parts with distinct body part characters, or multiple body parts with separate distinct body parts classified to a single body part value.

Insertion, Evacuating Port System, Subdural (SEPS)

Body System
Central Nervous System and Cranial Nerves

PCS Root Operation
Drainage

Root Operation Table
009 Central Nervous System and Cranial Nerves, Drainage

Body Part
Subdural Space, Intracranial

Approach
Percutaneous

Device
Drainage Device

Description
The placement of a subdural evacuating port system (SEPS) drain assists in evacuating chronic and subacute hematomas as well as hygromas from the brain. This minimally invasive procedure, which uses uniform negative pressure in a closed system, may be performed at a patient's bedside.

The ideal port site is identified with diagnostic imaging. Using a Percutaneous approach, a burr hole is created through the dura and subdural membrane; the evacuating port is inserted using a twisting motion. Silicone tubing and a bulb suction apparatus are attached to the metal evacuating port. Using the bulb, negative pressure is applied for a variable time period until there is no longer drainage of the subdural fluid. The system is then removed.

This procedure may also be documented as aspiration of subarachnoid or subdural space, cranial aspiration, puncture of anterior fontanel, subdural tap, subdural tap through fontanel, or placement of a subdural evacuating port system (SEPS).

> **Focus Point**
> Open approach would not be appropriate, as the surgical site is not directly exposed. The port is inserted through a small burr hole.

Coding Guidance
AHA: 2015, 3Q, 12

Insertion, Filter, Inferior Vena Cava (IVC)

Body System
Lower Veins

PCS Root Operation
Insertion

Root Operation Table
06H Lower Veins, Insertion

Body Part
Inferior Vena Cava

Approach
Percutaneous

Device
Intraluminal Device

Description
The inferior vena cava (IVC) filter is a small, cone-shaped device placed within the inferior vena cava with four legs with a small hook at the base of each for fixation. A hook at the top of the cone allows the filter to be retrieved if necessary. IVC filter placement is performed for patients with deep venous thrombosis (DVT) or pulmonary embolism (PE) who cannot be treated with anticoagulation therapy. The filter traps blood clots (embolisms) that have broken loose from the deep veins of the legs and prevents them from reaching the heart and lungs.

The patient is brought into the interventional radiology or vascular suite. Local anesthesia is administered, and the physician places an intravascular umbrella or tulip filter device using a Percutaneous (endovascular) (venous) approach. Under ultrasound guidance, the physician places a needle in the femoral (or internal jugular) vein, advances a guidewire through the needle, removes the needle over the wire, and advances an introducer sheath over the wire into the femoral vein. The physician advances the filter through the introducer sheath into the inferior vena cava under fluoroscopic guidance. The filter hooks are oriented but not released until the filter is in correct position. The wire is removed, and a contrast venography is performed to evaluate the placement of the filter. The physician removes the introducer sheath and compresses the femoral vein manually until hemostasis is achieved.

Medical and Surgical

© 2018 Optum360, LLC

Insertion, Hepatic Artery Infusion Device

See also Chemoembolization, Hepatic Artery

See also Insertion, Infusion Pump into Subcutaneous Tissue and Fascia

See also Introduction, Antineoplastic Agent, Hepatic Artery in the Medical and Surgical Related section, Administration

Body System
Lower Arteries

PCS Root Operation
Insertion

Root Operation Table
04H   Lower Arteries, Insertion

Body Part
Hepatic Artery

Approach
Open
Percutaneous
Percutaneous Endoscopic

Device
Infusion Device

Description
Insertion of hepatic artery infusion device is used for direct delivery of chemotherapy into the hepatic artery for patients with primary or metastatic liver cancer.

Via an Open laparotomy approach, the physician places the catheter for the chemoembolization into the hepatic artery. The hepatic artery is dissected out, and any small branches are ligated or cauterized. The catheter is then placed in the hepatic artery. The catheter is connected to a separately reportable infusion pump that is inserted into the subcutaneous tissue of the abdomen, and the incisions are closed. *See also* Insertion, Infusion Pump into Subcutaneous Tissue and Fascia.

If the gallbladder is still present, a separately reportable cholecystectomy is performed to remove the gallbladder from the operative field, allow identification of the common bile duct, and prevent

complications such as postoperative chemotherapy cholecystitis.

Alternatively, a Percutaneous Endoscopic (laparoscopic) approach may be used. The physician makes a 1 cm infraumbilical incision through which a trocar is inserted. Pneumoperitoneum is achieved by insufflating the abdominal cavity with carbon dioxide. A fiberoptic laparoscope fitted with a camera and light source is inserted through the trocar. Other incisions are made on the right side of the abdomen and in the subxiphoid area to allow other instruments or an additional light source to be passed into the abdomen. The hepatic artery is dissected out, and any small branches are ligated or cauterized. The catheter is then placed in the hepatic artery. The catheter is connected to an infusion pump inserted into the subcutaneous tissue of the abdomen.

Using a Percutaneous approach, referred to as a transarterial chemoembolization (TACE), under fluoroscopic guidance, the physician uses a peripheral artery (common femoral) to implant the catheter into the hepatic artery. The physician punctures the femoral artery and passes a guidewire via the needle through the aorta into the hepatic artery. The physician slides the infusion catheter over the guidewire into targeted arterial lumen with fluoroscopic guidance. A separately reportable subcutaneous pocket is created in the abdomen to place the infusion pump. The catheter is connected to the pump, and the incisions are closed.

Focus Point

Imaging guidance such as fluoroscopy or ultrasound used to help place the catheter can be reported separately using a code from the Ancillary section, Imaging, with the qualifier Guidance.

Focus Point

When coding the placement of the catheter part of an infusion device, report the body part for the site where the tip of the catheter ends up rather than the entry point.

Coding Guidance
AHA: 2015, 4Q, 26; 2014, 3Q, 5; 2013, 3Q, 18

Insertion, Infusion Pump into Subcutaneous Tissue and Fascia

See also Insertion, Central Line

Body System
Subcutaneous Tissue and Fascia

PCS Root Operation
Insertion

Root Operation Table
ØJH   Subcutaneous Tissue and Fascia, Insertion

Body Part
Refer to the ICD-10-PCS tabular list for a complete list of body parts.

Approach
Open

Device
Infusion Device, Pump

Description
An implantable infusion pump is a programmable self-contained device that controls the amount and timing of drugs delivered into the body from a pump implanted into subcutaneous tissue. Some drugs that are commonly delivered with an infusion pump include chemotherapy, pain medicine, insulin, or antispasmodics. Nutritional substances may also be delivered via an infusion pump.

There are three parts to an implantable infusion pump: the two part metal disc that contains the reservoir for the medication with a port for refilling, and a battery-powered programmable motor for the pumping action. This disc is attached to a catheter, which is threaded to the point of delivery. The pump is implanted in the subcutaneous tissue and can be refilled through the skin with a needle and syringe.

The location of the subcutaneous insertion is generally in the abdominal wall, chest, or back although locations can vary by patient.

The physician makes a midline incision overlying the placement site using an Open approach. A pocket is created in the subcutaneous tissue between the skin and muscles. The infusion pump housing (disc) is attached to a previously placed tunneled catheter, which is put into the pocket and sutured in place to the fascia. Layered sutures are used to close the incision.

Focus Point
An additional code may be added for the Administration of the specific drug.

Focus Point
Infusion pumps and vascular access devices are different; an implantable infusion pump is a self-contained pump that both stores and delivers its contents, whereas an implantable vascular access device is not a pump but is implanted into the body to provide an access point to the vascular system.

Focus Point
Two codes are required for the infusion pump, one for the pump implantation and another for the catheter; both are reported with the root operation Insertion. See also Insertion, Central Line.

Coding Guidance
AHA: 2014, 4Q, 40, 41

© 2018 Optum360, LLC

Medical and Surgical

Insertion, Intracranial Responsive Neurostimulator (RNS)

See also Insertion, Deep Brain Stimulator (DBS)

See also Insertion, Intracranial Responsive Neurostimulator or Deep Brain Stimulator Lead(s)

Body System
Head and Facial Bones

PCS Root Operation
Insertion

Root Operation Table
ØNH   Head and Facial Bones, Insertion

Body Part
Skull

Approach
Open

Device
Neurostimulator Generator

Description
The responsive neurostimulator (RNS) is specifically designed to treat adults with medically refractory localization-related (focal) (partial) epilepsy. Epilepsy is a chronic neurological condition characterized by abnormal electrical activity in the brain that causes seizures.

The responsive neurostimulator is a small, pacemaker-like curved device containing batteries, circuitry, and a radio for interrogation and programming that is implanted by craniectomy into the skull bone. The code for this stimulator is reported with the root operation Insertion using an Open

approach into the body part value Skull. The device is considered a Neurostimulator Generator.

Once leads are placed, the stimulator is anchored to the skull with bone screws. The scalp is replaced over the skull, covering the implanted neurostimulator, and the surgical site is sutured closed.

The entire procedure is performed in the hospital inpatient setting with patients under general anesthesia and takes approximately three hours to complete. The programmable, battery-powered, and microprocessor-controlled device delivers short bursts of mild electrical pulses to the brain through the implanted leads. The device continuously monitors brain electrical activity, detecting the abnormal electrical activity preceding seizure and responds by delivering brief and mild electrical stimulation to normalize brain activity. Stimulation parameters are programmed specifically to meet the patient's individual needs. Additionally, the RNS software allows the physician programmer to view the electrocorticogram, or ECoG, in real-time. Patients may transmit ECoG and system data remotely to their physicians.

Focus Point
Insertion of the leads is not included and must be coded in addition. See also Insertion, Intracranial Responsive Neurostimulator or Deep Brain Stimulator Lead(s).

Focus Point
Responsive neurostimulator (RNS) is not the same as a deep brain stimulator and is reported with different PCS values. See also Insertion, Deep Brain Stimulator (DBS).

Insertion, Intracranial Responsive Neurostimulator or Deep Brain Stimulator Lead(s)

See also Insertion, Deep Brain Stimulator (DBS)

See also Insertion, Intracranial Responsive Neurostimulator (RNS)

Body System
Central Nervous System and Cranial Nerves

PCS Root Operation
Insertion

Root Operation Table
00H   Central Nervous System and Cranial Nerves, Insertion

Body Part
Brain

Approach
Open

Percutaneous

Device
Neurostimulator Lead

Description

Deep brain stimulators (DBS) are used to control tremors in patients diagnosed with essential tremor, epilepsy, Parkinson's disease, or certain psychiatric diseases such as obsessive-compulsive disorder. Responsive neurostimulators (RNS) are specifically designed to treat adults with medically refractory localization-related (focal) (partial) epilepsy. Both of these neurostimulator devices consist of a generator connected to an electrode (lead) implanted into the brain. The specific area of the brain depends on the symptoms being treated.

For lead placement, depending on the location of the targeted area, different approach techniques such as twist drill, burr holes, craniectomy, or craniectomy may be used. If the brain is directly visualized, the approach is Open. However, if the brain is not directly visualized but the lead is placed with a small burr hole large enough only for a guidewire and aided by imaging, Percutaneous approach may be appropriate. The root operation reported for the placement of the lead/electrode is Insertion.

The physician uses a twist or burr drill, or performs a craniectomy or craniotomy to reach the site of the procedure. The physician incises the scalp and retracts it. Bone may be removed. Once the electrodes are placed into the target location, electrical impulses may be sent through the lead to make sure it is properly placed. The electrodes are connected to the generator by extension wires that are tunneled under the skin. Any bone that was removed is replaced, and any incisions are closed with no part of the wires, lead, or device on the outside of the body. The wires with attached electrodes are reported with the device value Neurostimulator Lead.

Focus Point

For the insertion of the generator, see Insertion, Deep Brain Stimulator (DBS) or Insertion, Intracranial Responsive Neurostimulator (RNS).

© 2018 Optum360, LLC

Medical and Surgical

Insertion, Limb Lengthening Device, Lower Extremity

Body System
Lower Bones

PCS Root Operation
Insertion

Root Operation Table
ØQH   Lower Bones, Insertion

Body Part
Upper Femur, Right
Upper Femur, Left
Femoral Shaft, Right
Femoral Shaft, Left
Lower Femur, Right
Lower Femur, Left
Tibia, Right
Tibia, Left
Fibula, Right
Fibula, Left

Approach
Open
Percutaneous

Device
External Fixation Device, Limb Lengthening

Description
Insertion of limb lengthening distraction devices is performed for congenital defects, previous injuries, or malunion of fractured bones and other bone diseases that lead to unequal limb lengths.

For femoral lengthening, two puncture wounds are made laterally in the distal and proximal femur. Two holes at each end are drilled in the bone, and a screw is inserted in each drill hole. In an Open approach, the physician makes a lateral longitudinal incision 6 to 8 cm long to expose the femur. The cortical surface of the bone may be cut, leaving the medullary surface intact. Osteotomy, if required, is performed with an oscillating saw at the metaphyseal-diaphyseal junction. The distraction apparatus is then attached to the two sets of screws, so that the apparatus is 1 to 2 cm lateral to the thigh. The incision is repaired in multiple layers. The device is then distracted up to 5 mm to 6 mm immediately. The apparatus is operated by a knob. Lengthening is about 1.5 mm or 1 cm per week. When the appearance of the femur is normal and the medullary has been reestablished, the plate and screws are removed.

A Percutaneous approach may be used, in which only the two puncture wounds are made laterally in the distal and proximal femur. Two holes at each end are drilled in the bone, and a screw is inserted in each drill hole. The distraction apparatus is then attached to the two sets of screws so that the apparatus is 1 cm to 2 cm lateral to the thigh. The puncture wounds are repaired. The device is then distracted up to 5 mm to 6 mm immediately. The apparatus is operated by a knob. Lengthening is about 1.5 mm or 1 cm per week. When the appearance of the femur is normal and the medullary has been reestablished, the plate and screws are removed.

Focus Point
In ICD-10-PCS a code for the root operation Division from the Medical and Surgical section would be assigned to report the osteotomy.

Focus Point
Subsequent procedures involving lengthening of the growing rods due to bone growth and/or malposition of the rods are reported with root operation Revision.

Insertion, Penile Prosthesis, Inflatable

Body System
Male Reproductive System

PCS Root Operation
Supplement

Root Operation Table
ØVU   Male Reproductive System, Supplement

Body Part
Penis

Approach
Open

Device
Synthetic Substitute

Description
Penile prosthesis surgery is performed to treat erectile dysfunction (ED) due to disease, scarring, other organic cause, or psychological impotence in patients who have failed other therapeutic, nonsurgical options, or for whom surgery is contraindicated.

Under general anesthesia, the patient is placed in frog-leg position, prepped, and draped. A Foley catheter is inserted into the bladder. The physician inserts an inflatable penile prosthesis made of three components: the reservoir, the pump, and two inflatable cylinders. Using an Open approach, a transverse incision is made at the base of the penis in the upper scrotum. With care to avoid the urethra and important nerves and blood vessels, dissection is carried down to the erectile tissues at the base of the

penis. The thick, fibrous membranes surrounding the two main erectile tissues are incised, and dilators are inserted to create space for the prostheses. Two inflatable cylinders are inserted into the two erectile tissue compartments down the length of the penis. A pouch is made in one side of the scrotum, and the pump mechanism and tubing are inserted into the space created. Using an index finger, the surgeon creates a tunnel from the pump to the space behind the pubic bone. The reservoir is placed behind the pubic bone with tubing running from it through the tunnel to the pump in the scrotum. The tubing between the reservoir and the pump is clamped and excess tubing cut. The connecting device is placed and the crimper used to secure the connection between the reservoir and the pump. The device is tested to ensure functionality. The incisions and tissues are closed in layers by suturing and dressings placed over the incisions. Temporary drains may be inserted. The operation can also be done in similar fashion using an incision just below the scrotum in the perineum to enter the erectile tissue and in the area above the pubic bone to gain access to place the reservoir.

Focus Point
A penile prosthesis consists of a single three-component device that augments the function of the penis without actually replacing it. This meets the definition of the root operation Supplement.

Coding Guidance
AHA: 2016, 2Q, 28; 2015, 3Q, 25

© 2018 Optum360, LLC

Insertion, Spinal Stabilization Device

Body System
Upper Joints
Lower Joints

PCS Root Operation
Insertion

Root Operation Table
ØRH Upper Joints, Insertion
ØSH Lower Joints, Insertion

Body Part
Cervical Vertebral Joint
Cervicothoracic Vertebral Joint
Thoracic Vertebral Joint
Thoracolumbar Vertebral Joint
Lumbar Vertebral Joint
Lumbosacral Joint

Approach
Open
Percutaneous

Device
Spinal Stabilization Device, Interspinous Process
Spinal Stabilization Device, Pedicle-Based
Spinal Stabilization Device, Facet Replacement

Description
Although spinal fusion has been the gold standard for the treatment of many pathologies of the spine, newer technologies are being continually tested and reviewed. Spinal stabilization devices, all relatively newer technologies, are constantly being updated and are most often used in the lumbar spine. A spinal stabilization device provides stability while allowing for some movement within the affected area of the spine. The root operation Insertion is used to report the use of these devices along with the appropriate device value.

There are three types of spinal stabilization devices, each reported with a specific PCS device value:

Spinal Stabilization Device, Interspinous Process. These devices act as spacers that open up space for nerve endings to pass through and are used to decompress spinal stenosis in lieu of spinal fusion.

With the patient under appropriate anesthesia and in prone (lying on the stomach) position, the patient's back is prepped and draped. Using an Open approach, the physician makes a small midline incision and lifts the paraspinal muscles, leaving the midline structures intact. The interspinous device is placed between the spinous processes while the patient is in a slight flexion position, protecting the supraspinous ligament. A dilator is placed between the spinous processes just posterior to the lamina. A sizing instrument is inserted between the spinous processes and expanded until the supraspinous ligament is taut. The appropriate interspinous device is then sized and inserted. The device is not attached to the osseous structures but is held in place by the supraspinous ligament posteriorly, by the lamina anteriorly, by the spinous processes cranially and caudally, and by the wings on each side of the device laterally. The wound is irrigated with sterile water containing antibiotics. The deep fascial layer and subcutaneous layers are closed with sutures, and the skin is closed with stitches or surgical staples. A sterile bandage is applied.

Spinal Stabilization Devices

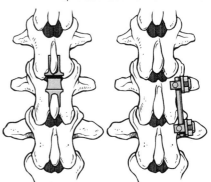

Interspinous Process Device   Pedicle-Based Device

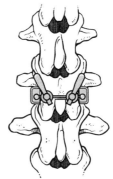

Facet Replacement Device

Insertion, Spinal Stabilization Device (continued)

Medical and Surgical

Spinal Stabilization Device, Pedicle-Based

These devices use flexible, movable, and even inflatable rods inserted into the pedicles to stabilize the spine. One of the most frequently employed systems currently in use is Dynesys, which uses screws and cords. It is used both adjunct to fusion and as a stand-alone procedure.

With the patient under appropriate anesthesia and in prone (lying on the stomach) position, the patient's back is prepped and draped. Using an Open approach, the physician makes a midline incision and exposes the lamina, facet joints, and transverse processes on both sides of the spinous processes. Titanium-alloy pedicle screws are placed bilaterally at the affected segments. After the pedicle screws are inserted, polyester cords or flexible rods or bands are connected between the pedicle screw heads, applying tension and compression as determined by the length of the bands. Once the devices are attached, the dynamic effect of the connection between the spacer and the band stabilizes the joints, keeping the vertebrae in normal anatomic position. The wound is irrigated with sterile water containing antibiotics. The deep fascial layer and subcutaneous layers are closed with sutures, and the skin is closed with stitches or surgical staples. A sterile bandage is applied.

Spinal Stabilization Device, Facet Replacement

These devices are used to reduce facet pain from spinal stenosis and replace facet joints while maintaining spinal movement. These devices are currently under FDA-regulated clinical trial.

With the patient under appropriate anesthesia and in prone (lying on the stomach) position, the patient's back is prepped and draped. Using an Open approach, the physician makes a posterior midline incision, exposing the spine. After spinal decompression, using special instruments, the inferior and superior articulating facet replacement implants are placed, aligned, and secured in anatomical position on the pedicle with pedicle screws and locking nuts. A crosslink is added to provide additional support and stability. The wound is irrigated with sterile water containing antibiotics. The deep fascial layer and subcutaneous layers are closed with sutures, and the skin is closed with stitches or surgical staples. A sterile bandage is applied.

> **Focus Point**
> Code separately any concurrent spinal fusion procedure.

Coding Guidance
AHA: 2017, 2Q, 23

© 2018 Optum360, LLC

Insertion, Tissue Expander, Breast

Body System
Skin and Breast

PCS Root Operation
Insertion

Root Operation Table
ØHH   Skin and Breast, Insertion

Body Part
Breast, Right
Breast, Left
Breast, Bilateral

Approach
Open

Device
Tissue Expander

Description
Tissue expansion is a medical process by which skin and subcutaneous tissue are stretched by traction applied to those tissues. In tissue expansion of the breast, the goal is to stretch the skin of the breast so that it can accommodate a later breast implant. The expansion often occurs in patients who are post-mastectomy.

Using an Open approach, the physician makes an incision in the skin of a patient who has undergone a mastectomy. A pocket is created using an existing chest wall muscle, and an expandable implant is placed into it at the site of the mastectomy. The port is placed by tunneling percutaneously to a site that is accessible to the skin surface. In some cases, the implant's button-shaped portal may be brought out through the skin so it is accessible by needle. Usually, the portal remains beneath the surface of the skin. The wound is closed over the expander and port. The physician injects saline into the access portal to expand the implant until it has stretched the surrounding tissue to a size slightly larger than the patient's existing breast. In some cases, the expander remains a permanent prosthesis, and small amount of fluid is aspirated until it duplicates the size of the existing breast. In other cases, a second surgery (reported separately) excises the implant and replaces it with a permanent breast prosthesis.

Focus Point
Some tissue expanders are designed to double as permanent breast prostheses, eliminating the need for a second surgery to complete the breast reconstruction. The insertion of these breast tissue expanders as prosthetic devices are reported with device Tissue Expander, as that is the function of the device.

Focus Point
Removal of an implanted tissue expander is reported with a code from table ØHP Removal, Skin and Breast.

Focus Point
The use of acellular dermal matrix in the creation of the tissue expander pocket is not reported separately.

Coding Guidance
AHA: 2014, 2Q, 12; 2013, 4Q, 96

Insertion, Tissue Expander, Subcutaneous Tissue

Medical and Surgical

Body System
Subcutaneous Tissue and Fascia

PCS Root Operation
Insertion

Root Operation Table
ØJH Subcutaneous Tissue and Fascia, Insertion

Body Part
Refer to the ICD-10-PCS tabular list for a complete list of body parts.

Approach
Open
Percutaneous

Device
Tissue Expander

Description
Tissue expansion is a medical process by which skin and subcutaneous tissue are stretched by traction applied to those tissues. This may be performed as a local function, to stretch the skin at the site adjacent to a skin defect that later will be excised and covered with this stretched skin. Tissue expansion is also performed on healthy skin for later use at a secondary site, where the excised, stretched skin will serve as a graft.

Tissue expanders are usually balloon-like devices inserted between the subcutaneous tissue and underlying muscle to enhance epithelial and collagen expansion by traction. For the scalp and forehead, the expander is placed subgaleally; in the neck, placement may be beneath the platysma.

The physician creates a subcutaneous pocket into which the skin expander is placed. The balloon-like expander is equipped with a port into which saline is injected over time, gradually increasing the balloon's size and stretching the surrounding skin. The port may be located directly on the balloon, or placed remotely, connected to the bladder by a subcutaneous tube. The port may be under the skin or externalized.

Using an Open approach, the physician makes an incision through the skin and places the expander under direct visualization. The port may be tunneled percutaneously. The wound is closed over the expander and port. Saline later is injected through a syringe into the port, which can be manually identified through the skin.

In a Percutaneous approach, the physician makes a small incision and undermines subcutaneous tissue through the small incision. The expander is folded, inserted through the incision, and expanded once placed between the undermined tissue layers. The port is secured percutaneously. This is performed without direct visualization. Saline later is injected through a syringe into the port, which can be manually identified through the skin.

Focus Point

The use of acellular dermal matrix in the creation of a tissue expander pocket is not reported separately.

Coding Guidance
AHA: 2013, 4Q, 96

© 2018 Optum360, LLC

Insertion, Vascular Access Device (CVAD, VAD, TIVAD, Port-A-Cath)

See also Insertion, Central Line

Body System
Subcutaneous Tissue and Fascia

PCS Root Operation
Insertion

Root Operation Table
ØJH   Subcutaneous Tissue and Fascia, Insertion

Body Part
Subcutaneous Tissue and Fascia, Chest
Subcutaneous Tissue and Fascia, Abdomen
Subcutaneous Tissue and Fascia, Right Upper Arm
Subcutaneous Tissue and Fascia, Left Upper Arm

Approach
Open (Vascular Access Device, Totally Implantable)
Percutaneous (Vascular Access Device, Tunneled)

Device
Vascular Access Device, Totally Implantable
Vascular Access Device, Tunneled

Description
Tunneled or totally implantable vascular access devices are indicated for patients in whom long-term (30 days) vascular access is anticipated for hemodialysis, for administering fluids, chemotherapy, antibiotics, blood, and parenteral nutrition, and for central venous pressure monitoring and blood sampling.

Central Venous Access Device, Tunneled (CVAD) (Vascular Access Device, Tunneled)
Tunneled central venous access devices (CVADs) such as Hickman, Broviac, Leonard, and Groshong catheters are inserted into a vein and subcutaneously tunneled to an external site away from the insertion site to prevent bacterial infections in the bloodstream and to provide a convenient, yet concealed, access point.

These tunneled central venous access device (CVAD) catheters are inserted by tunneling through the skin and subcutaneous tissue into either the subclavian vein (located beneath the collarbone) or into the internal jugular vein (located in the neck) and are long enough for the distal tip to reach the superior vena cava (central line). The proximal end is tunneled to an exit site on the chest or other site away from the insertion site. The external portion remains outside the skin and often consists of multiple lumens, which may be open-ended or valved. These external lumens are used to administer medications or draw blood. The device may be equipped with a Dacron cuff near the tunnel exit site that anchors the catheter and creates a barrier to prevent infection from entering the patient's bloodstream.

For insertion of a tunneled, centrally inserted CVAD without a subcutaneous port or pump, standard preparations are made and the site over the access vein (e.g., subclavian, jugular) is injected with local anesthesia and, using a Percutaneous approach, is punctured with a needle or accessed by cutdown using a small incision. A guidewire is inserted, and a subcutaneous tunnel is created using a blunt pair of forceps or sharp tunneling tools, under the clavicle from the anterior chest wall to the venotomy site, which is dilated to the right size. The central catheter is passed through this tunnel over the guidewire and into the target vein. Ultrasound guidance may be used to gain venous access and/or fluoroscopy may be employed to check the positioning of the catheter tip in the superior vena cava. The catheter is secured into position, and any incisions are sutured.

Totally Implantable Subcutaneous Central Vascular Access Device (TIVAD)
A totally implantable subcutaneous central vascular access device (TIVAD) is a device or port implanted into the subcutaneous tissue without any portion of it exiting the skin surface. It contains a single or double injection port with a catheter that connects the port to the central line with end placement in the superior vena cava. Central venous access is obtained through skin puncture into the port with a special needle. Totally implantable vascular devices facilitate safe and comfortable access for infusion of long-term or permanent therapies such as chemotherapy, antibiotics, or hemodialysis.

This procedure is a two-part process, with the first part involving the placement of the central venous line. *See also* Insertion, Central Line.

The second part of the procedure involves implanting the subcutaneous port or reservoir, reported with the root operation Insertion. The body part value depends on the insertion site of the port. The port may be placed in the chest in a subcutaneous pocket created through an incision in the chest wall, or in the arm through a small incision just above or halfway between the elbow crease and the shoulder on the inside of the arm. Less often, the abdomen is used. The approach value for the insertion is Open since the procedure requires cutting through the skin and subcutaneous layers to reach the insertion site.

For insertion of a centrally inserted TIVAD with a subcutaneous port or reservoir, the site is injected with local anesthesia. Using an Open approach, the physician creates a subcutaneous pocket for the port by incising through the skin into the subcutaneous tissue, using blunt dissection and cautery to create the pocket, and placing the port. A guidewire is inserted, and a subcutaneous tunnel is created using a blunt pair of forceps or sharp tunneling tools from the port

Medical and Surgical

Insertion, Vascular Access Device (CVAD, TIVAD, Port-A-Cath) (continued)

site to the venotomy site. The catheter is passed through this tunnel over the guidewire and into the target vein. The catheter is connected to the port and checked by injection. The catheter and port are secured into position, and any incisions are sutured.

Focus Point

Vascular access devices may be documented as:

Vascular access device, tunneled:

- *Hickman*
- *Broviac*
- *Leonard*
- *Groshong*

Vascular access device, totally implantable:

- *Port-A-Cath*
- *BardPort*
- *PassPort*
- *Medi-port*
- *Infusaport*

Coding Guidance

AHA: 2017, 4Q, 63; 2017, 2Q, 24, 26; 2017, 1Q, 31; 2016, 2Q, 14, 15; 2015, 4Q, 26; 2015, 2Q, 33; 2013, 4Q, 116

© 2018 Optum360, LLC

Insertion, Ventricular Assist Device

See also Implantation, Biventricular Heart Replacement System (Artificial Heart)

Body System
Heart and Great Vessels

PCS Root Operation
Insertion

Root Operation Table
Ø2H   Heart and Great Vessels, Insertion

Body Part
Heart

Approach
Open
Percutaneous

Device
Implantable Heart Assist System
Short-term External Heart Assist System

Qualifier
Intraoperative (Short-term External Heart Assist System)
Biventricular (Short-term External Heart Assist System)
No Qualifier

Description
A ventricular heart assist system is a mechanical support device with an internal or external circulation pump connected to the heart that provides temporary cardiac support for the left, right, or bilateral (biventricular) ventricles. It is most frequently used in the left ventricle and is called a left ventricular assist device (LVAD).

Unlike an internal biventricular artificial heart, which requires resection of the ventricles so the native heart is no longer intact, a ventricular assist device system is attached to the heart at the ventricle(s), leaving the heart intact. It may be used as a bridge to heart transplantation or in patients who are not candidates for heart transplantation. It may also be used in patients with reversible conditions affecting cardiac output in which the native heart may regain function. The components include an internal implantable pump or an external pump, inflow and outflow cannula, an external controller, which is a small computer that monitors the pump, a cable that connects the pump to the external controller, and power sources for the pump and controller.

Under general anesthesia, the physician inserts the VAD as temporary cardiac support for the left, right, or both left and right ventricles using an Open sternotomy approach to insert cannula attachments to the ventricle(s). An external blood pump is positioned outside the body and connected to the cannulas inserted into the heart, or for an implantable heart assist device, an internal pump may be placed in the left upper quadrant of the peritoneal cavity and connected to the cannulas inserted in the ventricles.

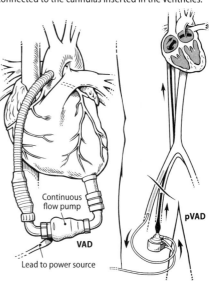

Continuous flow pump

VAD

Lead to power source

pVAD

Percutaneous ventricular assist devices (pVAD) are placed through the femoral artery or femoral vein using a Percutaneous approach. Two examples of pVADs are the TandemHeart and the Impella device. In the TandemHeart system, a catheter is introduced through the femoral vein and passed into the left atrium via transseptal puncture. Oxygenated blood is pumped from the left atrium into the arterial system via the femoral artery. The Impella device introduces a small pump through a femoral artery catheter into the left ventricle. The device(s) pumps blood into the ascending aorta from the left ventricle. If right ventricular assistance is required, a second Impella device is inserted through the femoral vein.

> **Focus Point**
> *Report qualifier Intraoperative for short-term external heart assist devices when the device is used only during the procedure. The ICD-10-PCS classification provides this qualifier for specific procedures involving clinically significant devices, where the device is to be used for a brief duration during the procedure. This qualifier is not used in procedures that involve a device that remains in the patient at the conclusion of the procedure and is removed anywhere from several hours to several days later. Report qualifier Biventricular for biventricular support or No Qualifier for single left or right ventricular support devices that remain in the patient at the conclusion of the procedure.*

Medical and Surgical

Insertion, Ventricular Assist Device (continued)

Focus Point

In addition to the code for Insertion of the Impella device, report an additional code from table 5A02 Assistance, Cardiac, to capture the cardiac output assistance with an impeller pump.

Coding Guidance
AHA: 2017, 1Q, 10; 2016, 4Q, 137-139

Intubation, Endotracheal

Body System
Respiratory System

PCS Root Operation
Insertion

Root Operation Table
0BH   Respiratory System, Insertion

Body Part
Trachea

Approach
Via Natural or Artificial Opening

Device
Intraluminal Device, Endotracheal Airway

Description
Endotracheal (ET) intubation is performed to ensure adequate ventilation in a patient in danger of respiratory failure or in respiratory failure. Endotracheal (ET) intubation is an emergency procedure performed on patients who are unconscious or unable to breathe on their own. The ET tube is placed into the trachea (windpipe) to maintain an open airway and prevent suffocation. The tube can be placed either orally or nasally.

The physician places an endotracheal tube to provide air passage in emergency situations. The patient is ventilated with a mask and bag and positioned by extending the neck anteriorly and the head posteriorly. The physician places the laryngoscope into the patient's mouth and advances the blade toward the epiglottis until the vocal cords are visible. An endotracheal tube is inserted between the vocal cords and advanced to the proper position. The cuff of the endotracheal tube is inflated.

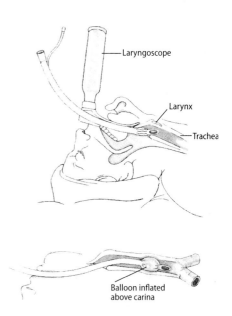

Laryngoscope

Larynx

Trachea

Balloon inflated above carina

Focus Point

In most cases, ET intubation associated with a surgical procedure is not reported. For the patient who remains on ET intubation following surgery (i.e., a complication of surgery), the mechanical ventilation would be reported but the ET intubation would not be reported.

Focus Point

Ongoing mechanical ventilation is reported with a code from root operation table 5A1 Performance, Respiratory. These codes are based on the duration of time the patient receives mechanical ventilation, beginning when the ET intubation is completed.

Coding Guidance
AHA: 2017, 1Q, 29; 2014, 4Q, 3

© 2018 Optum360, LLC

Jejunostomy, Percutaneous Endoscopic (PEJ)

See also Gastrostomy, Percutaneous Endoscopic (PEG)

See also Conversion, Gastrostomy to Jejunostomy (PEG-PEJ)

Body System
Gastrointestinal System

PCS Root Operation
Insertion

Root Operation Table
ØDH   Gastrointestinal System, Insertion

Body Part
Jejunum

Approach
Percutaneous

Device
Feeding Device

Description
A percutaneous jejunostomy (PEJ) is the surgical placement of a (feeding) tube directly into the midsection of the small intestine (jejunum) through the abdominal wall. Conversely the percutaneous gastrostomy (PEG) feeding tube is placed into the stomach (*see also* Gastrostomy, Percutaneous Endoscopic [PEG]). A gastrojejunostomy (PEGJ) is not a feeding device, but rather an anastomosis between the small intestine and stomach (Bypass).

A percutaneous (endoscopic assisted) jejunostomy tube can help patients continue to absorb nutrients through their small intestine without requiring the use of the mouth, esophagus, and stomach and is useful in preventing severe acid reflux. This is useful in patients with impaired swallowing function or those who are post-gastro-surgical procedures. Other candidates for PEJ tubes are patients in whom malignancies are blocking the stomach or esophagus, or those who have had esophageal reconstruction and need time to allow the esophagus to recover.

The physician passes an endoscope through the patient's mouth into the esophagus and advances it into the small intestine (jejunum) where it is transilluminated through the abdominal skin. Using a Percutaneous approach, a needle is placed through the skin on the exterior of the abdominal wall into the lumen of the jejunum under visualization of the endoscope. A wire is threaded through the needle into the bowel lumen. The needle is removed. A jejunostomy tube is placed over the wire, through the skin, into the jejunum, and secured into place. The endoscope is withdrawn.

The root operation Insertion is reported for the Insertion of the Feeding Device by a Percutaneous approach.

Focus Point
The endoscope is used to visualize the placement of a percutaneous jejunostomy tube and is considered inherent to the procedure and not coded separately. Fluoroscopy can also be used in conjunction with the percutaneous placement and does not have to be reported separately.

Focus Point
In some cases, a PEG is converted to a PEJ. This conversion procedure is reported with the same root operation as the performance of a new percutaneous (endoscopic assisted) jejunostomy (PEJ) but with a different approach. See also Conversion, Gastrostomy to Jejunostomy (PEG-PEJ).

Coding Guidance
AHA: 2013, 4Q, 117

Joint Replacement, Hip (Partial)

Body System
Lower Joints

PCS Root Operation
Replacement

Root Operation Table
ØSR   Lower Joints, Replacement

Body Part
Hip Joint, Acetabular Surface, Right
Hip Joint, Acetabular Surface, Left
Hip Joint, Femoral Surface, Right
Hip Joint, Femoral Surface, Left

Approach
Open

Device
Synthetic Substitute, Polyethylene (Acetabular Surface)
Synthetic Substitute, Metal
Synthetic Substitute, Ceramic
Synthetic Substitute

Qualifier
Cemented
Uncemented
No Qualifier

Description
Hip replacement surgery is a reconstructive procedure performed on patients with painful hips due to osteoarthritis, rheumatoid arthritis, hip fracture, avascular necrosis/osteonecrosis, and bone tumors.

Under general anesthesia, the patient is placed in a lateral decubitus position (lying on the side), and prepped and draped. The physician performs a repair of the femoral surface of a hip joint with a femoral prosthesis. Using an Open approach, the physician makes a posterolateral incision over the hip. The fascia lata is incised, and the muscles around the hip joint are retracted to visualize the capsule. The physician then incises the capsule, exposing the femoral neck. The diseased femoral head is surgically removed with a reciprocating saw and measured with a caliper to determine the appropriate size for replacement. The physician prepares the femoral shaft by enlarging the canal with a rasp and then selects the type of stem to be used. The stem is inserted and pounded into place

in the femoral shaft with an impactor. The physician then repositions the femoral stem prosthesis. Hip motion and stability are evaluated. The capsule is closed, and the incision is repaired in multiple layers.

Alternatively, only the acetabulum is replaced. Under general anesthesia, the patient is placed in a lateral decubitus position (lying on the side), and prepped and draped. The physician performs a repair of the acetabular surface of a hip joint with an acetabular prosthesis. Using an Open approach, the physician makes an incision along the posterior aspect of the hip with the patient in a lateral decubitus position. The short external rotator muscles are released by incision from their insertion point on the femur, exposing the joint capsule. The physician incises the capsule and dislocates the hip. The acetabulum is prepared, and any osteophytes are moved from around the rim with an osteotome. The acetabulum is reamed out with a power reamer, exposing both subchondral and cancellous bone. The acetabular component is measured and is inserted. The physician then repositions the hip. Any reflected muscles are reattached. The incision is then repaired in multiple layers with suction drains.

> **Focus Point**
> The root operation Replacement is reported for a total or partial hip arthroplasty and includes any explantation or excision of the body part being replaced.

> **Focus Point**
> In cases of significant bone loss, additional support may be required to secure a hip replacement. In these cases, it is appropriate to report an additional code for any Supplement procedure performed, as well as any autograft harvest from a different surgical location. Autograft tissue harvested from the operative site, however, is not reported separately, according to ICD-10-PCS guideline B3.9.

> **Focus Point**
> If the record documentation does not specify the type of bearing surface, use as the default the qualifier Synthetic Substitute or query the provider.

Coding Guidance
AHA: 2016, 3Q, 35; 2015, 3Q, 18; 2015, 1Q, 30

© 2018 Optum360, LLC

Joint Replacement, Hip (Total)

Body System
Lower Joints

PCS Root Operation
Replacement

Root Operation Table
ØSR   Lower Joints, Replacement

Body Part
Hip Joint, Right
Hip Joint, Left

Approach
Open

Device
Synthetic Substitute, Metal
Synthetic Substitute, Metal on Polyethylene
Synthetic Substitute, Ceramic
Synthetic Substitute, Ceramic on Polyethylene
Synthetic Substitute, Oxidized Zirconium on
Polyethylene
Synthetic Substitute
Articulating Spacer

Qualifier
Cemented
Uncemented
No Qualifier

Description

Hip replacement surgery is a reconstructive procedure
performed on patients with painful hips due to
osteoarthritis, rheumatoid arthritis, hip fracture,
avascular necrosis/osteonecrosis, and bone tumors.

The physician performs a total reconstruction of the
hip with replacement of both the femoral head and
acetabulum by prosthesis. Under general anesthesia,
the patient is placed in a lateral decubitus position
(lying on the side), and prepped and draped. Using an
Open approach, the physician makes an incision along
the posterior aspect of the hip. The short external
rotator muscles are released by incision from their
insertion point on the femur, exposing the joint
capsule. The physician incises the capsule and
dislocates the hip posteriorly. The physician surgically
removes the diseased femoral head with a
reciprocating saw. The physician removes any
osteophytes around the rim of the acetabulum with an
osteotome. The acetabulum is reamed out with a
power reamer, exposing both subchondral and
cancellous bone, and the acetabular component is
inserted. The femoral canal is then prepared using
either a hand or a power reamer. The excised femoral
head is measured with a caliper to determine the

appropriate size for replacement. The physician
prepares the femoral shaft by enlarging the canal with
a rasp and then selects the type of stem to be used.
The stem is inserted and pounded into place in the
femoral shaft with an impactor. The physician then
repositions the femoral stem prosthesis. The physician
may augment the area with an autograft or allograft.
The autograft may be harvested from the excised
femoral head. Donor bone (allograft) may be used
instead. The physician places the bone graft into the
canal and/or acetabulum. The hip is repositioned. The
external rotator muscles are reattached. The incision is
repaired in multiple layers with suction drains.

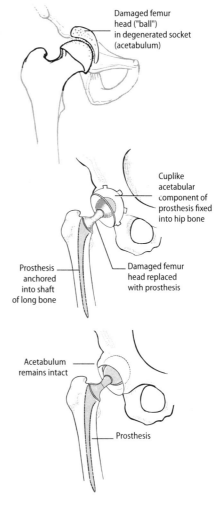

Damaged femur head ("ball") in degenerated socket (acetabulum)

Cuplike acetabular component of prosthesis fixed into hip bone

Prosthesis anchored into shaft of long bone

Damaged femur head replaced with prosthesis

Acetabulum remains intact

Prosthesis

© 2018 Optum360, LLC

Joint Replacement, Hip (Total) (continued)

Focus Point

The root operation Replacement is reported for a total or partial hip arthroplasty and includes any explantation of the body part being replaced.

Focus Point

In cases of significant bone loss, additional support may be required to secure a hip replacement. In these cases, it is appropriate to report an additional code for any Supplement procedure performed, as well as any autograft harvest from a different surgical location. Autograft tissue harvested from the operative site, however, is not reported separately, according to ICD-10-PCS guideline B3.9.

Focus Point

If the record documentation does not specify the type of bearing surface, use as the default the qualifier Synthetic Substitute or query the provider.

Focus Point

A newer bearing surface listed in the devices is Oxidized Zirconium, which is a metal alloy with a ceramic finish that combines the strength and durability of metal with the smoothness and reduced friction of a ceramic. Oxidized zirconium on polyethylene is reportedly longer wearing and less prone to metal allergic reactions.

Coding Guidance

AHA: 2016, 3Q, 35; 2015, 3Q, 18; 2015, 1Q, 30

© 2018 Optum360, LLC

Joint Replacement, Hip Resurfacing (Hip Resurfacing Arthroplasty)

Body System
Lower Joints

PCS Root Operation
Supplement

Root Operation Table
ØSU Lower Joints, Supplement

Body Part
Hip Joint, Right
Hip Joint, Left
Hip Joint, Acetabular Surface, Right
Hip Joint, Acetabular Surface, Left
Hip Joint, Femoral Surface, Right
Hip Joint, Femoral Surface, Left

Approach
Open

Device
Resurfacing Device

Description
In comparison to traditional hip replacement arthroplasty or revision arthroplasty, total or partial hip resurfacing arthroplasty involves the grinding away of only the worn surfaces of the femoral head and/or the acetabulum, retaining the greater part of the femoral head and the femoral neck and placing new bearing surfaces. A cobalt chrome cap is positioned over the smoothed surfaces of the femoral head, articulating with a metal cup that has been pressed into the reamed acetabulum; thus the articulation is metal on metal. Since the head of the femur is preserved, hip resurfacing conserves more of the bone. Intended as an initial joint replacement for patients who are likely to require more than one hip joint replacement in their lifetime, partial hip resurfacing is expected to delay total hip replacement and possibly eliminate the necessity of a revision hip replacement in patients who desire to continue a fairly active lifestyle.

Indications for total or partial resurfacing include osteoarthritis, traumatic arthritis, avascular necrosis, and dysplasia/developmental dislocation of the hip (DDH). Partial resurfacing is not recommended for treating inflammatory disease since the implants that are presently available have comparatively unpredictable pain relief. Mechanical failure of partial resurfacing is rare; however, inadequate pain relief can result in conversion of the partial resurfacing to a total hip replacement within a five-year period.

With the patient in a lateral position and using a posterior Open approach, the surgeon releases the external rotators from the piriformis to the gluteus maximus tendon. The surgeon performs a posterior capsulectomy and dislocates the femoral head. Anterior capsular release is accomplished, and the neck diameter is measured to determine the appropriate size of components to be used. The head is retracted anterosuperiorly, and the acetabulum is exposed with the aid of a retractor. Using hemispherical reamers, the surgeon shapes the acetabulum in 2 mm increments until the desired size is reached. The acetabular cup is fitted. The surgeon then prepares the femoral head in sequential steps to adapt to the resurfacing component. The surgeon reduces the components and fixes them into place using bone cement and then performs layered closure of the soft tissues. Drainage tubes may be left in place for a couple of days following the surgery.

Focus Point
The ICD-10-PCS Device Key lists two hip Resurfacing Devices: the Cormet Hip Resurfacing System and the CONSERVE® PLUS Total Resurfacing Hip System.

Focus Point
A total hip joint resurfacing involves the entire hip joint and includes both the femoral and acetabular surfaces. A partial hip joint resurfacing involves only one surface, either femoral or acetabular.

Joint Replacement, Hip Revision (Revision Arthroplasty)

Body System
Lower Joints

PCS Root Operation
Replacement

Root Operation Table
0SR   Lower Joints, Replacement

Body Part
Hip Joint, Right
Hip Joint, Left
Hip Joint, Acetabular Surface, Right
Hip Joint, Acetabular Surface, Left
Hip Joint, Femoral Surface, Right
Hip Joint, Femoral Surface, Left

Approach
Open

Device
Synthetic Substitute, Metal (Hip Joint)
Synthetic Substitute, Metal on Polyethylene (Hip Joint)
Synthetic Substitute, Ceramic (Hip Joint)
Synthetic Substitute, Ceramic on Polyethylene (Hip Joint)
Synthetic Substitute (Hip Joint)
Synthetic Substitute, Oxidized Zirconium on Polyethylene (Hip Joint)
Synthetic Substitute, Polyethylene (Hip Joint, Acetabular Surface)
Synthetic Substitute, Metal (Hip Joint, Acetabular Surface)
Synthetic Substitute, Ceramic (Hip Joint, Acetabular Surface)
Synthetic Substitute (Hip Joint, Acetabular Surface)
Synthetic Substitute, Metal (Hip Joint, Femoral Surface)
Synthetic Substitute, Ceramic (Hip Joint, Femoral Surface)
Synthetic Substitute (Hip Joint, Femoral Surface)
Articulating Spacer (Hip Joint)

Qualifier
Cemented
Uncemented
No Qualifier

Description
After an extended period of use, hip replacements can fail, necessitating revision surgery. Common reasons for revision joint replacement surgery include:

- Mechanical loosening of the prosthesis
- Wear of the weight-bearing surface
- Infection
- Dislocation and instability

- Fracture of the bone around the implant (peri-prosthetic fracture)
- Implant fracture
- Technical error
- Painful results with decrease in mobility
- Mechanical failure

Revision of Hip Replacement, Both Acetabular and Femoral Components
If both implants fail, revision of both the acetabular and femoral components may be necessary.

Using an Open approach with the patient in a lateral decubitus (lying on the side) position, the physician may access the hip through the previous hip surgery incision. Muscles are reflected. A trochanteric osteotomy may be performed with an oscillating saw. The physician incises the hip joint capsule and frees and removes any scar tissue. The physician manually dislocates the hip. Cement is removed from the upper portion of the femoral stem with a motorized or hand instrument. The stem may be removed. If the stem has fractured, the physician may drill a hole in the femoral shaft so that an instrument may remove the broken portion. Any remaining cement in the femoral shaft is removed. The physician removes scar tissue and cement from around the acetabular component with chisels and gouges. The acetabular component is removed from its bed. The physician reconstructs the acetabulum with or without cement. If the acetabulum is reconstructed without cement, the component is usually inserted and fixed with screws. If cement is used, it secures the new component in the acetabular bed. If significant bone loss is encountered, the physician may augment the area with an autograft or allograft, which is separately reported. The new femoral stem is inserted into the femoral shaft with or without cement. The physician reduces (repositions) the hip and closes the capsule. The greater trochanter is wired into place. Suction drains may be placed in the wound. The incision is repaired in multiple layers with sutures, staples, and/or Steri-Strips.

Revision of Hip Replacement, Acetabular Component
Revision of the acetabular component entails the removal and replacement of the entire acetabular component, including both the metal shell and the bearing surface (liner). The liner is a part of the acetabular component; if the liner alone is replaced, it is reported with the root operation Supplement rather than Replacement because only a part of the component is being replaced. Wearing of the modular bearing surface, loosening due to osteolysis, infection, or recurrent dislocations due to faulty positioning of the component are some of the most common indications for revision of the acetabular component. If the patient has sufficient remaining bone stock,

   © 2018 Optum360, LLC

Joint Replacement, Hip Revision (Revision Arthroplasty) (continued)

the replacement may be performed with an implant that is similar but slightly larger than the original implant.

If component malposition or osteolysis have resulted in a significant amount of bone destruction, specialized implants and a large amount of allograft bone or other bone substitutes may be required. Reconstruction in these cases is more complex, resulting in considerably prolonged surgery and recovery times and less predictable patient outcomes.

Using an Open approach with the patient in a lateral decubitus (lying on the side) position, the physician accesses the acetabular component through a previous hip surgery incision. Muscles are reflected. The physician may perform an osteotomy of the greater trochanter with an oscillating saw. The capsule is incised and the hip manually dislocated. Any scar tissue is removed from around the acetabulum. The physician removes cement from around the acetabular component with chisels and gouges. The acetabulum is levered out from its bed. The acetabulum may need to be reamed out in preparation for the new component. The physician reconstructs the acetabulum with or without cement. If the acetabulum is reconstructed without cement, the component is usually inserted and fixed with screws. Prior to the acetabulum component placement, the physician may harvest a bone graft from the patient's iliac crest and close the surgically created graft donor site. Donor bone (allograft) may be used instead. If cement is used, it secures the new component in the acetabular bed. Once the cement has dried, the hip is reduced (repositioned) and the capsule closed. The physician may place suction drains in the wound. The incision is repaired in multiple layers with sutures, staples, and/or Steri-Strips.

Revision of Hip Replacement, Femoral Component
Using an Open approach with the patient in a lateral decubitus position (lying on the side), the physician may access the femoral component through the previous hip surgery incision. Muscles are reflected. The physician may perform an osteotomy of the greater trochanter. The hip joint capsule is exposed

and incised. The physician dislocates the hip joint. If cement was used on the previous arthroplasty, the physician uses a motorized or hand instrument to remove it from around the upper portion of the femoral stem. If loose enough, the stem is removed with forceful blows. If the stem cannot be removed, additional cement may need to be removed from the femoral shaft so the stem can be extracted. The physician may place cement in the femoral shaft and insert the new femoral component. If the revision is cementless, donor bone (allograft) may be inserted as needed into the femoral shaft between the cortex and femoral component. The hip is reduced (repositioned). The physician reattaches the greater trochanter with wires. The incision is repaired in multiple layers with sutures, staples, and/or Steri-Strips.

Focus Point

When the objective of the procedure is to remove and replace the previously placed device, separate codes must be reported using the root operations Replacement and Removal. If the sole purpose of the procedure is to adjust the previously placed device without removal or replacement, the root operation Revision is used.

Focus Point

If the record documentation does not specify the type of bearing surface, use as the default the qualifier Synthetic Substitute or query the provider.

Focus Point

In cases of significant bone loss, additional support may be required to secure a hip replacement. In these cases, it is appropriate to report an additional code for any Supplement procedure performed, as well as any autograft harvest from a different surgical location. Autograft tissue harvested from the operative site, however, is not reported separately, according to ICD-10-PCS guideline B3.9.

Coding Guidance

AHA: 2016, 4Q, 110; 2016, 3Q, 35; 2015, 2Q, 19; 2015, 1Q, 30

Joint Replacement, Knee

See also Insertion, Intraoperative Knee Replacement Sensor, in the New Technology section

Body System
Lower Joints

PCS Root Operation
Replacement

Root Operation Table
ØSR   Lower Joints, Replacement

Body Part
Knee Joint, Right
Knee Joint, Left
Knee Joint, Femoral Surface, Right
Knee Joint, Femoral Surface, Left
Knee Joint, Tibial Surface, Right
Knee Joint, Tibial Surface, Left

Approach
Open

Device
Synthetic Substitute, Oxidized Zirconium on Polyethylene (Knee Joint, Right; Knee Joint, Left)
Synthetic Substitute
Synthetic Substitute, Unicondylar Medial (Knee Joint, Right; Knee Joint, Left)
Synthetic Substitute, Unicondylar Lateral (Knee Joint, Right; Knee Joint, Left)
Synthetic Substitute, Patellofemoral (Knee Joint, Right; Knee Joint, Left)
Articulating Spacer (Knee Joint, Right; Knee Joint, Left)

Qualifier
Cemented
Uncemented
No Qualifier

Description
Knee replacement surgery is most commonly performed on patients with osteoarthritis. The physician replaces severely damaged or worn bone and cartilage with a prosthetic implant in one (unicompartmental, or hemi-joint), two (bicompartmental), or three (tricompartmental) compartments.

Using an Open approach, a midline incision is made over the knee. Dissection is carried down to expose the knee joint. The physician may release soft tissues and/or ligaments to correct deformities and improve range

of motion. The physician uses a cutting-alignment jig placed on the upper tibia to remove the tibial joint surface (both medial and lateral compartments) by making a bone cut. A cutting-alignment jig is also used on the femoral condyles to make the appropriate bone cut. Depending on the integrity of the joint surface of the patella, the physician may also make a bone cut to remove damaged cartilage. If the joint surface is healthy, it is left intact. Peg holes are usually made, and the components of the prosthesis are placed into position on the tibia, femur, and, if needed, the patella. The surgeon may use an intraoperative knee replacement sensor, which is a sterile, disposable tibial insert used to help orthopaedic surgeons place prosthetic joint components during knee replacement surgery. After optimal range of motion and placement are confirmed, the components are secured with cement and/or bone screws. The incision is repaired in multiple layers with sutures, staples, and/or Steri-Strips.

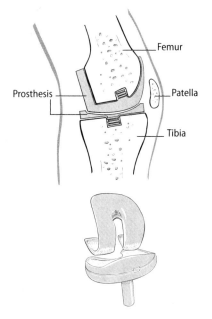

Focus Point
A replacement procedure includes removal of the body part being replaced; therefore, the removal or excision of the body part is not reported.

© 2018 Optum360, LLC

Joint Replacement, Knee (continued)

Focus Point

When coding knee replacement procedures, use the appropriate Body Part(s) depending on which components are replaced. A total knee replacement procedure includes both medial and lateral compartments of the tibia and femur. If the knee replacement involves both the femoral and tibial surfaces (medial, lateral, or both), use Knee Joint, Right or Knee Joint, Left. If the knee replacement involves only one surface—either the femoral or the tibial surface (full or partial)—use Knee Joint, Femoral Surface, Right; Knee Joint, Femoral Surface, Left; Knee Joint, Tibial Surface, Right; or Knee Joint, Tibial Surface, Left.

Focus Point

A unicondylar knee procedure replaces either the medial or the lateral portion of the knee joint, generally a femoral component and a tibial component with an insert that articulates against the femur; Synthetic Substitute, Unicondylar, Medial or Lateral, is reported.

Focus Point

Use of an intraoperative knee replacement sensor during the knee replacement is reported with an additional code from the ICD-10-PCS New Technology section X. See also Insertion, Intraoperative Knee Replacement Sensor.

Focus Point

A newer bearing surface listed in the devices is Oxidized Zirconium, which is a metal alloy with a ceramic finish that combines the strength and durability of metal with the smoothness and reduced friction of a ceramic. Oxidized zirconium on polyethylene is reportedly longer wearing and less prone to metal allergic reactions.

Coding Guidance

AHA: 2018, 2Q, 16; 2016, 4Q, 109, 110; 2016, 3Q, 35, 36; 2015, 2Q, 18, 19

Medical and Surgical

Joint Replacement, Shoulder (Partial)

See also Joint Replacement, Shoulder (Total)

See also Joint Replacement, Shoulder, Reverse (Reverse Shoulder Arthroplasty)

Body System
Upper Joints

PCS Root Operation
Replacement

Root Operation Table
ØRR   Upper Joints, Replacement

Body Part
Shoulder Joint, Right
Shoulder Joint, Left

Approach
Open

Device
Synthetic Substitute

Qualifier
Humeral Surface
Glenoid Surface

Description

Shoulder replacement surgery is a reconstructive procedure performed on patients with painful shoulders due to osteoarthritis or degenerative joint disease. Reduction in pain and restored range of motion are expected outcomes of shoulder replacement surgery. A total shoulder replacement is one in which both the humeral head (ball) and glenoid (socket) are replaced with a synthetic prosthesis; a partial shoulder replacement only involves one of the two components, most often the humeral head. The Qualifier value captures the body part being replaced.

Using an Open approach, the physician makes a long, curved incision from the superior aspect of the acromion along the deltopectoral interval to the deltoid insertion. The deltoid is retracted laterally and the pectoralis medially. The fascia between the pectoralis and the clavicle is divided, and the subacromial space is freed with a gloved finger or periosteal elevator. The coracoacromial ligament is freed, and often an acromioplasty is performed to allow for freedom of movement after surgery. The subscapularis tendon is tagged and removed from the capsule. The physician divides the anterior joint

capsule and dislocates the glenohumeral joint by further external rotation and extension of the arm. The joint is explored, and all loose bodies are removed. The humeral head is removed with a reciprocating saw or osteotome. A prosthesis is placed along the proximal humerus as a guide for proper inclination of the osteotomy. A horizontal cut (osteotomy) is made as previously determined, and a large curette is used to open the medullary canal for placement of the stem of the prosthesis. The canal is enlarged with a reamer to the appropriate size. The prosthesis is positioned in proper rotational alignment to articulate with the glenoid. Any remaining osteophytes (bone spurs) are removed. The joint is irrigated thoroughly. The prosthesis is reduced into the glenoid, and the subscapularis tendon is sutured in place with multiple interrupted nonabsorbable sutures with the shoulder in neutral position. The deltopectoral interval is closed loosely over drainage tubes. The arm is placed in a sling and swathe bandage.

> **Focus Point**
>
> Determine if the surgeon performed a total or partial replacement. See also Joint Replacement, Shoulder (Total).

> **Focus Point**
>
> If a reverse ball and socket technique is used, the device value is Synthetic Substitute, Reverse Ball and Socket. See also Joint Replacement, Shoulder, Reverse (Reverse Shoulder Arthroplasty).

> **Focus Point**
>
> Additional procedures—for example rotator cuff repair, tenodesis, and suture, and transfer of nearby muscles and tendons such as the latissimus dorsi—may be performed to complete the joint replacement procedure and achieve stability and functionality of the new joint. These procedures are included in the joint replacement and are not reported separately.

> **Focus Point**
>
> When a previously placed prosthesis needs to be removed and replaced, code both the Removal and the Replacement.

Coding Guidance
AHA: 2015, 3Q, 14

© 2018 Optum360, LLC

Joint Replacement, Shoulder (Total)

See also Joint Replacement, Shoulder (Partial)

See also Joint Replacement, Shoulder, Reverse (Reverse Shoulder Arthroplasty)

Body System
Upper Joints

PCS Root Operation
Replacement

Root Operation Table
ØRR   Upper Joints, Replacement

Body Part
Shoulder Joint, Right
Shoulder Joint, Left

Approach
Open

Device
Synthetic Substitute

Description

Shoulder replacement surgery is a reconstructive procedure performed on patients with painful shoulders due to osteoarthritis or degenerative joint disease. Reduction in pain and restored range of motion are expected outcomes of shoulder replacement surgery. A total shoulder replacement is one in which both the humeral head (ball) and glenoid (socket) are replaced with a synthetic prosthesis; a partial shoulder replacement involves only one of the two components.

A total shoulder replacement is done for the glenohumeral joint. Using an Open approach, a long, curved incision is made from the superior aspect of the acromion along the deltopectoral interval to the deltoid insertion. The deltoid is retracted laterally and pectoralis medially. The fascia between the pectoralis and the clavicle is divided, and the subacromial space is freed with a gloved finger or periosteal elevator. The coracoacromial ligament is freed, and often an acromioplasty is performed to allow for freedom of movement after surgery. The subscapularis tendon is tagged and removed from the capsule. The anterior joint capsule is divided, and the glenohumeral joint is dislocated by further external rotation and extension of the arm. The joint is explored, and all loose bodies

are removed. The humeral head is removed with a reciprocating saw or osteotome. In addition, a prosthetic device is placed proximally at the glenoid to articulate with the prosthetic humeral head. Before placement of the humeral prosthesis, the joint is opened to fully expose the glenoid surface. The surface cartilage of the glenoid is removed. A power drill is used to cut a slot into the glenoid the exact size of the holding device of the glenoid component. Small curettes are used to remove cancellous bone from the base of the coracoid bone. With a burr, articular cartilage is removed from the surface of the glenoid. A trial glenoid component is used to properly prepare the bone and fit the prosthesis. Once the glenoid preparation is complete, the glenoid vault is drilled and filled with polymethylmethacrylate (bone cement). The glenoid component is pushed into place and held until the cement is cured. Prior to final insertion of the humeral component, an anterior acromioplasty and acromioclavicular arthroplasty are performed, if necessary. If large rotator cuff tears are found, they are repaired at this time. The joint is brought through a full range of motion and fully irrigated. The subscapularis tendon is repaired to stabilize the joint; however, the joint capsule is not usually resutured. Drains are placed, and the deltopectoral interval is sutured closed. The arm is placed in a sling and swathe.

Focus Point
Determine if the surgeon performed a total or partial replacement. See also Joint Replacement, Shoulder (Partial).

Focus Point
If a reverse ball and socket technique is used, see also Joint Replacement, Shoulder, Reverse (Reverse Shoulder Arthroplasty).

Focus Point
Additional procedures—for example rotator cuff repair, tenodesis, and suture, and transfer of nearby muscles and tendons such as the latissimus dorsi—may be performed to complete the joint replacement procedure and achieve the stability and functionality of the new joint. These procedures are included in the joint replacement and are not reported separately.

Joint Replacement, Shoulder, Reverse (Reverse Shoulder Arthroplasty)

See also Joint Replacement, Shoulder (Partial)

See also Joint Replacement, Shoulder (Total)

Body System
Upper Joints

PCS Root Operation
Replacement

Root Operation Table
ØRR   Upper Joints, Replacement

Body Part
Shoulder Joint, Right
Shoulder Joint, Left

Approach
Open

Device
Synthetic Substitute, Reverse Ball and Socket

Description

Reverse total shoulder replacement is an alternative procedure for patients with certain diagnoses who cannot be treated effectively with conventional total shoulder replacement, the most common of which includes rotator cuff arthropathy. Other indications include certain complex humeral head fractures and advanced glenohumeral pathology. Since the reverse procedure may not restore full function, it is commonly performed for patients 65 to 70 years of age to relieve pain and restore basic function.

In a reverse total shoulder replacement, the ball is placed on the glenoid and the socket is placed on top of the humerus; this is the reverse position from conventional shoulder replacement, hence "reverse shoulder replacement." The deltoid muscle is employed to compensate for otherwise irreparable rotator cuff damage. The reverse shoulder prosthesis provides a fixed fulcrum for the shoulder joint, allowing the arm to be raised overhead. This configuration adds stability, enabling the deltoid muscle to elevate the shoulder. In some cases, transfer of nearby muscles and tendons such as the latissimus dorsi is also performed to help restore rotation and ensure stability of the joint postoperatively. Five or more implants are typically used: a baseplate screwed into a glenosphere, a metallic stem and neck implanted into the humerus that rests on a polyethylene liner or cup insert, with a spacer inserted for proper joint tensioning.

Focus Point

Additional procedures, for example rotator cuff repair, tenodesis, and suture, and transfer of nearby muscles and tendons such as the latissimus dorsi, may be performed to complete the joint replacement procedure and achieve the stability and functionality of the new joint. These procedures are included in the joint replacement and are not reported separately.

Coding Guidance

AHA: 2015, 1Q, 27

© 2018 Optum360, LLC

Keratoplasty, Penetrating

Body System
Eye

PCS Root Operation
Replacement

Root Operation Table
08R Eye, Replacement

Body Part
Cornea, Right
Cornea, Left

Approach
External

Device
Autologous Tissue Substitute
Synthetic Substitute
Nonautologous Tissue Substitute

Description
Keratoplasty is a surgical restoration of the cornea. The cornea is the clear tissue that forms a bulge overlying the pupil. Light enters the eye through the cornea and passes through aqueous humor, the ocular lens, and clear vitreous gel before it reaches the retina, where the image is captured and sent to the brain. The cornea is one of the components of refraction, or the focusing of the image. The cornea may be damaged by scarring, disease, or injury and may need to be restored. Restoration may consist of replacing a few layers of the cornea or replacing the entire cornea.

In a penetrating keratoplasty (PK), the physician, using an External approach, removes the entire cornea, except for a rim around the edge. Removal of the entire cornea compromises the structural integrity of the eye and also the eye's ability to focus. PK is reported as a Replacement of the cornea. The replacement is usually a button-shaped graft of Nonautologous Tissue Substitute cadaver cornea, but a Synthetic Substitute is possible. In rare instances, an Autologous Tissue Substitute taken from the patient's contralateral eye may be used.

The physician measures the patient's cornea to select the size of trephine that will be used to excise corneal tissue. The physician punches a circular hole in the cornea of the donor eye using the trephine. The physician removes the disk of corneal tissue, threads it with preplaced sutures, and sets it aside. In aphakic patients, vitreous and/or aqueous may be withdrawn from the eye before the cornea is removed. A metal ring may be sutured to the sclera of an aphakic patient to stabilize the operative field.

The defective cornea of the patient is removed with the trephine. The donor cornea is positioned with sutures, and then additional sutures secure it to the cornea. The physician may use a saline or air injection to restore proper intraocular pressure.

Focus Point
Restoration of aqueous humor in the anterior segment following keratoplasty is considered inherent in the operation and would not be separately reported.

Coding Guidance
AHA: 2015, 2Q, 24, 25

Kyphoplasty (Percutaneous Vertebral Augmentation)

See also Vertebroplasty

Body System
Upper Bones
Lower Bones

PCS Root Operation
Reposition

Root Operation Table
ØPS   Upper Bones, Reposition
ØQS   Lower Bones, Reposition

Body Part
Cervical Vertebra
Thoracic Vertebra
Lumbar Vertebra

Approach
Percutaneous

Device
No Device

Description
Percutaneous vertebral augmentation, commonly referred to as kyphoplasty, involves insertion of an inflatable balloon, bone tamps, or other device under fluoroscopic guidance to create a cavity, which is filled with a cement-like material to further stabilize the bone.

A percutaneous kyphoplasty is a two-step modification of the single-step percutaneous vertebroplasty. Both are performed for treating pain due to vertebral compression fractures from trauma or conditions such as neoplasm or osteoporotic pathological fractures (*see also* Vertebroplasty). This procedure has the added advantage of restoring vertebral body height and alignment.

The patient is placed in a prone, slightly flexed position. A 5 to 7 mm incision is made, and small cannulas are inserted into the vertebral body from both sides. Balloon catheters, called tamps, are inserted into the vertebra using a Percutaneous approach and are inflated. The tamps create a void in the soft trabecular bone and restore vertebral alignment and height. The intent of the first step of the procedure involves moving or realigning the bone tissue; Reposition is the root operation that describes this objective. Since the balloon tamps are then removed, No Device is reported for the device value for this first step, based on guideline B6.1a. After the balloon tamps are removed, bone cement is injected into the cavity, which is the second step—or the vertebroplasty portion—of the procedure. This step is reported separately with the root operation Supplement (*see also* Vertebroplasty).

Following the procedure, the patient may experience significant, almost immediate, pain relief.

Focus Point
To ensure accurate code assignment, carefully review the medical record documentation for specific information regarding the procedure performed. Both conventional vertebroplasty and vertebral augmentation are percutaneous procedures performed to treat fractured or diseased vertebrae using cement. They differ in that vertebral augmentation, or kyphoplasty, is a two-step procedure using a variety of techniques and devices to mechanically augment vertebral body height followed by injection of the cement filler.

© 2018 Optum360, LLC

Laminectomy, Decompressive (Hemilaminectomy)

See also Discectomy

See also Replacement, Intervertebral Disc, Artificial

Body System
Central Nervous System and Cranial Nerves
Peripheral Nervous System

PCS Root Operation
Release

Root Operation Table
ØØN Central Nervous System and Cranial Nerves, Release
Ø1N Peripheral Nervous System, Release

Body Part
Cervical Spinal Cord
Thoracic Spinal Cord
Lumbar Spinal Cord
Cervical Nerve
Thoracic Nerve
Lumbar Nerve
Sacral Nerve

Approach
Open

Description
Spinal stenosis may be caused by degenerative osteoarthritis of the spine, formation of osteophytes or bone spurs, or hypertrophy of the ligamentum flavum.

Decompressive laminectomy removes the lamina and enlarges the spinal canal, thus decompressing the spinal cord or spinal nerves. Under general anesthesia, the patient is placed face down on the operating table. Through an Open incision in the skin of the back over the affected vertebrae, the muscles are visualized and pushed to the sides with retractors or dilators to visualize the back of the vertebrae. The spinous processes, a portion of the vertebral lamina, and other soft tissues are removed in pieces with a rongeur, with care taken not to damage the surrounding structures such as the dura, as well as the spinal cord and spinal nerves. This allows more room for the spinal cord and spinal nerves. The incision is closed with staples or stitches. This procedure can be performed with a minimally invasive incision and a special surgical microscope.

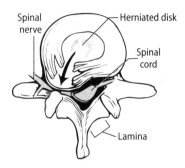
Laminectomy with Decompression

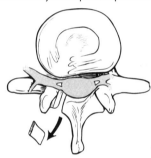
Laminectomy decompresses spinal nerve

Focus Point
When a physician removes the lamina (laminectomy and hemilaminectomy) and/or performs foraminotomies in conjunction with a spinal fusion, these procedures are considered a part of the operative approach for the spinal fusion and are not coded separately. However, decompressive foraminotomy/laminectomy performed specifically for spinal stenosis to release pressure on the spinal cord and/or nerve (root) is a distinct, separately reportable procedure, reported with root operation Release.

Focus Point
To report the correct ICD-10-PCS body part released, carefully review the record documentation for the site of spinal stenosis and compression. Radiculopathy is caused by compression of the spinal nerves or nerve roots. Myelopathy, however, occurs when the spinal cord, rather than the nerve root, is compressed.

Coding Guidance
AHA: 2018, 1Q, 7; 2017, 2Q, 23; 2016, 2Q, 16; 2015, 2Q 20; 2015, 2Q, 21; 2015, 2Q, 34

Lavage, Bronchoalveolar (BAL)

See also Washing, Bronchial
See also Suctioning, Bronchial (For Removal of Mucus Plug)

Body System
Respiratory System

PCS Root Operation
Drainage

Root Operation Table
ØB9   Respiratory System, Drainage

Body Part
Upper Lung Lobe, Right
Middle Lung Lobe, Right
Lower Lung Lobe, Right
Upper Lung Lobe, Left
Lung Lingula
Lower Lung Lobe, Left
Lung, Right
Lung, Left
Lungs, Bilateral

Approach
Via Natural or Artificial Opening Endoscopic

Device
No Device

Qualifier
Diagnostic

Description
Bronchoscopy with alveolar lavage, or bronchoalveolar lavage (BAL), is a diagnostic procedure that uses repeated instillation and aspiration of lavage fluid to obtain cells and noncellular components such as airway secretions from the epithelial surface of the lower respiratory tract for microbiological, cytological, or immunological analysis.

The physician views the airway using a flexible fiberoptic or rigid bronchoscope (a long, thin tube that has a close-focusing telescope on the end for viewing) introduced Via Natural or Artificial Opening Endoscopic approach through the nasal or oral cavity, or a tracheostomy stoma. The airway is anesthetized with a topical anesthetic. The bronchoscope is inserted and advanced through the nasal or oral cavity, or tracheostomy stoma past the larynx to inspect the bronchus. The procedure may employ fluoroscopic guidance.

After visualizing the bronchus, the practitioner samples alveolar lung tissue by irrigating with saline in small aliquots or subsets of the total fluid volume, followed by carefully suctioning the fluid. The bronchoscope is removed.

Focus Point
As BAL involves washing out and sampling the alveoli of the lung, the lung body part values more appropriately capture the objective of the procedure. This is also consistent with ICD-10-PCS guideline B4.1c, which states: "If a procedure is performed on a continuous section of a tubular body part, code the body part value corresponding to the furthest anatomical site from the point of entry."

Focus Point
Bronchial washing refers to the aspiration of secretions or small amounts of instilled saline from the larger airways within the lumen of the bronchus.

Focus Point
An additional code for fluoroscopic guidance may be reported, when performed.

Coding Guidance
AHA: 2017, 1Q, 51; 2016, 1Q, 26, 27

© 2018 Optum360, LLC

Medical and Surgical

Lengthening, Tendon

Body System
Tendons

PCS Root Operation
Division

Root Operation Table
ØL8   Tendons, Division

Body Part
Refer to the ICD-10-PCS tabular list for a complete list of body parts.

Approach
Open
Percutaneous

Description
Tendon lengthening (also known as tenotomy) is done to lengthen a tendon that has become shortened or is resistant to stretch. When a muscle becomes shortened, the tendon that attaches the muscle to bone can also shorten. The inability to move a joint through its full range of motion, whether due to chronic pain or due to a chronic condition, also may result in a tight (shortened) tendon. During a tenotomy, the tendon is surgically divided and allowed to expand and heal as a longer tendon.

In the traditional Open approach, an incision is made through the skin and subcutaneous tissue, and the tendon is transected. The skin and subcutaneous layers are closed with sutures. The area is then covered with a bandage to allow it to heal.

The physician uses a Percutaneous approach to insert a needle at the desired tenotomy level. The sharp edge of the needle transects the tendon with a sweeping back-and-forth motion. No sutures are needed for the minimally invasive Percutaneous approach.

Different techniques may be used to transect the tendon. They include making several small cuts in the tendon, notching the tendon, or making a Z-shaped incision in the tendon and stretching it to a particular length. Regardless of the technique used, the expected outcome is for the tendon to elongate as the wound heals.

Focus Point
The root operation Division is used since the body part (tendon) is being cut and separated to accomplish the procedure. Root operation Release is not appropriate since the cutting does not involve an abnormal constraint or attachment around the body part.

Medical and Surgical

Ligamentoplasty, Interspinous

Body System
Bursae and Ligaments

PCS Root Operation
Repair

Root Operation Table
ØMQ Bursae and Ligaments, Repair

Body Part
Upper Spine Bursa and Ligament
Lower Spine Bursa and Ligament

Approach
Open
Percutaneous
Percutaneous Endoscopic

Description
Interspinous ligamentoplasty (ILP) is a relatively new procedure that stabilizes mild degenerative lumbar instability with or without lumbar fusion. Since it is not inherent to the spinal fusion and has a distinctly different objective, a separate code is indicated for the ligamentoplasty. It is also being performed for stabilization post-decompression in lieu of a fusion. However, at this time, the root operation Insertion of a device is not recommended as the FiberWire that is used in between the spinous processes to tighten and stabilize the spine is a polyethylene suture material and not classified as a device. *AHA Coding Clinic* recommends the use of Repair as the root operation for ILP at this time.

Focus Point
Any concurrent procedures such as decompression, fusion, or discectomy are coded separately.

Coding Guidance
AHA: 2014, 3Q, 9

© 2018 Optum360, LLC

Ligation and Stripping, Varicose Veins

Body System
Lower Veins

PCS Root Operation
Extraction

Occlusion

Root Operation Table
06D   Lower Veins, Extraction
06L   Lower Veins, Occlusion

Body Part
Saphenous Vein, Right
Saphenous Vein, Left
Foot Vein, Right
Foot Vein, Left
Lower Vein

Approach
Percutaneous
Open

Description
Vein ligation and stripping are performed for superficial leg veins that have developed symptomatic varicosities. Veins return deoxygenated blood to the heart. While the heart actively pumps arterial blood into the extremities, the flow is strong and steady. The return flow is less controlled. In the legs, venous blood flows against gravity toward the heart as a result of pressure from arterial blood as it enters the venous system, and through the pumping action of the calf muscles, which act to squeeze leg veins when they are flexed. Unlike arteries, veins are equipped with a series of valves to prevent backflow of blood. While arteries have strong muscular walls to handle high arterial pressure, veins have thinner walls. When the venous valves break down, the patient may develop dilated and tortuous varicose veins and is at risk for chronic venous insufficiency (CVI).

CVI causes blood to pool in the veins of the legs in what is called venous stasis. Venous stasis can lead to stasis dermatitis and skin ulcers. When the problem lies within the superficial veins of the leg (the greater and lesser saphenous veins), the varicose veins may be removed. The deep veins of the leg (femoral, iliac, popliteal, and tibial) will assume the burden of return blood flow previously carried by the superficial veins.

Varicose veins may occur due to congenital defects or positional pressures associated with prolonged standing or sitting, and are often a complication associated with pregnancy in women. Surgical technique may vary depending on the anatomic site of the varicosity and the patient's state of cardiovascular health.

Extraction
In vein stripping, the physician extracts a length of faulty vein by pulling it through a small hole or series of small holes in the leg of the patient.

In vein stripping, the operation is Extraction. The physician makes a skin incision in the upper thigh or upper leg exposing the short saphenous vein or the long saphenous vein. Additional skin incisions are made at the knee and ankle and along the leg as necessary. Using a Percutaneous approach, a long wire is threaded through the length of the vein and brought out at the ankle. The vein is tied to the end of the wire and the wire is pulled out along with the vein, without direct visualization. Once the vein has been removed, the skin incisions are repaired with layered closures. The leg is wrapped with an elastic pressure dressing postoperatively.

Occlusion
In vein ligation, the root operation is Occlusion. The physician makes an incision in the skin overlying the short saphenous vein at its junction with the saphenopopliteal vein at the knee. The vessels are dissected under direct visualization using an Open approach, and ties are placed around the short saphenous vein, which is divided between the ties. Once the ties are in place and the vein has been divided, the vein is left in situ and the skin incision is repaired with a layered closure.

> **Focus Point**
> *Vein ligation and stripping may be performed bilaterally, in which case each side is reported separately. Surgical treatment of any stasis ulcer is reported in addition to the code for the vein ligation or stripping if it meets the reporting criteria for a separate procedure in ICD-10-PCS.*

> **Focus Point**
> *Any minor incisions used in vein stripping are inherent to meeting the objective of the root operation Extraction, which is to pull or strip out or off all or a portion of a body part by the use of force.*

© 2018 Optum360, LLC

Medical and Surgical

Ligation, Esophageal Varices

Body System
Lower Veins

PCS Root Operation
Occlusion

Root Operation Table
Ø6L   Lower Veins, Occlusion

Body Part
Esophageal Vein

Approach
Open
Via Natural or Artificial Opening Endoscopic

Device
Extraluminal Device
No Device

Description
Esophageal varices are dilated tortuous veins in the esophagus that can rupture, causing hemorrhage. Because ligation of varices involves the venous system below the diaphragm, the correct body system is Lower Veins. The intent of the procedure is to ligate, or "occlude," the abnormally enlarged esophageal veins; this is reported with root operation Occlusion.

The most common approach for ligation of esophageal varices, also called banding, is Via Natural or Artificial Opening Endoscopic. The physician passes a rigid or flexible esophagoscope through the patient's mouth and into the esophagus and visualizes the esophageal varices. The endoscopic band delivery device is positioned, and the rubber band is secured at the base of the varix. This is repeated until all varices have been banded.

Alternatively, the esophageal veins, also called the esophageal venous plexus, may be accessed via an Open approach, whereby the physician accesses the esophagus through a midline abdominal or thoracic incision and makes a longitudinal incision in the esophagus. The physician locates the varices (tortuous, dilated veins) and ligates them with sutures. The esophagotomy is closed with sutures, and the incision is sutured in layers. The sutures used to ligate the varices are integral to the procedure and are not reported as devices. Report these as No Device.

Focus Point
The bands are placed on the exterior of the varices so the correct device is Extraluminal Device.

Coding Guidance
AHA: 2013, 4Q, 121

© 2018 Optum360, LLC

Medical and Surgical

Ligation, Tubal (Sterilization)

Body System
Female Reproductive System

PCS Root Operation
Destruction

Excision

Occlusion

Root Operation Table
ØU5   Female Reproductive System, Destruction

ØUB   Female Reproductive System, Excision

ØUL   Female Reproductive System, Occlusion

Body Part
Fallopian Tube, Right

Fallopian Tube, Left

Fallopian Tubes, Bilateral

Approach
Open

Percutaneous Endoscopic

Via Natural or Artificial Opening Endoscopic

Device
Extraluminal Device (Occlusion)

Intraluminal Device (Occlusion)

Description
Tubal ligation is a method of female sterilization in which the fallopian tubes are tied, destroyed, or cut. It is considered a type of permanent birth control. Various methods are used and can be performed at any time, including after childbirth or during an abdominal surgery, including a C-section.

Destruction
Using an Open or Percutaneous Endoscopic (laparoscopic) approach, one or more of the fallopian tubes is destroyed using cautery. Destruction is the root operation to use when a body part is eradicated by the use of energy, force, or a destructive agent.

Excision
Using an Open or Percutaneous Endoscopic (laparoscopic) approach, one or both of the fallopian tubes is tied (or banded), and a segment of the tube is excised. Excision is the root operation to use when a portion of the fallopian tube is removed. An excision of a ligated portion of the fallopian tubes is also known as a Pomeroy operation. A Pomeroy sterilization technique involves the ligation of a loop of fallopian tube and subsequent resection of the tied loop.

Occlusion
Using an Open or Percutaneous Endoscopic (laparoscopic) approach, the physician blocks one or both of the fallopian tubes with a band, clip, or Falope ring. Qualifier Extraluminal Device is used when the device is placed on the outside of the tube.

Another method uses coils that are placed in the tubes at the point where they connect with the uterus. This type of occlusion procedure, otherwise known as hysteroscopic occlusion of the fallopian tubes, is performed using the Via Natural or Artificial Opening Endoscopic (through the cervix) approach and does not require an incision. The qualifier Intraluminal Device is used for the coils placed inside the tubes.

Focus Point
An Open approach is used when the patient is having an open abdominal surgery, including a C-section or within one to two days after childbirth.

Coding Guidance
AHA: 2015, 3Q, 31

Medical and Surgical

Lithotripsy, Direct Intracorporeal

See also Lithotripsy, Extracorporeal, Shock Wave (ESWL)

Body System
Hepatobiliary System and Pancreas
Urinary System

PCS Root Operation
Fragmentation

Root Operation Table
ØFF   Hepatobiliary System and Pancreas, Fragmentation

ØTF   Urinary System, Fragmentation

Body Part
Gallbladder
Hepatic Duct, Right
Hepatic Duct, Left
Hepatic Duct, Common
Cystic Duct
Common Bile Duct
Ampulla Of Vater
Pancreatic Duct
Pancreatic Duct, Accessory
Kidney Pelvis, Right
Kidney Pelvis, Left
Ureter, Right
Ureter, Left
Bladder
Bladder Neck
Urethra

Approach
Via Natural or Artificial Opening Endoscopic

Description
Lithotripsy is a method used to crush kidney, gallbladder, and other stones that are too large to pass naturally and are causing obstruction, infection, or bleeding while they are still inside the body.

Calculi in the urinary system usually are composed of calcium but may contain uric acid, cysteine, ammonium acid urate, xanthine, or dihydroxyadenine. Biliary calculi, conversely, contain cholesterol, bilirubin, or calcium. With lithotripsy, the urinary or biliary stones are pulverized and the small pieces pass out of the body, carried away by urine or feces.

Direct intracorporeal (within the body) lithotripsy using the approach Via Natural or Artificial Opening Endoscopic may be used for calculi that are lodged in a lumen—for example, the ureter or biliary duct. Urinary calculi may be targeted by a physician using a cystourethroscope. The physician threads a cystourethroscope into the urethral orifice and into the bladder, urethra, or kidney pelvis. The scope is used to transport an ultrasonic or electrohydraulic tool or a laser to fragment the calculus and to visualize the site. No fragments are removed. A physician may target biliary calculi in the gallbladder or ducts during endoscopic retrograde cholangiopancreatography (ERCP). The scope is used to transport an ultrasonic or electrohydraulic tool or a laser to fragment the calculus and to visualize the site. No fragments are removed.

Focus Point
The operation Fragmentation describes when force is applied to break solid matter up. By definition, Fragmentation requires that the shattered material not be removed from the patient's body. Extirpation would be the appropriate operation if the stones are removed in an Open or Percutaneous approach or when a basket retrieves the stone during endoscopy. Extirpation cannot be reported with Fragmentation, as Fragmentation is inherent to the Extirpation.

Focus Point
In some lithotripsy procedures, an intraluminal stent is placed to facilitate passage of larger stone fragments to avoid blocking the lumen. Code any stent insertion procedures in addition to the codes for fragmentation with the root operation Dilation and the device Intraluminal Device.

Coding Guidance
AHA: 2015, 2Q, 7; 2013, 4Q, 122

Medical and Surgical

© 2018 Optum360, LLC

Lithotripsy, Extracorporeal Shock Wave (ESWL)

See also Lithotripsy, Direct Intracorporeal

Body System
Hepatobiliary System and Pancreas
Urinary System

PCS Root Operation
Fragmentation

Root Operation Table
ØFF Hepatobiliary System and Pancreas, Fragmentation
ØTF Urinary System, Fragmentation

Body Part
Gallbladder
Hepatic Duct, Right
Hepatic Duct, Left
Hepatic Duct, Common
Cystic Duct
Common Bile Duct
Ampulla Of Vater
Pancreatic Duct
Pancreatic Duct, Accessory
Kidney Pelvis, Right
Kidney Pelvis, Left
Ureter, Right
Ureter, Left
Bladder
Bladder Neck
Urethra

Approach
External

Description
The use of shock waves delivered outside the body (extracorporeal) for the purpose of breaking up stones is called extracorporeal shock wave lithotripsy (ESWL). The treatment uses an External approach to break up the stones into tiny pieces so that they can pass out of the body spontaneously without being surgically removed.

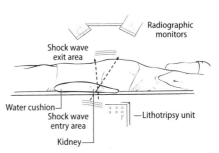

Extracorporeal Shock Wave Lithotripsy

The physician pulverizes a kidney stone (renal calculus), gallbladder stone, or calculus of other sites by directing shock waves through a liquid medium. The procedure is performed using one of two methods. In both, the physician first uses radiological guidance to determine the location and size of the calculus. In the first method, the patient is immersed in a liquid medium (degassed, deionized water), and shock waves are directed through the liquid to the stone. In the second, most common method, the patient is placed on a treatment table. A series of shock waves are directed through a water cushion or bellow placed against the patient's body at the location of the stone. Each shock wave is directed to the stone for only a fraction of a second, and the procedure generally takes from 30 to 50 minutes. The treatment table is equipped with video x-ray so the physician can view the pulverization process. Over several days or weeks, the tiny stone fragments pass harmlessly though the patient's system and are discharged during urination, digestion, or other process, depending on the site of the stone.

> **Focus Point**
> *When a stone does not pass spontaneously and needs to be surgically removed, Extirpation is the root operation reported.*

Coding Guidance
AHA: 2013, 4Q, 122

Medical and Surgical

Lobectomy, Lung

Body System
Respiratory System

PCS Root Operation
Excision

Resection

Root Operation Table
ØBB   Respiratory System, Excision

ØBT   Respiratory System, Resection

Body Part
Upper Lung Lobe, Right

Middle Lung Lobe, Right

Lower Lung Lobe, Right

Upper Lung Lobe, Left

Lung Lingula

Lower Lung Lobe, Left

Approach
Open

Percutaneous Endoscopic

Description

A lobectomy is a surgery to remove part or all of one of the lobes of the lungs and may be performed to remove diseased lung tissue for those with tuberculosis, lung abscess, emphysema, neoplasms, or fungal infections or to prevent spread of disease to the other lobes of the lungs.

The right lung has three lobes: upper, middle, and lower. Because the left lung shares space in the thorax with the heart, it has only two lobes: upper and lower. The left upper lobe, however, has two body parts designated in ICD-10-PCS: Upper Lung Lobe, Left and the Lung Lingula, which is a small area at the base of the upper lobe containing the inferior and superior bronchopulmonary segments. The lingula is differentiated from the upper left lobe in ICD-10-PCS because like the middle right lobe, the lingula is prone to infection and atelectasis. Its name is derived from its tongue-like shape. Lobectomy or lingulectomy may be performed using Open or Percutaneous Endoscopic approaches.

Most lobectomies/lingulectomies are performed using video-assisted thoracoscopy (VATS), reported as Percutaneous Endoscopic approach. In VATS, the physician removes an entire lobe or the lingula through a rigid or flexible fiberoptic endoscope. The physician makes a small incision between two ribs and by blunt dissection and the use of a trocar, enters the thoracic cavity. The endoscope is passed through the trocar and into the chest cavity. The lung is usually partially collapsed by instilling air into the chest through the trocar, or the lung may be collapsed through a double lumen endotracheal tube inserted through the mouth into the trachea. Under direct visualization through the endoscope, the physician manipulates the instruments inserted through secondary sites and clamps the blood vessels and bronchial tubes going to the lobe or lingula lobe to be removed. With the clamps in place, the lobe or lingula is removed by dividing the vessel and bronchial tubes isolated by the clamps. Any cut portions of the remaining lung tissue are repaired by suturing or clipping with surgical clips.

In an Open approach, the physician makes an incision in the chest overlying the targeted lobe and uses rib spreaders to access the lung.

Resection
Resection, which involves removal of all of a body part, is reported for the removal of the entire lobe or lingula.

Excision
If only a portion of the lobe or lingula is removed, the root operation is Excision. Excision may be performed for therapeutic or diagnostic purposes.

Focus Point
Resection includes all of a body part or any subdivision of the body part that has its own body part value. Removal of all of one of the body parts of the lung (Lobe or Lingula) is reported as Resection of the lobe or lingula rather than Excision of the right or left lung. Should two body parts (Lobe/Lingula) be removed from a single lung, report the Resection of each body part. If the entire lung is removed, report Resection of Lung, Right, or Resection of Lung, Left. See ICD-10-PCS guideline B3.8.

© 2018 Optum360, LLC

Lobectomy, Temporal, Brain (Epilepsy)

See also Electrocorticography (Intraoperative), under "Measurement and Monitoring" in the Medical and Surgical Related section.

Body System
Central Nervous System and Cranial Nerves

PCS Root Operation
Excision

Root Operation Table
00B   Central Nervous System and Cranial Nerves, Excision

Body Part
Cerebral Hemisphere

Approach
Open

Description
Temporal lobe epilepsy (TLE) is the most common form of localized epilepsy. It usually begins before adulthood following a fever with seizure or a brain injury, and in many cases, causes sclerosing of the hippocampus. In some patients, TLE with hippocampal sclerosis is resistant to anti-epileptic drugs (AEDs), creating a social hardship and difficulties with activities of daily living. Excision of the anterior temporal lobe is done in an attempt to control the drug-resistant seizures and reverse or decrease the risk of the neurologic effects of chronic epilepsy.

A temporal lobectomy is commonly performed for intractable epileptic seizures when the focal point of the seizures has been identified by previous exams. An access incision is made through the scalp and overlying muscle to reach the skull. Burr holes are drilled around the periphery of the bone flap area to be raised. Using a craniotome, the bone flap is freed and lifted to expose the dura, which is dissected and retracted out of the operative field. Electrodes are placed on the brain. The electrical activity of the brain is recorded and mapped while the cortex is kept irrigated. The recording grids may be moved a few times to gain enough information about various sites. After the electrocorticography, the electrodes are removed and markers are placed. Incisions are made into the cortex, and dissection is carried down deep into the cortex. The temporal horn of the lateral ventricle and hippocampus are identified. The pia is opened and the temporal lobe is removed, including any of the hippocampus, amygdala, and uncus that are identified to be removed with the temporal lobe.

In other cases, a selective amygdalohippocampectomy (SAH) is performed to spare the neocortex of the temporal lobe. During the excision, arteries are transected and coagulated, while preserving the main cerebral/choroidal arteries and the pia-arachnoid. Closure is done by suturing the dura and re-placing the bone flap into position. Screws or plates are placed to secure the bone flap to surrounding skull bone. The divided muscles are secured, and the galea aponeurotica and scalp are closed. Because the site of the surgery is accessed and directly visualized by cutting through all the body layers necessary to expose it, an Open approach is reported.

Focus Point
Because the body part is Cerebral Hemisphere, it is appropriate to use Excision even if the temporal lobe is completely resected. Individual lobes of the cerebrum are all reported with the body part Cerebral Hemisphere. The root operation Resection would be reported only if the entire body part (Cerebral Hemisphere) were removed.

Focus Point
During temporal lobectomy for intractable epilepsy, an electrocorticography is performed. Electrodes are placed on the brain. The electrical activity of the brain is recorded and mapped while the cortex is kept irrigated. The recording grids may be moved a few times to gain enough information about various sites. After the electrocorticography, the electrodes are removed and markers are placed. Electrocorticography is reported separately with root operation table 4A0 Measurement, Physiological Systems, and body system Central Nervous System. The function is Electrical Activity.

Coding Guidance
AHA: 2016, 2Q, 18

Lysis, Adhesions, Abdominal (Abdominal Adhesiolysis)

Body System
Gastrointestinal System

Hepatobiliary System and Pancreas

PCS Root Operation
Release

Root Operation Table
ØDN Gastrointestinal System, Release

ØFN Hepatobiliary System and Pancreas, Release

Body Part
Refer to the ICD-10-PCS tabular list for a complete list of body parts.

Approach
Open

Percutaneous Endoscopic

Description
Adhesions are fibrous bands of scar tissue that abnormally bind or connect body tissues and anatomical parts that are normally separate.

Abdominal adhesions may be caused by infection, appendicitis, injury, cancer, and/or inflammation. Past surgical procedures may also cause adhesions to form almost anywhere inside the body. Adhesions are most commonly formed in the abdomen (peritoneum) and in the gastrointestinal tract. They can cause intestinal obstruction by kinking, twisting, or pulling the intestines out of place.

Lysis of abdominal adhesions may be documented as lysis, division, or freeing of adhesions of the biliary tract, liver, peritoneum, or intestines.

Lysis of abdominal adhesions is primarily done intraoperatively during a separately reportable major procedure to remove abdominal organs like the gallbladder, appendix, or pancreas. For the physician to successfully operate and remove the organs, he may have to release them from the adhesions to other neighboring organs. Lysis of adhesions may also be performed as a primary procedure to release an intestinal blockage or to reduce chronic abdominal pain.

With the patient under anesthesia, using an Open approach, the physician enters the abdomen through a midline abdominal incision. The adhesions are divided, and any obstructed bowel is freed from its attachments to itself, the abdominal wall, and/or other abdominal organs. The abdominal incision is closed.

With the patient under anesthesia, using a Percutaneous Endoscopic (laparoscopic) approach, the physician places a trocar at the umbilicus into the abdominal or retroperitoneal space and insufflates the abdominal cavity. A laparoscope is placed through the umbilical incision, and additional trocars are placed into other small incisions in the abdomen. The abdominal adhesions are identified, and instruments are passed through to dissect and remove the adhesions, releasing any attachment to intestines, abdominal wall, or other intra-abdominal organs. The trocars are removed, and the incisions are closed with sutures.

Focus Point
In ICD-10-PCS, the root operation Release is used to code lysis of adhesion procedures. During a Release procedure, some of the constricting tissue may be removed but none of that body part is taken out. According to ICD-10-PCS guideline B3.13, the body part value coded is the body part being freed and not the tissue being manipulated or cut to free the body part. For example, lysis of intestinal adhesions is coded to the specific intestine body part being freed.

Focus Point
Adhesions are often a normal occurrence in abdominal procedures, and adhesiolysis is integral to performing the principal procedure. In these cases, adhesions and adhesiolysis are not reported separately. It is important that coders not code lysis of adhesions procedures and the diagnosis of adhesions based only on the operative report. The surgeon must clearly document both the clinical significance of the condition (adhesions) and the procedure performed (lysis of adhesions). Documentation by the surgeon may include such terms as numerous or dense adhesions requiring a significant/long time to lyse, extensive lysis, tedious lysis, etc. If the documentation is unclear or there is any uncertainty as to the clinical significance/complexity of the lysis of adhesions, query the provider.

Focus Point
Review the operative report for potential multiple lysis of adhesions procedure codes to be reported on different body parts, referring to ICD-10-PCS multiple procedures guideline B3.2a.

Focus Point
If a Percutaneous Endoscopic (laparoscopic) lysis of adhesions is converted to an Open procedure, code the Percutaneous Endoscopic Inspection and Open Release. See ICD-10-PCS guideline B3.2d.

Focus Point
If an Open lysis of adhesions is performed with Percutaneous Endoscopic (laparoscopic) assistance, it is reported as an Open procedure, according to ICD-10-PCS guideline B5.2.

Coding Guidance
AHA: 2017, 1Q, 35; 2014, 1Q, 3-6

© 2018 Optum360, LLC

Lysis, Adhesions, Female Pelvic (Pelvic Adhesiolysis)

Body System
Female Reproductive System

PCS Root Operation
Release

Root Operation Table
ØUN   Female Reproductive System, Release

Body Part
Ovary, Right
Ovary, Left
Ovaries, Bilateral
Uterine Supporting Structure
Fallopian Tube, Right
Fallopian Tube, Left
Fallopian Tubes, Bilateral
Uterus
Cervix
Cul-de-sac

Approach
Open
Percutaneous Endoscopic

Description
Adhesions are fibrous bands of scar tissue that abnormally bind or connect body tissues and anatomical parts that are normally separate. Pelvic adhesions may be caused by infection, appendicitis, injury, cancer, and/or inflammation. Past surgical procedures may also cause adhesions to form almost anywhere inside the body. Pelvic adhesions may cause obstructed fallopian tubes associated with infertility, pelvic tenderness, painful intercourse, and chronic pelvic pain.

Lysis of pelvic adhesions is primarily done intraoperatively during a major procedure on female pelvic organs. In order for the physician to successfully operate and remove the organs, the organs may need to be released from the restraint or adhesion to other neighboring organs. Lysis of pelvic adhesions may also be done as a primary procedure to treat infertility caused by adhesions or to reduce chronic pelvic pain.

With the patient under anesthesia, using an Open approach, the physician enters the pelvis through a horizontal incision just within the pubic hairline. The pelvic organs are freed of adhesions attaching to the organ itself, the pelvic wall, and/or other pelvic organs. The pelvic incision is closed.

With the patient under anesthesia, the physician may first insert an instrument through the vagina to grasp the cervix and manipulate the uterus during the surgery. Using a Percutaneous Endoscopic (laparoscopic) approach, the physician places a trocar just below the umbilicus into the pelvic space and insufflates the pelvic cavity. The physician places a laparoscope through the infra-umbilical incision, and additional trocars are placed into the pelvic cavity. Pelvic organ adhesions are identified, and instruments are passed through to dissect and remove the adhesions. The pelvic cavity is then deflated, the trocars are removed, and the incisions are closed with sutures.

Focus Point
Adhesions are often a normal occurrence in surgical procedures, and adhesiolysis is integral to performing the principal procedure. In these cases, adhesions and adhesiolysis are not reported separately.

It is important that coders not code lysis of adhesion procedures and the diagnosis of adhesions based only on the operative report. The surgeon must clearly document both the clinical significance of the condition (adhesions) and the procedure performed (lysis of adhesions). Documentation by the surgeon may include such terms as numerous or dense adhesions requiring significant/long time to lyse, extensive lysis, tedious lysis, etc. If the documentation is unclear or there is any uncertainty as to the clinical significance/complexity of the lysis of adhesions, query the provider.

Focus Point
In ICD-10-PCS, the root operation Release is used to code lysis of adhesion procedures. During a Release procedure, some of the constricting tissue may be removed, but none of that body part is taken out. According to ICD-10-PCS guideline B3.13, the body part value coded is the body part being freed and not the tissue being manipulated or cut to free the body part.

Focus Point
Review the operative report for potential multiple lysis of adhesion procedure codes to be reported on different body parts, referring to ICD-10-PCS multiple procedures guideline B3.2a.

Focus Point
If a Percutaneous Endoscopic (laparoscopic) lysis of adhesions is converted to an Open procedure, code the Percutaneous Endoscopic Inspection and Open Release. See ICD-10-PCS guideline B3.2d.

Focus Point
An Open lysis of adhesions performed with Percutaneous Endoscopic (laparoscopic) assistance is reported as an Open procedure, according to ICD-10-PCS guideline B5.2.

Coding Guidance
AHA: 2014, 1Q, 3-6

Mammoplasty, Reduction

Body System
Skin and Breast

PCS Root Operation
Alteration

Excision

Root Operation Table
ØHØ   Skin and Breast, Alteration

ØHB   Skin and Breast, Excision

Body Part
Breast, Right

Breast, Left

Breast, Bilateral

Approach
Open

Description
Reduction mammoplasty is reconstructive surgery to alter the size and appearance of or otherwise repair the breast. It is considered medically necessary when performed to improve functional limitations and to relieve the clinical signs and symptoms of hypertrophy of the breasts (macromastia and gigantomastia), such as chronic head, neck, and shoulder pain, poor blood circulation, impaired breathing, and skin chafing.

Alteration
Reduction mammoplasty for cosmetic purposes, performed solely to improve the patient's appearance, is assigned to the ICD-10-PCS root operation Alteration because it is performed to modify the natural anatomic structure of a body part without affecting its function. Alteration is coded for all procedures performed solely to improve appearance. All methods, approaches, and devices used for the objective of improving appearance are coded using the root operation Alteration. Because some surgical procedures can be performed for either medical or cosmetic purposes, coding for Alteration requires diagnostic confirmation that the surgery is in fact performed to improve appearance and is not medically necessary.

Excision
The physician reduces the size of the breast, removing wedges of skin and breast tissue from a female patient. The physician makes a circular skin incision above the nipple, in the position to which the nipple will be elevated. Another skin incision is made around the circumference of the nipple. Two incisions are made from the circular cut above the nipple to the fold beneath the breast, one on either side of the nipple, creating a keyhole shaped skin and breast incision. Wedges of skin and breast tissue are removed until the desired size is achieved. Bleeding vessels may be ligated or cauterized. The physician elevates the nipple and its pedicle of subcutaneous tissue to its new position and sutures the nipple pedicle with layered closure. The remaining incision is repaired with layered closure.

© 2018 Optum360, LLC

Medical and Surgical

Mapping, Cardiac

Body System
Heart and Great Vessels

PCS Root Operation
Map

Root Operation Table
Ø2K   Heart and Great Vessels, Map

Body Part
Conduction Mechanism

Approach
Open
Percutaneous

Description

Every heartbeat advances oxygen-rich blood out of the left ventricle and out to the peripheral arteries of the body. A heartbeat occurs when an impulse is sent along the heart's electrical pathways, essentially shocking the heart muscle and causing it to contract. Errors in the electrical pathways or impulses lead to heartbeat arrhythmias, including bradycardia, tachycardia, fibrillation, flutter, and blocks.

Cardiac mapping analyzes the conduction of electrical impulses along the pathways in the heart and records the results in what is called an electrophysiological study (cardiac EPS). Once the cause of an electrical problem is identified, corrective therapy may be considered.

The ICD-10-PCS root operation Map represents procedures that may be documented as cardiac mapping, cortical mapping, electrophysiological studies, or EP studies. In cardiac mapping, the correct body part is Conduction Mechanism, regardless of the different cardiac sites where the electrodes may be placed.

During an open-heart procedure with bypass, reported as an Open approach, the physician positions an electrode at the right ventricular apex, both for recording and stimulating the right atrium and the right ventricle. For mapping, additional electrodes are spaced at the specific site to be mapped. Tachycardia is induced by programmed electrical impulses. The earliest activation site is determined. Intraventricular electrograms with surface electrocardiograms are simultaneously displayed and recorded on a multichannel oscilloscopic photographic recorder.

For a Percutaneous approach, the physician inserts an electrode catheter percutaneously into the right subclavian vein and, under fluoroscopic guidance, positions the electrode catheter at the right ventricular apex, both for recording and stimulating the right atrium and the right ventricle. For mapping, additional electrode catheters are inserted percutaneously from the right femoral artery and advanced to the specific site to be mapped. Tachycardia is induced by programmed electrical impulses. The earliest activation site is determined, and the diastolic pressure is recorded on the endocardial activation map during the ventricular tachycardia. Intraventricular electrograms with surface electrocardiograms are simultaneously displayed and recorded on a multichannel oscilloscopic photographic recorder.

Focus Point
A documented cardiac mapping consisting of only an electrocardiogram is reported as root operation Measurement, Cardiac (see root operation table 4AØ).

Medical and Surgical

Mapping, Cortical

Body System
Central Nervous System and Cranial Nerves

PCS Root Operation
Map

Root Operation Table
00K   Central Nervous System and Cranial Nerves, Map

Body Part
Cerebral Hemisphere

Approach
Open
Percutaneous
Percutaneous Endoscopic

Description
The two major components of the brain are the upper cerebral cortex, which controls the thinking and reasoning functions, and the lower subcortex, which controls physiologic processes such as breathing and heart rate.

The cortical structures are the frontal lobe, parietal lobe, temporal lobe, and occipital lobe. According to the ICD-10-PCS Body Part Key, these structures are reported with the body part Cerebral Hemisphere.

Cortical mapping is performed to identify the relationship between areas of the brain and their function. Stimulation of an area of the brain with electricity (cortical stimulation mapping, CSM) will evoke a physical response. Mapping the anatomical

areas to sites on the cerebral hemisphere helps physicians preparing patients for brain surgery, for example, to determine what the outcome would be for a patient with epilepsy if the epileptogenic segment of brain were removed.

In a direct cortical stimulation (DCS) mapping via Open approach, electrodes are placed directly on the brain cortex and the brain is stimulated. The procedure maps the brain's surface to determine the focus of seizure or to identify vital brain structures. An open approach is usually limited to circumstances in which the brain is already exposed for another procedure.

In a Percutaneous approach, the physician uses a burr drill or trephine to create a hole in the cranium and the electrodes are threaded to the sites to be stimulated under radiologic guidance.

In a Percutaneous Endoscopic approach, the physician uses a burr drill or trephine to create a hole in the cranium and the electrodes are threaded to the sites to be stimulated with visualization through the scope.

Focus Point
If the cortical mapping is done at the time of another separately reportable procedure, report the cortical mapping in addition to the code for the other procedure performed. Craniotomy performed only as the approach to the cortical mapping procedure without another definitive procedure would not be reported separately.

© 2018 Optum360, LLC

Marsupialization, Bartholin's Gland Cyst

Body System
Female Reproductive System

PCS Root Operation
Drainage

Root Operation Table
ØU9   Female Reproductive System, Drainage

Body Part
Vestibular Gland

Approach
Open

Device
No Device

Qualifier
No Qualifier

Description
Bartholin's gland is at the end of the bulb of the vestibule of the vagina and is connected by a duct to the mucosa at the opening of the vagina. Marsupialization of Bartholin's gland is an incision of a large cyst in the gland and suturing it open.

The physician treats a Bartholin's gland cyst with marsupialization. Using an Open approach, the physician makes an elliptical incision over the center of the Bartholin's gland cyst and drains the contents of the cyst. The lining of the cyst is everted and approximated to the wall of the cyst in the vaginal mucosa with absorbable sutures, creating a pouch. The cyst site remains open and can drain freely. Marsupialization prevents recurrent cysts and infections.

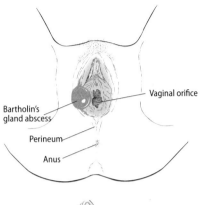

Bartholin's gland abscess
Vaginal orifice
Perineum
Anus

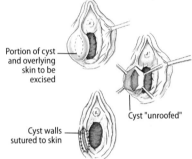

Portion of cyst and overlying skin to be excised
Cyst "unroofed"
Cyst walls sutured to skin

Focus Point

According to the ICD-10-PCS Body Part Key, Bartholin's gland is reported with the body part Vestibular Gland.

Focus Point

The approach for this procedure is Open, as it involves cutting through the skin or mucous membrane to expose the site of the procedure.

Focus Point

The body part Vestibular Gland is reported once whether one or both Bartholin's glands undergo marsupialization since the Vestibular Gland is classified to a single ICD-10-PCS body part value, without a specific body part for laterality.

Focus Point

The sutures placed in the marsupialization procedure are considered surgical supplies, not devices.

Medical and Surgical

Marsupialization, Pilonidal Cyst

Body System
Skin and Breast

Subcutaneous Tissue and Fascia

PCS Root Operation
Drainage

Excision

Root Operation Table
ØH9   Skin and Breast, Drainage

ØHB   Skin and Breast, Excision

ØJ9   Subcutaneous Tissue and Fascia, Drainage

ØJB   Subcutaneous Tissue and Fascia, Excision

Body Part
Skin, Back

Skin, Buttock

Subcutaneous Tissue And Fascia, Back

Subcutaneous Tissue And Fascia, Buttock

Approach
Open

External

Description
The term "pilonidal" is derived from the Latin words for hair and nest. A pilonidal cyst or sinus occurs when hair penetrates the subcutaneous tissue at the top of the gluteal cleft and is trapped there. The body undergoes a foreign-body type reaction that leads to granulation of tissue, the formation of a cyst, and potential for abscess. Pilonidal disease (PD) usually presents as a swelling, sometimes with drainage, in the sacrococcygeal area. PD can lead to the development of sinuses and chronic painful infection. Once infected, the pilonidal cyst becomes a pilonidal abscess.

Marsupialization of a pilonidal cyst is performed with two goals. The first is to clear out any existing infection. The second is to excise tissue and suture the edges of the pilonidal cavity so that the cavity becomes a permanent open pouch to allow continuous drainage. Marsupialization has a very low recurrence rate for pilonidal infection.

Drainage
Emergent care for pilonidal cyst infections usually involves incision and drainage of the infection and is reported with the root operation Drainage. The physician uses a scalpel to incise the roof of the pilonidal cyst. The edges of the wound are sutured to the surrounding skin, leaving the wound open for drainage. If the drainage involves only the skin, the approach is External, which is reported for procedures performed directly on the skin. If the incision and drainage extend into the subcutaneous tissue and/or fascia, the approach is Open.

Excision
The physician uses a scalpel to excise the pilonidal sinus cavity and any remaining hair or infection. The edges of the wound are sutured to the surrounding skin or presacral fascia to ensure the wound remains open. In some cases, the granulated lining of the cyst may also be excised. If the excision of the pilonidal cyst involves only the skin, the approach is External, which is reported for procedures performed directly on the skin. If the excision of the pilonidal sinus extends into the subcutaneous tissue and/or fascia, the approach is Open.

© 2018 Optum360, LLC

Mastectomy

Body System
Skin and Breast

PCS Root Operation
Excision
Resection

Root Operation Table
ØHB   Skin and Breast, Excision
ØHT   Skin and Breast, Resection

Body Part
Breast, Right
Breast, Left
Breast, Bilateral
Nipple, Right
Nipple, Left
Supernumerary Breast

Approach
Open
Percutaneous (Excision)
External (Excision, Nipple Right/Left)

Qualifier
Diagnostic (Excision)
No Qualifier

Description
Mastectomy is the partial or total removal of one or both breasts. A "simple" or "total" mastectomy involves removal of the entire breast, including the nipple. A radical mastectomy is the complete removal of the breast, including the nipple, the overlying skin, the muscles beneath the breast, and the axillary lymph nodes. A modified radical mastectomy involves removal of the entire breast, including the nipple, overlying skin, and the axillary lymph nodes, but leaves the chest muscles intact. In a double or bilateral mastectomy, both breasts are removed. During subcutaneous (nipple-sparing) mastectomy, all of the breast tissue is removed, but the nipple-areolar complex is preserved.

A partial mastectomy, or quadrantectomy, is a breast conserving method of removing only the cancerous part of the breast tissue with some normal tissue around it. A lumpectomy is technically a form of partial mastectomy but involves removal of less tissue than in a partial mastectomy.

The most common indications for mastectomy are breast cancer and prophylaxis to reduce the risk of breast cancer in patients with high risk of malignancy due to mutations in the BRCA1 or BRCA2 genes or a strong family history of breast cancer.

Excision
When the physician removes a portion of breast tissue, root operation Excision is reported. The physician performs a partial mastectomy by making an incision through the skin and fascia over a breast malignancy and clamping any lymphatic and blood vessels. The physician excises the mass along with a section of healthy tissue. A drainage tube may be placed through a separate stab incision to enhance drainage from the wound or lymphatic system. The incision is repaired with layered closure, and a dressing is applied.

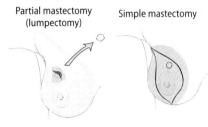

Partial mastectomy (lumpectomy)   Simple mastectomy

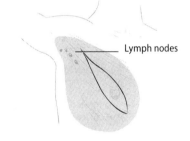

Radical mastectomy

Lymph nodes

Resection
The root operation Resection is reported when a radical or total mastectomy is performed. Using an Open approach, the physician makes an elliptical incision that includes the nipple and the tail of Spence, the extension of mammary tissue into the axillary region. The breast with or without the nipple, along with the overlying skin, pectoralis major and minor muscles, is removed as a single specimen. Some or all of the lymph nodes in the axilla may be removed. Bleeding vessels are ligated or electrocauterized. In large-breasted patients, adequate skin may be available for primary closure. Patients with insufficient skin for coverage may require skin grafts or myocutaneous flaps. If no prosthesis is to be inserted, a closed wound suction catheter may be inserted. The wound is closed, and a pressure dressing is applied.

Focus Point
Excision (sentinel or partial) or Resection (entire chain) of lymph nodes is reported with an additional code from the Lymphatic and Hemic Systems body system.

Medical and Surgical

Mastectomy (continued)

Focus Point

If the mastectomy is immediately (in the same episode) followed by a reconstructive procedure using the root operation Replacement, the Excision or Resection is not coded separately as it is included in the Replacement root operation definition.

Coding Guidance
AHA: 2016, 1Q, 30; 2014, 4Q, 34

Meniscectomy, Knee

Body System
Lower Joints

PCS Root Operation
Excision

Root Operation Table
ØSB   Lower Joints, Excision

Body Part
Knee Joint, Right
Knee Joint, Left

Approach
Open
Percutaneous Endoscopic

Description
The meniscus is made up of cartilage that cushions the joint and provides a smooth surface for motion and rotation of the knee joint. The knee has two menisci, located on either side, that cushion the knee joint to facilitate weight bearing and joint movement. A meniscectomy is performed on patients with damaged or torn meniscus cartilage that usually occurs due to trauma but can be caused by degeneration and weakening of the tissue.

Under general anesthetic, using an Open approach, the physician makes an incision along the anteromedial or anterolateral aspect of the knee, depending on which cartilage is torn. Dissection is carried down to the cartilage. The patella is shifted to the side, and the knee joint is exposed. The torn cartilage is removed, and the roughened edges are smoothed. A partial synovectomy and release or excision (partial or total) of plica may be performed. Plica is a fold, pleat, band, or shelf of synovial tissue (e.g., transverse suprapatellar, medial suprapatellar, mediopatellar, and infrapatellar). Debridement of the chondral surface of the patella may be performed as well. A temporary drain may be applied. The incision is repaired in layers with sutures, staples, and/or Steri-Strips.

For a Percutaneous Endoscopic meniscectomy, the physician makes 1 cm-long portal incisions on either side of the patellar tendon for arthroscopic access into the knee joint. Once the meniscal tear is identified, additional portal incisions may be made to provide easier access to the area. There may be a tear on either the medial or lateral meniscus or on both. The procedure is the same for medial or lateral meniscal tears. Angled scissors, a motorized cutter, or punch forceps remove torn fragments. The remaining intact meniscus is trimmed and contoured. A temporary drain may be applied and the incisions closed with sutures and Steri-Strips.

Focus Point

If both medial and lateral meniscectomies are performed on the same knee joint, report two procedures, with the laterality as appropriate. The medial and lateral menisci are identified as separate and distinct body parts classified to a single ICD-10-PCS body part value. These body parts have separate, distinct entries in the Body Part Key. This is consistent with ICD-10-PCS guideline B3.2.b.

Focus Point

If excision of other knee joint structures is performed at the same time as the meniscectomy, report in addition codes for any procedures performed on different body parts as defined by distinct values of the body part character. For example, the anterior cruciate ligament (ACL) and the lateral collateral ligament (LCL) are classified to the body parts Knee Bursa and Ligament, Left and Knee Bursa and Ligament, Right. This is consistent with ICD-10-PCS guideline B3.2.a.

Focus Point

There is no bilateral body part value in ICD-10-PCS for the knees. Therefore, if identical procedures are performed on both knee joints, report two codes using the body part values Knee Joint, Right and Knee Joint, Left.

Coding Guidance
AHA: 2015, 1Q, 34

© 2018 Optum360, LLC

Medical and Surgical

Myomectomy, Uterine

Body System
Female Reproductive System

PCS Root Operation
Excision

Root Operation Table
ØUB   Female Reproductive System, Excision

Body Part
Uterus

Approach
Open
Percutaneous Endoscopic
Via Natural or Artificial Opening, Endoscopic

Description
Myomas, also called leiomyomas and uterine fibroids, are benign smooth muscle tumors commonly occurring in the wall of the uterus. They may appear within the muscle (intramural), near the surface of the outside wall of the uterus (subserosal), or near the surface on the inside wall of the uterus (submucosal). They may be pedunculated, with a mass inside the uterus or within the peritoneal cavity. Myomectomy is an option for patients who have symptomatic myomas and wish to preserve their fertility.

The physician performs an Open myomectomy, removing a fibroid tumor or tumors from the wall of the patient's uterus through a transverse abdominal incision under direct visualization. The anterior sheath of the rectus abdominus muscle is dissected, and the muscles are retracted. Vasoconstrictors are injected, and a tourniquet is applied to encompass the uterine mass and the adnexa to limit blood flow. The physician incises the uterus through the myometrium to expose the myoma, which is dissected free from surrounding myometrium. The pedicle is isolated, clamped, and ligated, and the myoma is dissected from the pedicular blood supply. Other myomas are identified by palpating the uterine wall through the defect created by the already excised myoma. Any adjacent myomas may be reached by tunneling and removed through the initial incision. Additional incisions may be required for more distant myoma sites in the uterus. The uterus is closed with layered suturing. Anti-adhesion prophylaxis may be instilled in the abdominal cavity, and the operative wound is closed.

Alternatively, the physician may perform a laparoscopic myomectomy via a Percutaneous Endoscopic approach, removing a fibroid tumor or tumors from the wall of the patient's uterus. The patient is placed in the dorsal lithotomy position. A trocar is inserted periumbilically, and the abdomen is insufflated with gas. Additional trocars are placed in the right and left lower quadrants. The physician incises the uterus through the myometrium to expose the myoma, which is dissected free from surrounding myometrium. The pedicle is isolated, clamped, and ligated, and the myoma is dissected from the pedicular blood supply. Any adjacent myomas may be reached by tunneling and removed through the initial incision. Additional incisions may be required for more distant myoma sites in the uterus. Morcellation (division into smaller pieces or fragments) may be required to remove the myomas via a collection bag through the laparoscopic incision. The uterus is closed with layered suturing. The laparoscopic instruments are removed, and the operative wounds are closed.

A hysteroscopic myomectomy involves removing the fibroids with electricity or laser through the vagina, which is Via Natural or Artificial Opening, Endoscopic approach. The physician vaginally inserts a resectoscope equipped with a small light and advances through the cervix and into the uterus where a saline solution is instilled to expand the cavity for better visualization and access. The resectoscope using laser beams resects the fibroids from the uterine wall. The resectoscope is removed and the cavity drained. The excised fibroid particles are washed out with the saline fluid.

Focus Point
Excision of multiple uterine myomas is reported only once, as only one body part, the Uterus, is the site of the excision. According to ICD-10-PCS Multiple Procedure guidelines, the operation is reported multiple times only when performed on multiple body parts defined by distinct body part values or separate and distinct body parts classified to a single ICD-10-PCS body part value. The uterus has only one body part value and no other distinct body parts classified in ICD-10-PCS.

Coding Guidance
AHA: 2014, 4Q, 16

Myringotomy with Tubes (Tympanostomy)

Body System
Ear, Nose, Sinus

PCS Root Operation
Drainage

Root Operation Table
Ø99   Ear, Nose, Sinus, Drainage

Body Part
Tympanic Membrane, Right
Tympanic Membrane, Left

Approach
Via Natural or Artificial Opening
Via Natural or Artificial Opening Endoscopic

Device
Drainage Device
No Device

Qualifier
Diagnostic
No Qualifier

Description

Myringotomy is a small incision in the tympanic membrane (eardrum), which separates the external ear from the middle ear. Myringotomy is sometimes done to facilitate inflation of Eustachian tubes or to decompress a fluid-filled middle ear. More commonly, myringotomy is followed by placement of a small ventilation tube in an operation called tympanostomy.

Tympanostomies are most commonly performed on young children with immature Eustachian tubes. Eustachian tubes are critical to the health of the middle ear. These canals lead from the middle ear to the pharynx, draining secretions and debris from the middle ear space and providing circulating air to it. In young children, Eustachian tubes are short and easily blocked, leading to a buildup of fluid in the middle ear. Short Eustachian tubes also provide a pathway for pathogens when patients have an upper respiratory infection. Pathogens within the middle ear can lead to otitis media (OM) or chronic otitis media with effusion (COME). Eustachian tube dysfunction (ETD) and chronic OM may be treated with tympanostomy.

The placement of a ventilation tube in the ear restores the flow of air, encourages the opening of any Eustachian tube blockage, and allows any debris or effusion to drain from the middle ear into the outer ear canal. Tympanostomy is commonly a pediatric procedure but may be performed on a patient of any age who has ETD or chronic OM. Most ventilation tubes, which may be documented as pressure equalization tubes (PE tubes), are temporary and usually dislodge from the patient's ears within a year.

Rarely, more permanent T-tubes may be placed. PE tubes are about the size of a wooden match head.

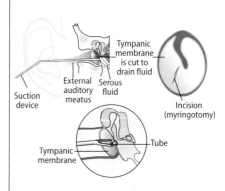

Using a microscope outside the ear canal for guidance, the physician inserts the instruments through the ear canal and makes a small incision in the tympanic membrane (eardrum). Any middle ear fluid is suctioned and may be reserved for analysis. The physician inserts a ventilating tube into the incised eardrum in tympanostomy, which is reported as a Drainage Device. In myringotomy only, reported with No Device, the physician aspirates fluid from the middle ear and inflates the Eustachian tubes by infusing the middle ear with air. This is usually performed to decompress the middle ear and is reported with No Qualifier. However, if the purpose of the fluid aspiration is stated to be diagnostic, report the qualifier Diagnostic. No other treatment is required. This approach is reported as Via Natural or Artificial Opening.

In an endoscopic procedure, the physician advances a rigid otoendoscope into the external ear canal, visualizing the surgical field. The otoendoscope is held against one wall of the external ear so that hand-held tools may be advanced along the other wall. The physician makes a small incision in the tympanic membrane (eardrum). Any middle ear fluid is suctioned and may be reserved for analysis. The physician inserts a ventilating tube into the incised eardrum in tympanostomy (Drainage Device). In myringotomy only, reported with No Device, the physician aspirates fluid from the middle ear and inflates the Eustachian tubes by infusing the middle ear with air. This is usually performed to decompress the middle ear and is reported with No Qualifier. However, if the purpose of the fluid aspiration is stated to be diagnostic, report the qualifier Diagnostic. No other treatment is required. This approach is reported as Via Natural or Artificial Opening Endoscopic.

© 2018 Optum360, LLC

Myringotomy with Tubes (Tympanostomy) (continued)

<table>
<tr><td>

Focus Point

Report the root operation Drainage for both diagnostic and therapeutic drainage procedures. When a drainage device is placed and remains in situ at the completion of the procedure, assign the device value Drainage Device.

</td><td>

Focus Point

By definition, in the approach Via Natural or Artificial Opening Endoscopic, the endoscope must enter the natural or artificial opening. An operating microscope remains outside the ear canal. Therefore, myringotomy/tympanostomy using an operating microscope is reported with the approach Via Natural or Artificial Opening, without any mention of endoscopy. Endoscopy would require an otoendoscope to enter the ear canal.

</td></tr>
</table>

Nephrolithotomy, Percutaneous

See also Nephrolithotripsy, Percutaneous

Body System
Urinary System

PCS Root Operation
Extirpation

Root Operation Table
ØTC   Urinary System, Extirpation

Body Part
Kidney, Right
Kidney, Left
Kidney Pelvis, Right
Kidney Pelvis, Left

Approach
Percutaneous
Percutaneous Endoscopic

Description
Kidney stones may block the natural flow of urine from the kidney to the ureters. Removing the stones is one method to alleviate this condition. Percutaneous nephrolithotomy is a surgical procedure in which a nephrostomy tube is inserted into the kidney through which the stones are removed.

After appropriate anesthesia and with the patient in prone position, a small incision is made in the patient's back. With the assistance of radiological guidance, a nephrostomy tube is placed in the kidney. A nephroscope, which contains a fiberoptic camera, is inserted through the tube to locate the stone(s). Additional instruments are inserted through the nephroscope, and the stone(s) are removed. The nephrostomy tube is secured to the skin, and an external drainage bag is attached.

Since the objective of this procedure is to remove the stone(s) regardless of whether they are broken up or not, the root operation Extirpation (defined as taking or cutting out solid matter from a body part) is reported.

Focus Point

The breaking up of stones before they are removed is referred to as nephrolithotripsy. See also Nephrolithotripsy, Percutaneous.

Medical and Surgical

Nephrolithotripsy, Percutaneous

See also Nephrolithotomy, Percutaneous

See also Nephrostomy (with Fragmentation), Percutaneous

Body System
Urinary System

PCS Root Operation
Extirpation

Root Operation Table
ØTC   Urinary System, Extirpation

Body Part
Kidney, Right
Kidney, Left
Kidney Pelvis, Right
Kidney Pelvis, Left

Approach
Percutaneous
Percutaneous Endoscopic

Description
Kidney stones may block the natural flow of urine from the kidney to the ureters. Removing the stones is one method to alleviate this condition. Percutaneous nephrolithotripsy is a surgical procedure in which a nephrostomy tube is inserted into the kidney through which the stones are broken up and removed.

After appropriate anesthesia and with the patient in prone position, a small incision is made in the patient's back. With the assistance of radiological guidance, a nephrostomy tube is placed in the kidney. A nephroscope, which contains a fiberoptic camera, is inserted through the tube to locate the stone(s). Ultrasonic energy or laser lithotripsy is applied to break up the stone(s). The stones are removed through the tube. The nephrostomy tube is secured to the skin, and an external drainage bag is attached.

Since the objective of this procedure is to remove the stone(s) regardless of whether they are broken up or not, the root operation Extirpation (defined as taking or cutting out solid matter from a body part) is reported. The fragmentation is inherent in the Extirpation of the stone(s) and not coded separately.

Focus Point

Removing the stones without breaking them up is referred to as nephrolithotomy. See also Nephrolithotomy, Percutaneous.

Focus Point

When the stones are broken up (fragmented) without removal, Fragmentation is the appropriate root operation. See also Nephrostomy (with Fragmentation), Percutaneous.

Coding Guidance
AHA: 2015, 2Q, 7

© 2018 Optum360, LLC

Nephrostomy (with Fragmentation), Percutaneous

See also Nephrolithotripsy, Percutaneous

Body System
Urinary System

PCS Root Operation
Fragmentation

Root Operation Table
ØTF   Urinary System, Fragmentation

Body Part
Kidney Pelvis, Right
Kidney Pelvis, Left

Approach
Percutaneous
Percutaneous Endoscopic

Description
Kidney stones block the natural flow of urine from the kidney to the ureters. Breaking up the stones is one method to remove this obstruction; small fragments of stone can be left to spontaneously pass without being surgically removed.

During a percutaneous nephrostomy with fragmentation, a physician inserts a tube through the skin into the kidney and breaks up stones without removing them. The nephrostomy creates an opening from the kidney to the exterior of the body and is used to drain urine.

Using radiologic guidance, the physician determines where to place the nephrostomy tube. After appropriate anesthesia with the patient in a prone position, a small incision is made in the back through which a needle is passed into the kidney. A guidewire is placed through the needle into the kidney. The nephrostomy tube is passed over the guidewire and placed into the kidney. A nephroscope is placed through this tube to visualize the stone or stones, and then ultrasonic energy or laser lithotripsy is applied to break them up. The nephrostomy tube is secured to the skin, and a drainage bag is used to collect urine.

Focus Point
When the stones are broken up and removed, Extirpation is the appropriate root operation to use. See also Nephrolithotripsy, Percutaneous.

Nephrostomy (without Fragmentation), Percutaneous

Body System
Urinary System

PCS Root Operation
Drainage

Root Operation Table
ØT9   Urinary System, Drainage

Body Part
Kidney, Right
Kidney, Left
Kidney Pelvis, Right
Kidney Pelvis, Left

Approach
Percutaneous

Device
Drainage Device

Description
Urine flows from the kidney through the ureters, into the bladder, and out through the urethra. When this normal flow is disrupted and urine is retained in the kidneys, a nephrostomy tube is temporarily placed in the kidney to remove the urine.

During a percutaneous nephrostomy, a physician inserts a tube through the skin into the kidney without breaking up stones. The nephrostomy creates an opening from the kidney to the exterior of the body and is used to drain urine.

The first step in performing a percutaneous nephrostomy is to select the suitable location for inserting the nephrostomy tube using radiological guidance. After appropriate anesthesia and using a Percutaneous approach with the patient in a prone position, a small incision is made in the back through which a needle is passed into the kidney. A guidewire is placed through the needle into the kidney. The nephrostomy tube is passed over the guidewire and placed into the kidney. Placement of the tube is confirmed with ultrasound guidance, CT, or fluoroscopy. A drainage bag is used to collect the urine, and the catheter is fixed to the skin.

Focus Point
The objective of this procedure is to drain the urine from the obstructed kidney. The procedure is therefore reported with root operation Drainage with device value Drainage Device according to guideline B6.2.

Nephroureterectomy

Body System
Urinary System

PCS Root Operation
Resection

Root Operation Table
ØTT Urinary System, Resection

Body Part
Kidney, Right
Kidney, Left
Ureter, Right
Ureter, Left

Approach
Open
Percutaneous Endoscopic

Description
A nephroureterectomy is the surgical removal of all of a kidney along with its associated ureter. Nephroureterectomy is often used to treat patients who have cancer of the urinary system. The procedure can be accomplished using various approaches and techniques.

The root operation Resection is reported when a total nephroureterectomy is performed. The physician removes the entire kidney and the entire ureter using an Open approach. To access the kidney and ureter, the physician usually makes an incision in the skin of the flank, cuts the muscles, fat, and fibrous membranes (fascia) overlying the kidney, and sometimes removes a portion of the 11th or 12th rib. After mobilizing the kidney and ureter, the physician clamps, ligates, and severs the ureter and major renal blood vessels (renal pedicle). The physician removes the kidney and all of the ureter but does not remove the adrenal gland, surrounding fatty tissue, or Gerota's fascia. After controlling bleeding, the physician irrigates the site with normal saline and places a drain tube, bringing it

out through a separate stab incision in the skin. The physician removes the clamps and performs layered closure.

When performing a Percutaneous Endoscopic nephroureterectomy, the physician removes the entire kidney and all of the ureter using a laparoscope to visualize the site of the procedure. The physician makes a 1 cm periumbilical incision and inserts a trocar. The abdominal cavity is insufflated with carbon dioxide. A fiberoptic laparoscope fitted with a camera and light source is inserted through the trocar. Other incisions (ports) are made in the abdomen or flank to allow other instruments or an additional light source to be passed into the abdomen or retroperitoneum. The colon is mobilized, and the laparoscope is advanced to the operative site. The physician mobilizes the kidney and clamps, ligates, and severs all of the ureter at the ureterovesical junction and major renal blood vessels (renal pedicle). The kidney and ureter are bagged and brought through one of the port sites (e.g., periumbilical) that have been slightly enlarged. The instruments are removed, and the small abdominal or flank incisions are closed with staple or suture.

Focus Point
A hand-assisted laparoscopic nephroureterectomy using an Open incision with assistance via laparoscopy is reported with an Open approach. See ICD-10-PCS guideline B5.2.

Focus Point
If only a portion of a kidney and/or ureter is removed, report root operation Excision, rather than Resection.

Focus Point
A nephroureterectomy may include a separately reportable Excision of a portion (cuff) of the bladder.

Coding Guidance
AHA: 2014, 3Q, 16

© 2018 Optum360, LLC

Neurolysis, Trigeminal (Trigeminal Nerve Decompression)

Body System
Central Nervous System and Cranial Nerves

PCS Root Operation
Release

Root Operation Table
ØØN Central Nervous System and Cranial Nerves, Release

Body Part
Trigeminal Nerve

Approach
Open

Description

Trigeminal neurolysis is performed on patients with trigeminal neuralgia. Trigeminal neuralgia causes extreme, sudden facial pain that can be caused by a compression on the trigeminal nerve or with patients with multiple sclerosis.

Under general anesthesia, using an Open approach, the physician makes an incision overlying the nerve and dissects it free of the surrounding tissue. If the nerve is in bone and must be decompressed, freed, or moved, the overlying bone is first removed using drills and/or osteotomes. The physician makes an incision in the area of nerve tension and locates the nerve. Surrounding soft tissues are dissected from the nerve to release pressure on the nerve.

Microvascular decompression (MVD) surgery is performed under general anesthesia, through an Open incision, and microsurgical instruments are used to mobilize the offending vessels away from the trigeminal nerve root.

Focus Point

In ICD-10 PCS, the correct code depends on the root operation that describes the main objective of the procedure. When the objective is to free the body part, Release is the root operation. Division is coded when the objective of the procedure is to transect or separate a body part.

In the root operation Release, the body part value coded is the body part being freed and not the tissue being manipulated or cut to free the body part.

Focus Point

Alcohol injection or radiofrequency neuroablation using a Percutaneous approach to reduce pain is reported with root operation Destruction.

Neuroplasty, Peripheral

Body System
Peripheral Nervous System

PCS Root Operation
Repair

Supplement

Root Operation Table
Ø1Q   Peripheral Nervous System, Repair

Ø1U   Peripheral Nervous System, Supplement

Body Part
Refer to the ICD-10-PCS tabular list for a complete list of body parts.

Approach
Open

Percutaneous

Percutaneous Endoscopic

Device
No Device

Autologous Tissue Substitute (Supplement)

Synthetic Substitute (Supplement)

Nonautologous Tissue Substitute (Supplement)

Description
Neuroplasty is a surgical technique used to restore or repair damaged nerve tissue. The peripheral nerves consist of those outside the central nervous system. Comprising the nerves that exit the brain and spinal cord, the peripheral nervous system serves the limbs and organs of the body.

Repair
The physician repairs a cranial or peripheral nerve. The physician locates the damaged nerve in a previously opened incision or wound. The nerve is sutured to restore sensory or motor function. Restoring a body part to its normal function meets the definition of the root operation Repair.

Supplement
The physician obtains and places a nerve graft to restore innervation to the head, neck, arm, leg, hand, or foot. A typical graft harvest is obtained from the sural nerve. To harvest the graft, the physician makes a lateral incision of the lateral malleolus of the ankle. The nerve is identified and freed. The physician cuts the nerve to obtain the length needed for the graft, elongating the incision as necessary. The proximal and distal sural nerve endings are anastomosed. The physician makes an incision over the damaged nerve and dissects the tissues to locate the nerve. The damaged area of the nerve is resected and removed. Innervation is restored by suturing the graft to the proximal and distal ends of the damaged nerve. A single nerve strand or multiple nerve strands (cable) may be grafted. Supplement is the appropriate root operation since the graft is reinforcing the damaged nerve tissue.

Focus Point

If an Autologous Tissue Substitute is harvested from a different body part, report a code for the Excision of the graft tissue in addition to the Supplement procedure, according to guideline B3.9.

© 2018 Optum360, LLC

Nuss Procedure

See also Ravitch Procedure (Repair of Pectus Deformity)

Body System
Upper Bones

PCS Root Operation
Reposition

Root Operation Table
ØPS   Upper Bones, Reposition

Body Part
Sternum

Approach
Percutaneous Endoscopic

Device
Internal Fixation Device

Description
The Nuss procedure is a surgical technique that involves using a convex steel bar placed beneath the pectus deformity to correct pectus excavatum. It is considered a minimally invasive repair of the pectus excavatum (MIRPE) as compared with the Ravitch procedure (*see* Ravitch Procedure [Repair of Pectus Deformity]), which is also used to correct pectus excavatum.

The chest is first marked at strategic points, and the length of a curved steel bar, called the Lorenz pectus bar, to be inserted into the sternum is measured and shaped to fit the individual's chest. Midaxillary line incisions are made on the right and left sides aligned with the deepest depression point. A skin tunnel is raised from the incisions, and another small lateral incision is made for insertion of a thoracoscope. The skin incisions are elevated, and a long introducer instrument is inserted through the right intercostal space at the top of the pectus ridge and slowly advanced across the anterior mediastinal space with videoscopic guidance. The sternum is forcefully lifted as the introducer is passed to the other side. Once behind the sternum, the tip is pushed through the intercostal space at the top of the pectus ridge on the left side and brought out through that skin incision. Umbilical tape is pulled through the tunnel and used to guide the prepared bar. The bar is inserted with the convex curve facing posteriorly and rotated with a flipping instrument until the convex curve faces anteriorly. The bar can be pulled back out and bent in a more ideal curvature for correction as many times as needed. Usually only one bar is placed. With the bar in position, a stabilizing bar is sutured around the pectus bar and to the muscle. Sutures are placed in the lateral chest wall musculature, as well as one other fixation point to the side of the sternum around one rib and the pectus bar.

> **Focus Point**
> *The intent of both the Nuss and Ravitch procedure is to move the sternum into normal position; Reposition is the appropriate root operation.*

Coding Guidance
AHA: 2015, 4Q, 33

Orchiectomy

Body System
Male Reproductive System

PCS Root Operation
Excision

Resection

Root Operation Table
ØVB   Male Reproductive System, Excision

ØVT   Male Reproductive System, Resection

Body Part
Testis, Right

Testis, Left

Testes, Bilateral

Approach
Open

Percutaneous

Percutaneous Endoscopic

Qualifier
Diagnostic

No Qualifier

Description
The testes manufacture male hormones and spermatozoa. Because spermatozoa are temperature sensitive, the testes reside in the scrotum, which is covered in skin rugae that retract and relax based on ambient and body temperatures.

Excisional orchiectomy (also, orchidectomy) may be performed to remove a benign or malignant lesion, or to remove a sample for biopsy. Resection usually is associated with a malignancy or with undescended testis.

The testes in a developing fetus do not descend into the scrotum until shortly before or after birth. In some males, one or both testes may remain undescended (cryptorchidism). This is usually detected and corrected in childhood. The undescended testis of an adult may be resected due to an increased risk of developing cancer in the undescended testis.

Excision
In an Excision, only a portion of one or both testes is removed. An Open approach involves an incision made in the scrotal skin or the inguinal skin, and the separation of tissues to expose the spermatic cord. If the testis is to be preserved, the portion to be excised is removed and the excision site and operative wound are closed in layers by suturing.

In a Percutaneous approach, the physician obtains a sample of testicular tissue by needle biopsy. While the testis is held firmly with the scrotal skin stretched tightly over the testis and the epididymis positioned away from the biopsy site, a biopsy needle is guided into the targeted area of the testis. The needle biopsy sheath is advanced over the needle and twisted to shear off the enclosed sample and withdrawn with the sample enclosed. The scrotal wound may be closed by suturing.

Resection
An Open approach involves an incision made in the scrotal skin or the inguinal skin and the separation of tissues to expose the spermatic cord. The spermatic cord is opened, and the individual bundles making up the cord (vein, artery, spermatic nerve, epididymis, vas deferens) are cross-clamped, cut, and secured with nonabsorbable suture material. The entire testis is removed through the incision. The wound is closed in layers by suturing.

In a Percutaneous Endoscopic approach, the physician removes the testis, which may be undescended, injured, or diseased, using a laparoscope. The physician places a trocar at the umbilicus into the abdominal or retroperitoneal space and insufflates the abdominal cavity. The physician places a laparoscope through the umbilical incision and additional trocars in the abdomen. The testis and all its associated structures are pushed up from the scrotum or freed from their undescended intra-abdominal location and removed through the abdominal or retroperitoneal space via the trocar port. Packing may be placed in the empty scrotum. Care is taken to avoid important nerves and vessels in the area. The trocars are removed, and the incisions are closed with sutures.

Focus Point
If a prosthetic testis is implanted during the concurrent surgery, report the root operation Replacement rather than Excision or Resection with a code from root operation table ØVR Replacement Male Reproductive System, with the qualifier Synthetic Substitute. Replacement involves putting in or on biological or synthetic material that takes the place and/or function of all or a portion of a body part, which may be taken out during the Replacement procedure. Excision and Resection are by definition without replacement.

Focus Point
In cases of testicular cancer, the scrotal sac may be emptied and portions of the spermatic cord excised in addition to the testis. Report resection or excision of the epididymis, scrotal skin, and/or other body part(s) in addition to the excision or resection of the testis. This is consistent with advice in ICD-10-PCS guideline B3.2.a.

Focus Point
If a bilateral orchiectomy is performed, report one code with the body part value Testes, Bilateral rather than two codes with a Right and Left body part value. See ICD-10-PCS guideline B4.3

© 2018 Optum360, LLC

Orchiopexy

Body System
Male Reproductive System

PCS Root Operation
Repair

Reposition

Root Operation Table
ØVQ   Male Reproductive System, Repair

ØVS   Male Reproductive System, Reposition

Body Part
Testis, Right

Testis, Left

Testes, Bilateral

Approach
Open

Percutaneous Endoscopic

Description
The testes manufacture male hormones and spermatozoa. Because spermatozoa are temperature sensitive, normal testes reside in the scrotum, which is covered in skin rugae that retract and relax based on ambient and body temperatures.

The testes in a developing fetus do not descend into the scrotum until shortly before or after birth. In some males, one or both testes may remain undescended (cryptorchidism). This is usually detected and corrected in childhood.

Orchiopexy (also called orchidopexy, cryptorchidopexy, orchidorrhaphy, orchiorrhaphy) is performed to reposition and surgically fixate an undescended testicle into the scrotum. It can also refer to surgery performed to anchor a testicle susceptible to torsion in the scrotum.

Repair
Orchiopexy is performed to prevent recurrent testicular torsion by surgically anchoring the testicle into the scrotum. Torsion occurs when the testicle rotates, thus reducing blood flow and causing severe pain and swelling.

In an Open scrotal approach, the physician makes an incision in the scrotum. The tissues are separated by dissection. In the scrotum, the testis is sutured in place to prevent recurrent torsion and/or retraction into the inguinal canal. The incision is closed in layers by suturing.

Reposition
Orchiopexy is performed to surgically fixate an undescended testicle into the scrotum. Using an Open abdominal approach, an incision is made in the inguinal area from the pubic bone to the upper lateral pelvic area in the skin fold made by the thigh and the lower abdomen. The physician searches the abdominal cavity for a testis that failed to descend into the scrotum during development. The tissues are separated by dissection to find the testis in the area. At this point several surgical options are available. The one chosen depends on the mobility of the testis and how far it can be brought down through the inguinal canal and into the scrotum. The procedure may take two stages approximately six to 12 months apart. Eventually, the spermatic cord is mobilized sufficiently to allow positioning of the testis in the scrotum. In the scrotum, a small pouch is created for the testis where the testis is sutured in place to prevent retraction back into the inguinal canal or abdominal cavity. The incision is closed in layers of suturing.

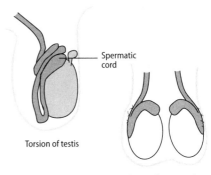

Spermatic cord

Torsion of testis

Testes after correction showing bilateral fixation

In an Open inguinal or scrotal approach, the physician makes an incision in the scrotum or the inguinal area from the pubic bone to the upper lateral pelvic area in the skin crease made by the thigh and the lower abdomen. If the orchiopexy is performed to treat an undescended testicle, the physician searches for a testis that failed to descend into the scrotum during development. The tissues are separated by dissection to find the testis in the inguinal canal area. The spermatic cord is mobilized to allow positioning of the testis in the scrotum. In the scrotum, a small pouch is created for the testis where the testis is sutured in place to prevent retraction back into the inguinal canal. The incision is closed in layers by suturing.

© 2018 Optum360, LLC

Orchiopexy (continued)

In a Percutaneous Endoscopic approach, the physician performs an orchiopexy (the surgical fixation of an undescended testicle into the scrotum) with the assistance of a fiberoptic laparoscope. A para-umbilical port is created by placing a trocar at the level of the umbilicus. The abdominal wall is insufflated. The laparoscope is advanced through the umbilical port, and additional trocars are placed into the abdominal cavity. The physician uses the laparoscope fitted with a fiberoptic camera and/or an operating instrument to search the abdominal cavity for the undescended testis. The physician may have several surgical options depending on the mobility of the testis and how far it can be brought down through the inguinal canal into the scrotum. The procedure may take two stages approximately six to 12 months apart. The spermatic cord is mobilized sufficiently to allow positioning of the testis in the scrotum (which often occurs during the first and perhaps only operative session). A small pouch is created for the testis where the testis is sutured in place to prevent retraction back into the inguinal canal or into the abdominal cavity. The small abdominal incisions are closed by staple or suture in the usual fashion.

Focus Point

If a bilateral orchiopexy is performed, report one code with the body part value Testes, Bilateral rather than two codes with a Right and Left body part value. See ICD-10-PCS guideline B4.3.

Focus Point

If there is a concomitant hernia, it is often repaired at the same time through the same incision. The hernia present in the inguinal canal is repaired by folding and suturing tissues to strengthen the abdominal wall and correct the weakness responsible for the hernia. Report an additional code for inguinal hernia repair if performed.

Osteosynthesis, Rotational Tibial (Tibial Rotationplasty)

Body System
Lower Bones

PCS Root Operation
Reposition

Root Operation Table
0QS   Lower Bones, Reposition

Body Part
Tibia, Right
Tibia, Left

Approach
Open

Device
Internal Fixation Device
Internal Fixation Device, Intramedullary

Description
Rotational tibial osteosynthesis is usually performed to treat defects created from resection of malignant neoplasms such as osteosarcoma of the distal femur or proximal tibia.

Under general anesthesia, the lower limb is prepped and draped. Using an Open approach, the physician makes two circumferential incisions, which are then connected by longitudinal incisions medially and laterally. The sciatic nerve is isolated and preserved. Vessels and muscles are transected at the level of the planned bone resection. Osteotomies of the tibia and femur are completed, removing the malignant neoplasm and surrounding tissues. The lower section of the tibia is rotated 180 degrees back to front with the pivot at the knee. Osteosynthesis using a plate or intramedullary fixation is carried out between the proximal ends of the femur and tibia. This allows the ankle joint to bend forward somewhat like a knee, thus creating an effective weight-bearing stump. A prosthesis can be attached to the foot to make up the difference in leg length.

Circulation is reestablished to the distal part of the limb. The muscles are then reattached by suturing. Skin flaps are then trimmed and closed.

Focus Point

Reposition is the appropriate root operation for rotational osteosynthesis. Osteotomies of the tibia are included in the Reposition procedure. Code any additional procedures separately that are performed for distinct objectives or on distinct body parts, such as excision of the femur and/or knee joint.

Coding Guidance
AHA: 2014, 4Q, 29

© 2018 Optum360, LLC

Panniculectomy, Cosmetic

Body System
Subcutaneous Tissue and Fascia
Anatomical Regions, General

PCS Root Operation
Alteration

Root Operation Table
ØJØ Subcutaneous Tissue and Fascia, Alteration
ØWØ Anatomical Regions, General, Alteration

Body Part
Subcutaneous Tissue and Fascia, Abdomen
Abdominal Wall

Approach
Open
Percutaneous

Description
The objective of panniculectomy when performed as a cosmetic procedure is to reduce tissue size by removing excessive skin and at times subcutaneous tissue from the pannus, which is the overhanging tissue or apron in the abdomen for aesthetic purposes.

Panniculectomy/lipectomy: To reduce a pendulous abdomen, the physician uses an Open approach to make an incision traversing the abdomen below the belly button in a horizontal fashion. Excessive skin and subcutaneous tissue are elevated off the abdominal wall, and excess tissue and fat are excised. The flaps are brought together and sutured in at least three layers. The physician may also suture the rectus abdominis muscles together in the midline to reinforce the area.

This is documented as abdominoplasty and is included in the Alteration, Anatomical Regions, General procedure.

Liposuction: When liposuction is performed for cosmetic purposes, the root operation Alteration is reported. A liposuction cannula is inserted through a regional incision using a Percutaneous approach, and the physician moves the cannula through the fat deposits, creating tunnels and removing excess deposits. The incisions are closed simply.

The root operation Alteration is used to report all aspects of the cosmetic procedure regardless of the type of surgical technique used.

Focus Point
A panniculectomy performed for medical purposes rather than cosmetic purposes should not be reported with the root operation Alteration but depends on the objective and type of technique employed.

Focus Point
When tightening of muscles is also involved, it is referred to as an abdominoplasty. If the procedure is performed for cosmetic body contouring purposes, the root operation Alteration is used.

Focus Point
The physician may remove excess skin and subcutaneous tissue on the thigh, leg, hip, buttock, arm, submental fat pad (inferior to the chin), or other area in a similar fashion. Each uniquely different body part is reported with an Alteration code.

Medical and Surgical

Paracentesis, Peritoneal Cavity

Medical and Surgical

Body System
Anatomical Regions, General

PCS Root Operation
Drainage

Root Operation Table
0W9   Anatomical Regions, General, Drainage

Body Part
Peritoneal Cavity

Approach
Percutaneous
Percutaneous Endoscopic

Device
Drainage Device
No Device

Qualifier
Diagnostic
No Qualifier

Description

The peritoneal cavity is a closed sac that normally contains a small amount of lubricating fluid. Excess fluid can accumulate in the peritoneal cavity as a result of blockage or disease. Ascites is the abnormal collection of fluid in the peritoneum. This fluid may be aspirated for therapeutic reasons, i.e., to make the patient more comfortable. The fluid may also be aspirated to undergo pathological examination to determine the extent of disease or the cause of the ascites. Paracentesis of peritoneal fluid may be documented as an ascitic tap.

The physician inserts a needle or catheter into the peritoneal cavity via a Percutaneous approach and withdraws fluid, reported with root operation Drainage, for diagnostic or therapeutic purposes. If the needle or catheter is removed at the completion of the procedure, report No Device. If the drainage device is left in the patient at the end of the procedure for ongoing drainage of ascites, report Drainage Device.

Endoscopic ultrasound guided paracentesis (EUS-P) may be performed in cases of suspected malignancy because the guidance allows the needle to localize and accurately sample minimal peritoneal fluid when there is little or no ascites. It is also useful in the staging of a malignancy of a patient with minimal or no ascites. EUS-P is performed during an upper endoscopy for diagnostic purposes. The endoscope is advanced into the patient's mouth and down the throat, into the stomach or duodenum. The EUS-P device contains a needle attachment that is able to pierce the wall of the stomach or duodenum to enter the peritoneal cavity where a pocket of peritoneal fluid has been identified. The fluid is aspirated into a reservoir in the scope through the needle. The scope is withdrawn.

Focus Point
EUS-P is performed using an upper gastrointestinal endoscopic approach via a natural (mouth) or artificial opening (gastrostomy). However, this is not an option in the root operation table 0WD Drainage, Anatomical Regions, General in ICD-10-PCS. As the Percutaneous Endoscopic approach most closely describes the procedure performed, use this approach, and because this is a diagnostic procedure, report the qualifier Diagnostic.

Focus Point
ICD-10-PCS code assignment depends on the objective of the procedure (therapeutic or diagnostic). If paracentesis is documented as both therapeutic and diagnostic, the more definitive (therapeutic) treatment is reported. However, if the diagnostic procedure uses a different approach or obtains samples from a different site from the therapeutic procedure, both the diagnostic and the therapeutic procedures are reported. Surgical specimens are routinely sent to pathology for study without necessarily being considered diagnostic. If the documentation is unclear, query the physician.

Focus Point
If peritoneal fluid is obtained from the pouch of Douglas (cul-de-sac, rectouterine pouch) via a needle inserted into the vagina (culdocentesis), report 0U9 Drainage, Female Reproductive System, with the body part Cul-de-sac, instead.

Coding Guidance
AHA: 2017, 3Q, 12; 2014, 4Q, 11

© 2018 Optum360, LLC

Parathyroidectomy

See also Reimplantation, Parathyroid
(Autotransplantation)

Body System
Endocrine System

PCS Root Operation
Excision
Resection

Root Operation Table
ØGB Endocrine System, Excision
ØGT Endocrine System, Resection

Body Part
Superior Parathyroid Gland, Right
Superior Parathyroid Gland, Left
Inferior Parathyroid Gland, Right
Inferior Parathyroid Gland, Left
Parathyroid Glands, Multiple
Parathyroid Gland

Approach
Open
Percutaneous Endoscopic

Device
No Device

Qualifier
Diagnostic (Excision)
No Qualifier

Description
The parathyroid glands consist of four, small,
pea-shaped glands, two superior and two inferior,
located in the neck on either side of the trachea next to
the thyroid gland. These glands control the calcium
level in the blood by secreting parathyroid hormone
(PTH) that increases the calcium level when it is too
low.

Parathyroidectomy is the removal of part or all of one
or more of the parathyroid glands, usually performed
for primary hyperparathyroidism. The most common
cause of primary hyperparathyroidism is parathyroid
adenoma. Primary hyperparathyroidism occurs when
the PTH level is elevated in relation to the serum
calcium level.

In an Open approach, the physician directly exposes
the parathyroid via a low cervical incision in the skin.
The platysma muscles are divided, and the strap
muscles are separated and flaps are raised. A
localization scan is done, and, depending on which
side has the abnormality, the thyroid is mobilized on
that side, rotating it until the parathyroid gland to be
removed is isolated. Using blunt dissection of the
tissue in this area, the physician locates both normal
and abnormal parathyroid glands. The fascia covering
the gland is divided, vessels serving the diseased gland
are ligated, and the parathyroid gland is excised.
During the procedure, care is taken to identify and
preserve the superior and recurrent laryngeal nerves.
When the excision or resection is complete, the thyroid
gland is repositioned, the muscles are reapproximated,
and the skin incision is closed.

In a Percutaneous Endoscopic approach, the physician
makes a small incision and dissects through the
platysma and strap muscles until locating the thyroid,
at which point the endoscope is inserted and a
minimally invasive video-assisted parathyroidectomy
is performed using endoscopic dissector and aspirator
tools. The physician isolates the parathyroid tissue to
be excised and ligates the vessels serving the gland.
When the excision or resection is complete, the
instruments are removed and the muscles are
reapproximated. The skin incision is closed.

Focus Point
*If only a portion of any of the named parathyroid gland
body part is removed (Superior Parathyroid Gland,
Right; Superior Parathyroid Gland, Left; Inferior
Parathyroid Gland, Right; Inferior Parathyroid Gland,
Left; Parathyroid Glands, Multiple; Parathyroid Gland),
the root operation is Excision. Excision may be
performed for therapeutic and/or diagnostic purposes.
Parathyroid gland excision for diagnostic purposes
is reported with the qualifier Diagnostic.*

Focus Point
*Resection, which involves removal of all of a body part,
is reported when the entire named parathyroid gland
body part is removed (Superior Parathyroid Gland,
Right; Superior Parathyroid Gland, Left; Inferior
Parathyroid Gland, Right; Inferior Parathyroid Gland,
Left; Parathyroid Glands, Multiple; Parathyroid Gland).*

Parotidectomy

See also Sialoadenectomy

Body System
Mouth and Throat

PCS Root Operation
Excision
Resection

Root Operation Table
ØCB   Mouth and Throat, Excision
ØCT   Mouth and Throat, Resection

Body Part
Parotid Gland, Right
Parotid Gland, Left

Approach
Open
Percutaneous

Qualifier
Diagnostic (Excision)
No Qualifier

Description

The parotid glands are bilateral salivary glands situated high in the neck just below and anterior to the ears. They are the largest salivary glands. Salivary glands are stimulated by autonomic nerves to secrete saliva that aids in digestion of food and lubrication of the mouth. Saliva also has natural antibacterial properties that protect the mouth.

Neoplasms are the most common diagnosis associated with parotidectomy, although excision or resection may be performed for chronic inflammation, calculi, or infection. About 80 percent of neoplasms of the parotid gland are benign. Because the facial nerve and its branches traverse the parotid glands bilaterally, surgery to remove all or part of the parotid gland is usually accompanied by intraoperative nerve testing.

The physician excises a portion or all of the parotid gland with or without facial nerve preservation and unilateral neck dissection. Using an Open approach to directly visualize the operative site, the physician makes a preauricular incision into the skin with a curved cervical extension to the midpoint of the mandible. The anterior and posterior skin flaps are retracted, and the tissues are retracted to expose the parotid gland. If a facial nerve dissection is performed, the main trunk of the facial nerve is visualized, and the lateral (superficial) lobe of the parotid gland may be freed and excised, depending on the extent of excision, or the facial nerve may be identified and the lateral lobe lifted off the branches of the nerve using

dissection. The facial nerve is dissected free of the parotid gland. A nerve stimulator is used to test nerve integrity. The facial nerve may be retracted so the deep parotid gland can be removed without damaging the facial nerve, if necessary. The physician removes all or part of the left and/or right parotid gland, and the operative incision is closed in layers.

Excision
Parotidectomy excises a portion of the right or left parotid gland in the root operation Excision. A superficial parotidectomy removes only the superficial lobe and is reported with root operation Excision. The deep lobe is not removed. An excisional biopsy is reported with the qualifier Diagnostic.

Resection
Parotidectomy excises the entire right or left parotid gland (both the superficial and deep lobes) in the root operation Resection.

Focus Point
Excision of the parotid duct(s) and/or local lymph nodes would be reported separately.

Focus Point
Because parotid gland body parts are not currently listed in the Extraction root operation table, needle biopsy of the parotid gland is reported using root operation Excision and approach Percutaneous, with the qualifier Diagnostic.

Focus Point
To protect the patient's facial nerve function, ongoing intraoperative neurophysiologic monitoring (IOM) may be performed by a technologist present during parotidectomy. This is a dedicated monitoring, much more intense than the intermittent nerve testing as described above, and would be reported from the root operation table 4A1 Monitoring Physiological Systems (repetitive over a period of time).

Focus Point
Resection of the specific body part is coded whenever all of the body part is cut out or off, rather than coding Excision of a less specific body part. The root operation Resection is assigned only when the entire right or left parotid gland is resected, including the superficial and deep lobes. The parotid gland has distinct anatomic designations for the right and left gland. If both right and left sides of the parotid gland are resected, report two codes. See ICD-10-PCS guideline B3.8.

Coding Guidance
AHA: 2016, 2Q, 12; 2014, 3Q, 9, 21

© 2018 Optum360, LLC

Pleurectomy, Parietal, with Decortication

Body System
Respiratory System

PCS Root Operation
Extraction

Root Operation Table
ØBD Respiratory System, Extraction

Body Part
Pleura, Right
Pleura, Left

Approach
Open
Percutaneous Endoscopic
No Device

Qualifier
Diagnostic
No Qualifier

Description
Pleurectomy is the removal of the pleura and usually involves the parietal pleura. Decortication is the removal of visible pleural tumors in the chest area. A pleurectomy with decortication may be performed to treat mesothelioma, pleural metastases, or persistent or recurrent pleural effusions, including malignant pleural effusions.

The physician removes the membranous tissue lining the inside surface of the chest cavity (the parietal pleura).

Using an Open approach, the physician opens the chest cavity widely to gain access to the inside surface of the chest. Using a scalpel, the surgeon makes a long incision around the side of the chest between two of the ribs. The incision is carried through all the tissue layers into the chest cavity. Rib spreaders are inserted into the wound, and the ribs are spread apart, exposing the lung. The parietal pleura is stripped from the inside surface of the chest. The chest wall incision is then sutured closed in layers. A chest tube may be used to provide drainage for the chest cavity.

Alternatively, the chest cavity can be opened and the operation performed through a vertical incision in the center of the chest through the sternum. The skin incision is carried down to the sternum bone, and then a saw is used to split the sternum. With the sternum split in half, the chest is entered by spreading the sternum apart with a set of rib spreaders. When the procedure is complete, the wound is closed by using wires to bring the two halves of the sternum together. A chest tube is placed through the incision to evacuate fluid and air, and the skin is closed over the sternum by suturing.

In a Percutaneous Endoscopic approach, the physician uses two small incisions along with a thoracoscope and video to access and excise the pleura.

Focus Point
Extraction is used as the root operation since tissue is being stripped (use of force) from the inside surface of the chest.

Focus Point
The term decortication has two unique definitions, each of which is reported with a different root operation. One meaning of decortication is removing the cortex (outer layer) of a structure or organ such as the pleura of the lung. This is represented with the root operation Extraction, which is the stripping off all or a portion of that cortex. The other definition of decortication is removal of the fibrous bands or tissues that prevent lung expansion, which is best represented by the root operation Release.

Plication, Emphysematous Bleb

Body System
Respiratory System

PCS Root Operation
Repair

Root Operation Table
ØBQ   Respiratory System, Repair

Body Part
Upper Lung Lobe, Right
Middle Lung Lobe, Right
Lower Lung Lobe, Right
Upper Lung Lobe, Left
Lung Lingula
Lower Lung Lobe, Left
Lung, Right
Lung, Left
Lungs, Bilateral

Approach
Open
Percutaneous Endoscopic

Description

Emphysematous lungs may develop areas of damaged tissues called blebs or bullae. Usually located in the upper lung regions, these thin, air-filled blisters can rupture, causing spontaneous pneumothorax. Surgical treatment includes plication, which is folding or pleating, to reduce the size of a bleb by making folds or tucks in its walls.

The physician opens the chest cavity using an Open approach to plicate one or more lung bullae (large nonfunctional air sacs). Using a scalpel, the surgeon makes a long incision around the side of the chest between two of the ribs. The incision is carried through all of the tissue layers into the chest cavity. Rib spreaders are inserted into the wound, and the ribs are spread apart to expose the lung. Alternatively, the chest cavity can be opened and the operation performed through a vertical incision in the center of the chest through the sternum. The skin incision is carried down to the sternum bone, and a saw is used to split the sternum. With the sternum split in half, the chest is entered by spreading the sternum apart with a set of rib spreaders. Space is made in the chest by packing the uninvolved lung away from the operative field using large, moist, gauze sponges. To perform the procedure, the pleural surface may require an

operative procedure such as pneumonolysis (separation of the surface of the lung that has become adherent to the inside surface of the chest cavity). The lung bulla is located, and the lung tissue is rolled and folded in a plication technique. A noncutting stapler is positioned over the plicated lung tissue, and the grasping mechanism is withdrawn. The stapler is fired, and the lung tissue remains in place, but the bleb has been sealed or the volume of the lung has been reduced without removing any tissue. When the procedure is complete, the instruments and gauze sponges are removed. A temporary chest tube(s) may be used to provide drainage for the chest cavity. If applicable, the sternotomy is repaired using wires to bring the two halves of the sternum together, and the operative wound is closed by sutures or staples.

Using a Percutaneous Endoscopic approach, the physician examines the inside of the chest cavity with a rigid or flexible fiberoptic endoscope and plicates one or more lung bullae. The physician makes a small incision between two ribs and by blunt dissection and uses a trocar to enter the thoracic cavity. The endoscope is passed through the trocar and into the chest cavity. The lung is usually partially collapsed by instilling air into the chest through the trocar, or the lung may be collapsed through a double lumen endotracheal tube inserted through the mouth into the trachea. The contents of the chest cavity are examined by direct visualization and/or by the use of a video camera. Still photographs may be taken as part of the procedure. A second and/or third trocar and instruments may be inserted into the chest cavity through a second and/or third wound in the chest. Under visualization through the endoscope, the physician manipulates the instruments inserted through the secondary sites and localizes the bulla. The lung tissue is rolled, folded, and sutured in a plication technique. The lung tissue remains in place, but the bleb has been sealed or the volume of the lung has been reduced without removing any tissue. At the conclusion of the procedure, the endoscope and the trocars are removed. A temporary chest tube for drainage and re-expansion of the lung is usually inserted through the wound used for the thoracoscopy.

Focus Point
Postoperative drainage devices are considered inherent in the procedure and not coded separately according to guideline B6.1b.

  © 2018 Optum360, LLC

Proctectomy

See also Resection, Abdominoperineal (APR)

Body System
Gastrointestinal System

PCS Root Operation
Excision

Resection

Root Operation Table
ØDB   Gastrointestinal System, Excision
ØDT   Gastrointestinal System, Resection

Body Part
Rectum

Approach
Open

Qualifier
Diagnostic (Excision)
No Qualifier

Description
Proctectomy may be defined as surgical removal of a damaged or dysfunctional portion of the rectum. Indications for rectal resection include:

- Disease (e.g., diverticulitis, neoplasm, inflammatory conditions)
- Injury
- Obstruction
- Ischemia

Rectal resections remove damaged portions of the rectum to restore function. Disease or injury can result in scar tissue formation, obstruction, and impairment of the mechanisms that facilitate normal elimination of feces. Some disease processes can cause perforations in the bowel, which can cause serious intra-abdominal infections. Surgical techniques vary, but complete removal is reported with the root operation Resection regardless of technique. The root operation Excision is used when only a portion of the rectum is removed. If a colostomy is formed, an additional Bypass procedure is reported.

The physician removes all or a portion of the rectum through an Open transsacral approach. The physician makes a posterior incision at the junction of the sacrum and coccyx. The coccyx is excised.

Dissection is continued posteriorly, and the rectum and distal colon are mobilized. The rectum is transected proximally and distally, and a portion of the rectum is removed. The distal end of colon is approximated to the remaining rectal stump with sutures or staples. The incision is closed.

The proctectomy may also be performed using an Open abdominal approach. The physician removes the diseased rectal segment and performs an anastomosis of the colon and anus. The physician makes an abdominal incision. The rectum and distal colon are mobilized, and the colon is divided just proximal to the diseased rectal segment. The rectal segment is removed and the distal colon pulled through the sphincter complex and approximated to the anus with sutures from a perineal approach. The incision is closed.

Focus Point
Any anastomosis performed to re-establish intestinal continuity is considered inherent in the Resection or Excision procedure and is not coded separately based on guideline B3.1b.

Coding Guidance
AHA: 2016, 1Q, 22; 2014, 4Q, 40

Prostatectomy

Body System
Male Reproductive System

PCS Root Operation
Destruction
Excision
Resection

Root Operation Table
ØV5	Male Reproductive System, Destruction
ØVB	Male Reproductive System, Excision
ØVT	Male Reproductive System, Resection

Body Part
Prostate

Approach
Open
Percutaneous Endoscopic
Via Natural or Artificial Opening Endoscopic

Qualifier
Diagnostic (Excision)
No Qualifier

Description
Prostatectomy is a surgical technique used to treat prostate cancer or benign prostatic hyperplasia (enlarged prostate) that involves removing all or part of the prostate.

Destruction
Benign prostatic hyperplasia (BPH) may be treated with transurethral resection of the prostate (TURP), which is performed Via Natural or Artificial Opening Endoscopic approach. A resectoscope is passed through the penis into the urethra to the level of the prostate. The inner part of the prostate gland that surrounds the urethra is destroyed with electrical heat or laser. A Foley catheter is placed and left in the bladder. No incisions are made during this procedure.

Excision
When the physician removes a portion of prostatic tissue, this is reported with the root operation Excision. Using an Open approach, an incision is made to access the diseased or damaged prostate tissue. The tissue or lesion is identified and removed. Bleeding is controlled, and the dissected tissues and skin incision are closed in layers by suturing. The procedure may also be done via Percutaneous Endoscopic (laparoscopic) approach.

Alternatively, a transurethral resection of the prostate (TURP) is performed Via Natural or Artificial Opening Endoscopic approach. A resectoscope is passed through the penis into the urethra to the level of the prostate, and the obstructing prostatic tissue is trimmed or excised and removed.

Resection
The root operation Resection is reported when a total prostatectomy is performed. Using an Open approach to access the prostate, the physician makes an incision in the skin between the base of the scrotum and the anus. If the internal diameter of the urethra is not adequate, the opening of the urethra is enlarged (meatotomy) and the diameter of the penile urethra is enlarged with an instrument (internal urethrotomy). A curved instrument (Lowery Tractor) is advanced into the urethra to the prostate to aid in the dissection. Through the perineal incision and with manipulation of the tractor, the tissues are dissected to expose the prostate. The curved tractor instrument in the urethra is replaced with a straight tractor. The entire gland is removed. The bladder outlet is revised and bleeding controlled by ligation or cautery. Local lymph nodes may also be removed for analysis. A Foley catheter is placed and left in the bladder. A rubber drain may be placed in the site of the operative wound and brought out through a separate stab wound. The dissected tissues and the skin incision are closed in layers by suturing.

The physician resects the prostate using a resectoscope

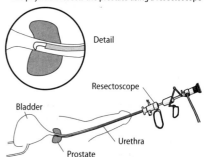

In a minimally invasive Percutaneous Endoscopic approach, several small incisions along with laparoscope are used to access the prostate. The Percutaneous Endoscopic approach employs the same principles of the Open approach. Robotic assistance is often employed and is coded additionally with a code from Other Procedures table (8E0). The minimally invasive surgery constitutes the majority of the total or radical prostatectomies.

Focus Point
In a radical prostatectomy, the surgery may involve removal of the prostate, epididymis, and vas ampullae. Code separately any organs or structures that are removed and for which there is a distinctly defined body part in ICD-10-PCS.

Coding Guidance
AHA: 2014, 4Q, 33

© 2018 Optum360, LLC

Medical and Surgical

Pyloromyotomy

Body System
Gastrointestinal System

PCS Root Operation
Division

Root Operation Table
ØD8   Gastrointestinal System, Division

Body Part
Stomach, Pylorus

Approach
Open
Percutaneous Endoscopic

Description
The pylorus is the lower part of the stomach that empties into the small intestine. Hypertrophy of the pylorus results in narrowing (stenosis) of the opening in the stomach to the small intestine, causing projectile vomiting. Pyloromyotomy is a surgical procedure used to treat pyloric stenosis in which an incision is made in the pylorus to loosen the muscle, allowing the stomach to empty and food to pass easily into the small intestine.

The physician incises the pyloric muscle. Using an Open approach, the physician makes a small subcostal incision over the pyloric olive. The peritoneum is incised, the tissues are retracted, and the pylorus is identified. The serosa is incised, and the tension of the pyloric muscle is released with longitudinal incisions. The peritoneum is sutured closed, and the operative site is sutured in layers.

In a Percutaneous Endoscopic approach, the pyloromyotomy is accomplished by making two small incisions and using a periumbilical port for visualization. The Percutaneous Endoscopic approach employs the same principles as the Open approach.

Focus Point
The intent of the procedure is to expand the opening of the stenotic pylorus by incising the circular muscle fibers around the opening, relaxing them, and restoring the pylorus to its normal function, which is best described by the root operation Division. Root operation Release would not be appropriate because the body part being freed was cut. Assignment of the most appropriate root operation depends on the intent of the procedure.

Rastelli Procedure (Right Ventricular-Pulmonary Artery Conduit)

See also Repair, Ventricular Septal Defect (VSD)

Body System
Heart and Great Vessels

PCS Root Operation
Bypass

Occlusion

Root Operation Table
Ø21   Heart and Great Vessels, Bypass

Ø2L   Heart and Great Vessels, Occlusion

Body Part
Right Ventricle (Bypass)

Pulmonary Valve (Occlusion)

Approach
Open

Device
Zooplastic Tissue (Bypass)

Synthetic Substitute (Bypass)

Nonautologous Tissue Substitute (Bypass)

No Device (Occlusion)

Qualifier
Pulmonary Trunk (Bypass)

No Qualifier (Occlusion)

Description
The Rastelli procedure is an extensive corrective operation, performed to repair congenital defects such as transposition of the great vessels with pulmonary stenosis or atresia and ventricular septal defects.

Occlusion
The patient is placed under general anesthesia and on cardiopulmonary bypass. Using an Open approach, a median sternotomy incision is made. The aorta is cross-clamped. An incision is made through the right ventricle to access the ventricular septal defect (VSD), and a patch or baffle is sutured into place, closing the VSD and redirecting the blood flow from the left ventricle to the aorta. *See also* Repair, Ventricular Septal Defect (VSD).

Bypass
Incisions are then made on the pulmonary artery and right ventricle. A right ventricular outflow tract (RVOT) valved conduit is created using graft material to supply blood flow to the lungs. One end of the conduit graft is sewn onto the incision on the main pulmonary artery, and the other end of the graft is sewn onto the incision on the right ventricle. The anomalous pulmonary valve is oversewn with sutures along with the stump of the pulmonary artery. A previously placed modified Blalock-Taussig shunt is no longer needed with the new conduit in place and is ligated and divided. The ligation and division of the redundant modified Blalock-Taussig shunt is not coded separately.

> **Focus Point**
> Conduit grafts may be Synthetic Substitutes such as Gore-Tex, Nonautologous Tissue Substitute cadaver graft, or Zooplastic tissue (bovine jugular vein or porcine valves).

> **Focus Point**
> Bypass procedures require clarification of the body part bypassed "from" and body part bypassed "to," according to guideline B3.6a.

> **Focus Point**
> Effective October 1, 2016, the body part value H, Pulmonary Valve, was added to table Ø2L, Occlusion, Heart and Great Vessels, to report the oversewing of the pulmonary valve. No code is reported for the the ligation and division of a modified Blalock-Taussig shunt.

> **Focus Point**
> Cardiopulmonary bypass is an exception to the usual practice of not reporting supporting procedures that are components of a larger operation. When a surgical procedure is performed with cardiopulmonary bypass, it is coded as an additional procedure using table 5A1.

Coding Guidance
AHA: 2016, 4Q, 104; 2015, 4Q, 22

© 2018 Optum360, LLC

Ravitch Procedure (Repair of Pectus Deformity)

See also Nuss Procedure

Body System
Upper Bones

PCS Root Operation
Reposition

Root Operation Table
ØPS   Upper Bones, Reposition

Body Part
Sternum

Approach
Open

Device
Internal Fixation Device, Rigid Plate
Internal Fixation Device
No Device

Description
The Ravitch procedure is performed on patients with congenital deformities of the chest wall such as pectus excavatum and pectus carinatum. This procedure is used for deformities that are quite complex and is more invasive than the Nuss procedure (*see also* Nuss Procedure), which is also performed to correct pectus excavatum.

Under general anesthesia, the patient is placed in a supine position. Preoperative placement of epidural catheter or paravertebral nerve blocks may be used to help control significant postoperative pain. Using an Open approach, the physician removes the ends of the ribs and costal cartilages that are attached to the sternum, while preserving the lining of cartilage. The sternum is detached and flattened into a more normal position. Using sutures or a temporary metal chest strut (bar) the physician secures the sternum in the desired position. The bar remains in place until the costal cartilage grows back in approximately six months. Drains are inserted on either side of the chest to remove fluid from the surgical site, as seromas are a common complication of this procedure.

> **Focus Point**
> As the intent of this procedure is to move the deformed sternum into a more normal anatomic position, this is reported with root operation Reposition.

Coding Guidance
AHA: 2015, 4Q, 33

Recession, Extraocular Muscle

Medical and Surgical

Body System
Eye

PCS Root Operation
Reposition

Root Operation Table
08S   Eye, Reposition

Body Part
Extraocular Muscle, Right
Extraocular Muscle, Left

Approach
Open

Description
Recession of the extraocular muscle(s) is performed to correct strabismus or misaligned eyes, which interferes with normal binocular vision. Common types of strabismus are esotropia, exotropia, hypotropia, and hypertropia. During a recession, the extraocular muscle is detached and moved posteriorly along the surface of the eye. This lengthens the muscle, resulting in better eye alignment.

Using an Open Approach, the physician makes incisions in the conjunctiva about 7 mm posterior to the juncture of the sclera and cornea (the limbus) in the superior nasal quadrant of the globe. An incision is made to expose the sclera, and a muscle hook is used to engage the extraocular muscle initially. The tendon of the superior oblique may be located about 12 mm behind the medial or nasal edge of the insertion of the superior rectus. The physician recesses the muscle by detaching it and moving it posteriorly. The muscle is secured with sutures. The operative wound is closed with layered sutures.

During strabismus surgery, the extraocular muscle is isolated far posterior to its insertion. The borders or edges of the muscle are sutured to the eye posterior to the original insertion point in what is commonly called the Faden procedure. The surgical wound is closed with sutures. This posterior fixation suturing technique on an extraocular muscle is done in conjunction with the strabismus surgery.

> **Focus Point**
> There is no body part value for bilateral extraocular muscle recession. If the procedure is performed bilaterally, two codes must be assigned using the appropriate body part values (Right, Left).

© 2018 Optum360, LLC

Reconstruction, Breast (Transverse Rectus Abdominis Myocutaneous (TRAM) Free Flap)

Body System
Skin and Breast

PCS Root Operation
Replacement

Root Operation Table
ØHR   Skin and Breast, Replacement

Body Part
Breast, Right
Breast, Left
Breast, Bilateral

Approach
Open

Device
Autologous Tissue Substitute

Qualifier
Transverse Rectus Abdominis Myocutaneous Flap

Description
The TRAM flap is the most frequent procedure performed for autologous breast reconstruction. In the free TRAM technique, the flap and the inferior vascular pedicle are dissected free and detached; the flap is then brought to the mastectomy site, and the deep inferior epigastric vessels are reconnected to vessels in the chest. The flap is completely detached from the blood and nervous supply and is transplanted to the mastectomy site. This is reported with the root operation Replacement.

Using an Open approach, the physician excises skin and fatty tissue from the abdominal wall. The flap to the mastectomy site is transplanted by completely detaching the blood supply and then reattaching it to recipient vessels using microvascular surgery. The

inferior epigastric artery and vein(s) are used to supply circulation to the flap. The physician adjusts the flap for the most aesthetically pleasing appearance and secures it with sutures to the chest wall, adjacent muscles, and skin. Temporary postoperative suction drains are also placed.

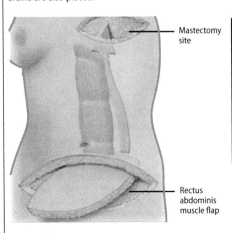

Mastectomy site

Rectus abdominis muscle flap

Focus Point
A Replacement procedure includes removal of the body part being replaced; therefore, the removal or excision of the body part is not reported. In the case of a mastectomy with immediate TRAM flap reconstruction, no code is assigned for the mastectomy, as the intent of the procedure is Replacement of the breast.

Focus Point
The transverse rectus abdominus muscle (TRAM) flap is coded for each flap developed.

Reconstruction, Breast (Transverse Rectus Abdominis Myocutaneous (TRAM) Pedicle Flap)

Body System
Muscles

PCS Root Operation
Transfer

Root Operation Table
ØKX   Muscles, Transfer

Body Part
Abdomen Muscle, Right
Abdomen Muscle, Left

Approach
Open

Qualifier
Transverse Rectus Abdominis Myocutaneous Flap
No Qualifier

Description
The TRAM flap is the most frequent procedure performed for autologous breast reconstruction. In a pedicled TRAM, the flap of muscle, fat, and skin is dissected free and rotated through a subcutaneous tunnel into the mastectomy defect, where it is shaped into the form of a breast and sutured in place. This type of flap is pedicled, remains connected to its vascular and nervous supply, and is reported with root operation Transfer.

The physician may cut a skin island flap on the lower abdominal wall. A superior skin and fat flap is elevated off the rectus abdominis muscle. A transverse incision is made in the rectus sheath, and the muscle is divided and elevated, keeping the superior epigastric arteries intact for blood supply. Once the muscle is elevated, the physician makes an incision through the chest skin. This is also elevated, creating a pocket for the muscle flap. A connecting tunnel is made between the elevated chest skin and the inferiorly positioned flap. The flap is passed superiorly under the tunnel of tissue, placed into its new position and sutured, after contouring a breast. The abdominal wall is closed by reapproximating the remaining anterior rectus muscle to the remaining lateral muscle and sheath. Skin edges are brought together and sutured in layers. Temporary postoperative suction drains are also placed.

Focus Point
If muscle only, rather than a composite flap that includes skin and muscle, is used for the flap, report with No Qualifier.

Focus Point
The transverse rectus abdominus muscle (TRAM) flap is coded for each flap developed.

Coding Guidance
AHA: 2014, 2Q, 10

© 2018 Optum360, LLC

Medical and Surgical

Reconstruction, Lateral Ulnar Collateral Ligament (LUCL)

Body System
Bursae and Ligaments

PCS Root Operation
Supplement

Root Operation Table
ØMU Bursae and Ligaments, Supplement

Body Part
Elbow Bursa and Ligament, Left
Elbow Bursa and Ligament, Right

Approach
Open

Device
Autologous Tissue Substitute
Synthetic Substitute
Nonautologous Tissue Substitute

Description
The lateral collateral ligament complex (LCLC) of the elbow is made up of the radial collateral ligament (RCL), lateral ulnar collateral ligament (LUCL), annular ligament, and accessory lateral collateral ligament.

The LUCL arises from the lateral humeral epicondyle and inserts on the supinator crest of the ulna, connecting the distal end of the humerus to the proximal end of the ulna, providing lateral stability to the elbow joint. Injury or repetitive stress to the LUCL

can lead to joint instability or elbow dislocation, resulting in the need for reconstruction.

The LUCL of the elbow is reconstructed with a graft. Under general anesthesia, the patient is placed in supine position and the arm is positioned on an arm board. After prepping and draping, the physician administers a local anesthetic block and using an Open approach, makes a skin incision and dissects to the damaged LUCL. The damaged ligament may be repaired with autologous palmaris longus tendon graft, or other autologous grafts, including triceps fascia, semitendinosus, gracilis, plantaris, and Achilles tendons. Cadaver nonautologous grafts or synthetic graft materials may also be used.

A guidewire is placed into the humerus center of rotation and drilled with a reamer perpendicular to the surface of the lateral epicondyle. A second guidewire is placed on the supinator crest of the ulna and then drilled with a reamer. Any bone fragments are removed with irrigation. The graft is placed into the hole in the ulna and secured. The graft is then secured through the hole in the lateral epicondyle. Any remaining tendon graft is cut off or sutured to the annular ligament. The incision is closed in layers.

Focus Point
If an Autologous Tissue Substitute is harvested from a different body part, report a code for the Excision of the graft tissue in addition to the Supplement procedure, according to guideline B3.9.

Reconstruction, Urethra, Male (Urethroplasty)

See also Repair, Hypospadias

See also Release, Chordee

Body System
Urinary System

PCS Root Operation
Supplement

Root Operation Table
ØTU   Urinary System, Supplement

Body Part
Urethra

Approach
Open

Device
Autologous Tissue Substitute
Synthetic Substitute
Nonautologous Tissue Substitute

Description
Urethral reconstruction may be performed to remove a stricture, repair trauma, or correct a prolapse. It may

also be performed in conjunction with repair of hypospadias, a congenital abnormality of the urethral opening. Hypospadias is corrected by penile chordee resection and by repositioning and/or supplementing the urethra so that it is in a normal position and of adequate caliber and length.

Using an Open approach, an incision is made over the area and carried through the skin, fat, and other tissues (fascia). A closed urethra is created by reapproximating the tissues and by using skin, tube, or free tissue grafts, or a combination of techniques depending on the extent of the defect. The physician cuts around the urethral defect, using the graft to make a urethra. The right size urethra must be constructed to allow a catheter and prevent obstructions. The physician pulls the loose skin around the urethra and closes the incisions.

Focus Point
Urethral reconstruction is often performed in conjunction with repair of hypospadias. According to ICD-10-PCS multiple procedures guideline B3.2c, multiple procedures with distinct objectives may be reported separately.

© 2018 Optum360, LLC

Medical and Surgical

Reduction, Fracture, Closed with Percutaneous Pinning

Body System
Head and Facial Bones
Upper Bones
Lower Bones
Upper Joints
Lower Joints

PCS Root Operation
Reposition

Root Operation Table
ØNS   Head and Facial Bones, Reposition
ØPS   Upper Bones, Reposition
ØQS   Lower Bones, Reposition
ØRS   Upper Joints, Reposition
ØSS   Lower Joints, Reposition

Body Part
Refer to the ICD-10-PCS tabular list for a complete list of body parts.

Approach
Percutaneous

Device
Internal Fixation Device

Description
Reduction is the restoring of displaced bone segments or joints to their normal position. Closed reduction

means that the fracture site or dislocated joint is not surgically opened (exposed to the external environment and directly visualized).

After appropriate anesthesia, sedative, or nerve block, the provider performs external manipulation to realign the fracture or dislocation. This manipulation can be performed with or without traction. The reduction is verified by clinical tests or radiology.

To stabilize the fracture, metal pins (e.g., Steinmann pin, Kirschner wires) are immediately inserted through the skin into bone fragments across the fracture line. These pins are usually left in place until the fracture has healed.

Focus Point
The manipulation is done externally while the placement of the pin is directly through the skin; Percutaneous approach is used for the coding of these procedures.

Focus Point
An intramedullary pin, also referred to as IM nail or IM rod, consists of a longer pin, nail, or rod percutaneously inserted down into the medullary cavity of the bone and held in place by interlocking screws. The device value Internal Fixation Device, Intramedullary, denotes this specific fracture reduction (Reposition) with internal fixation technique.

Reduction, Fracture, Open, with Internal Fixation (ORIF)

Medical and Surgical

Body System
Head and Facial Bones
Upper Bones
Lower Bones

PCS Root Operation
Reposition

Root Operation Table
ØNS   Head and Facial Bones, Reposition
ØPS   Upper Bones, Reposition
ØQS   Lower Bones, Reposition

Body Part
Refer to the ICD-10-PCS tabular list for a complete list of body parts.

Approach
Open

Device
Internal Fixation Device
Internal Fixation Device, Rigid Plate (Reposition, Upper Bones, Sternum)
Internal Fixation Device, Intramedullary (Reposition, Upper Bones and Lower Bones)

Description
An open reduction internal fixation (ORIF) procedure is performed to Reposition severe bone fractures, with the technique differing based on the location and type of fracture.

Under general anesthesia, an Open incision is made at the site of the fracture. The physician first identifies and realigns the fractured bone to its normal position. The appropriate internal fixation devices, including steel rods, screws, or plates, are inserted into the bone to hold the fracture together and stabilize the fracture site. The fixation devices can be permanent or temporary, to be removed after healing takes place. An x-ray confirms successful reduction and fixation of the fracture. Once the fracture is stabilized, the wound is irrigated. The soft tissues are repositioned and sutured in place. The skin is sutured, and the wound is covered with a soft dressing. A cast or splint is usually applied.

Focus Point
Open reduction performed with percutaneous endoscopic-assisted techniques to help in visualization is reported as an Open approach. See guideline B5.2.

Focus Point
Application of a cast or splint in conjunction with the Reposition procedure is not coded separately. See guideline B3.15.

Focus Point
Irrigation and/or debridement to clean the wound in conjunction with the Reposition procedure are not coded separately.

Coding Guidance
AHA: 2016, 3Q, 34; 2014, 4Q, 32

© 2018 Optum360, LLC

Reduction, Joint Dislocation

Body System
Upper Joints
Lower Joints

PCS Root Operation
Reposition

Root Operation Table
ØRS   Upper Joints, Reposition
ØSS   Lower Joints, Reposition

Body Part
Refer to the ICD-10-PCS tabular list for a complete list of body parts.

Approach
Open
External

Description
Reduction is the restoring of displaced joint segments to their normal position using manipulation or traction. Closed reduction means that the dislocation site is not surgically opened (exposed to the external environment and directly visualized). Open treatment is used when the dislocation site is surgically opened (exposed to the external environment). Open reduction may be used following an unsuccessful attempt at a closed reduction.

Closed Reduction of Dislocation
The physician performs a manipulative reduction of a displaced joint without an incision, with or without external traction. Using an External approach, the physician treats a closed joint dislocation using manipulation; anesthesia may be used if necessary. The physician determines the dislocated position of the joint and uses external manipulation to relocate the joint. The reduction is verified by clinical tests or radiology. In order to rest the joint, slings or braces are often placed.

Open Reduction of Dislocation
The physician performs reduction of a displaced joint via an Open approach. Using appropriate anesthesia, an Open incision is made at the site of the dislocation. The physician first identifies and realigns the dislocated joint to its normal position. An x-ray is performed to confirm successful reduction of the dislocation. The skin is sutured, and the wound is covered with a soft dressing. A cast or splint is usually applied.

Focus Point
Application of a sling, brace, cast, or splint in conjunction with the Reposition procedure is not coded separately. See guideline B3.15.

Focus Point
Careful review of the operative report is needed to verify that the manipulation is taking place on a joint versus a fractured bone.

Coding Guidance
AHA: 2014, 4Q, 32

Reimplantation, Parathyroid (Autotransplantation)

See also Parathyroidectomy

Body System
Endocrine System

PCS Root Operation
Reposition

Root Operation Table
ØGS   Endocrine System, Reposition

Body Part
Superior Parathyroid Gland, Right
Superior Parathyroid Gland, Left
Inferior Parathyroid Gland, Right
Inferior Parathyroid Gland, Left
Parathyroid Glands, Multiple
Parathyroid Gland

Approach
Open

Device
No Device

Qualifier
No Qualifier

Description
The parathyroid glands consist of four, small, pea-shaped glands, two superior and two inferior, located in the neck on either side of the trachea next to the thyroid gland. These glands control the calcium level in the blood by secreting parathyroid hormone (PTH) that increases the calcium level when it is too low.

Following radical surgery on the thyroid gland, the development of hypocalcemia, osteomalacia with severe bone pain, and multiple fractures is noted in many patients. Parathyroid autotransplantation, or placement of a parathyroid tissue graft into another functional site, is often indicated to treat these conditions in patients who have undergone operations on the head and neck organs in which the parathyroid glands have been damaged or have questionable viability.

A separately reportable parathyroidectomy is performed, during which all four parathyroid glands are completely resected.

Using an Open approach, a small pocket is made in the muscle in the neck, forearm, or upper arm. The previously resected parathyroid tissue is cut into one or more small 1–2 mm pieces, which are inserted into the muscle pocket. The incision is closed in layers. The autotransplanted parathyroid gland will develop a new blood supply and start functioning within four to six weeks after implantation.

Focus Point
A parathyroid autotransplantation procedure involves moving a portion of a parathyroid gland to another functional location. This meets the ICD-10-PCS definition of Reposition, which is "moving to its normal location, or other suitable location, all or a portion of a body part."

Focus Point
Code separately the parathyroidectomy. See also Parathyroidectomy.

© 2018 Optum360, LLC

Release, Achilles' Tendon (Achillotenotomy) (Achillotomy)

Body System
Tendons

PCS Root Operation
Division

Root Operation Table
ØL8 Tendons, Division

Body Part
Lower Leg Tendon, Right
Lower Leg Tendon, Left

Approach
Open
Percutaneous

Description
Achilles tendon release is performed for contractures or developmental deformity of the tendon leading to muscle shortening. Tenotomy is performed to lengthen the Achilles tendon, which allows the muscle to return to its normal length and allows the ankle joint to straighten.

Using either a Percutaneous approach directly through the skin, or an Open approach directly visualizing the Achilles tendon, the physician performs a tenotomy of the Achilles tendon. The physician infiltrates the skin and Achilles tendon with a local anesthetic about 1 cm above the insertion into the calcaneus. A knife blade or tenotome held vertically is inserted through the skin and subcutaneous tissue into the Achilles tendon. The blade is turned medially and laterally and swept back forth, creating a nick in the tendon, until the foot can be dorsiflexed at the ankle. Pressure is applied over the incision for about five minutes. A dressing and long leg cast are applied with the ankle in 10 degree dorsiflexion and the knee in maximal extension.

Focus Point
Although the documentation may state that a "release" operation was performed, the coder must consult the operative report to confirm surgical technique. A Division is defined as cutting into a body part in order to separate or transect it, whereas a Release is the freeing of a body part by cutting into the tissues and attachments surrounding the body part. The body part itself is not cut. In this case, the Achilles tendon was transected.

Focus Point
There is no specific body part value for Achilles tendon. The ICD-10-PCS Body Part Definitions and Body Part Key direct the coder to use Lower Leg Tendon, Right, or Lower Leg Tendon, Left, as the body part value.

Release, Carpal Tunnel

Body System
Peripheral Nervous System

PCS Root Operation
Release

Root Operation Table
01N   Peripheral Nervous System, Release

Body Part
Median Nerve

Approach
Open
Percutaneous
Percutaneous Endoscopic

Description
The carpal tunnel is a tight canal, or "tunnel," at the base of the palm through which tendons and nerves must pass on their way from the forearm to the hand and fingers. The median nerve passes through this narrow tunnel to reach the hand. Swelling and inflammation of the tendons or bursa surrounding the median nerve can cause the nerve to be compressed, causing pain, numbness, and tingling. The most common cause of carpal tunnel syndrome is repetitive strain injuries (RSI). This is caused by long periods of steady hand movement. Nonsurgical methods such as a brace, nonsteroidal anti-inflammatories, or corticosteroids, may be used initially to treat the condition, but severe or persistent symptoms may require surgical treatment.

Using an Open approach, the physician decompresses or transposes a portion of the ulnar or median nerve to restore feeling to the hand. The physician makes a horizontal incision in the wrist at the metacarpal joints and locates the affected nerve. Soft tissues are resected, and the nerve is freed from the underlying bed. Care is taken to ensure tension is released, and the incision is closed in sutured layers.

In a Percutaneous Endoscopic approach, the patient is placed supine with the arm positioned on a hand table. Endoscopic release may be accomplished by a one- or two-portal technique. In a single-portal technique, a small, 1 1/2 cm, horizontal incision is made at the wrist. Using a two-portal technique, two small incisions are made: one in the palm and one at the wrist. The palmar

skin, underlying cushioning fat, protective fascia, and muscle are not cut. The endoscope is introduced underneath the transverse carpal ligament. The endoscope allows the physician to view the procedure on a monitor. A special blade attached to the arthroscope is then used to incise the transverse carpal ligament from the inside of the carpal tunnel. The instruments are removed and the portal(s) closed with sutures or Steri-Strips. A splint may be applied.

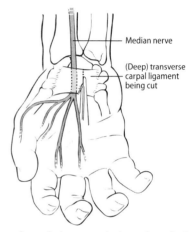

Median nerve

(Deep) transverse carpal ligament being cut

A carpal tunnel release may also be performed using a Percutaneous approach. The patient is given a local anesthetic, and the physician uses a minimally invasive cutting device along with ultrasound guidance to incise the carpal ligament, releasing the median nerve.

Focus Point
In the root operation Release, the body part value coded is the body part being freed and not the tissue being manipulated or cut to free the body part.

Focus Point
In ICD-10 PCS, coders must remember to identify the root operation that describes the main objective of the procedure. When the objective is to free the body part, Release is the root operation. Division is coded when the objective of the procedure is to transect or separate a body part.

© 2018 Optum360, LLC

Release, Chordee

See also Repair, Hypospadias

Body System
Male Reproductive System

PCS Root Operation
Release

Root Operation Table
ØVN   Male Reproductive System, Release

Body Part
Penis

Approach
Open

Description
Chordee is a condition in which the penis curves downward. In most cases, chordee is associated with hypospadias, a congenital abnormality of the urethral opening.

The physician corrects downward displacement of the penis. To help plan the surgery, an artificial erection may be produced by placing a band around the base of the penis and injecting saline into the body of the penis. The area of deformity is determined, and by using an Open approach, with a combination of incisions and excisions of abnormal fibrous tissue and occasionally normal tissue, the defect is corrected. Care is taken to dissect around nerves and blood vessels. Sometimes the urethra is dissected free of its position and retracted temporarily away from the operative site. The separate tissues of the penis are closed in layers with absorbable suture material. An artificial erection may again be produced to test and demonstrate the adequacy of the repair.

Focus Point
Release of chordee is often performed in conjunction with repair of hypospadias. According to ICD-10-PCS multiple procedures guideline B3.2c, multiple procedures with distinct objectives may be reported separately.

Focus Point
Root operation Release is defined as "Freeing a body part from an abnormal physical constraint by cutting or by the use of force."

Release, Coracoacromial Ligament

See also Decompression, Subacromial, Rotator Cuff Tendon

See also Repair, Rotator Cuff (Shoulder)

Body System
Bursae and Ligaments

PCS Root Operation
Release

Root Operation Table
ØMN Bursae and Ligaments, Release

Body Part
Shoulder Bursa and Ligament, Right
Shoulder Bursa and Ligament, Left

Approach
Open
Percutaneous Endoscopic

Description

The coracoacromial ligament (CAL) is a wide, strong band extending between the acromion and the coracoid process of the scapula. Coracoacromial ligament release is performed to correct shoulder impingement syndrome caused by hypertrophy (thickening) or calcification of the coracoacromial ligament. It may also be performed in conjunction with other procedures for shoulder impingement syndrome as well as rotator cuff tears, bursitis, and tendinitis.

The patient is positioned on his or her side with the affected side up. Using an Open approach, the physician makes an incision centered over the acromioclavicular joint. The soft tissues are reflected,

and the ligament between the coracoid and the acromion is released. Following completion, the joint is irrigated and the incisions are closed with sutures or Steri-Strips.

Using a Percutaneous Endoscopic approach, the physician makes two to four small portal incisions, and the anterior, lateral, and posterior arthroscopic portals are established. The posterior portal is used to view the subacromial space, the lateral portal is used for instrumentation, and anterior portal is used for outflow or inflow. The arthroscope is inserted into the posterior portal into the subacromial space for visualization of the subacromial joint. A limited bursectomy may be performed and, if necessary, the physician clears the undersurface of the anterolateral acromion of soft tissue using intra-articular cautery. The coracoacromial ligament is released. A long-acting local anesthetic may be injected into the joint to help with postoperative pain. The joint is irrigated and the incisions are closed with sutures or Steri-Strips. The area is covered with a dressing, and the arm is positioned in a sling or shoulder immobilizer, and movement is restricted to allow for proper healing.

Focus Point
Coracoacromial release may be performed in conjunction with other procedures to correct impingement syndrome, such as subacromial decompression using acromioplasty or acromionectomy where the underside of the acromion is reduced to allow more room for the rotator cuff tendons. ICD-10-PCS guidelines on multiple procedures should be followed when assigning codes for these procedures.

© 2018 Optum360, LLC

Removal, Esophageal Foreign Body

Body System
Gastrointestinal System

PCS Root Operation
Extirpation

Root Operation Table
ØDC   Gastrointestinal System, Extirpation

Body Part
Esophagus, Upper
Esophagus, Middle
Esophagus, Lower
Esophagogastric Junction
Esophagus

Approach
Via Natural or Artificial Opening
Via Natural or Artificial Opening Endoscopic

Description
If food or another foreign body becomes lodged in the esophagus, the immediate result is that food and fluid may encounter a disrupted pathway to the stomach. Secondary infections can occur, with or without perforation of the esophageal wall.

Foreign bodies in the gastrointestinal tract usually occur by intentional or accidental swallowing. Children and psychiatric patients may purposefully swallow nonfood items that become lodged in the esophagus. Occasionally bones are inadvertently swallowed and may become lodged. Older patients with gastric esophageal reflux disease may be at risk for a narrowing esophagus due to scarring from long-time exposure of the esophagus to acidic fluids. Food that isn't thoroughly chewed may become lodged in the stenotic esophagus, and this, too, is classified as a foreign body. An edentulous patient would be at risk due to unchewed food.

In some cases, the approach may be through the mouth, into the esophagus, with the approach Via Natural or Artificial Opening. If the foreign body is radiopaque and can be seen on x-ray, it may be possible for the physician to grasp it by inserting the tip of Magill forceps in the patient's mouth and directing the forceps to the site of the foreign body. The foreign body is grasped and removed.

More commonly, the foreign body is removed using an endoscopic approach, Via Natural or Artificial Opening Endoscopic. The scope may be rigid or flexible. In either case, the physician advances the scope through the patient's mouth and into the esophagus and locates the foreign body. It may be suctioned or grasped with forceps and retracted through the scope. An alternative technique is to pass a balloon beyond the foreign body, inflate the balloon, and withdraw it, capturing the foreign body.

> **Focus Point**
> If the foreign body is not successfully removed, the operation Inspection is reported instead of Extirpation.

> **Focus Point**
> Foreign bodies in the oropharynx are reported with codes from the Mouth and Throat body system.

Coding Guidance
AHA: 2015, 1Q, 23

© 2018 Optum360, LLC

Removal, Ingrown Toenail

Medical and Surgical

Body System
Skin and Breast

PCS Root Operation
Excision

Extraction

Resection

Root Operation Table
ØHB   Skin and Breast, Excision

ØHD   Skin and Breast, Extraction

ØHT   Skin and Breast, Resection

Body Part
Toe Nail

Approach
External

Description
An ingrown toenail (onychocryptosis) occurs when the skin along the side of the toenail grows over the nail edge to cover it. This may cause inflammation, infection, and pain at the distal corner of the nailbed. If the ingrown nail fails to respond to nonsurgical treatment, if the ingrowth recurs, or if the patient has underlying comorbidities that make an ingrown nail unacceptable (i.e., diabetes), surgery may be required.

The goal of surgery for chronic ingrown toenail is to prevent recurrence. Therefore, matrix tissue under the skin at the proximal base of the toenail is destroyed, and the exposed toenail distal to the matrix is removed. Any site in which the matrix is removed can no longer generate nail tissue distal to it.

The physician removes all or part of a toenail. The nail plate (toenail) is bluntly dissected and lifted away from the nailbed. The nail plate is detached from the matrix using a scalpel. The matrix is destroyed using chemical ablation, CO_2 laser, or electrocautery. The wound is dressed loosely.

Excision
When only a portion of the toenail is excised and a portion of the matrix is destroyed, report the operation Excision.

Resection
When the entire toenail is excised and the entire matrix is destroyed, report the operation Resection.

Extraction
In cases of advanced disease, the toenail may be surgically pulled away from the nailbed without cutting. In this case, the nail is removed and matrix is destroyed using chemical ablation, CO_2 laser, or electrocautery. The wound is dressed loosely. The root operation Extraction is reported.

Focus Point

In some patients, acute ingrown toenail is treated with what is called a wedge resection. This "resection" is reported with the operation Excision. The physician excises a wedge of restrictive skin from the nail fold to free an ingrown nail but does not excise the nail itself. Wedge resection of the skin around the ingrown nail would be reported with the root operation table ØHB, with the body parts Skin, Right Foot or Skin, Left Foot.

© 2018 Optum360, LLC

Removal, Internal Fixation Device, Bone

Body System
Head and Facial Bones

Upper Bones

Lower Bones

PCS Root Operation
Removal

Root Operation Table
ØNP Head and Facial Bones, Removal

ØPP Upper Bones, Removal

ØQP Lower Bones, Removal

Body Part
Refer to the ICD-10-PCS tabular list for a complete list of body parts.

Approach
External

Open

Percutaneous

Percutaneous Endoscopic

Device
Internal Fixation Device

Description
In some cases, a splint or cast is insufficient to stabilize a bone fracture. A stainless steel or titanium internal fixation device may be inserted to hold pieces of bone in place while they knit. The bone fragments are returned to their normal position, and the internal fixation device secures the bones in place. In some cases, internal fixation devices may be removed once healing has occurred or due to pain or irritation from the hardware. The site of the device placement and the type of device determine the approach for removal.

Various types of procedures are performed to remove implanted devices from bone. The physician makes an incision overlying the site of the implant. Deep dissection is carried down to visualize the implant, which is usually below the muscle level and within bone. The physician uses instruments to remove the implant from the bone. The incision is repaired in multiple layers using sutures, staples, and/or Steri-Strips. In some cases, the physician removes the external fixation frame and pulls pins out manually while the patient is under anesthesia. In other cases, the physician uses instruments to remove the implant from the bone.

An Open approach is used if removal includes removal of multiple screws or pins, or if the device is implanted in deep tissue; for example, within the pelvic girdle or anywhere below the muscle layer. In some cases, an Open approach is used for superficial pins or screws, to allow for direct visualization of the implant.

For single pins or wires, a Percutaneous approach, with or without radiological guidance, may be possible; for example, removal of a pin from the thumb. In this case, a small stab incision allows the physician to grasp the wire or pin and pull it out without direct visualization.

Occasionally, a Percutaneous Endoscopic approach is employed; for example, for a stabilization device placed in a lumbar vertebra. The device is retrieved through the endoscope placed percutaneously.

Coding Guidance
AHA: 2015, 3Q, 12; 2014, 4Q, 28; 2013, 2Q, 39

© 2018 Optum360, LLC

Removal, Intracranial Responsive Neurostimulator (RNS) Generator

See also Removal, Intracranial Responsive Neurostimulator (RNS) or Deep Brain Stimulator (DBS) Lead

Body System
Head and Facial Bones

PCS Root Operation
Removal

Root Operation Table
ØNP   Head and Facial Bones, Removal

Body Part
Skull

Approach
Open

Device
Neurostimulator Generator

Qualifier
No Qualifier

Description
The responsive neurostimulator system (RNS) is specifically designed to treat adults with medically refractory localization-related (focal) (partial) epilepsy. The device continuously monitors brain electrical activity, detecting the abnormal electrical activity preceding seizure, and responds by delivering brief and mild electrical stimulation to normalize brain activity. Battery life of a cranially implanted neurostimulator is approximately three years, at which time the battery may be surgically replaced. When battery replacement is necessary, removal of a cranially implanted neurostimulator requires surgical replacement.

A physician removes an intracranial neurostimulator generator by using an Open approach to cut open a flap of skull to locate the generator. The generator is removed, the dura is closed, and the scalp is reapproximated and closed in sutured layers.

Focus Point

According to multiple procedures guideline B3.2c, a code using the root operation Removal is reported as well as a code for Insertion of a new device if applicable.

Focus Point

Removal of an intracranial responsive neurostimulator (RNS) generator is not the same as Removal of a deep brain stimulator (DBS) generator. The deep brain stimulator generator is removed from a subcutaneous pocket that is created in the chest wall.

Medical and Surgical

© 2018 Optum360, LLC

Removal, Intracranial Responsive Neurostimulator (RNS) or Deep Brain Stimulator (DBS) Lead

See also Removal, Intracranial Responsive Neurostimulator (RNS) Generator

See also Insertion, Deep Brain Stimulator (DBS)

Body System
Central Nervous System and Cranial Nerves

PCS Root Operation
Removal

Root Operation Table
ØØP   Central Nervous System and Cranial Nerves, Removal

Body Part
Brain

Approach
Open

Device
Neurostimulator Lead

Qualifier
No Qualifier

Description
Intracranial neurostimulator devices are implanted into the brain for deep brain stimulation (DBS) to control tremors in patients diagnosed with essential tremor, epilepsy, or Parkinson's disease or responsive neurostimulator system (RNS) for the treatment of epileptic seizures The devices consist of a generator unit implanted either in the skull for RNS or in a subcutaneous pocket for DBS and flexible thin wires that are connected to the generator on one end and to electrodes (leads) on the other end that are implanted either on the surface of or deep within the brain.

The leads are typically considered permanent with the exception of a complication. If removal is necessary, different approach techniques such as twist drill, burr holes, craniotomy, or craniectomy may be used to remove the electrodes, depending on the location of the targeted area. The root operation reported for the removal of the lead/electrode is Removal. An additional code is required if reinsertion of the lead is performed.

To remove intracranial neurostimulator leads, using an Open approach the physician incises and retracts the scalp and drills a burr hole in the cranium to locate the electrode. The electrode is removed, the dura is closed, and the scalp is reapproximated and closed in sutured layers.

Medical and Surgical

Repair, Aneurysm, Abdominal Aorta, Endovascular with Stent Graft (EVAR)

Body System
Lower Arteries

PCS Root Operation
Restriction

Root Operation Table
Ø4V   Lower Arteries, Restriction

Body Part
Abdominal Aorta

Approach
Percutaneous

Device
Intraluminal Device

Intraluminal Device, Branched or Fenestrated, One or Two Arteries

Intraluminal Device, Branched or Fenestrated, Three or More Arteries

Qualifier
Bifurcation

No Qualifier

Description
Endovascular stent grafting or endovascular aneurysm repair (EVAR) is less invasive than the traditional open approach under general anesthesia. Endovascular procedures may be performed using local or regional anesthesia, decreasing the risks associated with general anesthesia. The term "endovascular" describes a procedure that is contained within the blood vessel, usually by access through a catheter placed in an access vessel such as the femoral artery. Radiological imaging assists in guiding the catheter to the aneurysm to insert the stent graft inside the vessel. Endovascular procedures have been successful in treating aneurysms with less surgical trauma to the patient, while expediting healing time.

A catheter-guided stent graft, reported with ICD-10-PCS device value Intraluminal Device, is deployed via Percutaneous approach into the abdominal aorta to prevent continued blood flow into the weakened, aneurysmal portion of the vessel while maintaining blood flow through the vessel. Since only the aneurysm is occluded, not the artery itself, the ICD-10-PCS root operation is Restriction, which is defined as partially closing an orifice or lumen of a tubular body part.

Two small incisions are made into the femoral arteries by cut-down. With radiological guidance and imaging, the delivery sheath that contains the folded and

compressed graft components is guided through the femoral artery to the aorta. Once properly positioned at the site of aneurysm, the endograft is deployed and expands to fit the arterial wall excluding the aneurysm sac. The stent is secured into position, and the catheter is removed.

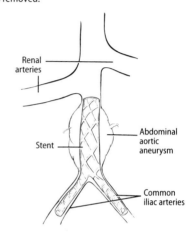

Fenestrated and branched endograft repair is a new technology for repairing abdominal aortic aneurysms in patients who are not candidates for standard endovascular repair. These include the elderly, those with high-risk comorbid conditions, and those with complicated aneurysms that involve either large aneurysms, those of overlapping chest and abdominal sites, or those affecting the complex anatomy (e.g., juxtarenal, perivisceral, hypogastric, aortic arch). The term "fenestration" refers to the specialized reinforced openings that allow the physician to custom fit and position the stent into vessel branches or bifurcations at complex anatomic sites (e.g., renal or mesenteric artery bifurcations) and to align openings with the branch vessels of the aorta. The stents are composed of small, flexible metal tubes that are modular and adjustable. The components of the stent graft are custom made to each patient's specific anatomy and presentation. Computed tomographic angiography (CTA) is used to map the targeted area for repair and tailor construct the device. Once the customized endograft components are assembled, they are delivered to the site of the aneurysm via a catheter inserted into the femoral artery and threaded into the aorta. The fenestrated stent is delivered over a guidewire to the anatomic site of repair, where it is positioned and deployed. Patency is then tested and the catheter removed.

© 2018 Optum360, LLC

Repair, Aneurysm, Abdominal Aorta, Endovascular with Stent Graft (EVAR) (continued)

Medical and Surgical

Focus Point

The device values in table 02V provide options to report specialized fenestrated or branched stents. Report Intraluminal Devices, Branched or Fenestrated, One or Two Arteries or Intraluminal Devices, Branched or Fenestrated, Three or More Arteries depending on the number of arteries involved. Use the qualifier value Bifurcation if the stent spans the bifurcation of two or more vessels.

Coding Guidance
AHA: 2016, 4Q, 89; 2016, 3Q, 39

Repair, Aneurysm, Cerebral, Craniotomy with Clipping

Body System
Upper Arteries

PCS Root Operation
Occlusion

Restriction

Root Operation Table
03L   Upper Arteries, Occlusion
03V   Upper Arteries, Restriction

Body Part
Intracranial Artery

Approach
Open

Device
Extraluminal Device

Description
Clipping the vessels of a brain aneurysm is performed via a craniotomy, which is considered an Open procedure. This surgical technique is used to treat brain aneurysms or arterial wall weaknesses that result in dilation and ballooning of a cerebral blood vessel. Left untreated, an aneurysm may lead to stroke or death.

An access incision is made through the scalp and overlying muscle to reach the skull. Burr holes are drilled around the periphery of the bone flap area to be raised. Using a craniotome, the bone flap is freed and lifted to expose the dura, which is dissected and retracted out of the operative field. An incision is made over the affected vessel, and the aneurysm is isolated.

The affected vessel is dissected from adjacent critical structures. The aneurysm is then obliterated with a tiny metal clip, which is reported as an Extraluminal Device. The clip prevents blood from entering the aneurysm, and future bleeding is prevented, protecting the surrounding tissues and organs. The appropriate ICD-10-PCS root operation is determined by whether the blood flow is totally obstructed (Occlusion) or if the blood is allowed to continue to flow freely with only the bulging of the vessel obstructed (Restriction).

Closure is done by suturing the dura meticulously and replacing the bone flap into position. Screws or plates are placed to secure the bone flap to surrounding skull bone. The divided muscles are sutured and the galea and the scalp are closed. The craniotomy and closure are an inherent part of the procedure and are not reported separately according to guideline B3.1b.

Focus Point

If the aneurysmal section of the intracranial vessel is excised instead of clipped, the correct root operation is Excision with the device value of No Device.

Focus Point

If there is swelling and the bone flap is placed in the subcutaneous tissue of the abdomen for storage to be replaced at a later date, it is reported separately with the root operation of Reposition, which is defined as moving to its normal or other suitable location, all or a portion of a body part.

Coding Guidance
AHA: 2016, 2Q, 30

Repair, Aneurysm, Cerebral, Endovascular

Body System
Upper Arteries

PCS Root Operation
Occlusion

Restriction

Root Operation Table
Ø3L   Upper Arteries, Occlusion

Ø3V   Upper Arteries, Restriction

Body Part
Intracranial Artery

Approach
Percutaneous

Device
Intraluminal Device

Intraluminal Device, Bioactive

Description
Endovascular coil embolization is a minimally invasive procedure used to treat brain aneurysms or arterial wall weaknesses that result in dilation and ballooning of a cerebral blood vessel. Left untreated, an aneurysm may lead to stroke or death.

The appropriate ICD-10-PCS root operation is determined by whether the blood flow is totally obstructed (Occlusion) or more commonly, if the blood is allowed to continue to flow freely with only the bulging of the vessel obstructed (Restriction). Using a Percutaneous approach, a catheter is inserted into the femoral artery and guided to the site of the aneurysm in the brain with fluoroscopic assistance. Endovascular restriction or occlusion of the cerebral or neck vessels does not differentiate between the use of bare platinum coils (BPC), microspheres (beads), and liquid tissue adhesive (glue); they are all considered intraluminal devices. Filling the aneurysm with coils, microspheres, or adhesive initiates a healing response and prevents rupture of the aneurysm. There is a more specific device value for Intraluminal Device, Bioactive, which refers to coils that are coated with an active biological agent such as polyglycolic (PGA) or polyglycolic/polylactic acid (PGLA). These coated coils have shown improved clinical outcomes for treating cerebral aneurysms with enhanced occlusion and thrombus formation due to the amplified inflammatory response as well as increasing packing density.

Focus Point
The Intracranial Artery body part encompasses all of the cerebral arteries in the Occlusion and Restriction root operation tables. Separate body part values are available for the intracranial portion of the carotid and vertebral arteries.

Coding Guidance
AHA: 2016, 1Q, 19

© 2018 Optum360, LLC

Repair, Atrial Septal Defect (ASD) (Atrioseptoplasty) (Repair of Foramen Ovale (Patent))

Body System
Heart and Great Vessels

PCS Root Operation
Repair

Supplement

Root Operation Table
Ø2Q   Heart and Great Vessels, Repair

Ø2U   Heart and Great Vessels, Supplement

Body Part
Atrial Septum

Approach
Open

Percutaneous

Percutaneous Endoscopic

Device
No Device (Repair)

Autologous Tissue Substitute (Supplement)

Zooplastic Tissue (Supplement)

Synthetic Substitute (Supplement)

Nonautologous Tissue Substitute (Supplement)

Description
An atrial septal defect (ASD) is a hole in the septum that divides the left and right atria. It is a common congenital defect that often does not present until adulthood. This can be repaired by many techniques. Although the intention of the procedure is to close or occlude the defect, the root operation Occlusion in the ICD-10-PCS tables does not currently offer a body part for atrial septum. The root operations depend on the type of technique used.

Open Approach
In an Open procedure, the physician performs a sternotomy and splits the sternum. Cardiopulmonary bypass is established. Two venous tubes are placed for the bypass machine: one draining the superior caval vein and one draining the inferior caval vein. The right atrium is isolated by placing tourniquets around the superior and inferior vena cava and their corresponding tubes. The right atrium is opened, and the size and location of the arterial septal defect is assessed. The defect can often be closed with sutures, which is coded as the root operation Repair with No Device. To avoid atrium distortion, larger defects are best closed using a patch sewn to the edge of the defect for closure, which is reported with the root operation Supplement. The type of patch can vary from an Autologous Tissue such as harvested pericardium tissue or a Synthetic Substitute such as Dacron poly polymer or polytetrafluoroethylene (PTFE). If autologous pericardium tissue is used, add

code Ø2BNØZZ for the harvesting of the pericardial tissue.

Percutaneous Approach
Recently, transcatheter technique reported as Percutaneous approach has become more widely performed. This transcatheter procedure describes closure of an atrial septal defect by percutaneous technique and is reported with the root operation Supplement. This may be performed on infants or adults, usually under conscious sedation. After heparinization is induced, a combined right and left heart catheterization is first undertaken through the existing septal opening. Contrast material is injected for atrial and ventricular angiograms to map the anatomy. Using a specialized catheter, the atrial defect is crossed from the right atrium into the left. The catheter is threaded into the upper left pulmonary vein. A guidewire is inserted, the catheter is removed, and a balloon is threaded over the guidewire into position across the defect and inflated with low pressure. The stretched diameter of the defect is measured. Testing is carried out to ensure that the repair will remain hemodynamically stable by occluding the defect temporarily with the balloon while taking right-side pressures and saturation measurements. A dilator and sheath holding the device are advanced over the guidewire and positioned in the left atrium. Positioning is checked using echocardiography or fluoroscopy before releasing the device. The implant is deployed across the atrial opening, and positioning is checked again. Any leaks, abnormal placement, or an improperly sized device may require removal of the implant and placement of a second device. The catheters and guidewires are removed. The device implant is reported with device value Synthetic Substitute; some of the current devices on the market include Amplatzer septal occluder (ASO) which is the most widely used, followed by CardioSEAL, HELEX septal occluder, or Sideris patch.

Percutaneous Endoscopic
Using a Percutaneous Endoscopic approach, the femoral veins are accessed and several ports (incisions) are created in the chest into which cannulas for instrumentation and endoscopic trocars for visualization can be inserted. Cardiopulmonary bypass is established. The myocardium is incised, and the endoscopic tool is advanced to the right atrium site of the defect. Depending on its size, the defect is repaired with sutures, which is reported with the root operation Repair, or a Dacron poly patch, pericardium, other tissue graft, or plug implant, which are all reported with the root operation Supplement. The defect is closed, the endoscope is removed, and access incisions are sutured in layers. If autologous pericardium tissue

Repair, Atrial Septal Defect (ASD) (Atrioseptoplasty) (Repair of Foramen Ovale (Patent)) (continued)

is used, add code Ø2BN4ZZ for the harvesting of the pericardial tissue.

Percutaneous Endoscopic repairs may be performed with or without the use of robotic assistance.

Focus Point

Cardiopulmonary bypass is used in both the Open and Percutaneous Endoscopic techniques and is reported separately with 5A1221Z Performance of Cardiac Output, Continuous.

Other procedures that may be performed during this atrial septal defect repair that are separately coded include:

- Transesophageal echocardiogram (TEE), reported with a code from Imaging, Heart, Ultrasonography, table B24
- Heart cath, reported with a code from Measurement and Monitoring, Measurement, Cardiac, table 4A02
- Coronary angiography, reported with a code from Imaging, Heart, Fluoroscopy, table B21
- Cardiac ventriculography, reported with a code from Imaging, Heart, Fluoroscopy, table B21

Focus Point

Assign an additional code for Autologous Tissue Substitute (graft) harvested from a separate incision site, according to ICD-10-PCS guideline B3.9.

Focus Point

If robotic assistance is used, a code from table 8EØ Other Procedures, is added. Review the record carefully for the appropriate approach for the root operation performed. If the robotic assistance was used only for visualization but incisions were extended beyond the trocars to perform the procedure, report Open approach, according to guideline B5.2. If the trocars were used to perform and visualize the entire procedure, Percutaneous Endoscopic approach is appropriate.

Coding Guidance

AHA: 2016, 4Q, 103-107; 2015, 4Q, 23

© 2018 Optum360, LLC

Medical and Surgical

Repair, Bronchopleural Fistula, Autologous Graft, Omentum

Body System
Respiratory System

PCS Root Operation
Supplement

Root Operation Table
ØBU   Respiratory System, Supplement

Body Part
Main Bronchus, Right
Upper Lobe Bronchus, Right
Middle Lobe Bronchus, Right
Lower Lobe Bronchus, Right
Main Bronchus, Left
Upper Lobe Bronchus, Left
Lingula Bronchus
Lower Lobe Bronchus, Left

Approach
Open

Device
Autologous Tissue Substitute

Description
A bronchopleural fistula is an abnormal passageway between the remaining end of a bronchial tube and the chest pleura that occurs sometimes after the removal of a lung or portion of a lung. This can be a life-threatening condition that is difficult to manage. Treatment includes surgery to close a bronchopleural fistula.

Using an Open approach, a thoracotomy incision is made into the chest cavity. After the removal of infected and necrotic tissue, the pleural space is filled with antibiotic solution, and the vascularized pedicle of greater omentum is transposed into the hemithorax through the diaphragm. The omental flap is fixed in place over the bronchial stump using sutures and biological glue. After the repair of the fistula, a chest tube and subcutaneous drainage tube are placed and the thoracic incision is sutured closed.

Focus Point
While the root operation Transfer is the most appropriate for a pedicled graft that retains its vasculature, there is no omental body part available in the Transfer, Gastrointestinal System table. In ICD-10-PCS, root operation Supplement can function as a Repair with device option when a more specific code is not available.

Coding Guidance
AHA: 2015, 1Q, 28

© 2018 Optum360, LLC

Repair, Cleft Lip (Cheiloplasty)

See also Repair, Cleft Palate, Alveolar

Body System
Mouth and Throat

Muscles

PCS Root Operation
Repair

Transfer

Root Operation Table
ØCQ   Mouth and Throat, Repair

ØKX   Muscles, Transfer

Body Part
Upper Lip (Repair)

Facial Muscle (Transfer)

Approach
Open

Device
No Device

Qualifier
No Qualifier (Repair)

Skin and Subcutaneous Tissue (Transfer)

Description
Cleft lip (cheiloschisis) is a common birth defect that occurs early in fetal development. There are several types of cleft lip, ranging from a minor, small groove on the border of the upper lip to a major, larger deformity that extends into the floor of the nostril and part of the upper jawbone. Cleft lip repair (cheiloplasty) is performed to restore functions such as breathing, speaking, and eating and to restore a more normal appearance.

Repair
The physician surgically corrects a partial or complete unilateral developmental cleft lip deformity. A cleft lip may range in appearance from a "notch" in the upper lip to a complete separation running into the nose. Using an Open approach, the physician incises the cleft margins on either side from the mouth toward the nostril and through the full-thickness layers of mucosa,

muscle, and skin. The vermilion border of the cleft lip is turned downward to restore the normal shape of the lip; the muscle and skin are brought together to close the cleft separation and preserve muscle function. The nasal deformity often caused by the cleft lip may be repaired in a separately reportable procedure. The incisions are closed in layers from the intraoral mucosa through the muscle, with final closure of the skin.

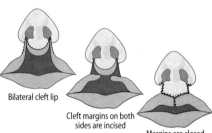

Bilateral cleft lip

Cleft margins on both sides are incised

Margins are closed, correcting cleft

Transfer
Using an Open approach, the physician makes an incision on each side of the cleft from the lip to the nostril, with the length of the incision depending upon the size of the defect. A rotation and advancement flap of muscle with attached skin and subcutaneous tissue is lifted up and rearranged to fill the cleft, and the two sides of the lip are sutured together, closing the lip and realigning the muscle of the upper lip. The nasal deformity often caused by the cleft lip may be repaired in a separately reportable procedure. The incisions are closed in layers from the intraoral mucosa through the muscle, with final closure of the skin.

> **Focus Point**
> *The rotation advancement technique, also known as the Millard technique, is reported with root operation Transfer, as the body part transferred is moved to a new location but remains attached to its vascular supply.*

Coding Guidance
AHA: 2017, 1Q, 20; 2015, 3Q, 33

© 2018 Optum360, LLC

Medical and Surgical

Repair, Cleft Palate, Alveolar

See also Repair, Cleft Lip (Cheiloplasty)

Body System
Mouth and Throat

Head and Facial Bones

PCS Root Operation
Repair

Supplement

Root Operation Table
ØCQ   Mouth and Throat, Repair

ØNQ   Head and Facial Bones, Repair

ØNU   Head and Facial Bones, Supplement

Body Part
Hard Palate (Mouth and Throat)

Soft Palate (Mouth and Throat)

Maxilla (Head and Facial Bones)

Approach
Open

Device
No Device (Repair)

Autologous Tissue Substitute (Supplement)

Synthetic Substitute (Supplement)

Nonautologous Tissue Substitute (Supplement)

Description
Cleft palate (palatoschisis), along with cleft lip (cheiloschisis), is a common birth defect that occurs early in fetal development. Surgical techniques and root operations reported for cleft palate repair may vary depending on the characteristics of the cleft and necessary repair. Multiple root operations may be performed concomitantly.

Repair
The physician repairs the developmental cleft opening of the palate. The cleft size and location dictate the type of repair to be performed. The physician closes the opening between the oral and nasal cavities with a partition of soft tissue. Typically, using an Open approach, incisions are made in the palatal mucosa adjacent to the alveolar (tooth-bearing) bone. The mucosa is elevated and loosened from the bony palate. The margins of the cleft are incised and dissected to develop mucosal and muscular layers. These incised midline margins are closed in layers, thus cutting off the communication between the oral and nasal cavities. This is reported using table ØCQ Repair, Mouth and Throat.

The physician repairs the developmental cleft opening of the palate, which extends through the alveolar ridge (tooth-bearing region) of the maxilla. The cleft size and location dictate the type of repair performed. The physician closes the opening between the oral and nasal cavities with a partition of soft tissue. Closure of the alveolar ridge facilitates development of both the maxilla and the teeth. Typically, incisions are made in the palatal mucosa adjacent to the alveolar bone. The mucosa is elevated and loosened from the bony palate. The midline margins of the cleft are incised and dissected to develop mucosal and muscular layers. The physician closes the midline margins in layers. This is reported using table ØNQ Repair, Head and Facial Bones.

Supplement
The physician repairs the developmental cleft opening of the palate and reconstructs the alveolar ridge (tooth-bearing region) of the maxilla. The cleft size and location dictate the type of repair performed. The physician closes the opening between the oral and nasal cavities with a partition of soft tissue. Bony reconstruction of the alveolar ridge can stabilize maxillary segments, benefit development of the teeth, and aid dental rehabilitation of chewing functions.

Typically, the physician uses an Open approach to make incisions in the palatal mucosa adjacent to the alveolar bone. The mucosa is elevated and loosened from the bony palate. The midline margins of the cleft mucosa and gingiva are incised and dissected to develop mucosal and muscular layers. In a separately reportable procedure, through a separate Open incision, the physician harvests bone from the hip or the skull and closes the incision. The bone is placed in the alveolar cleft, re-establishing normal contours of the maxilla. The physician closes all midline incisions in layers and gingival incisions in a single layer. This is reported using table ØNS Supplement, Head and Facial Bones.

> **Focus Point**
> Procedures to correct congenital anomalies may require that multiple procedures be performed concomitantly. According to ICD-10-PCS multiple procedures guideline B3.2c, multiple procedures with distinct objectives may be reported separately. See also *Repair, Cleft Lip (Cheiloplasty)*.

> **Focus Point**
> Harvesting of an autograft from a different procedure site is coded separately, according to guideline B3.9.

Coding Guidance
AHA: 2017, 1Q, 20; 2016, 3Q, 29; 2015, 2Q, 26

Repair, Complete Common Atrioventricular Canal Defect

See also Repair, Atrial Septal Defect (ASD)
(Atrioseptoplasty) (Repair of Foramen Ovale [Patent])

See also Repair, Ventricular Septal Defect (VSD)

Body System
Heart and Great Vessels

PCS Root Operation
Creation

Root Operation Table
Ø24   Heart and Great Vessels, Creation

Body Part
Mitral Valve
Tricuspid Valve

Approach
Open

Device
Autologous Tissue Substitute
Zooplastic Tissue
Synthetic Substitute
Nonautologous Tissue Substitute

Qualifier
Common Atrioventricular Valve

Description
Complete common atrioventricular canal defect, also
known as an endocardial cushion defect, has three
features: an atrial septal defect (ASD), a ventricular
septal defect (VSD), and a single common
atrioventricular (AV) valve rather than separate mitral
and tricuspid valves. Surgical treatment includes repair
of each of the three defects.

The physician corrects a complete common
atrioventricular canal defect. The patient is placed
under general anesthesia and on cardiopulmonary
bypass. The physician uses an Open approach to make

an opening in the right atrium. The competency of the
single common AV valve is assessed, as is the
imaginary line where the plane extending upward
from the ventricular septal defect intersects the valve.
The valve leaflets are divided along this line. The
ventricular septal defect patch is placed. The valve
leaflets are resuspended by sewing them to the
ventricular septal defect patch. The competency of the
valves is assessed. The atrial septal defect is closed with
a patch sewn in place, and the valve leaflets are
resuspended by sewing them to the atrial septal defect
patch. The competency of the valves is assessed. With
this technique, new mitral and tricuspid valves are
created. The incisions are closed, and cardiopulmonary
bypass is discontinued when cardiac function has
returned.

Focus Point
*Procedures to correct congenital anomalies may require
that multiple procedures be performed concomitantly.
According to ICD-10-PCS multiple procedures guideline
B3.2c, multiple procedures with distinct objectives may
be reported separately.*

Focus Point
*Cardiopulmonary bypass is an exception to the usual
practice of not reporting supporting procedures that are
components of a larger operation. When a surgical
procedure is performed with cardiopulmonary bypass,
it is coded as an additional procedure using table 5A1.*

Focus Point
*Closure of the VSD and closure of the ASD are coded
separately. See also Repair, Atrial Septal Defect (ASD)
(Atrioseptoplasty) (Repair of Foramen Ovale [Patent])
and Repair, Ventricular Septal Defect (VSD).*

Coding Guidance
AHA: 2016, 4Q, 104; 2015, 4Q, 22

© 2018 Optum360, LLC

Repair, Hypospadias

See also Release, Chordee

See also Reconstruction, Urethra, Male (Urethroplasty)

Body System
Male Reproductive System

PCS Root Operation
Transfer

Root Operation Table
ØVX   Reproductive System, Transfer

Body Part
Prepuce

Approach
Open
External

Device
No Device

Qualifier
Urethra
Penis

Description
Hypospadias is a congenital abnormality of the penis in which the urethral opening is positioned along the shaft of the penis on its underside or on the scrotum or perineum instead of being located at the tip of the penis. With increasing degrees of severity, the penis is curved downward (referred to as chordee). Distal hypospadias, with the urethral meatus on the glans penis or distal penile shaft, is the most common location.

The physician corrects hypospadias in a one-stage procedure. The physician uses an Open approach to make an incision on the surface of the penis and around the urethral opening, taking care to avoid injuring the urethra. Any chordee present is corrected in a separately reportable procedure. Skin in the area is pulled up to the glans and fashioned into an opening by suturing in the head of the penis. In some cases,

considerable dissection is required to mobilize the urethra. An island flap of skin may be created from the foreskin and sutured together to form a tube to be used as a segment of urethra. A closed urethra may also be created by using skin, tube, or free tissue grafts, or a combination of techniques depending on the extent of the defect. This is separately reported as a Supplement procedure. *See also* Reconstruction, Urethra (Urethroplasty). This formed urethral tube flap is sutured in place between the urethral opening at the base of the shaft of the penis and an opening created in the head of the penis. The foreskin and skin overlying the shaft are further divided and dissected free and sutured over the defect left by the flap on the ventral surface of the penis. A circumcision is usually the result of the procedure.

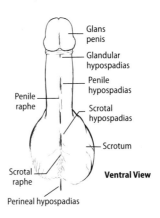

Glans penis
Glandular hypospadias
Penile hypospadias
Penile raphe
Scrotal hypospadias
Scrotum
Scrotal raphe
Ventral View
Perineal hypospadias

Focus Point
Release of chordee and urethroplasty are often performed in conjunction with repair of hypospadias. According to ICD-10-PCS multiple procedures guideline B3.2c, multiple procedures with distinct objectives may be reported separately.

© 2018 Optum360, LLC

Repair, Labral Tear (Shoulder)

Body System
Upper Joints

PCS Root Operation
Repair

Root Operation Table
ØRQ   Upper Joints, Repair

Body Part
Shoulder Joint, Right
Shoulder Joint, Left

Approach
Open
Percutaneous Endoscopic

Description
The glenoid labrum is the fibrocartilaginous supporting structure that surrounds the shoulder socket joint (glenoid). Tears in the labrum can result due to injury or overuse. Surgical procedures on the shoulder are performed using various surgical approaches and techniques, including open and arthroscopic methods. The Percutaneous Endoscopic approach is the most common.

In a Percutaneous Endoscopic approach, an arthroscope and surgical instruments are inserted into the shoulder joint through small incisions. Using suture anchors, the surgeon repairs the torn part of the labrum to the glenoid.

In an Open approach, the surgeon makes an incision in the front of the shoulder to access the labral tear. The Open approach employs the same principles of the Percutaneous Endoscopic approach.

© 2018 Optum360, LLC

Repair, Obstetrical Laceration/Episiotomy Extension

Body System
Gastrointestinal System

Skin and Breast

Subcutaneous Tissue and Fascia

Muscles

Urinary System

Female Reproductive System

Anatomical Regions, General

PCS Root Operation
Repair

Root Operation Table
0DQ Gastrointestinal System, Repair

0HQ Skin and Breast, Repair

0JQ Subcutaneous Tissue and Fascia, Repair

0KQ Muscles, Repair

0TQ Urinary System, Repair

0UQ Female Reproductive System, Repair

0WQ Anatomical Regions, General, Repair

Body Part
Rectum

Anus

Anal Sphincter

Skin, Perineum

Skin, Genitalia

Subcutaneous Tissue and Fascia, Perineum

Perineum Muscle

Bladder

Urethra

Vagina

Clitoris

Vulva

Perineum, Female

Approach
External

Open

Description
During childbirth, the emergence of the infant head through the vaginal canal may stretch the perineal tissue to the point that it tears. Alternatively, the physician attending the delivery may incise the perineum with scissors or a scalpel to accommodate the crowning head, or extend a laceration to prevent further trauma. The incision (episiotomy) may be midline or mediolateral. If the physician extends an episiotomy, it remains an episiotomy and is coded as such; the repair is not reported separately. An episiotomy that extends spontaneously is considered a laceration.

After the delivery of the placenta, the laceration and incision are repaired. The apex of the incision or laceration is identified, and the tissue is reapproximated and sutured. A deeper laceration repair may require submucosal and muscle sutures. Physician documentation of the degree of obstetric laceration or the tissue level repaired is required for accurate code assignment. If the documentation of the specific degree or tissue level repaired is unavailable, the default general anatomical region Female Perineum may be reported as a last resort.

Perineal tears are classified by degrees indicating the size and effect:

First degree—Involves the skin of the perineum and may include the vaginal mucosa. These tears usually do not require repair.

Second degree—Involves the perineal skin, vaginal mucosa, vaginal wall, perineal muscles and fascia but not the anal sphincter. These tears usually require suture closure.

Third degree—Involves vaginal mucosa, perineal skin, perineal muscles, and fascia and extends partially or completely through the anal sphincter but without involvement of the anal/rectal mucosa beneath. These tears require suture repair.

Fourth degree—Extends through the external and internal anal sphincter into the rectal mucosa. These tears require suture repair.

> **Focus Point**
> The root operation reported for obstetric laceration repair, regardless of the body site, is Repair: "Restoring, to the extent possible, a body part to its normal anatomic structure and function." When there are overlapping body layers involved in the laceration, report only the deepest layer of repair, according to ICD-10-PCS guideline B3.5.

> **Focus Point**
> Code also the episiotomy (root operation Division) if performed.

Coding Guidance
AHA: 2018, 2Q, 25; 2016, 1Q, 6; 2014, 4Q, 18; 2014, 4Q, 43; 2013, 4Q, 120

Medical and Surgical

Repair, Rotator Cuff (Shoulder)

See also Decompression, Subacromial, Rotator Cuff Tendon

See also Joint Replacement, Shoulder (Partial)

See also Joint Replacement, Shoulder (Total)

See also Joint Replacement, Shoulder, Reverse (Reverse Shoulder Arthroplasty)

Body System

Tendons

PCS Root Operation

Repair

Root Operation Table

ØLQ   Tendons, Repair

Body Part

Shoulder Tendon, Right
Shoulder Tendon, Left

Approach

Open
Percutaneous Endoscopic

Description

The rotator cuff comprises tendons and muscles that provide stability to the shoulder and allow the shoulder to rotate. By surrounding the shoulder joint, the rotator cuff helps to keep the humerus in place. Overuse or injury may result in a rotator cuff tear, which may need to be surgically repaired. Rotator cuff repairs are performed using various surgical techniques and approaches.

In a Percutaneous Endoscopic approach, small incisions are made around the shoulder through which the arthroscopic instruments are inserted. A solution is pumped through one of these incisions to cleanse and expand the joint for better visualization. The physician first performs a diagnostic arthroscopic exam to assess the joint. A limited bursectomy may be performed with a subacromial decompression in which the undersurface of the anterolateral acromion is cleared of soft tissue, if necessary. The frayed tendon edges are removed. Suture anchors are placed and the tendon repaired by passing sutures through the anchors. The arthroscope and instruments are removed, and the arm is placed in a sling to maintain abduction.

Using an Open approach, a longitudinal incision is made along the anterior portion of the shoulder, and the skin is reflected. The distal frayed edges of the tendon are removed. Suture anchors are placed and the tendon repaired by passing sutures through the anchors. The incision is closed, and a soft dressing is applied. The patient then follows a regime of a specific progression of exercises with protected motion.

Focus Point

Review the operative report carefully to determine the true objective of the procedure(s) performed in order to report the appropriate root operation. For example, rotator cuff repair performed in conjunction with a reverse total shoulder replacement to achieve functionality of the replacement joint is integral to the shoulder replacement surgery and would not be reported separately.

Coding Guidance

AHA: 2016, 3Q, 32; 2015, 1Q, 27; 2013, 3Q, 20

© 2018 Optum360, LLC

Repair, Superior Labrum Anterior and Posterior (SLAP)

See also Repair, Labral Tear (Shoulder)

Body System
Upper Joints

PCS Root Operation
Repair

Root Operation Table
ØRQ   Upper Joints, Repair

Body Part
Shoulder Joint, Right
Shoulder Joint, Left

Approach
Open
Percutaneous Endoscopic

Description
Superior labrum anterior and posterior (SLAP) lesions are injuries to the top (superior) part of the labrum that occur both in front (anterior) and back (posterior) of where the bicep tendon attaches to the labrum. The severity of the tear determines the SLAP classification. A type II SLAP tear is the most common and involves detachment of the superior labrum from the glenoid fossa. Repair of a type II SLAP tear involves reattaching the torn labrum.

Using a Percutaneous Endoscopic approach, the physician makes three incisions: one for the arthroscope, a second for the suture hook, and a third for a cannula. The surgeon prepares the bony bed with a small ball burr and drills or punches a hole at the cartilage bone junction of the superior labrum. A hook is passed through the anterior superior portal, and the inside limb is grasped with a suture retrieval forceps. The physician sets an anchor into the drill hole by mounting the suture anchor on the inserter and sliding it down the suture. The physician closes the loop with a slipknot that is tied and tightened outside the cannula. A knot pusher secures the knot under arthroscopic control. A long-acting local anesthetic may be injected into the joint to help with postoperative pain. The joint is irrigated and sutures or Steri-Strips close the incisions. The area is covered with a dressing, and a sling or shoulder immobilizer is applied.

In an Open approach, the surgeon makes an incision in the front of the shoulder to access the labral tear. The Open approach employs the same principles of the Percutaneous Endoscopic approach.

Focus Point
Glenoid ligament (labrum) in the ICD-10-PCS Body Part Key directs the user to Shoulder Joint, Right and Shoulder Joint, Left. No table exists for the root operation Reattachment; Repair is the most appropriate option.

Coding Guidance
AHA: 2013, 3Q, 20

Repair, Tendon (Tenorrhaphy)

Body System
Tendons

PCS Root Operation
Repair

Root Operation Table
ØLQ   Tendons, Repair

Body Part
Refer to the ICD-10-PCS tabular list for a complete list of body parts.

Approach
Open
Percutaneous
Percutaneous Endoscopic

Description
If a tendon has ruptured, surgery may be required to repair the ruptured tendon. Tenorrhaphy is the term used to describe the surgical suture or repair of a torn tendon.

Using an Open approach, an incision is made to expose the tendon, and all scar tissue is removed. The ruptured ends of the tendon are then debrided. Sutures are passed through the ruptured ends to bring them together. The incision is closed with sutures and staples or Steri-Strips.

The Percutaneous and Percutaneous Endoscopic approaches employ the same principles as the Open approach.

Focus Point
Surgical procedures on the tendon are performed using various surgical techniques and approaches. Review the documentation for specific information regarding the procedure before final code selection to ensure accurate code assignment.

Focus Point
A tendon repair with a graft would be reported with root operation Supplement. Supplement is used for repairs that involve devices.

Medical and Surgical

© 2018 Optum360, LLC

Repair, Truncus Arteriosus with Aortic Valve Creation

See also Rastelli Procedure (Right Ventricular-Pulmonary Artery Conduit)

See also Repair, Ventricular Septal Defect (VSD)

Body System
Heart and Great Vessels

PCS Root Operation
Creation
Repair
Supplement

Root Operation Table
024   Heart and Great Vessels, Creation
02Q   Heart and Great Vessels, Repair
02U   Heart and Great Vessels, Supplement

Body Part
Aortic Valve (Creation)
Thoracic Aorta, Descending (Repair, Supplement)
Thoracic Aorta, Ascending/Arch (Repair, Supplement)

Approach
Open

Device
Autologous Tissue Substitute
Zooplastic Tissue
Synthetic Substitute
Nonautologous Tissue Substitute
No Device (Repair)

Qualifier
Truncal Valve (Creation)
No Qualifier (Repair, Supplement)

Description
Truncus arteriosus, also known as common truncus, is a congenital defect. Patients with this defect have a single, large great vessel that failed to divide into the aorta and the pulmonary artery during fetal development. This vessel has a single common valve (truncal valve) that controls blood flow out of the heart, resulting in unrestricted left-to-right shunting of blood and pulmonary overcirculation. In addition, these patients usually have a large ventricular septal defect (VSD). Surgery to correct the truncus arteriosus involves the creation of a right ventricular outflow conduit from the right ventricle to the pulmonary arteries and creation of a functioning aortic valve with a single truncal valve.

The physician gains access to the mediastinum using an Open approach through a median sternotomy incision (through the sternum). The physician places the patient on cardiopulmonary bypass and stops the heart by infusing cardioplegia solution into the coronary circulation. The aorta is cross-clamped. In a separately reportable procedure, the physician applies a large Dacron patch to direct oxygenated blood from the left ventricle through the large VSD into the aortic valve and ascending aorta. *See* Repair, Ventricular Septal Defect (VSD).

The physician ligates the proximal main pulmonary artery or oversews the pulmonic valve. In an additional, separately reportable procedure, the physician creates a right ventricle-pulmonary artery (RV-PA) valved conduit using a graft to direct unoxygenated blood from the right ventricle to the branch pulmonary arteries after they are separated from the truncal root. *See* Rastelli Procedure (Right Ventricular-Pulmonary Artery Conduit).

The single great truncal vessel is then repaired as necessary; it may be closed directly in a Repair or with a patch graft in a Supplement to convert the truncal vessel to the new aorta. The single truncal valve is repaired as necessary to create a new aortic valve; Creation is used as the root operation with body part Aortic Valve and qualifier Truncal Valve.

The physician closes the cardiac incisions, takes the patient off cardiopulmonary bypass, closes the remaining surgical incisions, and dresses the sternal or chest wall wound. Chest tubes and mediastinal drainage tubes may be left in place following the procedure.

Focus Point

Procedures to correct congenital anomalies may require that multiple procedures be performed concomitantly. According to ICD-10-PCS multiple procedures guideline B3.2c, multiple procedures with distinct objectives may be reported separately.

Focus Point

Cardiopulmonary bypass is an exception to the usual practice of not reporting supporting procedures that are components of a larger operation. When a surgical procedure is performed with cardiopulmonary bypass, it is coded as an additional procedure using table 5A1.

Coding Guidance
AHA: 2016, 4Q, 104; 2015, 4Q, 22

Repair, Ventricular Septal Defect (VSD)

Body System
Heart and Great Vessels

PCS Root Operation
Repair

Supplement

Root Operation Table
0Q Heart and Great Vessels, Repair

0U Heart and Great Vessels, Supplement

Body Part
Ventricular Septum

Approach
Open

Percutaneous

Percutaneous Endoscopic

Device
No Device

Autologous Tissue Substitute (Supplement)

Zooplastic Tissue (Supplement)

Synthetic Substitute (Supplement)

Nonautologous Tissue Substitute (Supplement)

Description
A ventriculoseptal defect (VSD) is a defect or hole in the wall that divides the left and right ventricles of the heart. It can be either a congenital or a post-myocardial infarction complication. This can be repaired using many techniques. Although the intention of the procedure is to close or occlude the defect, the root operation Occlusion in the ICD-10-PCS tables does not currently offer a body part for ventricular septum. The root operations depend on the type of technique performed.

Open Approach
A thoracotomy is performed in this open heart procedure. Cardiopulmonary bypass is established with tubes in both the caval veins. The ventricular septal defect can almost always be accessed and repaired through an incision in the right atrium, except in the case of a supracristal VSD, in which the ventricle is higher in the outflow part of the right ventricle. This type of VSD is most often accessed and repaired through an incision in the pulmonary artery. All types of ventricular septal defects can be accessed and repaired through an incision in the muscle of the right

ventricle, but this causes more damage and is avoided if possible. The defect is usually repaired with a patch of Dacron or pericardium, which is reported with the root operation Supplement, but may be closed using only sutures, which is coded with the root operation Repair. After the ventricular septal defect is closed, the hole that has been created in the right atrium, right ventricle, or pulmonary artery is closed. The chest incision is repaired. Cardiopulmonary bypass is discontinued when heart function returns. If autologous pericardium tissue is used, add code 02BN0ZZ for the harvesting of the pericardial tissue.

Percutaneous Approach (Transcatheter)
Various techniques are used but a very simplified explanation of a common method is described here. Percutaneous access is obtained in the femoral vein, the femoral artery, and the right internal jugular vein. A heart catheterization is performed, and a guidewire is advanced through the site into the pulmonary artery, where it is snared by another guidewire that is exteriorized through the sheath in the internal jugular forming a stable rail in which to transport the device. An Fr sheath is then advanced from the internal jugular on the guide rail to the left ventricle. The implant device, most commonly Amplatzer device, is screwed into a delivery cable and advanced through the sheath slowly into the defect and deployed. The root operation is Supplement with a device value Synthetic Substitute.

Percutaneous Endoscopic Approach
Using a Percutaneous Endoscopic approach, the femoral veins are accessed and several ports (incisions) are created in the chest through which cannulas for instrumentation and endoscopic trocars for visualization can be inserted. Cardiopulmonary bypass is established. The myocardium is incised, and the endoscopic tool is advanced through the right atrium and to the site of the ventricular defect. Depending on its size, the defect is repaired with sutures, which is reported with the root operation Repair, or a Dacron poly patch, pericardium, other tissue graft, or plug implant, which are all reported with the root operation Supplement. The defect is closed, the endoscope is removed, and access incisions are sutured in layers. If autologous pericardium tissue is used, add code 02BN4ZZ for the harvesting of the pericardial tissue.

Percutaneous Endoscopic repairs may be performed with or with the use of robotic assistance.

© 2018 Optum360, LLC

Repair, Ventricular Septal Defect (VSD) (continued)

Focus Point

Cardiopulmonary bypass is used in both the Open and Percutaneous Endoscopic techniques and is reported separately with 5A1221Z Performance of Cardiac Output, Continuous.

Other procedures that may be performed during this ventricular septal defect repair that are separately coded include:

- Transesophageal Echocardiogram (TEE), reported with a code from Imaging, Heart, Ultrasonography, table B24
- Heart cath, reported with a code from Measurement and Monitoring, Measurement, Cardiac, table 4A02
- Coronary angiography, reported with a code from Imaging, Heart, Fluoroscopy, table B21
- Cardiac ventriculography, reported with a code from Imaging, Heart, Fluoroscopy, table B21

Focus Point

Assign an additional code for Autologous Tissue Substitute (graft) harvested from a separate incision site, according to ICD-10-PCS guideline B3.9.

Focus Point

If robotic assistance is used, a code from table 8E0 Other Procedures, is added. Review the record carefully for the appropriate approach for the root operation performed. If the robotic assistance was used only for visualization but incisions were extended beyond the trocars to perform the procedure, report Open approach, according to guideline B5.2. If the trocars were used to perform and visualize the entire procedure, Percutaneous Endoscopic approach is appropriate.

Coding Guidance

AHA: 2016, 4Q, 104-107; 2015, 4Q, 24

Medical and Surgical

Replacement, Intervertebral Disc, Artificial

Body System

Upper Joints

Lower Joints

PCS Root Operation

Replacement

Root Operation Table

ØRR   Upper Joints, Replacement

ØSR   Lower Joints, Replacement

Body Part

Cervical Vertebral Disc

Cervicothoracic Vertebral Disc

Lumbar Vertebral Disc

Lumbosacral Disc

Approach

Open

Device

Synthetic Substitute

Description

Intervertebral discs, which are contained between each of the spinal joints, are made up of a strong outer fibrous ring called the annulus fibrosus, which protects and absorbs compression, and the softer inner center, called the nucleus pulposus, which acts as a shock absorber. Artificial disc replacement (ADR), also referred to as total disc replacement (TDR), is a newer technology performed in lieu of fusion to replace a severely damaged or diseased intervertebral disc, most often caused by degenerative disc disease. This technology is not yet available for thoracic discs.

ICD-10-PCS includes the intervertebral cervical and lumbar disc body part values in the Upper Joints and Lower Joints body systems. Artificial discs are manufactured from synthetic materials such as metal and rubber polyethylene, which are considered Synthetic Substitute for ICD-10-PCS device value reporting. The root operation Replacement is reported and is defined as putting in or on a biological or synthetic material that physically takes the place and/ or function of all or a portion of a body part. Either the entire disc or just the nucleus can be replaced. The PCS explanation of the root operation Replacement

includes the removal of the body part being replaced; therefore discectomy is *not* reported.

For the replacement of a cervical disc, the physician uses an anterior approach to reach the damaged cervical vertebrae by making an incision through the neck, avoiding the esophagus, trachea, and thyroid. For a lumbar disc, an anterior approach to reach the damaged lumbar vertebrae is made with an incision through the abdomen. Some implants require only minimal access, approximately 7 cm long, for a mini-retroperitoneal approach. Retractors separate the intervertebral muscles. The intervertebral disc space to be replaced is cleaned out with a rongeur, removing the cartilaginous material in preparation for inserting the implant.

Preparation may include discectomy, osteophytectomy for nerve root or spinal cord decompression, and/or microdissection, all of which are inherent in the replacement surgery. One type of implant for total disc replacement has two endplates made of a metal alloy and a convex weight-bearing surface made of ultra-high molecular weight polyethylene. The endplates are inserted in a collapsed form and seated into the vertebral bodies above and below the interspace. Minimal distraction is applied to open the intervertebral space, and the polyethylene disc material is snap-fitted into the lower endplate. With the disc assembly complete, the wound is closed, and a drain may be placed.

Focus Point

When an intervertebral disc is removed and replaced, do not report the root operation Excision or Resection; only the root operation Replacement is reported.

Focus Point

Even when minimally invasive is documented, an Open approach is still used to access and visualize the site. There is no specific approach value for minimally invasive surgery and no current guidelines addressing them. Each operative report must be carefully reviewed and the ICD-10-PCS approach definitions applied to determine the correct approach value.

Coding Guidance

AHA: 2013, 4Q, 108

© 2018 Optum360, LLC

Medical and Surgical

Replacement, Pacemaker Generator (End of Life)

See also Insertion, Cardiac Pacemaker Generator

Body System
Subcutaneous Tissue and Fascia

PCS Root Operation
Removal

Root Operation Table
ØJP   Subcutaneous Tissue and Fascia, Removal

Body Part
Subcutaneous Tissue and Fascia, Trunk

Approach
Open

Device
Cardiac Rhythm Related Device

Description
Pacemaker generators run on batteries that last anywhere from five to 15 years. When the battery has reached the end of its life, the pacemaker generator must be replaced.

Removal
The existing pacemaker generator pocket is incised, reported with Open approach, into the subcutaneous tissue of the chest or abdomen depending on the location of the existing pacemaker generator. The generator is disconnected from the existing leads and removed. The root operation for the removal of the previously placed device is captured with the root operation Removal. In the Removal table, both chest and abdominal locations are captured in the body part Subcutaneous Tissue and Fascia, Trunk. The device value used for the removal of the generator only is the more generic Cardiac Rhythm Related Device. This generic device value is used for the removal of all such devices, including cardiac defibrillators and CRT-P and CRT-D.

Insertion
The existing pacer wires or wires are connected to the new generator and tested. The new device is inserted, and the pocket is closed. A second code is needed for the insertion of the new generator, which is reported with the root operation Insertion (*see also* Insertion, Cardiac Pacemaker Generator). The insertion of the new generator uses a more specific device value that indicates the precise type of cardiac device being used.

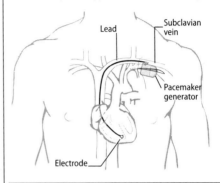

Focus Point
The root operation Revision is used only when the existing generator or lead(s) are displaced and moved but not replaced. The root operation Replacement is also not appropriate as it is not a body part or a previously placed replacement of a body part that is involved.

Focus Point
If any leads are replaced, additional codes for Removal of and Insertion of cardiac leads would be reported from the Heart and Great Vessel body system.

Coding Guidance
AHA: 2012, 4Q, 104

© 2018 Optum360, LLC

Replacement, Transcatheter Aortic Valve (TAVR)

See also Filtration, Cerebral Embolic, in the New Technology section

Body System
Heart and Great Vessels

PCS Root Operation
Replacement

Root Operation Table
Ø2R   Heart and Great Vessels, Replacement

Body Part
Aortic Valve

Approach
Percutaneous

Device
Zooplastic Tissue

Qualifier
Transapical
No Qualifier

Description

Transcatheter aortic valve replacement or implantation (TAVR/TAVI) is performed on patients with symptomatic aortic stenosis that are high risk or not eligible for traditional open chest surgery. This minimally invasive procedure uses a catheter instead of open surgery to replace a damaged aortic valve by inserting a fully collapsible valve replacement through a catheter. The new Zooplastic Tissue valve, which is made from cow or pig heart tissue, is wedged into the damaged valve and once it is expanded, takes over the function of the valve. Access is usually through the femoral artery but can also be through the subclavian artery, or through a small incision in the chest directly through the ascending aorta (transaortic) or through the bottom of the heart (Transapical).

The patient receives general anesthesia prior to the procedure. Using a Percutaneous approach, the physician places a guidewire through the femoral artery through an incision in the groin (transfemoral), through a small incision in the upper chest (transaortic), or through a small incision in the chest between the ribs (Transapical). The guidewire is manipulated into the left ventricle with the use of imaging. A catheter is inserted following the guidewire to the aortic valve, and a balloon is inflated to compress the native valve. A replacement valve attached to an expandable stent is deployed over the compressed native valve. Following confirmation that the valve is properly placed, the catheter and guidewire are removed. All approaches are closed using standard surgical techniques.

Focus Point
Although the damaged valve is not being removed, it is considered nonfunctional and replaced with the new valve; Replacement is used as the root operation.

Focus Point
A separate code is needed when cerebral embolic filtration is done in conjunction with TAVR/TAVI. See Filtration, Cerebral Embolic.

Focus Point
In TAVR procedures performed via a small incision in the chest, the body part value of the code specifies the aortic valve, which is not visualized directly. The procedure is performed via a catheter inserted into the heart, so the appropriate approach value is Percutaneous.

Coding Guidance
AHA: 2016, 4Q, 115; 2013, 3Q, 26

© 2018 Optum360, LLC

Medical and Surgical

Replantation, Scalp

Body System
Skin and Breast

PCS Root Operation
Reattachment

Root Operation Table
ØHM Skin and Breast, Reattachment

Body Part
Skin, Scalp

Approach
External

Description
Scalp replantation is performed in cases of severe trauma resulting in partial or complete scalp avulsions.

In ICD-10-PCS, this is reported with root operation Reattachment.

The physician uses a surgical microscope to reconnect the arteries and veins of the scalp, and reattaches the scalp to the cranium using complex, layered suturing of torn, crushed, or deeply lacerated scalp tissue. The physician debrides the wound by removing foreign material or damaged tissue. The wound is irrigated , and antimicrobial solutions are used to decontaminate and cleanse the wound. The physician may trim skin margins with a scalpel or scissors to allow for proper closure. The wound is closed in layers. Stents or retention sutures may also be used in complex repair of a wound.

Reposition, Uterus, Transvaginal

See also Version, External Cephalic (ECV) in the Medical and Surgical Related section, Obstetrics

Body System
Female Reproductive System

PCS Root Operation
Reposition

Root Operation Table
ØUS Female Reproductive System, Reposition

Body Part
Uterus

Approach
Via Natural or Artificial Opening

Device
No Device

Qualifier
No Qualifier

Description
A retroverted or tilted uterus curves in a backwards position at the cervix instead of the normal anteverted (forward) position. Generally, this is not symptomatic and requires no intervention or can be corrected with exercises. However, in some patients, a retroverted uterus can become symptomatic and the uterus may need to be repositioned. In pregnant patients, the most common malpresentation seen is retroversion with incarceration, which means the uterus remains retroverted as the pregnancy advances and the uterus becomes wedged in the pelvic cavity. This can complicate the pregnancy and cause bladder outlet obstruction and urinary retention.

The bladder is drained with a Foley catheter. The patient may be placed in a knee-chest or all-fours position. Using a Via Natural or Artificial Opening approach, and real-time ultrasound guidance, an open-sided speculum is inserted into the vagina, and the anterior lip of the cervix is grasped with a long clamp. The speculum is then removed, and the surgeon inserts a finger into either the vagina or rectum and applies pressure to the uterus, while applying gentle constant traction to the cervix with the long clamp. In this technique, the uterus is slowly rotated into a normal position. The instruments are removed. The patient may be instructed to do repositioning exercises several times a day and sleep in the prone position.

Focus Point
Fetal repositioning within the uterus is reported with a code from table 1ØS Obstetrics, Pregnancy, Reposition. See also Version, External Cephalic (ECV), in the Medical and Surgical Related section, Obstetrics.

Focus Point
Even if a uterine reposition procedure is performed on a pregnant patient, no code is assigned from the obstetrics section because it is repositioning the mother's uterus, not the fetus (Products of Conception). ICD-10-PCS guideline C1 states: "Procedures performed on the pregnant female other than the products of conception are coded to the appropriate root operation in the Medical and Surgical section."

Coding Guidance
AHA: 2016, 1Q, 9

Resection, Abdominoperineal (APR)

See also Creation, Colostomy

Body System
Gastrointestinal System

PCS Root Operation
Resection

Root Operation Table
ØDT   Gastrointestinal System, Resection

Body Part
Sigmoid Colon
Rectum
Anus

Approach
Open
Percutaneous Endoscopic

Description
An abdominoperineal resection (APR), formerly referred to as abdominoperineal resection of the rectum, is performed for conditions such as malignancies of the rectum or anus. The root operation Resection is reported with either an Open or Percutaneous Endoscopic (laparoscopic) approach. Three separate codes are necessary to report the resections since the Sigmoid Colon, Rectum, and Anus all have individual body part values in ICD-10-PCS.

In an abdominoperineal resection (APR), the physician removes the entire sigmoid colon, rectum, and anus through either an Open or Percutaneous Endoscopic (laparoscopic) technique using both an abdominal and perineal operative approach and then forms a colostomy.

Abdominoperineal pull-through resection involves incising around the anus and excising the anus and rectum. Through the abdominal incision, the rectum and sigmoid are mobilized, and the sigmoid is divided from the remaining large intestine. The sigmoid and rectum are removed. Using the perineal incision, the anus is divided and removed. Anastomosis is not involved in this type of abdominoperineal resection because all of the anal structures are excised. A stoma site is prepared, and the remaining open end of the large intestine is pulled through the incision to the skin and sutured into place for the colostomy.

Focus Point
The creation of the stoma or colostomy is coded separately using root operation Bypass. See also Creation, Colostomy.

Coding Guidance
AHA: 2015, 1Q, 38; 2014, 4Q, 40, 41

© 2018 Optum360, LLC

Resection, Lymph Node

Body System
Lymphatic and Hemic Systems

PCS Root Operation
Resection

Root Operation Table
Ø7T Lymphatic and Hemic Systems, Resection

Body Part
Lymphatic, Head
Lymphatic, Right Neck
Lymphatic, Left Neck
Lymphatic, Right Upper Extremity
Lymphatic, Left Upper Extremity
Lymphatic, Right Axillary
Lymphatic, Left Axillary
Lymphatic, Thorax
Lymphatic, Internal Mammary, Right
Lymphatic, Internal Mammary, Left
Lymphatic, Mesenteric
Lymphatic, Pelvis
Lymphatic, Aortic
Lymphatic, Right Lower Extremity
Lymphatic, Left Lower Extremity
Lymphatic, Right Inguinal
Lymphatic, Left Inguinal

Approach
Open
Percutaneous Endoscopic

Description
The lymphatic system picks up clear fluid that naturally leaks from blood vessels in the extremities and carries the fluid toward the chest, where it reenters blood circulation at the subclavian veins. Along the lymphatic channels are lymph nodes, which act as spongy filters to collect potentially dangerous cells to prevent spread of disease. Infectious agents and cancer cells may be captured by the lymph nodes. Often, when a cancerous organ is excised, the regional lymph nodes also are excised to reduce or eradicate metastatic cells. In other cases, the lymphatic system itself may be the origin of the disease—for example in lymphoma—and the lymph nodes may be removed to reduce or eradicate the disease.

Lymph nodes exist along lymphatic chains that include lymphatic channels and the nodes. In Resection, an entire lymph node chain is removed. If the intent is to remove all of the lymph nodes in an area, this is also reported as Resection. The lymphatic resection may be performed alone or as part of a more extensive operation. Report the lymphatic resection code(s) in addition to the codes for separately reportable procedures.

In lymphadenectomy with an Open approach, the physician makes an incision in the skin overlying the lymphatic chain. The surrounding tissues, nerves, and blood vessels are dissected away, and the lymph nodes are visualized. One or more complete lymphatic chains are removed, and the wound is closed with sutures or staples.

In lymphadenectomy with a Percutaneous Endoscopic approach, the physician performs a laparoscopic resection of the lymphatic chain or chains. The physician places a trocar at the umbilicus into the abdominal or retroperitoneal space and insufflates the peritoneal or retroperitoneal space. The laparoscope is placed through the umbilical trocar, and additional trocars are placed in the insufflated cavity. The lymphatic chain or chains are identified, and the surrounding tissues, nerves, and blood vessels are dissected away so that the lymphatic tissue can be removed. The trocars are removed, and the incisions are closed.

Focus Point
Lymph node sampling, sentinel node biopsy, or "selective" lymph node removal, are reported as the root operation Excision. If a partial removal of a lymph node chain is done, it is coded as Excision. Lymph node dissection, resection, and radical or modified radical lymph node excision usually describe complete removal of a chain of lymphatic tissue, which is Resection. In radical procedures, everything within a designated anatomic boundary is resected.

Focus Point
Removal of one or more entire chains of lymph nodes plus one or more partial chains of lymph nodes or isolated lymph nodes of a single, named body part meets the definition of the root operation Resection of the single body part. Therefore, report only Resection without an additional code for Excision.

Focus Point
The neck is a structure dense with lymph nodes, which are classified by levels in the staging of squamous cell carcinoma. If the entire lymphatic chain of one level of the neck (right or left) is documented as removed, report this removal as Resection even though all lymphatic chains (levels) in the body part were not removed.

Coding Guidance
AHA: 2018, 1Q, 22; 2016, 2Q, 12; 2016, 1Q, 30; 2014, 3Q, 9

Resection, Stapled Transanal Rectal (STARR) (Rectorectostomy)

Body System
Gastrointestinal System

PCS Root Operation
Excision

Root Operation Table
ØDB   Gastrointestinal System, Excision

Body Part
Rectum

Approach
Via Natural or Artificial Opening
Via Natural or Artificial Opening Endoscopic

Description
Obstructed defecation syndrome (ODS), which is associated with formation of pouches (rectoceles), intussusception (telescoping of the intestinal walls), and mucosal prolapse, is one cause of chronic constipation. Bowel movements become difficult with these rectal abnormalities, and incomplete evacuation may occur. The stapled transanal rectal resection (STARR) procedure is performed to reduce the deformities.

After the administration of anesthesia, the patient is placed in lithotomy position. An anal dilator is inserted into the anal canal. Two circular staplers are inserted and used to remove excess tissue from the anterior and posterior rectal wall. The tissue removed is delivered through the stapler housing and sent to pathology. Hemostasis of the staple line is controlled with sutures. The entire procedure is minimally invasive, performed directly through the anus, and requires no external incisions.

Coding Guidance
AHA: 2016, 1Q, 22

© 2018 Optum360, LLC

Revision, Graft, Arteriovenous (AV)

See also Graft, Arteriovenous (AV)

Body System
Upper Arteries

PCS Root Operation
Revision

Root Operation Table
03W Upper Arteries, Revision

Body Part
Upper Artery

Approach
Open
Percutaneous

Device
Synthetic Substitute

Qualifier
No Qualifier

Description
A hemodialysis arteriovenous graft can be complicated by malfunction due to stenosis or thrombosis, requiring thrombectomy and/or revision of the graft.

Open
Using an Open approach, the physician makes an incision in the skin of the extremity overlying the graft and dissects around any muscle, vessels, or other structures to access the graft site. The physician dissects around the vessel, applies vessel clamps above and below the graft, and excises above and below the existing malfunctioning graft. The graft is opened, and thrombectomy is performed. A portion of the existing graft may be excised and replaced with a new section of graft. The new graft is anastomosed to the old graft with sutures. After the repair has been made, the vessel clamps are removed, and the incision is closed in layers.

Percutaneous
Under radiologic guidance, using a Percutaneous approach, a catheter is advanced to the site of a thrombus or clot that has formed in a previously created arteriovenous graft. The catheter is inserted into the clot, and the clot is fragmented. Injection of urokinase may be required to dissolve the clot, or percutaneous pharmacomechanical thrombolysis may be performed. Pharmacomechanical thrombolysis involves both injection of urokinase and mechanical fragmentation of the clot. Suction is applied, and the clot fragments are removed from the graft through the catheter. A balloon may be used, which is inserted via the catheter and inflated beyond the clot. The balloon is slowly pulled out, capturing and retrieving the clot. Once the clot is dissolved or retrieved, the catheter is removed, and pressure and/or suture is applied at the insertion site.

Focus Point
The intent of this procedure is to correct a malfunctioning or displaced graft without replacing it; therefore, the appropriate root operation is Revision. Revision is defined as "correcting, to the extent possible, a portion of a malfunctioning or the position of a displaced device."

Focus Point
If the entire graft is excised and replaced with a new arteriovenous graft, report the root operation Bypass.

Focus Point
The arteries of the upper extremities are classified to the Upper Arteries body system in ICD-10-PCS, since the upper extremities are above the level of the diaphragm. See ICD-10-PCS guideline B2.1b.

Coding Guidance
AHA: 2016, 3Q, 39

Medical and Surgical

Revision, Shunt, Transjugular Intrahepatic Portosystemic (TIPS)

See also Shunt, Transjugular Intrahepatic Portosystemic (TIPS)

Body System
Lower Veins

PCS Root Operation
Revision

Root Operation Table
06W Lower Veins, Revision

Body Part
Lower Vein

Approach
Percutaneous

Device
Intraluminal Device

Qualifier
No Qualifier

Description

A transjugular intrahepatic portosystemic shunt (TIPS) is a shunt created within the liver between the portal and hepatic veins. This involves percutaneous placement of a stent to manage the complications of portal hypertension and control variceal bleeding and ascites. If an existing shunt/stent becomes occluded with clots, a declotting procedure is performed.

Once the patient is under general anesthesia or conscious sedation, the right internal jugular vein is accessed in a Percutaneous approach, and a catheter is placed into the right hepatic vein. Catheter placement is verified with separately reportable venography. A needle is advanced through the catheter into the wall of the right hepatic vein to access the right portal vein. A guidewire and catheter are advanced along this route into the portal vein, and venography again is performed to verify placement.

Clots are removed with a mechanical thrombectomy device or pulse-spray thrombolysis, and the occluded stent may be reopened by placing another stent within the lumen of the original stent using a balloon catheter. In some cases, the flow may need to be reduced with a smaller diameter stent inserted into the existing stent, thus narrowing the diameter of the shunt. Venography and pressure measurements confirm adequate stent position and flow through the shunt. The balloon, catheter, and other instruments are removed, and pressure is applied to the insertion site, which may require suture.

Focus Point
The intent of this procedure is to correct a malfunctioning or displaced intraluminal device; therefore, the appropriate root operation is Revision. Revision is defined as "correcting, to the extent possible, a portion of a malfunctioning or the position of a displaced device."

Focus Point
The veins of the liver are classified to the Lower Veins body system in ICD-10-PCS, since the liver is below the level of the diaphragm. See ICD-10-PCS guideline B2.1b.

Coding Guidance
AHA: 2018, 1Q, 10; 2014, 3Q, 25

© 2018 Optum360, LLC

Rhinoplasty, Augmentation

Body System
Ear, Nose, Sinus

PCS Root Operation
Alteration

Root Operation Table
Ø9Ø   Ear, Nose, Sinus, Alteration

Body Part
Nasal Mucosa and Soft Tissue

Approach
Open

Device
Autologous Tissue Substitute
Synthetic Substitute
Nonautologous Tissue Substitute
No Device

Description
Augmentation rhinoplasty, otherwise known as a "nose job," is a popular cosmetic surgery performed to reshape the nose. The desired look is achieved by sculpting the cartilage and nose. Alteration is the root operation used when the intent of a procedure is to improve appearance.

The physician performs surgery to reshape or enlarge the external nose. No surgery to the nasal septum is necessary. This surgery is performed via an Open approach either with external skin incisions or intranasal incisions. Topical vasoconstrictive agents are applied to shrink the blood vessels, and local anesthesia is injected in the nasal mucosa. After incisions are made, dissections expose the external nasal cartilaginous and bony skeleton. The cartilages may be reshaped by trimming or may be augmented by grafting. Local grafts from adjacent nasal bones and cartilage are not reported separately. The physician may reshape the dorsum with files and may fracture the lateral nasal bones with chisels. Fat also may be removed from the subcutaneous regions. When the reshaping process is complete, incisions are closed in single layers. Steri-Strip tape is used to support cartilaginous surgery of the nasal tip. An external splint or cast supports changes in bone position.

Focus Point
If rhinoplasty is performed for functional reasons such as a correction of birth defects or to improve breathing difficulty, Alteration would not be used as the root operation.

Focus Point
Graft material may include material from the patient's own body (autologous), a synthetic implant such as silicone, or material from another living or biologic source (nonautologous). The device value in the Alteration code indicates the type of implanted material.

Focus Point
If graft material is obtained from another site of the patient's body, a code for the separate harvesting of a graft is required, according to guideline B3.9.

Rhinoscopy

Body System
Ear, Nose, Sinus

PCS Root Operation
Inspection

Root Operation Table
Ø9J   Ear, Nose, Sinus, Inspection

Body Part
Nasal Mucosa and Soft Tissue

Approach
Via Natural or Artificial Opening Endoscopic

Description
Rhinoscopy may be used to determine whether there are any fixed blockages such as a deviated septum, nasal polyps, or enlarged adenoids and tonsils. The test may also be performed to identify anatomic factors contributing to a sleep disorder or stability of the upper airway, and to determine treatments.

An endoscope, used to perform an intranasal examination, allows for both increased visualization and magnification of internal anatomy. Topical vasoconstrictive agents are applied to the nasal mucosa, and nerve blocks with local anesthesia are administered. The endoscope is placed into the nose, and the physician thoroughly inspects the internal nasal structures.

A rhinoscopy procedure may also be used to examine the nasopharynx. With the patient lying in prone position, a local anesthetic with topical Lidocaine is sprayed onto the back of the throat and into the nasal passages. The endoscope is introduced through the nose and advanced into the pharynx.

Rhizotomy, Spinal Nerve Root

Body System
Peripheral Nervous System

PCS Root Operation
Division

Root Operation Table
Ø18   Peripheral Nervous System, Division

Body Part
Cervical Nerve
Thoracic Nerve
Lumbar Nerve
Sacral Nerve

Approach
Open
Percutaneous Endoscopic

Description
A rhizotomy is performed on the anterior spinal nerve roots to stop involuntary spasmodic movements associated with paraplegia or torticollis. It is also performed on the posterior spinal nerve roots to eliminate pain in a restricted area. Severing a nerve root to stop involuntary movements or to relieve pain is coded to the root operation Division.

The patient is placed prone. Using an Open approach, the physician makes a midline incision overlying the affected vertebrae. The fascia is incised, and the paravertebral muscles are retracted. Laminectomy is performed. The physician identifies the anterior or posterior spinal nerve roots to be divided. Each is lifted with a nerve hook and severed. Fascia, muscles, and ligaments are allowed to fall back into place. The incision is closed with layered sutures.

A Percutaneous Endoscopic rhizotomy is a minimally invasive surgical procedure that allows direct visualization of the spinal nerve roots with the use of a cannula and endoscope to divide the nerve.

Focus Point
Multiple spinal nerve root rhizotomies performed at the same spinal level are reported only once. The spinal nerve roots are not classified in ICD-10-PCS as separate and distinct body parts but as single body parts: Cervical Nerve, Thoracic Nerve, Lumbar Nerve, and Sacral Nerve. See Multiple Procedures guideline B3.2.b

Focus Point
Laminectomy performed only as the approach to a rhizotomy is not reported separately.

© 2018 Optum360, LLC

Rupture, Shoulder Joint Adhesions (Arthrolysis) (Manual)

Body System
Upper Joints

PCS Root Operation
Release

Root Operation Table
ØRN   Upper Joints, Release

Body Part
Shoulder Joint, Right
Shoulder Joint, Left

Approach
External

Description
Manipulation of the shoulder under anesthesia may be necessary to regain the loss of motion that occurs in the case of frozen shoulder or adhesions following a surgical procedure.

The patient is positioned supine and given general anesthesia. In manual rupture of shoulder joint adhesions, the physician applies gradual pressure in the desired direction, forcibly releasing adhesions or scar tissue to restore mobility. No incision is required to perform manual rupture.

Focus Point
Freeing scar tissue or adhesions in a joint to increase mobility or reduce pain is reported with the root operation Release. In Release, the body part being freed is the body part that is coded. Therefore, for manual rupture of a joint adhesion, the joint would be reported since the joint is the body part being freed. The approach is External because the application of external force through the skin overlying the joint is sufficient to release the adhesions within the joint (manual rupture).

Sacroplasty

Body System
Lower Bones

PCS Root Operation
Supplement

Root Operation Table
ØQU   Lower Bones, Supplement

Body Part
Sacrum

Approach
Percutaneous

Device
Synthetic Substitute

Description
Sacroplasty is a minimally invasive procedure for treating pain from vertebral compression fractures, which involves a cement-like material injected into the collapsed bone to stabilize the fracture. The PCS root operation used for this procedure is Supplement, which is defined as putting in or on biological or synthetic material that physically reinforces and/or augments the function of a portion of a body part.

Using a Percutaneous approach, a needle is inserted into the sacrum, and a cement mixture is injected. CT or fluoroscopy is used to guide the percutaneous placement of the needle during the procedure and to monitor the injection procedure. Sterile biomaterial such as polymethyl methacrylate is injected along the fracture lines and acts as a bone cement to reinforce the fractured sacrum. The procedure does not restore the original shape to the sacrum, but it does stabilize the bone, preventing further fracture or collapse. Following the procedure, the patient may experience significant, almost immediate, pain relief.

Septoplasty, Deviated Nasal Septum

Body System
Ear, Nose, Sinus

PCS Root Operation
Reposition

Root Operation Table
Ø9S   Ear, Nose, Sinus, Reposition

Body Part
Nasal Septum

Approach
Open
Percutaneous Endoscopic

Description

Nasal septoplasty is a surgical procedure done to straighten a deviated or crooked nasal septum. The nasal septum separates the nasal passageways into right- and left-sided cavities and helps to support the nose. A deviated septum may be congenital or the result of trauma. When the septum is deviated (crooked), breathing can be difficult and result in snoring and sleep apnea. The intent of the procedure is to straighten the septum, which meets the root operation definition of Reposition.

With the patient under appropriate anesthesia, topical vasoconstrictive agents are applied to shrink the blood vessels, and local anesthesia is injected in the nasal mucosa. Using an Open approach, the physician makes an incision on one side of the nose, then makes a

vertical incision in the septal mucosa and elevates the mucoperichondrium from the septal cartilage. The deviated portion of the bony and cartilaginous septum is moved into appropriate position, removing any extra bone or cartilage. If the cartilaginous septum remains bowed, partial- or full-thickness incisions are made in the cartilage to straighten the septum. The septal mucosa is repositioned, and the incisions are closed in single layers. Transseptal sutures are placed. Septal splints may support the septum during healing.

Alternatively, a Percutaneous Endoscopic approach may be used. The physician reshapes the nasal septum, correcting airway obstruction. Topical vasoconstrictive agents are applied to shrink the blood vessels, and local anesthesia is injected in the nasal mucosa. The physician inserts the sinus endoscope, makes a vertical incision in the septal mucosa, and elevates the mucoperichondrium from the septal cartilage. The deviated portion of the bony and cartilaginous septum is repositioned. Excess cartilage is excised from the bone-cartilage junction. Incisions are closed in single layers. Transseptal sutures are placed. Septal splints may support the septum during healing.

Focus Point

The excision of excess septal bone or cartilage is inherent to the repositioning of the septum and is not reported separately.

© 2018 Optum360, LLC

Septostomy, Percutaneous, Atrial Balloon (Rashkind Procedure)

Body System
Heart and Great Vessels

PCS Root Operation
Bypass

Root Operation Table
021 Heart and Great Vessels, Bypass

Body Part
Atrium, Right

Approach
Percutaneous

Device
No Device

Qualifier
Atrium, Left

Description
Certain congenital heart defects, particularly those involving transposition of the great vessels, require surgical creation of a shunt, or opening in the interatrial septum (wall) that separates the upper right and left chambers of the heart.

Atrial balloon septostomy is usually performed as an emergency intervention to allow planning for further surgery. It involves making a small hole in the wall between the left and right atria of the heart using a balloon introduced via a thin flexible tube, which is inserted into the chambers of the heart. This reduces the pressure in the right side of the heart, allowing the heart to pump more efficiently. This improves blood flow to the lungs.

The physician places two catheters through small incisions: a central venous catheter and a second, special balloon-tipped catheter introduced from the femoral vein or the umbilical vein and threaded up to the heart. After vascular access is obtained and heparin is administered, the balloon catheter containing the deflated balloon is advanced into the right atrium through the femoral vein and inferior cava. From the right atrium, the catheter is advanced into the left atrium. The balloon is then inflated with diluted contrast material. Using fluoroscopic and endocardiographic guidance, the position of the balloon is then checked, making sure that it is in the appropriate position. The inflated balloon is drawn sharply back into the right atrium, and deflated. This inflation and deflation may be repeated several times, each time increasing the volume of the balloon until the created interatrial septal defect reaches the desired dimension. The balloon is then deflated and withdrawn through the catheter. The catheters are removed. Pressure is placed over the incision for 20 to 30 minutes to stem bleeding. A cardiac catheterization may be included. The patient is observed for a period afterward.

Focus Point
The approach value Percutaneous was added to table 021 Heart and Great Vessels, Bypass, for the body part value Atrium, Right, with the qualifier Atrium, Left, to capture percutaneous septostomy procedures.

Coding Guidance
AHA: 2017, 4Q, 55

Shunt, Endolymphatic

Body System
Ear, Nose, Sinus

PCS Root Operation
Bypass

Root Operation Table
Ø91   Ear, Nose, Sinus, Bypass

Body Part
Inner Ear, Right
Inner Ear, Left

Approach
Open

Device
Synthetic Substitute

Qualifier
Endolymphatic

Description
Meniere's disease (or syndrome), also known as endolymphatic hydrops, is an inner ear condition that can cause vertigo, tinnitus, a feeling of fullness or pressure in the ear, and hearing loss. The hearing loss can become permanent.

In endolymphatic shunt surgery, a very small silicone shunt is placed in the inner ear to drain excess endolymphatic fluid in patients with Meniere's disease, bypassing the endolymphatic sac, relieving the

pressure and the vertigo and preventing the progression of hearing loss.

Under general anesthesia, the patient is placed on the operating table with the head turned to one side with the affected ear exposed. Using an Open approach through a postauricular incision, the physician opens the mastoid bone and drills out the mastoid cavity. The posterior ear canal wall remains intact. The horizontal and posterior semicircular canals are visualized. Drilling is continued until the endolymphatic sac is identified. The physician may use a diamond burr to remove the bone around the sac (i.e., decompression). A hole is made in the outer layer of the endolymphatic sac, and a shunt, usually made of silicone, is inserted through the hole into the sac. The mastoid cavity is packed with absorbable packing, the outer incision is sutured, and a pressure dressing is applied.

Focus Point
This procedure is reported with the root operation Bypass because it uses a shunt (Synthetic Substitute) to alter the route of the passage of the endolymphatic fluid from the endolymphatic sac to the inner ear. Table Ø91 Ear, Nose, Sinus, Bypass, with the body part values Inner Ear, Right, and Inner Ear, Left, along with the qualifier value Endolymphatic, differs slightly from guideline B3.6a for bypass procedures, which normally are coded by identifying the body part bypassed "from" and the body part bypassed "to."

Medical and Surgical

© 2018 Optum360, LLC

Shunt, Transjugular Intrahepatic Portosystemic (TIPS)

See also Measurement, Portal Venous Pressure, under "Measurement and Monitoring" in the Medical and Surgical Related section

Body System
Lower Veins

PCS Root Operation
Bypass

Root Operation Table
061   Lower Veins, Bypass

Body Part
Portal Vein

Approach
Percutaneous

Device
Synthetic Substitute

Qualifier
Hepatic Vein

Description
Shunts are placed percutaneously to manage the complications of portal hypertension and control variceal bleeding and ascites that are caused by liver damage. Liver damage causes the blood to back up into the portal vein. The transjugular intrahepatic portosystemic shunt (TIPS) procedure alleviates this by routing the blood directly from the portal vein into the hepatic vein, bypassing the liver.

This Bypass procedure begins with the patient under general anesthesia or conscious sedation. The right internal jugular vein is accessed via Percutaneous approach, and a catheter is placed into the right hepatic vein. A needle is advanced through the catheter into the wall of the right hepatic vein to access the right portal vein. A guidewire and catheter are advanced along this route into the portal vein. A self-expanding metallic shunt is deployed through the catheter and dilated using an angioplasty balloon to the desired diameter where it bridges the portal and hepatic veins. Post-placement venography and portal pressure measurements confirm adequate position and flow through the TIPS (*see also* Measurement, Portal Venous Pressure). The balloon, and catheters are removed, and pressure is applied to the insertion site, which may require sutures, which are inherent to the procedure.

Focus Point
If an existing shunt becomes occluded and is declotted, the root operation Revision is used, defined as correcting, to the extent possible, a portion of a malfunctioning or the position of a displaced device. The only body part option available is the generic Lower Vein.

Coding Guidance
AHA: 2017, 4Q, 66; 2014, 3Q, 25

Sialoadenectomy

See also Parotidectomy

Body System
Mouth and Throat

PCS Root Operation
Excision

Resection

Root Operation Table
ØCB   Mouth and Throat, Excision

ØCT   Mouth and Throat, Resection

Body Part
Sublingual Gland, Right

Sublingual Gland, Left

Submaxillary Gland, Right

Submaxillary Gland, Left

Minor Salivary Gland

Approach
Open

Qualifier
Diagnostic (Excision)

No Qualifier

Description
Using an Open approach, the physician removes a portion or all of a salivary gland. Indications for surgery include an infected or blocked salivary gland, injured gland, or tumor. Depending on the specific gland (submaxillary [submandibular], sublingual) excised and the extent of the excision (partial or complete), surgical technique may vary:

- **Submaxillary (submandibular) gland:** The physician removes all or a portion of a diseased, infected, blocked, or injured submandibular gland. The physician makes an incision in the skin of the neck below the inferior border of the mandible and near the angle of the mandible. The underlying tissues are dissected to the submandibular gland. The gland is exposed, freed from the surrounding tissue, and removed. The incision is closed with sutures.

- **Sublingual gland:** The physician removes all or a portion of a diseased, infected, blocked, or injured sublingual gland. The physician makes an intraoral incision in the mucosa overlying the gland. Tissues are dissected down to the gland. The gland is exposed, freed from surrounding tissue, and removed. The incision is closed with sutures.

Focus Point
The qualifier Diagnostic is assigned when the documented purpose of the partial sialoadenectomy is diagnostic.

Focus Point
A partial sialoadenectomy is coded using root operation Excision, and a complete sialoadenectomy is coded using Resection. Resection of a specific body part is coded whenever all of that body part is cut out or off. The salivary glands have specific body parts for anatomical subdivisions and laterality. If the entire right parotid gland is removed, report Resection of the right parotid gland.

Focus Point
Review the operative report carefully to determine the full extent of areas excised or resected. Excision or Resection of the facial nerve or lymph nodes, for example, is not integral to the procedure and may be reported separately.

Focus Point
In ICD-10-PCS, the submandibular glands are included in the Submaxillary Gland, Left or Submaxillary Gland, Right body parts.

Coding Guidance
AHA: 2016, 2Q, 12; 2014, 3Q, 21

Medical and Surgical

© 2018 Optum360, LLC

Sialodochoplasty, Parotid Duct

Body System
Mouth and Throat

PCS Root Operation
Dilation

Repair

Root Operation Table
ØC7   Mouth and Throat, Dilation
ØCQ   Mouth and Throat, Repair

Body Part
Parotid Duct, Right
Parotid Duct, Left

Approach
Open

Device
Intraluminal Device (Dilation)
No Device (Repair)

Description

Sialodochoplasty is a surgical procedure that repairs the salivary duct by shortening it or enlarging the outflow opening to alleviate ductal outflow obstruction caused by stenosis or injury. It is often performed during a sialolithotomy.

Dilation
Using the appropriate anesthesia, the physician repairs a salivary duct by inserting a hollow plastic or silicone tube into the duct. Using an Open approach, either via an incision in the oral buccal mucosa or an incision via the face, the tube is threaded through the duct. The duct is allowed to heal and may be sutured around the tube. The tube is later removed, and patency is restored.

Repair
Another method of repair is to simply stitch the duct open. This permits shortening of the duct and enlarging the salivary outflow. After appropriate anesthesia, using either a transoral or facial Open approach, under loupe magnification the physician sutures the edges of the duct mucosa to the surrounding oral mucosa. An approach through the face may require insertion of temporary postoperative drains, which are not reported as devices.

> **Focus Point**
> See *Sialolithotomy for the removal of a stone causing obstruction.*

> **Focus Point**
> The ICD-10-PCS index lists multiple root operation cross-references under the main term "Sialodochoplasty." While the root operation Dilation is not included, this may be coded from the appropriate table without consulting the index if the intent of the procedure meets the definition of the root operation Dilation, which is expanding an orifice or the lumen of a tubular body part. Review the operative report, and select the appropriate root operation from the ICD-10-PCS tables.

© 2018 Optum360, LLC

Sialolithotomy

Body System
Mouth and Throat

PCS Root Operation
Extirpation

Root Operation Table
ØCC Mouth and Throat, Extirpation

Body Part
Parotid Duct, Right
Parotid Duct, Left
Parotid Gland, Right
Parotid Gland, Left
Sublingual Gland, Right
Sublingual Gland, Left
Submaxillary Gland, Right
Submaxillary Gland, Left
Minor Salivary Gland

Approach
Open
Percutaneous

Description
Sialolithotomy is a surgical procedure used to remove stones from a salivary gland or duct. Depending on the specific anatomic location (parotid, submaxillary [submandibular], sublingual), surgical technique and approach may vary.

In an Open approach, the physician makes an incision in the gland to remove a sialolith (a stone). An incision is made intraorally or extraorally in the skin overlying the gland and dissected to reach the stone, or the intraoral mucosa overlying the duct is incised. Tissue is dissected to the gland. The physician removes the stone. The incision may be sutured closed.

In a Percutaneous approach, a sialoendoscope is advanced to the gland. Once the stone has been located, a basket is used to remove the stone.

Focus Point
The removal of solid matter from a body part is coded using the root operation Extirpation. In Extirpation procedures, the body part itself is not the focus of the procedure. The objective is to remove solid material (an abnormal byproduct of a biological function or a foreign body) such as a foreign body, thrombus, or calculus from a body part.

Focus Point
As ICD-10-PCS does not provide a Percutaneous Endoscopic approach value for salivary gland procedures; Percutaneous approach is reported as the closest available equivalent.

Coding Guidance
AHA: 2016, 2Q, 20

© 2018 Optum360, LLC

Medical and Surgical

Sinuplasty (Balloon Sinuplasty, Balloon Sinus Dilation (BSD))

Body System
Ear, Nose, Sinus

PCS Root Operation
Repair

Root Operation Table
Ø9Q   Ear, Nose, Sinus, Repair

Body Part
Maxillary Sinus, Right
Maxillary Sinus, Left
Frontal Sinus, Right
Frontal Sinus, Left
Sphenoid Sinus, Right
Sphenoid Sinus, Left

Approach
Percutaneous Endoscopic

Description
Balloon sinuplasty is a minimally invasive treatment that provides relief of chronic sinusitis symptoms by opening blocked sinus passageways in the frontal, sphenoid, and maxillary sinuses with a small, flexible sinus balloon catheter. No tissue is removed, and there is minimal bleeding during the procedure.

The physician uses an endoscope for surgical access to perform balloon dilation of the sinuses. Following application of a vasoconstrictor and with the patient under appropriate anesthesia, the physician inserts a sinus guide cannula and positions it near the entrance of the involved sinus under endoscopic visualization. Using fluoroscopic guidance, the physician inserts a sinus guidewire through the cannula and into the sinus ostium. The physician advances a catheter with an attached balloon over the guidewire, through the cannula, and into the targeted sinus. Once correct placement is confirmed, the balloon is inflated using a radiopaque fluid. The balloon is left inflated for several seconds and then deflated; repositioning and reinflation may be necessary. Following deflation and removal of the balloon, the endoscope is used to inspect the sinus.

Focus Point
Repair is the most appropriate root operation to use for this procedure, as there is no specific code for dilation of the sinus. There is no sinus body part in the Ø97 Dilation, Ear, Nose and Sinus table.

Focus Point
If balloon sinuplasty procedures are performed on more than one designated sinus body part, a procedure code for each body part is reported separately using all appropriate body part values, according to guideline B4.3.

Coding Guidance
AHA: 2013, 4Q, 114

Sling Suspension, Urethral (Pubovaginal Sling)

Body System
Urinary System

PCS Root Operation
Reposition

Root Operation Table
ØTS   Urinary System, Reposition

Body Part
Urethra

Approach
Open
Percutaneous Endoscopic

Description
Pubovaginal sling procedures are performed to treat female urinary incontinence by providing support to the urethra, restoring the normal position of the urethra. This is reported with root operation Reposition.

Using an Open approach, incisions are made in the abdomen and vaginal walls. A sling, formed out of synthetic material or from fascia harvested from the sheath of the rectus abdominus muscle, is placed under the bladder and urethra. The sling is attached to the abdominal wall. The abdominal and vaginal incisions are closed in layers by suturing.

Using a Percutaneous Endoscopic approach, the physician inserts an instrument through the cervix into the uterus to manipulate the uterus. A small incision is made just below the umbilicus through which a fiberoptic laparoscope is inserted. A second incision is

made, and a second instrument is passed into the abdomen. The physician manipulates the tools so that the pelvic organs can be observed through the laparoscope. A sling, formed out of synthetic material or from fascia harvested from the sheath of the rectus abdominus muscle, is placed under the bladder and urethra. The sling is attached to the abdominal wall. The incisions are sutured closed.

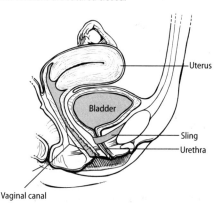

Focus Point
The sling repositions the angle of the misplaced urethra, restoring anatomic position, and thus meets the definition of root operation Reposition.

Coding Guidance
AHA: 2016, 1Q, 15

© 2018 Optum360, LLC

Sphincteroplasty, Pancreatic

Body System
Hepatobiliary System and Pancreas

PCS Root Operation
Repair

Root Operation Table
ØFQ   Hepatobiliary System and Pancreas, Repair

Body Part
Ampulla of Vater

Approach
Open

Percutaneous Endoscopic

Description
Pancreatic sphincteroplasty is performed on patients with chronic and acute pancreatitis as well as postcholecystectomy pain. It is also performed as a method to widen the distal bile duct to allow for passage of stones from the ampulla of Vater.

The physician performs a transduodenal pancreatic sphincteroplasty, which is the division of muscle around common bile and pancreatic ducts. Using an Open approach, the physician exposes the second portion of the duodenum via a subcostal or upper midline incision through skin, fascia, and muscle. The duodenum is opened using a longitudinal incision. The pancreatic sphincter is identified, and an incision is made at the two o'clock position. Sutures are placed on both sides of the incision. The common bile duct mucosa may be reapproximated to the duodenal mucosa and the duodenum transversely closed with interrupted sutures. The abdominal incision is closed.

In a Percutaneous Endoscopic approach, the sphincteroplasty is accomplished by making two small incisions through which the laparoscope and instruments are placed. The Percutaneous Endoscopic approach employs the same principles as the Open approach and is more widely used.

Sphincterotomy, Papillotomy Endoscopic Retrograde Cholangiopancreatography

Body System
Hepatobiliary System and Pancreas

PCS Root Operation
Drainage

Root Operation Table
ØF9   Hepatobiliary System and Pancreas, Drainage

Body Part
Ampulla of Vater

Approach
Via Natural or Artificial Opening Endoscopic

Device
Drainage Device

No Device

Description
An endoscopic retrograde cholangiopancreatography (ERCP) is an imaging procedure that uses a lighted endoscope and fluoroscopy to visualize the bile and pancreatic ducts. Bile duct obstructions in the ampulla of Vater, found during ERCP, are treated with sphincterotomy/papillotomy, which involves cutting into the bile duct to allow small gallstones and bile to drain.

The physician performs an ERCP with a sphincterotomy/papillotomy. Following administration of anesthesia, the physician passes the endoscope through the patient's oropharynx, esophagus, stomach, and into the small intestine (Via Natural or Artificial Opening Endoscopic approach). The ampulla of Vater is cannulated and filled with contrast. The common bile duct and the whole biliary tract, including the gallbladder, are visualized. The sphincter is cannulated using a sphincterotome. The sphincter is divided by making a small cut, allowing bile to drain, using electrocautery to control bleeding. A stent (Drainage Device) may be placed to allow continuous drainage. The endoscope is removed from the patient.

Focus Point
When ERCP is used to help perform a specific therapy, it is considered inherent in the procedure and not coded separately.

Focus Point
Code also any additional procedures performed with sphincterotomy, following ICD-10-PCS multiple procedures guidelines.

Spinal Tap (Lumbar Puncture)

Medical and Surgical

Body System
Central Nervous System and Cranial Nerves

PCS Root Operation
Drainage

Root Operation Table
009   Central Nervous System and Cranial Nerves, Drainage

Body Part
Spinal Canal

Approach
Percutaneous

Device
Drainage Device
No Device

Qualifier
Diagnostic
No Qualifier

Description
The spinal column and brain are encased in a sheath called the meninges. Within the meninges flows the cerebrospinal fluid (CSF), which circulates between the spine and brain, acting as a cushion and supplying nutrients.

A spinal tap or lumbar puncture can be a diagnostic and/or therapeutic procedure. For diagnostic assessment of the brain or spinal column, CSF may be aspirated for pathological examination. Often, the physician is looking for infective agents (indicating meningitis or encephalitis) or blood (indicating intracranial or spinal injury). Alternatively, CSF may be aspirated for therapeutic reasons; for example, to lower intracranial pressure (ICP).

The lumbar region of the spine is the usual site for spinal tap. Lumbar puncture (LP) is preferred due to the anatomical structure of the lumbar spine.

For LP, the patient is usually seated, leaning forward, but may be lying on one side with the knees drawn up to the chest, with the back flexed to widen the spaces between the vertebrae. The L3 and H4 vertebrae are located, and local anesthesia is administered. The lumbar puncture needle is inserted. In diagnostic cases, CSF is drawn through the needle into a syringe. In therapeutic cases, a catheter may be inserted and the fluid emptied into a reservoir. Pressure reading is performed with a manometer. When the tap is completed, the needle is removed and the wound is

dressed. In many cases, the patient lies prone to prevent fluid leakage.

Occasionally, in a therapeutic lumbar puncture, serial or repeated drainage may need to be performed. In these cases, to avoid the need for repeated punctures, a lumbar drainage catheter is left in place until it is no longer needed. Multiple pressure measurements may be obtained, depending on the type of drainage needed: draining a specified level or volume, or to keep a specific pressure. If the drainage device remains at the conclusion of the lumbar puncture procedure, report Drainage Device. If all catheters and tubes are removed at the conclusion of the procedure, report No Device.

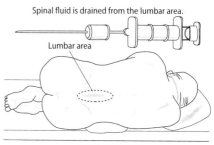

Spinal fluid is drained from the lumbar area.

Lumbar area

Spinal tap position

For both diagnostic and therapeutic spinal tap, the appropriate root operation is Drainage, which involves taking or letting out fluids and/or gases from a body part. The approach is Percutaneous, as the instrumentation (needle or catheter) is inserted through the skin and other body layers to reach the site of the procedure (spinal canal). For a diagnostic spinal tap, report the qualifier Diagnostic, and for a therapeutic tap report No Qualifier.

Focus Point
Fluid is drained from the spinal canal in a spinal tap. Therefore, the correct body part is Spinal Canal, not the Spinal Cord.

Focus Point
Documentation of a "dry" tap means no CSF was obtained. Root operation Inspection is coded when drainage is attempted and no cerebrospinal fluid can be obtained, because the full definition of the root operation Drainage is not met.

Coding Guidance
AHA: 2017, 1Q, 50; 2014, 1Q, 8

© 2018 Optum360, LLC

Splenectomy, Partial

Body System
Lymphatic and Hemic Systems

PCS Root Operation
Excision

Root Operation Table
Ø7B   Lymphatic and Hemic Systems, Excision

Body Part
Spleen

Approach
Open
Percutaneous Endoscopic

Qualifier
Diagnostic
No Qualifier

Description
In a partial splenectomy, the physician removes only a portion of the spleen, usually to treat pain caused by an enlarged spleen. A portion of the spleen may need to be removed for splenic cysts, benign tumors, metastases, splenic infarction, injury to the spleen, or congenital hemolytic anemias.

Using an Open approach, the physician makes a midline incision and dissects tissue around the spleen. The short stomach vessels are doubly ligated and cut. The splenic recess is dissected, the splenic artery and vein are divided and cut individually as needed, and the physician removes a portion of the spleen. A drain may be placed, and the wound is irrigated. The

physician closes the incision with sutures or staples and applies a dry sterile dressing.

In an alternative technique, the physician performs a splenectomy using a Percutaneous Endoscopic (laparoscopic) approach. With the patient under anesthesia, the physician makes a small incision in the abdominal wall and inserts a trocar just below or above the umbilicus. The physician insufflates the abdominal cavity and places the laparoscope through the umbilical incision. Additional small incisions are performed, and trocars are placed into the peritoneal space to be used as ports for instruments, video camera (the camera allows the physician to operate both by viewing through the laparoscope and on a video monitor), and/or an additional light source. Dissection is carried down to the level of the spleen with care taken to identify the tail of the pancreas. A portion of the spleen is excised using special instruments to ensure hemostasis. The freed splenic tissue is isolated and pouched. Pieces of the spleen are then suctioned from the pouch through a trocar. The laparoscope and trocars are removed. The incisions are closed with sutures.

Focus Point
If the spleen is partially removed for pathologic or histologic evaluation for diagnostic purposes, the qualifier Diagnostic is used. If the biopsy is obtained using fine needle aspiration (FNA), use root operation Extraction.

Focus Point
If the entire spleen is removed, see Splenectomy, Total.

Splenectomy, Total

Body System
Lymphatic and Hemic Systems

PCS Root Operation
Resection

Root Operation Table
Ø7T   Lymphatic and Hemic Systems, Resection

Body Part
Spleen

Approach
Open
Percutaneous Endoscopic

Description
Total splenectomy is a surgical procedure that removes the entire spleen. Indications for the removal of the spleen may include injury that has caused the spleen to rupture, cancer involving the spleen, or a blood disorder called idiopathic thrombocytopenic purpura (ITP).

There are two operative approaches to access the spleen for a total splenectomy. In an Open procedure, which is performed under general anesthesia, the physician makes an incision in the abdomen, ties the artery to the spleen, detaches the ligaments holding the spleen in place, and removes the spleen. A drain may be placed, and the wound is irrigated. The incision is closed with sutures or staples, and a dry sterile dressing is applied.

A laparoscopic splenectomy, using Percutaneous Endoscopic approach, is another alternative. The patient is placed in a right lateral decubitus position, left arm over the head. With the patient under anesthesia, the physician makes a small incision in the abdominal wall and inserts a trocar just below or above the umbilicus. The physician insufflates the abdominal cavity and places the laparoscope through the umbilical incision. Additional small incisions are performed, and trocars are placed into the peritoneal space to be used as ports for instruments, video camera (the camera allows the physician to operate both by viewing through the laparoscope and on a video monitor), and/or an additional light source. Dissection is carried down to the level of the spleen with care taken to identify the tail of the pancreas. Electrocautery is used to divide ligaments, and the spleen is mobilized. Short gastric vessels may be transected to gain additional exposure. The splenic vessels are transected, and the spleen is resected using special instruments to ensure hemostasis. The freed spleen is isolated and pouched. Pieces of the spleen are then suctioned from the pouch through a trocar. The laparoscope and trocars are removed. The incisions are closed with sutures.

Focus Point
Removal of only a portion of the spleen is reported with root operation Excision. See Splenectomy, Partial.

Focus Point
Resection of the entire spleen to stop acute bleeding is coded to Resection instead of Control. See ICD-10-PCS guideline B3.7.

Coding Guidance
AHA: 2015, 4Q, 13

© 2018 Optum360, LLC

Stapedectomy, with Prosthesis

Body System
Ear, Nose, Sinus

PCS Root Operation
Replacement

Root Operation Table
Ø9R   Ear, Nose, Sinus, Replacement

Body Part
Auditory Ossicle, Right
Auditory Ossicle, Left

Approach
Open

Device
Synthetic Substitute

Description
Stapedectomy is performed to correct the conductive type of hearing loss caused by otosclerosis, an abnormal growth of bone around the stapes bone that fixes the bone in place, limiting motion and sound transmission (conduction).

Stapedectomy with prosthesis is the removal of all or part of the fixed stapes (stirrup), one of the bones in the middle ear that conducts sound vibrations to the incus, a bone in the inner ear. The stapes is replaced with a tiny prosthesis, which can be made from many different materials, including Teflon, platinum, gold, stainless steel, and nitinol, a nickel titanium alloy. The most common type of stapes prosthesis is a piston with a wire loop on one end that is secured by crimping it around the incus. The prosthesis allows sound vibrations to be transmitted properly to the inner ear for hearing.

Under appropriate anesthesia, the patient is prepped and draped. The tympanic membrane is examined to ensure that there are no perforations. With the use of the operating microscope, using an Open approach through an ear canal incision, the eardrum is elevated and turned forward. The hearing bones are palpated, confirming the diagnosis of otosclerosis. A laser is used to vaporize parts of the stapes, freeing it from all attachments, including any adhesions, to allow placement of the prosthesis. The remainder of the stapes is removed with a curette. A small opening is made in the footplate of the stapes. The distance from the incus to the footplate is measured for the appropriate prosthesis size, and the prosthesis is placed into the opening and connected to the incus. Once the prosthesis is in place, the ossicular chain is tested for adequate mobility. Small pieces of Gelfoam may be placed around the prosthesis to ensure it remains in proper place. The eardrum is then returned to its normal position. The incision is closed, and packing is placed in the ear canal.

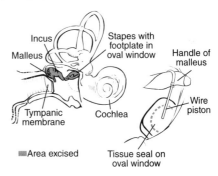

■Area excised   Tissue seal on oval window

Focus Point
According to the ICD-10-PCS Body Part Key, the stapes is included in the body parts Auditory Ossicle, Right and Auditory Ossicle, Left.

Suctioning, Bronchial (For Removal of Mucus Plug)

See also Lavage, Bronchoalveolar (BAL)

See also Washing, Bronchial

Body System
Respiratory System

PCS Root Operation
Extirpation

Root Operation Table
ØBC   Respiratory System, Extirpation

Body Part
Main Bronchus, Right
Upper Lobe Bronchus, Right
Middle Lobe Bronchus, Right
Lower Lobe Bronchus, Right
Main Bronchus, Left
Upper Lobe Bronchus, Left
Lingula Bronchus
Lower Lobe Bronchus, Left

Approach
Via Natural or Artificial Opening Endoscopic

Device
No Device

Qualifier
No Qualifier

Description
Bronchial washing is commonly performed to facilitate removal of unusually thick (inspissated) forms of mucus that accumulate within the airways, known as mucus plugs, or other debris that can partially or completely obstruct the bronchial airways and cause lung collapse. Mucus plugs can occur in diseases such as chronic obstructive bronchitis, bronchiectasis and asthma, and usually cannot be removed with forceps because they are too soft, but they are also often too thick to suction. Removal in these cases is done with bronchoscopic irrigation and suction.

After administering a mucolytic to loosen the secretions, the physician views the airway using a flexible fiberoptic or rigid bronchoscope (a long, thin tube that has a close-focusing telescope on the end for viewing) introduced Via Natural or Artificial Opening Endoscopic approach through the nasal or oral cavity, or a tracheostomy stoma. The airway is anesthetized with a topical anesthetic. The bronchoscope is inserted and advanced through the nasal or oral cavity, or the tracheostomy stoma, and past the larynx to inspect the bronchus. This procedure may employ fluoroscopic guidance.

After visualizing the bronchus, the physician removes the mucus plugs or debris by irrigating the bronchial tubes with saline followed by carefully suctioning the fluid. The bronchoscope is removed.

Focus Point
Root operation Extirpation, defined as "taking or cutting out solid matter from a body part," is reported, as the removal of the mucus plug is the intent of the procedure. A separate code is not required for the irrigation/washing done to facilitate the removal.

Focus Point
An additional code for fluoroscopic guidance may be reported, when performed.

Coding Guidance
AHA: 2017, 3Q, 14

© 2018 Optum360, LLC

Switch, Duodenal (Biliopancreatic Diversion)

See also Gastrectomy, Vertical Sleeve (VSG)

Body System
Gastrointestinal System

PCS Root Operation
Bypass

Root Operation Table
ØD1 Bypass, Gastrointestinal System

Body Part
Duodenum

Approach
Open
Percutaneous Endoscopic

Qualifier
Ileum

Description
The duodenal switch (DS), also known as biliopancreatic diversion with duodenal switch, is the second part of a weight-loss surgery that helps the patient feel full sooner and absorb fewer calories from the food that they eat. The first part is the vertical sleeve gastrectomy, which is the restrictive aspect and the second part is the duodenal switch, the malabsorptive portion. The entire procedure can be performed in conjunction with the gastrectomy in a one-encounter or two-stage surgery for patients with severe morbid obesity. In the two-stage procedure, the patient is required to lose a significant amount of weight after the first gastrectomy surgery before the patient undergoes the duodenal switch procedure.

After the first part of the surgery during which the vertical sleeve gastrectomy is performed, the pylorus-preserving duodenoileostomy and ileoileostomy is done to combine gastric restriction with limited intestinal absorption for weight loss. *See also* Gastrectomy, Vertical Sleeve (VSG).

The intent of the duodenal switch procedure is to make two separate, shorter channels and one common channel from one long piece of intestine. The shorter of the two separate pieces is the digestive loop that moves food from the stomach to the common channel. The longer piece is the biliopancreatic loop and carries bile from the liver to the common channel. In the common channel, the food from the digestive loop mixes with the bile from the biliopancreatic loop and empties into the large intestine. This configuration allows food to bypass the duodenum to the ilium,

reducing the amount of time during which calories and fat are absorbed into the body.

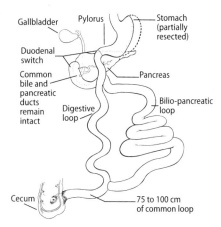

To perform this procedure, the provider divides the duodenum near the pyloric valve. The small intestine is also divided. The distal end of the small intestine in continuity with the large intestine is brought up and anastomosed to the short duodenal segment on the stomach. The other end of the small intestine—the duodenal segment in connection with the gallbladder and pancreas, or the biliopancreatic loop—is attached to the newly anastomosed other limb further down near the large intestine. This forms a 75 cm to 100 cm common loop where the contents of both these segments channel together before dumping into the large intestine.

Because this is a complex procedure, it is generally reserved for the super obese (BMI > 50kg/m2). The preferred method is laparoscopic, which is reported as Percutaneous Endoscopic, although it can be performed by Open approach or a combination of endoscopic and open, which is also reported as Open approach based on guideline B5.2. Since the contents of the body are being rerouted, the root operation Bypass is reported for this procedure with body part Duodenum and qualifier Ileum.

Focus Point
Per guideline B3.6a, for Bypass procedures, the body part describes the part bypassed "from" (Duodenum) and the qualifier represents the body part bypassed "to" (Ileum).

Coding Guidance
AHA: 2016, 2Q, 31

Switch Procedure, Arterial

Body System
Heart and Great Vessels

PCS Root Operation
Reposition

Root Operation Table
Ø2S   Heart and Great Vessels, Reposition

Body Part
Pulmonary Trunk

Thoracic Aorta, Ascending/Arch

Coronary Artery, Two Arteries

Approach
Open

Description
The arterial switch surgery is used to treat transposition of the great arteries. This congenital heart condition is characterized by a flip in the relationship of the great arteries, the aorta and pulmonary artery, to the right and left ventricles.

The physician gains access to the mediastinum using an Open approach via sternotomy. The physician places cardiopulmonary bypass catheters through incisions in the low inferior vena cava, the superior vena cava, and aorta or femoral artery. The physician stops the heart by infusing cardioplegia solution into the coronary circulation. The physician removes the pulmonary artery band placed during a previous surgery and dilates the pulmonary artery to normal size. If this is not possible, the physician removes the pulmonary band and constricted area of pulmonary artery and applies a woven Dacron patch over the hole. The physician removes the coronary ostia from the aortic root and sews them into the root of the pulmonary trunk. The pulmonary trunk and aortic root are each transected and interchanged to direct blood from the pulmonary veins through the left ventricle to the aorta, and the systemic venous drainage to the pulmonary trunk via the right ventricle.

The physician closes the cardiac incisions, takes the patient off cardiopulmonary bypass, closes the remaining surgical incisions, and dresses the sternal or chest wall wound. The physician may leave chest tubes and/or a mediastinal drainage tube in place following the procedure.

Focus Point
Concomitant repair of PDA and ASD are coded separately, and additional codes are assigned if a patch is used to reconstruct the aorta and/or the pulmonary trunk.

Focus Point
This procedure involves "switching" the aorta and pulmonary trunk and connecting them to the correct ventricles. The ostia of the coronary arteries, also called buttons, are also repositioned to the new aortic root.

Coding Guidance
AHA: 2016, 4Q, 102; 2015, 4Q, 22

© 2018 Optum360, LLC

Medical and Surgical

Sympathectomy, Thoracic Endoscopic (ETS)

Body System
Peripheral Nervous System

PCS Root Operation
Division

Excision

Root Operation Table
Ø18 Peripheral Nervous System, Division

Ø1B Peripheral Nervous System, Excision

Body Part
Thoracic Sympathetic Nerve

Approach
Percutaneous Endoscopic

Device
No Device

Qualifier
No Qualifier

Description
Endoscopic thoracic sympathectomy (ETS) is usually performed for hyperhidrosis (abnormal, excessive sweating) in the hands, armpits, and feet but can also be performed less commonly for chronic regional pain syndrome (CRPS)/reflex sympathetic dystrophy (RSD), Raynaud's disease, upper extremity ischemia, and other conditions. Using very small incisions and endoscopic instruments, the physician cuts or excises the sympathetic nerve chain to eradicate the excessive sympathetic nerve activity causing the condition.

Under general anesthesia, the patient is placed on the operating table and ventilated in one lung with an endobronchial tube. A small incision is made in the sixth intercostal space, and a port with an operative thoracoscope is inserted. The procedure is performed through the thoracoscope using a Percutaneous Endoscopic approach. If needed, two to three more ports may be placed for better visualization. Carbon dioxide insufflation is used to aid in deflating and retracting the lung for visualization. The sympathetic nerve chain is identified under the parietal pleura.

Sympathectomy is performed, starting on either side. Either the sympathetic chain is cut using cautery (Division), or a small segment of the nerve chain is excised (Excision). The cut ends of the sympathetic nerve chain are separated and cauterized to prevent regrowth of the nerve and recurrence of symptoms. Usually division is done at levels T2, T3 or T2-T5 for patients with hyperhidrosis, and at levels T1-T3 for RSD. A small chest tube is left in the chest and the subcutaneous tissue is sutured closed. After both lungs are expanded with positive pressure ventilation, the chest tube is quickly removed at positive pressure to avoid pneumothorax, and the opening is closed with sutures. The procedure may be repeated on the other side. Postoperative imaging is done to confirm complete expansion of the lungs.

Focus Point
Thoracic sympathectomy for CRPS/RSD may be done in conjunction with thoracic outlet decompression, but it is a separately reportable procedure. The thoracic outlet decompression is reported using root operation Release and body part Brachial Plexus.

Focus Point
Performance of the procedure with thoracoscopic assistance via a mini-thoracotomy approach is considered an Open approach even though it is minimally invasive. Procedures that are performed using the Open approach with percutaneous endoscopic assistance are coded to the approach Open, according to ICD-10-PCS guideline B5.2.

Focus Point
According to ICD-10-PCS guideline B4.3, if an identical procedure is performed on contralateral body parts and no bilateral body part value exists, each procedure is coded separately using the appropriate body part value.

Coding Guidance
AHA: 2017, 2Q, 19; 2017, 1Q, 36

Thoracentesis

Body System
Anatomical Regions, General

PCS Root Operation
Drainage

Root Operation Table
0W9 Anatomical Regions, General, Drainage

Body Part
Pleural Cavity, Right
Pleural Cavity, Left

Approach
Percutaneous

Qualifier
Diagnostic
No Qualifier

Description
Thoracentesis is the surgical drainage of the pleural cavity with a specialized needle or hollow tubing to aspirate air or fluid from within the pleural space for diagnostic or therapeutic reasons.

Two layers of pleura cover the lungs. The inner, visceral layer follows the fissures between the lobes of each lung. The outer, parietal layer overlies the fissures. Normally, fluid between the two pleural layers acts as a lubricant to absorb the motion of breathing so that the lungs do not rub against other structures in the chest. Fluid may be removed for pathologic examination for patients suspected of having pneumonia, empyema, cancer, or other disorders. Fluid also may be removed to reduce an overload of fluid in the pleural space that is a result of heart failure, cirrhosis of the liver, or other pathologies. In some cases, thoracentesis is performed to remove air from the pleural space. When air escapes from the lungs into the pleural space (pneumothorax), the lung collapses. Removal of the air allows the lung to reinflate. Thoracentesis is also called thoracocentesis or pleurocentesis.

In thoracentesis, a needle or catheter is inserted into the pleural cavity through the space between the ribs, and fluid or air is removed via negative pressure of a syringe or vacuum bottle. With the end of the needle in

the pleural space, the physician withdraws the fluid by pulling back on the plunger of the syringe. The patient is usually seated upright, leaning forward, during thoracentesis. Ultrasonography may be performed to localize the site and help with guiding the needle between two ribs and into the narrow space between pleural layers.

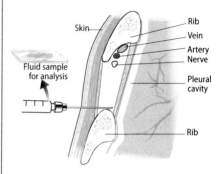

The root operation Drainage is coded for both diagnostic and therapeutic thoracentesis procedures. The approach value is Percutaneous.

Focus Point
ICD-10-PCS code assignment depends on the objective of the procedure (therapeutic or diagnostic). If a thoracentesis is documented as both therapeutic and diagnostic, the more definitive (therapeutic) treatment is reported.

Focus Point
When drainage is accomplished by putting in a catheter or tube that remains at the end of the procedure (thoracostomy), the device value Drainage Device is reported.

Focus Point
Thoracentesis is sometimes performed on a fetus, in which case the ICD-10-PCS section is Obstetrics and the body system is Products of Conception. The qualifier Fetal Fluid, Other is used to report pleural fluid.

© 2018 Optum360, LLC

Thoracoscopy (Diagnostic)

Body System
Anatomical Regions, General

PCS Root Operation
Inspection

Root Operation Table
ØWJ   Anatomical Regions, General, Inspection

Body Part
Pleural Cavity, Right
Pleural Cavity, Left

Approach
Percutaneous Endoscopic

Description
A diagnostic thoracoscopy uses an endoscope to visually examine the pleural cavity and its contents.

The physician examines the pleural cavity through the serous membrane using either a rigid or flexible fiberoptic endoscope. The procedure can be done under local or general anesthesia. The surgeon makes a small incision between two ribs and by blunt dissection and the use of a trocar enters the thoracic cavity. The endoscope is passed through the trocar and into the chest pleural cavity. The lung is usually partially collapsed by instilling air into the chest through the trocar, or if general anesthesia is used, the lung may be collapsed through a special double lumen endotracheal tube inserted through the mouth into the trachea. The contents of the chest cavity are examined by direct visualization and/or the use of a video camera. Still photographs may be taken as part of the procedure. At the conclusion of the procedure, the endoscope and the trocar are removed. A separately reportable chest tube for drainage and re-expansion of the lung is usually inserted through the wound used for the thoracoscopy.

Coding Guidance
AHA: 2015, 2Q, 31

Thoracostomy, Tube

Body System
Anatomical Regions, General

PCS Root Operation
Drainage

Root Operation Table
ØW9   Anatomical Regions, General, Drainage

Body Part
Pleural Cavity, Right
Pleural Cavity, Left

Approach
Percutaneous

Device
Drainage Device

Description
Two layers of pleura cover the lungs. The inner, visceral layer follows the fissures between the lobes of each lung. The outer, parietal layer overlies the fissures. Normally, fluid between the two pleural layers acts as a lubricant to absorb the motion of breathing so that the lungs do not rub against other structures in the chest. Fluid may be removed for pathologic examination for patients suspected of having pneumonia, empyema, cancer, or other disorders. Fluid also may be removed to reduce an overload of fluid in the pleural space that is a result of heart failure, cirrhosis of the liver, or other pathologies. In some cases, air may need to be removed from the pleural space. When air escapes from the lungs into the pleural space (pneumothorax), the lung collapses. Removal of the air allows the lung to reinflate.

In tube thoracostomy, a catheter is inserted into the pleural cavity and air or fluid is removed via a drainage system into a vacuum bottle. To enter the chest cavity, the physician makes an incision in the space between two ribs using a trocar and enters the pleural cavity. With the end of the trocar in the chest cavity, the physician advances the plastic tube into the chest cavity. The sharp trocar is removed, leaving one end of the plastic catheter in place within the chest cavity. A large syringe may be attached to the outside end of the catheter, and the air or fluid (blood, pus, or pleural fluid) is removed from the chest cavity by pulling back on the plunger of the syringe. The outside end of the tube may be connected to a drainage system, such as a water seal, to prevent air from being sucked into the chest cavity and to allow continuous or intermittent repeated removal of air or fluid. A chest x-ray is usually taken after the tube is inserted to confirm correct placement.

Because the thoracostomy tube remains in place at the end of the procedure, report Drainage Device.

Focus Point
In tube thoracostomy, a tube is placed to drain the pleural cavity. In thoracentesis, a syringe or catheter is used to aspirate from the pleural cavity.

Thrombectomy, Percutaneous Mechanical (Pharmacomechanical) (PMT)

Body System
Heart and Great Vessels
Upper Arteries
Lower Arteries
Upper Veins
Lower Veins

PCS Root Operation
Extirpation

Root Operation Table
02C   Heart and Great Vessels, Extirpation
03C   Upper Arteries, Extirpation
04C   Lower Arteries, Extirpation
05C   Upper Veins, Extirpation
06C   Lower Veins, Extirpation

Body Part
Refer to the ICD-10-PCS tabular list for a complete list of body parts.

Approach
Percutaneous

Description
Thrombectomy is performed to remove a thrombus, a stationary blood clot causing vessel obstruction. Percutaneous mechanical thrombectomy (PMT) involves the use of a catheter system with a mechanical attachment. It may be performed with devices categorized as rheolytic, using a high-pressure saline jet (AngioJet), or rotational (Trerotola, Amplatz) thrombectomy devices. These devices can be used alone or in combination.

Access to the occluded vessel is obtained using a Percutaneous approach. The physician isolates the targeted vessel and under radiologic guidance advances a percutaneously placed catheter into the vessel to the site of a thrombus or clot. Angiography is performed to confirm the location of the thrombus. Transcatheter removal of the thrombus is performed using suction, a snare basket, or a mechanical thrombectomy device under fluoroscopic guidance. Thrombolytic injections may also be used during the procedure. Pharmacomechanical thrombolysis involves both injection of thrombolytic and mechanical fragmentation of the clot. Suction is applied, and the clot fragments are removed through the catheter. The catheter is removed, and pressure is applied at the insertion site.

AngioJet thrombectomy uses a thin, flexible catheter tunneled to the site of the thrombus. High-speed water jets pull the thrombus into the catheter, crushing it into tiny fragments. The fragments are evacuated from the body through the catheter. The catheter is removed, and the incision is closed.

Focus Point
If a thrombus extends through two distinct tubular body parts and the thrombectomy is performed on a continuous section of one vessel into another, code the body part value corresponding to the furthest anatomical site from the point of entry. See ICD-10-PCS guideline B4.1c.

Coding Guidance
AHA: 2015, 1Q, 36; 2013, 4Q, 115

© 2018 Optum360, LLC

Medical and Surgical

Thyroidectomy

Body System
Endocrine System

PCS Root Operation
Excision
Resection

Root Operation Table
ØGB Endocrine System, Excision
ØGT Endocrine System, Resection

Body Part
Thyroid Gland Lobe, Left
Thyroid Gland Lobe, Right
Thyroid Gland, Isthmus
Thyroid Gland (Resection)

Approach
Open
Percutaneous Endoscopic

Qualifier
No Qualifier
Diagnostic (Excision)

Description
Thyroidectomy describes the removal of all or part of the thyroid gland. As an endocrine organ, the thyroid gland manufactures hormones and secretes them into the bloodstream. These hormones regulate metabolic functions, including heart rate, digestion, and body temperature. The average thyroid gland is approximately the size of a business card, with a half-inch thickness. The thyroid gland wraps around the trachea at the level of the fifth cervical vertebra. It is divided into two lobes that are connected by a small band, the isthmus.

Thyroidectomy may be indicated if the patient has a malignancy or if a benign disorder causes symptoms. Symptoms of a benign disorder include dysphagia, dyspnea, or vocal changes related to compression of the esophagus, trachea, or larynx due to thyroid hyperplasia. Hypersecretion of hormones also can cause metabolic symptoms and may lead to thyroidectomy, as in the case of refractory Graves' disease.

In an Open approach, the physician directly exposes the thyroid via a transverse cervical incision in the skin. The platysma muscles are divided, and the strap muscles are separated in the midline. The thyroid lobe to be excised is isolated, the vessels serving the lobe are ligated, and the isthmus is severed. The parathyroid glands are preserved. The thyroid tissue is divided in the midline of the isthmus over the anterior trachea. The thyroid lobe is resected, or a portion is excised. When the excision or resection is complete, the muscles are reapproximated and the skin incision is closed.

In a Percutaneous Endoscopic approach, the physician makes a small incision and dissects through the platysma and strap muscles until the superior pole of the thyroid is located, at which point the endoscope is inserted and minimally invasive video-assisted thyroidectomy (MIVAT) is performed using endoscopic dissector and aspirator tools. The thyroid tissue to be excised is isolated, the vessels serving the lobe are ligated, and the isthmus is severed. The parathyroid glands are preserved, and the thyroid tissue is cut and aspirated. When the excision or resection is complete, the instruments are removed and the muscles are reapproximated. The skin incision is closed.

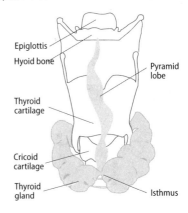

Both lobes of the thyroid gland are removed along with any tissues associated with the isthmus

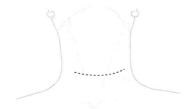

Typical incision for total thyroidectomy

Excision
If only a portion of the thyroid gland lobe is removed (body part Thyroid Gland Lobe, Right, Thyroid Gland Lobe, Left, or Thyroid Gland, Isthmus), the root operation is Excision. Excision may be performed for therapeutic and/or diagnostic purposes. Thyroid gland excision for diagnostic purposes is reported with the qualifier Diagnostic.

Thyroidectomy (continued)

Resection

Resection, which involves removal of all of a body part, is reported for the removal of the entire lobe of the thyroid gland (Thyroid Gland Lobe, Right, Thyroid Gland Lobe, Left, or Thyroid Gland, Isthmus) or the entire Thyroid Gland.

Focus Point

Resection includes all of a body part or any subdivision of the body part that has its own body part value. Removal of all of one of the Body Parts of the thyroid (right or left lobe or isthmus) is reported as Resection of the lobe or isthmus. If both the right and left thyroid lobes are removed, along with the isthmus, report Resection of Thyroid Gland. See ICD-10-PCS guideline B3.8.

Focus Point

If a thyroid biopsy is obtained using needle aspiration, use root operation Extraction, approach Percutaneous, and qualifier Diagnostic. If a diagnostic Extraction is followed by a therapeutic Excision or Resection at the same procedure site, both procedures are reported, according to ICD-10-PCS guideline B3.4b.

Focus Point

ICD-10-PCS classifies three body parts for the thyroid gland in the Excision table: Thyroid Gland Lobe, Right, Thyroid Gland Lobe, Left and Thyroid Gland, Isthmus. The Resection table also includes the body part Thyroid Gland. The thyroid gland also contains the isthmus, a small band of tissue that joins the right and left lobes. In less than a third of the population, there is a third "lobe" of the thyroid gland called the pyramidal. It is very small and arises from the medial anterior aspect of the isthmus. Excision or Resection of the pyramidal lobe or the isthmus is reported as an Excision, Thyroid Gland Isthmus.

Coding Guidance

AHA: 2017, 2Q, 20

© 2018 Optum360, LLC

Medical and Surgical

Tonsillectomy, Lingual

See also Epiglottopexy, Transoral Endoscopic

See also Excision, Lingual, Submucosal Minimally Invasive (SMILE)

Body System
Mouth and Throat

PCS Root Operation
Destruction

Excision

Root Operation Table
ØC5   Mouth and Throat, Destruction
ØCB   Mouth and Throat, Excision

Body Part
Pharynx

Approach
Via Natural or Artificial Opening Endoscopic

Qualifier
Diagnostic (Excision)
No Qualifier

Description
The lingual tonsils are lymphatic tissue located at the base of the tongue. Enlarged lingual tonsils may obstruct breathing airways, resulting in sleep apnea. Lingual tonsillectomy is a surgical procedure to remove or destroy the lingual tonsils.

Destruction
Lingual tonsillectomy is performed under general anesthesia, using the approach Via Natural or Artificial Opening Endoscopic with direct laryngoscopy. The physician uses electrocautery or laser ablation to destroy the lingual tonsils.

Excision
Lingual tonsillectomy is performed under general anesthesia, using the approach Via Natural or Artificial Opening Endoscopic with direct laryngoscopy. The physician removes one or both of the lingual tonsils using a scalpel, cold knife, or coblation wand. The

lingual tonsil tissue is removed, and bleeding controlled.

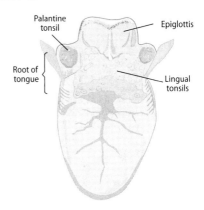

The lingual tonsils are surgically destroyed, usually by laser method via intraoral approach

Focus Point
According to the ICD-10-PCS Body Part Key, the lingual tonsils are included in body part Pharynx.

Focus Point
If the lingual tonsils are removed for pathologic or histologic evaluation for diagnostic purposes (e.g., neoplasm), the qualifier Diagnostic is used.

Focus Point
A coblation wand excises tissue with precision while minimizing heat to the surrounding tissue.

Focus Point
Lingual tonsillectomy is frequently performed with epiglottopexy. An additional code for the epiglottopexy is listed. See also Epiglottopexy, Transoral Endoscopic. For excision of base of tongue, see Excision, Lingual, Submucosal Minimally Invasive (SMILE).

Coding Guidance
AHA: 2016, 3Q, 28

Medical and Surgical

Tonsillectomy (Without Adenoidectomy)

Body System
Mouth and Throat

PCS Root Operation
Destruction

Excision

Resection

Root Operation Table
ØC5   Mouth and Throat, Destruction

ØCB   Mouth and Throat, Excision

ØCT   Mouth and Throat, Resection

Body Part
Tonsils

Approach
External

Qualifier
Diagnostic

No Qualifier

Description
During a tonsillectomy, the physician removes all or a portion of the tonsils. The tonsillectomy can be the first the patient has undergone, or a secondary procedure to remove tonsil regrowth since the primary procedure. In rare cases, a tonsillectomy may be performed to diagnose and/or remove neoplasms of the tonsils.

Destruction
Electrocautery (use of high-frequency electrical current to produce heat) or laser ablation is used to eradicate the tonsils via an External approach.

Excision
Using an External (intraoral) approach, the physician removes a portion of one or both of the tonsils by grasping the tonsil with a tonsil clamp and dissecting only the inflamed or diseased tonsil tissue. The tonsil tissue is removed, and bleeding vessels are clamped and tied. Bleeding may also be controlled using silver nitrate and gauze packing.

Resection
Using an External (intraoral) approach, the physician removes both of the tonsils completely by grasping each tonsil with a tonsil clamp and dissecting the capsule of the tonsil. The tonsils are removed, and bleeding vessels are clamped and tied. Bleeding may also be controlled using silver nitrate and gauze packing.

> **Focus Point**
> If the tonsils are removed for pathologic or histologic evaluation for diagnostic purposes (e.g. neoplasm), the qualifier Diagnostic is used.

> **Focus Point**
> The body part Tonsil is reported once whether one or both tonsils are removed. The tonsils are classified to a single ICD-10-PCS body part value, without a specific body part for anatomical subdivisions. If any tonsil tissue remains at the end of the procedure, report Excision rather than Resection. An Excision is coded when any portion of tonsil tissue is left behind.

> **Focus Point**
> When the procedure is performed in conjunction with an adenoidectomy, a separate code is needed for the adenoidectomy.

> **Focus Point**
> An External approach is used on procedures within an orifice on structures that are visible without the aid of instrumentation. See guideline B5.3a.

© 2018 Optum360, LLC

Tonsillectomy with Adenoidectomy

Body System
Mouth and Throat

PCS Root Operation
Destruction

Excision

Resection

Root Operation Table
ØC5   Mouth and Throat, Destruction

ØCB   Mouth and Throat, Excision

ØCT   Mouth and Throat, Resection

Body Part
Tonsils

Adenoids

Approach
External

Qualifier
Diagnostic

No Qualifier

Description
Tonsillectomy and adenoidectomy (T&A), the removal of both tonsils and adenoids, is a common and frequently performed procedure. It is often done to prevent recurrent infections, improve breathing, mitigate sleep apnea and snoring issues. In rare cases, a tonsillectomy and/or adenoidectomy may be performed to diagnose and/or remove neoplasms of the tonsils/adenoids.

Destruction
Electrocautery (use of high frequency electrical current to produce heat) or laser ablation is used to eradicate the tonsils and adenoids via an External approach.

Excision
Using an External (intraoral) approach, the physician removes a portion of one or both tonsils by grasping the tonsil with a tonsil clamp and dissecting only the inflamed or diseased tonsil tissue. The tonsil tissue is removed, and bleeding vessels are clamped and tied. Bleeding may also be controlled using silver nitrate and gauze packing. Using a mirror or nasopharyngoscope for visualization, the physician

uses an adenotome or a curette and basket punch to excise a portion of one or both of the adenoids.

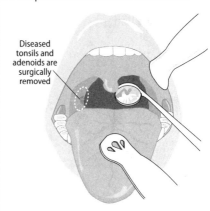

Diseased tonsils and adenoids are surgically removed

Resection
Using an External (intraoral) approach, the physician removes both tonsils completely by grasping each tonsil with a tonsil clamp and dissecting the capsule of the tonsil. The tonsils are removed, and bleeding vessels are clamped and tied. Bleeding may also be controlled using silver nitrate and gauze packing. Using a mirror or nasopharyngoscope for visualization, the physician uses an adenotome or a curette and basket punch to excise the adenoids.

> **Focus Point**
> If the tonsils and adenoids are removed for pathologic or histologic evaluation for diagnostic purposes, (e.g., neoplasm) the qualifier Diagnostic is used.

> **Focus Point**
> Two codes are needed, one for the removal of the tonsils and one for the removal of the adenoids. When both tonsils and/or adenoids are removed by either Excision or Resection, only one procedure is reported for each body part. Both the tonsils and adenoids are classified to single ICD-10-PCS body part values, without specific body parts for anatomical subdivisions. If any tonsil or adenoid tissue remains at the end of the procedure, report the root operation Excision rather than Resection. An Excision is coded when only part of the tonsil or adenoid is removed and there is a portion left behind.

> **Focus Point**
> An External approach is used on procedures within an orifice on structures that are visible without the aid of instrumentation. See guideline B5.3a.

© 2018 Optum360, LLC

Trabeculectomy Ab Externo

Body System
Eye

PCS Root Operation
Bypass

Root Operation Table
Ø81 Eye, Bypass

Body Part
Anterior Chamber, Right
Anterior Chamber, Left

Approach
Percutaneous

Device
No Device

Qualifier
Sclera

Description

Trabeculectomy ab externo (from the outside), or ab externo trabeculectomy (AET), also known as fistulization of sclera, is a common surgical procedure performed to treat refractory primary open-angle glaucoma (POAG) by lowering intraocular pressure (IOP) of aqueous humor (clear, watery fluid circulating in the chamber of the eye between the cornea and the lens). A portion of the blocked drainage channels of the trabecular mesh is removed, creating a new opening that bypasses the blocked portion and allowing the fluid to drain into a new channel in the space between the conjunctiva and the sclera or cornea.

Under appropriate anesthesia, the patient is prepped and draped appropriately. The physician places an ocular speculum in the patient's eye and accesses the anterior chamber through a small incision through the limbus (the corneal-scleral juncture).To promote better drainage of fluid, the physician removes a partial-thickness portion of the ring of meshlike tissue at the iris-scleral junction (the trabecular meshwork). A scleral trap door is left open so that aqueous may flow through the new channel into the space between the conjunctiva and the sclera or cornea (bleb). The route of passage of the fluid is thus altered to a new location in the body. The physician closes the incision with

sutures and may restore the intraocular pressure with an injection of water or saline. A topical antibiotic or pressure patch may be applied.

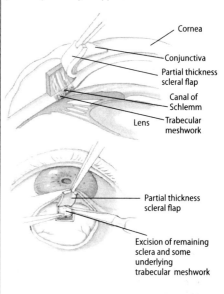

Focus Point

ICD-10-PCS categorizes the body parts Anterior Chamber, Right and Anterior Chamber, Left as tubular body parts included in the bypass tables. The root operation Bypass is defined as "Altering the route of passage of the contents of a tubular body part." Bypass procedures require that the body part bypassed from (anterior chamber) and body part bypassed to (sclera) be specified, according to guideline B3.6a.

Focus Point

The anterior chamber is the fluid-filled cavity behind the cornea. A Percutaneous approach is used since the anterior chamber is reached by going through the corneal-scleral juncture.

Coding Guidance

AHA: 2016, 4Q, 22

© 2018 Optum360, LLC

Medical and Surgical

Trabeculoplasty, Laser

Body System
Eye

PCS Root Operation
Drainage

Root Operation Table
Ø89   Eye, Drainage

Body Part
Anterior Chamber, Right
Anterior Chamber, Left

Approach
Percutaneous

Description
Laser trabeculoplasty is used for the treatment of glaucoma. This procedure uses a laser to selectively burn the ring of meshlike tissue at the iris-scleral junction (the trabecular meshwork) to improve the drainage of fluids in the anterior segment. After application of a topical anesthetic, a special contact lens is placed on the patient's eye. This lens allows the physician to view the angle structures of the eye and the trabecular network while using the laser. The laser is focused on the iris, and multiple short bursts of laser light create holes in the iris. This procedure allows fluids in the eye to pass from behind the iris through the openings into the space between the iris and the cornea (the anterior chamber) and lowers intraocular pressure.

Though the trabecular network runs along the entire circumference of the iris, holes are burned in only a portion of that circumference during a single treatment session. In this way, the effects of each treatment upon the eye's fluid can be measured and treatment suspended once the proper intraocular fluid pressure is reached. No incision is made during this procedure.

There are two general types of laser trabeculoplasty: argon laser trabeculoplasty (ALT) and selective laser trabeculoplasty (SLT). The laser used in SLT works at lower power levels than an argon laser. It treats only "selective" cells while leaving the trabecular meshwork intact, which allows for repeat application and results in less scarring.

Focus Point
The anterior chamber is the fluid-filled space behind the cornea. A Percutaneous approach is used since the anterior chamber is reached by going through the cornea.

Coding Guidance
AHA: 2016, 2Q, 21

Tracheostomy

Medical and Surgical

Body System
Respiratory System

PCS Root Operation
Bypass

Root Operation Table
ØB1   Respiratory System, Bypass

Body Part
Trachea

Approach
Open
Percutaneous
Percutaneous Endoscopic

Device
Tracheostomy Device

Qualifier
Cutaneous

Description

In respiration, air is inhaled through the nose or mouth and carried into the trachea, leading to the bronchial tubes for an oxygen exchange in the lungs. In tracheostomy, a stoma is surgically created as an air conduit for the trachea to the exterior through an incision in the skin of the neck. In this way, the cervical trachea and oropharynx are bypassed and air can pass directly through the stoma and into the distal trachea for respiration.

A tracheostomy may be performed on a patient who is on mechanical ventilation long-term or one who has suffered trauma or neurological damage. In some cases, infection or malignancy may lead to tracheostomy.

In an Open approach, the physician creates a tracheostomy by making a horizontal neck incision and dissecting the muscles to expose and visualize the trachea. The thyroid isthmus is cut if necessary. The trachea is incised, and an airway is inserted. After bleeding is controlled, a stoma is created by suturing the skin to the tissue layers. This may be a planned or an emergency procedure.

The physician creates a tracheostomy by inserting a needle using a Percutaneous approach through the skin of the neck and into the trachea. A cannula is threaded over the needle. The cannula is secured with sutures. One type of percutaneous tracheostomy is percutaneous transtracheal jet ventilation (PTJV). In PTJV, a catheter is inserted through the cricothyroid

membrane. The catheter is attached to a high-pressure oxygen supply.

Percutaneous dilatational tracheostomy (PDT) is typically performed at the bedside as opposed to a tracheostomy done in the operating room using the traditional open surgical approach. Percutaneous dilatational tracheostomy involves making an incision in the skin over the tracheal cartilage and inserting a needle and guide wire into the trachea. The physician uses a dilator to enlarge the opening, then inserts a standard tracheostomy tube. Bronchoscopy may be performed synchronously to visualize and confirm the placement of the needle, guide wire, and dilator.

Report a Percutaneous Endoscopic approach if the tracheostomy tube is inserted with visualization of the operative site via an endoscope inserted percutaneously through the skin into the trachea.

Regardless of the approach, report tracheostomy tube insertion with the device Tracheostomy Device and the qualifier Cutaneous to show that the root operation Bypass is performed from the trachea to the skin.

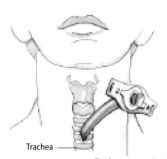

Trachea

Tracheostomy tube

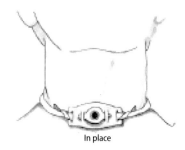

In place

© 2018 Optum360, LLC

Tracheostomy (continued)

Focus Point

Tracheostomy is defined as a permanent or semipermanent airway established into the trachea through the skin of a patient's neck, while tracheotomy is defined as a temporary incision into the trachea. Report a code from root operation table 0B1 when tracheostomy is performed (Bypass). Report a code from root operation table 0B9 when tracheotomy is performed (Drainage).

Focus Point

Review documentation of the tracheostomy procedure carefully. Do not report a new tracheostomy insertion procedure when the tracheostomy tube is only being replaced or changed. Report instead code 0B21XFZ Change Tracheostomy Device in Trachea, External Approach.

Focus Point

If a laryngoscope or bronchoscope is used only to confirm the placement of a percutaneous tracheostomy, do not code the endoscopic guidance (inspection) separately. Inspection of a body part(s) performed to achieve the objective of a procedure is not coded separately. See ICD-10-PCS guideline B3.11a.

Coding Guidance
AHA: 2014, 4Q, 3

Tracheostomy Revision (Stomaplasty)

See also Tracheostomy

See also Tracheostomy Tube Change

Body System
Anatomical Regions

PCS Root Operation
Repair

Root Operation Table
0WQ Anatomical Regions, General, Repair

Body Part
Neck

Approach
External

Qualifier
Stoma

Description
During a tracheostomy, a stoma is surgically created as an air conduit for the trachea to the exterior through an incision in the skin of the neck, and a tracheostomy tube is inserted. In this way, the cervical trachea and oropharynx are bypassed and air can pass directly through the stoma and into the distal trachea for respiration. For patients with longer-term presence of a tracheostomy, complications such as narrowing (stenosis) of the stoma due to scar tissue or the development of bumps (granulation tissue) can arise that require repair of the stoma.

The physician revises a tracheal stoma. Using an External approach, the physician incises the stoma area and resects redundant scar or granulation tissue. The skin is re-anastomosed and sewn to the stoma in sutured layers.

Focus Point

For initial insertion of the tracheostomy or creation of a new tracheostomy stoma, see Tracheostomy.

Focus Point

See Tracheostomy Tube Change when the procedure performed is a change of the tracheostomy tube.

Tracheostomy Tube Change

See also Tracheostomy

See also Tracheostomy Revision (Stomatoplasty)

Body System
Respiratory System

PCS Root Operation
Change

Root Operation Table
ØB2   Respiratory System, Change

Body Part
Trachea

Approach
External

Device
Tracheostomy Device

Description
During a tracheostomy, a stoma is surgically created as an air conduit for the trachea to the exterior through an incision in the skin of the neck, and a tracheostomy tube is inserted. In this way, the cervical trachea and oropharynx are bypassed and air can pass directly through the stoma and into the distal trachea for respiration. The first tracheostomy tube change is usually performed by a surgeon a few days after placement of the original tube to confirm that the tracheostomy site is healing properly. Additional tube changes are needed if the tube falls out or becomes plugged.

Using an External approach, the physician gently removes the indwelling tracheostomy tube. A new tube is inserted, taking care not to damage the trachea. The skin around the tube is cleaned.

Focus Point

Root operation Change is used when a device is exchanged for another device that is the same or similar, without making an incision or puncturing the skin or mucous membrane. Except in the Obstetrics section, root operation Change is always coded using an External approach.

Focus Point

For the initial insertion of a tracheostomy, see Tracheostomy.

Medical and Surgical

© 2018 Optum360, LLC

Transfer, Lymph Node (LNT)

Body System
Lymphatic and Hemic Systems

PCS Root Operation
Repair

Root Operation Table
07Q   Lymphatic and Hemic Systems, Repair

Body Part
Lymphatic, Head
Lymphatic, Right Neck
Lymphatic, Left Neck
Lymphatic, Right Upper Extremity
Lymphatic, Left Upper Extremity
Lymphatic, Right Axillary
Lymphatic, Left Axillary
Lymphatic, Thorax
Lymphatic, Internal Mammary, Right
Lymphatic, Internal Mammary, Left
Lymphatic, Mesenteric
Lymphatic, Pelvis
Lymphatic, Aortic
Lymphatic, Right Lower Extremity
Lymphatic, Left Lower Extremity
Lymphatic, Right Inguinal
Lymphatic, Left Inguinal

Approach
Open

Device
No Device

Qualifier
No Qualifier

Description
The lymphatic system is a network of vessels that carry lymphatic fluid throughout the body, draining from the tissues into the blood. Lymphedema is a progressive, painful disorder in which excessive lymph fluid is unable to drain normally and accumulates in the tissues, causing swelling, usually in the arms and legs.

Postmastectomy syndrome is a form of lymphedema that occurs after excision of the axillary lymphatic structures during mastectomy. Edema in the arms and hands develops from pooling of interstitial fluids due to reduced lymphatic circulation. Lymphedema can often be treated with nonsurgical interventions, such as medications, compression, massage therapy, and diet modification, to reduce the swelling and discomfort. To treat chronic lymphedema or as a preventative measure, surgical intervention such as lymph node transfer (LNT) may be performed.

LNT involves moving lymph nodes with an attached blood supply. These newly transferred lymph nodes then drain the obstructed lymphatic fluid and promote new growth of lymphatic vessels (lymphangiogenesis).

With the patient under general anesthesia, the surgeon injects a fluorescent indocyanine green (ICG) dye through a central venous line. The dye lights up, mapping the pathway of the lymphatic system in the affected area. The lymphatic vessels are identified, and using an Open approach, the surgeon harvests the lymph nodes along with the attached vessels from an area of the body such as the abdomen, groin, or supraclavicular area. Accurate location of the recipient site is determined using intraoperative ICG lymphangiography to detect lymphatic leakage. The surgeon also uses a second Open approach in this area by creating an incision and excising any scar tissue to repair the recipient site. The surgeon, using microscopic instruments and suture techniques, connects the new lymph vessels and blood vessels in the area of lymphatic obstruction. Patency is confirmed with dye and imaging, and the incisions are closed under the microscope to avoid damaging the anastomoses. Blood loss is minimal.

Focus Point
The intent of a lymph node transfer is to move a lymph node with attached vasculature from one location in the body to another location, restoring lymphatic drainage to the affected body part. This would more appropriately meet the root operation definition of Reposition, which is "moving to its normal location, or other suitable location, all or a portion of a body part." There are, however, no lymph node body part options available in table 07S Lymphatic and Hemic Systems, Reposition. The root operation Repair is used instead, as the closest available alternative.

Coding Guidance
AHA: 2017, 1Q, 34

Transplant, Heart

Body System
Heart and Great Vessels

PCS Root Operation
Transplantation

Root Operation Table
Ø2Y   Heart and Great Vessels, Transplantation

Body Part
Heart

Approach
Open

Qualifier
Allogeneic
Syngeneic
Zooplastic

Description
Heart replacement procedures are reserved for patients suffering from end-stage heart disease, recalcitrant to other treatment options. This is reported with the root operation Transplantation as it involves taking a living heart from another individual or an animal to physically take the place and/or take over all or part of the function of the patient's heart. The recipient heart does not have to be removed, and the donor heart does not have to entirely take over the recipient's heart's function to report the root operation Transplantation.

The patient is placed on cardiopulmonary bypass. Other supportive measures such as temporary pacing wires, intra-aortic balloon pump, or transfusion catheters may be used during the procedure.

Cardiac transplantation may be performed by one of two techniques: total orthotopic heart replacement or heterotopic implantation. A total orthotopic heart replacement is the most common and involves excising the ventricles, atrial appendages, and most of the coronary sinus from the donor heart. It involves removing the recipient heart and replacing it with the donor heart. A heterotopic transplant involves leaving the recipient heart in place and connecting the donor

heart to the recipient heart to act as a support to the donor heart.

Under general anesthetic, using an Open approach via a median sternotomy, the recipient heart is opened. The atria, aorta, and pulmonary artery of the recipient heart are anastomosed to the donor heart. The sinoatrial nodes of both the donor and recipient heart are left intact. The recipient heart is removed and replaced with the donor heart in a total orthotopic heart replacement. In a heterotopic implantation, the donor's organs are placed by sewing the left atrium of the donor heart to the left atrium of the recipient and sewing together the atrial septum and the right atrium. The donor aorta is trimmed to an appropriate length and sewn to the ascending aorta of the recipient. Immunosuppressive drugs may be given to the patient before, during, and after the operation. Cardiopulmonary bypass and temporary auxiliary procedures are discontinued when the donor heart begins functioning in the recipient.

Orthotopic heart transplant using a porcine or other animal heart is reported with the qualifier Zooplastic. The qualifier Allogenic is used when the donor heart comes from another person who may or may not be related. The qualifier Syngeneic would be reported only when the donor heart comes from a person who is genetically identical to the recipient, such as an identical twin.

Focus Point
Auxiliary procedures such as the use of transfusion catheters, intra-aortic balloon pumps, and temporary pacing that are routinely done to support the heart transplant procedure are not coded separately, with the exception of cardiopulmonary bypass, which is reported as Performance of Cardiac Output, Continuous. However, when continued after surgery, these procedures are considered more extensive than the temporary support required during the procedure and may be separately reported.

Coding Guidance
AHA: 2013, 3Q, 18

© 2018 Optum360, LLC

Transplant, Kidney

Body System
Urinary System

PCS Root Operation
Transplantation

Root Operation Table
ØTY   Urinary System, Transplantation

Body Part
Kidney

Approach
Open

Qualifier
Allogenic
Syngeneic

Description
Kidney transplantation is the replacement of a nonfunctioning kidney with a healthy kidney from a donor. It is often used to treat chronic renal failure or end-stage renal disease. Donor kidneys can be obtained from a living or nonliving (cadaveric) kidney donor. Since this procedure involves taking a functioning, living kidney from another individual to physically take the place and/or function of the patient's kidney, the root operation of Transplantation is reported.

The removal of a living donor's kidney is typically performed laparoscopically since traditional open surgery requires a larger incision in the side between the ribs and the hip and also involves the removal of a donor's rib. Once the donor kidney has been removed, the transplant procedure is the same for either a living or a cadaveric kidney donor.

During kidney transplant surgery, an Open approach is used to make an incision in the transplant recipient's abdomen, usually on the lower right side, and the donor kidney is placed near the bladder on the right side of the recipient's pelvis. The recipient's own kidneys are often not removed. The physician attaches the donor ureter to the recipient's bladder, allowing urine to flow normally from the new kidney, and restores the blood supply to the donor kidney by connecting it to the recipient's blood vessels.

Focus Point
The qualifier Allogenic is used when the donor kidney comes from another person who may or may not be related. The qualifier Syngeneic is reported only when the donor kidney comes from a person who is genetically identical to the recipient, such as an identical twin.

Transplant, Liver

Body System
Hepatobiliary System and Pancreas

PCS Root Operation
Transplantation

Root Operation Table
ØFY Hepatobiliary System and Pancreas, Transplantation

Body Part
Liver

Approach
Open

Qualifier
Allogeneic
Syngeneic
Zooplastic

Description
Liver transplant procedures are performed on patients with end-stage liver disease. Since this procedure involves taking a functioning, living liver from another individual or an animal to physically take the place of and/or function as the patient's liver, the root operation of Transplantation is reported.

The physician performs a partial or whole liver transplantation using an Open approach. With the patient under general anesthesia, the physician makes an abdominal incision. The hepatic arteries, bile duct, cystic duct, and hepatic duct are all ligated. The donor liver is placed in an acceptable position in the upper abdominal cavity that is not the normal liver bed location. Anastomoses are created between the donor hepatic vessels and the appropriate recipient vessels. The donor bile duct is approximated to the recipient

bile duct or to a limb of small bowel for drainage. The physician then places drains and closes the abdominal incision.

The qualifier Allogenic is used when the donor liver comes from another person who may or may not be related. The qualifier Syngeneic would be reported only when the donor liver comes from a person who is genetically identical to the recipient, such as an identical twin. Orthotopic liver transplant using a porcine or other animal liver is reported with the qualifier Zooplastic.

Focus Point
The orthotopic technique is used in the majority of liver transplants. Division of all ligaments attached to the liver along with the common bile duct, hepatic artery, portal vein, and the hepatic vein are part of the liver resection. The retrohepatic portion of the inferior vena cava is also removed during this resection. The new donor liver involves the anastomoses of the inferior vena cava, portal vein, and hepatic artery, and bile duct anastomosis to the native bile duct or small intestine. The anastomoses are not coded separately because they are considered components of the surgery.

In a domino liver transplant, the patient with familial amyloidosis receives a liver transplant to treat his or her condition. Since the patient's explanted liver function is good and with no cirrhosis, the liver can be transplanted in another patient. There is no specific ICD-10-PCS code to describe a domino liver transplant. To indicate that a domino liver transplant was performed, assign a code for Transplantation of Liver and a code for Resection of Liver.

Coding Guidance
AHA: 2014, 3Q, 13; 2012, 4Q, 99

© 2018 Optum360, LLC

Transplant, Lung

See also Transplant, Heart

See also Perfusion, Respiratory Donor Organ (EVLP) (ex-vivo lung perfusion), under "Extra-corporeal or Systemic Therapies" in the Medical and Surgical Related section

Body System
Respiratory System

PCS Root Operation
Transplantation

Root Operation Table
ØBY   Respiratory System, Transplantation

Body Part
Upper Lung Lobe, Right
Middle Lung Lobe, Right
Lower Lung Lobe, Right
Upper Lung Lobe, Left
Lung Lingula
Lower Lung Lobe, Left
Lung, Right
Lung, Left
Lungs, Bilateral

Approach
Open

Qualifier
Allogeneic
Syngeneic
Zooplastic

Description
A lung transplant is performed to replace diseased lung(s) with healthy lung(s) from an organ donor. Lung transplantations may involve two lungs, a single lung, or a lobe of a lung. Bilateral lung transplantation is also referred to as double-lung transplantation or en bloc transplantation and involves sequential excision and implantation of both lungs.

Most donated lungs are taken from deceased donors. In a living transplant, however, a living, healthy person donates one lung lobe. Most lobar transplantations involve one lobe from each of two living donors. Lung transplants may be performed for diseases such as chronic obstructive pulmonary disease (COPD) including emphysema, cystic fibrosis, idiopathic pulmonary fibrosis, and sarcoidosis.

An allogeneic transplant comes from a nonidentical donor of the same species who is compatibility matched for blood and tissue. The donor can be a family member or an unrelated person. A syngeneic transplant involves an organ from a genetically identical member of the same species, usually an identical twin, but can be a sibling who is a close enough match genetically to be immunologically compatible. Zooplastic transplants involve transplanting living organs from one species to another.

Depending on the transplant procedure being performed, various incision sites can be used to access the operative site. The physician may make a long, midline vertical incision through all of the layers of the skin down to the sternum bone. The sternum is split and the chest cavity entered. For a single lung transplant, the incision might be made on the side of chest where the lung will be replaced. For a bilateral sequential transplant, the incision could also be made horizontally across the chest below the breasts. The recipient's original lung is deflated, the root of the lung is isolated, and the major arteries and veins that carry blood to and from the heart are identified and divided. The main bronchial tube to that lung or lobe is severed and the lung or lobe is removed. The donor lung or lobe is placed in the chest cavity, and the bronchial tube and arteries and veins are sutured to the patient where the lung or lobe was attached. Circulation and functioning of the donor organ are ensured, and the chest is closed. The incision is closed with sutures and surgical staples in layers. A sternal incision is closed with sternal wires. Chest tubes are inserted into the chest cavity for drainage and to allow the transplanted lungs to fully expand.

Focus Point
Lung transplants are commonly performed in conjunction with heart transplants. Combined heart-lung transplantation requires a code for each body part defined by distinct values of the body part character, according to ICD-10-PCS guideline B3.2.a.

Focus Point
Cardiopulmonary bypass is an exception to the usual practice of not reporting supporting procedures that are components of a larger operation. When a surgical procedure is performed with cardiopulmonary bypass, it is coded as an additional procedure from table 5A1. Any other auxiliary procedures done to support the surgical procedure are not reported unless they are continued beyond the operative episode.

Focus Point
ICD-10-PCS contains multiple specific body parts for anatomical subdivisions of the lungs. Follow multiple procedure guideline B3.2.a to assign the appropriate code or code combinations for lung transplantation.

Transplant, Meniscus

See also Meniscectomy, Knee

Body System
Lower Joints

PCS Root Operation
Replacement

Root Operation Table
ØSR   Lower Joints, Replacement

Body Part
Knee Joint, Right
Knee Joint, Left

Approach
Open

Device
Nonautologous Tissue Substitute

Description
The meniscus is made up of cartilage that cushions the joint and provides a smooth surface for motion and rotation of the knee joint. The knee has two menisci, located on either side, that cushion the knee joint to facilitate weight bearing and joint movement. Damaged or torn meniscus cartilage can result in wear of the articular cartilage, causing pain and eventually osteoarthritis. As an alternative to knee replacement surgery after other surgical methods have failed, a meniscus transplant is performed to replace torn meniscal cartilage in the knee using cadaver donor meniscus. Meniscus transplant is typically performed on younger patients who do not exhibit symptoms of arthritis.

Imaging is done to size-match the donor meniscus to the recipient knee. The physician makes 1 cm-long portal incisions on either side of the patellar tendon for arthroscopic access into the knee joint. The arthroscope and a tibial guide are placed through portal holes. The native meniscal cartilage is removed, including resectioning the native horns. Pins are placed at posterior and anterior horn locations, suture tunnels are drilled over the pins, and sutures are passed. The anterior portal is widened, and both the anterior and posterior sutures are brought out together. The donor meniscus is brought in through the widened incision, and sutures are placed through each horn of the donor meniscus. The posterior and

anterior horn sutures are drawn out through the tibial tunnel and secured to the tibial bone. Meniscal repair techniques are used to suture the donor meniscus securely to the capsule, placing knots directly over the capsule. Routine closure is performed.

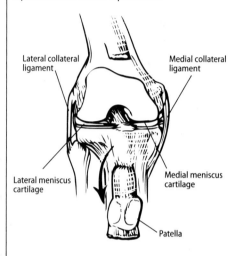

Focus Point

Focus Point
According to the ICD-10-PCS Body Part Key, the meniscus is included in the body parts Knee Joint, Right and Knee Joint, Left.

Focus Point
There is no bilateral body part value in ICD-10-PCS for the knees. Therefore, if identical procedures are performed on both knees, report two codes using the body part values Knee Joint, Right and Knee Joint, Left.

Focus Point
Although this procedure is done arthroscopically, Open is the only approach option in ICD-10-PCS for root operation Replacement in the Lower Joints body system. The intent of this procedure is to replace torn meniscal cartilage in the knee using cadaver donor meniscus.

Focus Point
When the meniscus is removed but not replaced, see Meniscectomy, Knee.

© 2018 Optum360, LLC

Transplant, Uterus

Body System
Female Reproductive System

PCS Root Operation
Transplantation

Root Operation Table
ØUY   Female Reproductive System, Transplantation

Body Part
Uterus

Approach
Open

Device
No Device

Qualifier
Allogeneic
Syngeneic

Description
Uterine transplantation is currently being performed in clinical trials with the goal of providing fertility to women of childbearing age (between ages of 21 to 39) who have absolute uterine factor infertility (AUFI). Women with AUFI have a malformation of the uterus or a complete absence of the uterus that prevents embryo implantation or completion of pregnancy to term and have no other options to give birth to their own child.

When a uterine transplant is performed, the uterus, but not the fallopian tubes, from a living or deceased donor is implanted. Recipients require in vitro fertilization before the transplant, with the embryos cryopreserved, ready for transfer to the transplanted uterus after recovery, healing, organ stability, and menstrual function are achieved. Unlike during a typical menstrual cycle, the unfertilized egg released by the ovary does not travel to the uterus because the fallopian tubes are not connected. Instead, the previously cryopreserved embryo is placed into the uterus for the woman to become pregnant.

The recipient starts antirejection medications to prepare for the transplant and remains on a reduced dosage of these medications, which are monitored during the pregnancy. The patient's pregnancy is also monitored by a high-risk obstetrics team, and delivery is done by cesarean section. The patient may need monthly cervical biopsies to test for organ rejection.

These types of transplants are intended to be temporary, as the uterus is not a life-sustaining organ. After one or two successful pregnancies, the transplant recipient has a hysterectomy to avoid the need for lifetime antirejection medications.

With the patient under general anesthesia, using an Open approach, the surgeon makes an incision into the pelvic cavity. Depending on the patient's anatomy, the malformed uterus and cervix may be removed. The supporting pedicles containing the ligaments and arteries are clamped and cut free. The donor uterus arteries and veins are connected via end-to-side vascular anastomoses to the external iliac arteries and veins. The fallopian tubes and nerves are not connected; sensation is absent in the uterus. The vaginal tissues of the donor uterus are connected to the recipient's vagina with sutured anastomosis, and the uterus is securely sewn into the pelvis for stability for future pregnancies. The abdomen is closed in layers, and temporary surgical drains may be placed.

Focus Point
The qualifier Allogenic is used when the donor uterus comes from another person who may or may not be related. The qualifier Syngeneic is reported only when the donor uterus comes from a person who is genetically identical to the recipient, such as an identical twin. The qualifier Zooplastic is an available option in the ICD-10-PCS table, but currently uterine transplants from animals to humans are not being performed.

Focus Point
In transplant procedures, the native body part may or may not be taken out, and the transplanted body part may take over all or a portion of its function.

Medical and Surgical

Transposition, Nerve

Body System
Central Nervous System and Cranial Nerves
Peripheral Nervous System

PCS Root Operation
Reposition

Root Operation Table
00S Central Nervous System and Cranial Nerves, Reposition
01S Peripheral Nervous System, Reposition

Body Part
Refer to the ICD-10-PCS tabular list for a complete list of body parts.

Approach
Open
Percutaneous Endoscopic

Description
Pain and numbness can result from a nerve being compressed or irritated. Nerve transplantation or transposition is one technique used to alleviate these symptoms whereby a nerve is moved to another location.

The physician moves an intact nerve to a new position (transposition). Nerve transplantation or transposition can be performed using either an Open or Percutaneous Endoscopic (laparoscopic) approach. When the procedure employs open surgery, an incision is made overlying the nerve. The laparoscopic technique involves only small incisions, just large enough for trocars and instrumentation to fit that enable the physician to visualize the site and perform the procedure. The physician dissects the nerve free from the surrounding tissue and moves the nerve to a new position. If the nerve is in bone and must be decompressed, freed, or moved, the overlying bone is first removed using drills and/or osteotomes. Reposition is the root operation used when a body part is moved to its normal location or to another suitable location.

Focus Point
If the partially attached nerve is being moved to another location to be anastomosed to a damaged or diseased nerve to take over the function of that nerve, the root operation is Transfer. If another body part is compressing the nerve and that body part is removed or altered to decompress the nerve, the root operation Release is reported.

Coding Guidance
AHA: 2014, 4Q, 35

© 2018 Optum360, LLC

Turbinectomy, Submucous Resection

Body System
Ear, Nose, Sinus

PCS Root Operation
Destruction

Excision

Root Operation Table
095   Ear, Nose, Sinus, Destruction

09B   Ear, Nose, Sinus, Excision

Body Part
Nasal Turbinate

Approach
Open

Qualifier
Diagnostic (Excision)

No Qualifier

Description
A submucous turbinectomy is removal of the turbinate bones and/or soft tissue. The nasal turbinates are scrolled, spongy bones covered with mucosa in the nasal passages. There are three pairs of nasal turbinates on each side, divided by the nasal septum—the inferior (largest), middle, and superior. Turbinectomy is most often performed on the inferior nasal turbinates.

Turbinectomy, also called turbinate reduction surgery, is often performed to treat chronic sinusitis but may also be indicated in the presence of neoplasm or other structural abnormalities that obstruct the airway (e.g., obstructive sleep apnea). The intent of the procedure is to reduce the size of the turbinate(s) and open up the nasal airway, regardless of the surgical method used.

Destruction
This code describes turbinectomy by electrocautery, laser, diathermy, or cryosurgery. The physician removes a part or all of the inferior turbinate bone through a submucous incision using an Open approach. The physician places vasoconstrictive drugs on the turbinate to shrink the blood vessels. A full-thickness incision is made over the anterior-inferior surface of the turbinate and continued deep to bone. The physician lifts the mucoperiosteum with an elevator to expose the bony

turbinate. The bony turbinate is destroyed using laser (ablation), high-frequency electrical current (diathermy), or freezing (cryosurgery). The turbinate mucosa may be closed in a single layer, or electrocautery may be used to control the bleeding. The nasal mucosa may be sutured in single layers. The nasal cavity may be packed with gauze.

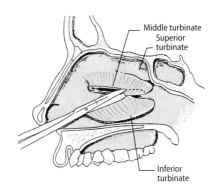

Middle turbinate
Superior turbinate
Inferior turbinate

Excision
The physician removes a part or all of the inferior turbinate bone through a submucous incision in an Open approach. The physician places vasoconstrictive drugs on the turbinate to shrink the blood vessels. A full-thickness incision is made over the anterior-inferior surface of the turbinate and continued deep to bone. The physician lifts the mucoperiosteum with an elevator to expose the bony turbinate. A chisel or forceps is used to remove portions of the bony turbinate. Electrocautery may control bleeding. The turbinate mucosa is closed in a single layer.

Focus Point
When the nasal turbinates are completely removed, Resection is used as the root operation. This is not routinely done as it often results in empty nose syndrome.

Focus Point
Turbinectomy is commonly performed in conjunction with other, separately reportable procedures, such as rhinoplasty, septoplasty, or sinus surgery.

Ureteroneocystostomy

Body System
Urinary System

PCS Root Operation
Bypass

Root Operation Table
ØT1   Urinary System, Bypass

Body Part
Ureter, Right
Ureter, Left
Ureters, Bilateral

Approach
Open
Percutaneous Endoscopic

Device
No Device

Qualifier
Bladder

Description
Ureteroneocystostomy is a surgical procedure that removes diseased or damaged portions of the distal ureter close to the ureteral orifice and reimplants the remaining ureter into a new site in the bladder. It is often performed to treat vesicoureteral reflux (VUR), as well as injury, stricture, or obstruction of the distal ureter.

Using an Open approach to access the bladder and ureters, the physician makes a midline incision in the skin of the abdomen and cuts the corresponding muscles, fat, and fibrous membranes (fascia). The physician mobilizes the bladder, ureter(s), and the major vesical blood vessels. The ureter is transected proximal to the damaged area. The physician brings the cut end of the ureter through a stab wound in the bladder and sutures the ureter to a new section of the bladder. To provide support during healing, the physician inserts a ureteral catheter, bringing the tube end out through the urethra or a bladder incision. The physician inserts a temporary drain tube and performs layered closure.

In a Percutaneous Endoscopic approach, the physician makes a midline lower abdominal incision and uses a laparoscope/cystoscope to access the bladder and ureters. The Percutaneous Endoscopic approach employs the same principles as the Open approach.

Focus Point
Bypass procedures require that the body part bypassed from and body part bypassed to be specified, according to guideline B3.6a.

Focus Point
A temporary drain is not coded as a device, according to guideline B6.1b.

Focus Point
This alteration of the site reroutes the passage of contents to a new (neo) but similar route using the same body part. This fits the definition of Bypass and in this example, since part of the remaining ureter was used for the conduit, No Device value is appropriate.

Coding Guidance
AHA: 2015, 3Q, 34

© 2018 Optum360, LLC

Ureteroplasty

Body System
Urinary System

PCS Root Operation
Excision

Replacement

Root Operation Table
ØTB   Urinary System, Excision
ØTR   Urinary System, Replacement

Body Part
Ureter, Right
Ureter, Left

Approach
Open
Percutaneous Endoscopic

Device
No Device (Excision)
Autologous Tissue Substitute (Replacement)
Synthetic Substitute (Replacement)
Nonautologous Tissue Substitute (Replacement)

Qualifier
Diagnostic (Excision)
No Qualifier

Description
Ureteroplasty is a surgical procedure used to treat urethral strictures. Scar tissue from previous surgeries, trauma, or another medical condition can form in the ureters, restricting urine flow. This can cause urine to collect in the kidneys, resulting in urinary tract and kidney infections.

When performing ureteroplasty, the physician uses plastic surgery to correct an obstruction or defect in the ureter. Ureteroplasty can be performed using either an Open or Percutaneous Endoscopic (laparoscopic) approach. For open surgery, an incision is made in the side over the ribs or in the abdomen. The laparoscopic technique involves only small incisions, just large enough for trocars and instrumentation to fit, that enable the physician to visualize the site and perform the procedure.

Excision
After appropriate anesthesia is administered to the patient and the physician gains entry to the operative site using either an Open or a Percutaneous Endoscopic (laparoscopic) approach, a catheter is inserted into the bladder through the ureter to drain urine. The physician removes the narrowed portion of the ureter, and absorbable sutures are used to stitch the cut end of the ureter together. A slender tube (stent) may be inserted into the ureter to provide support during healing. The physician may place a drain tube, bringing it out through a separate stab incision in the skin, and performs layered closure.

> **Focus Point**
> Although the PCS index lists Repair as a root operation, Excision best fits the description of the procedure since a portion of the body part is removed. The root operation Repair is used only when the method to accomplish the repair is not one of the other root operations.

> **Focus Point**
> If the ureter is removed for pathologic or histologic evaluation for diagnostic purposes, the qualifier Diagnostic is used.

Replacement
If a large portion of the ureter is removed, autograft tissue taken from another part of the body (often the bladder) may be used to replace the excised portion of the ureter. Anastomosis is done using absorbable sutures. Use the appropriate device values for Autologous Tissue Substitute, Synthetic Substitute or Nonautologous Tissue Substitute, depending upon the device used in the Replacement procedure.

> **Focus Point**
> If an autograft is obtained from a different body part, a separate procedure is coded, according to guideline B3.9.

> **Focus Point**
> Anastomosis of a tubular body part is considered integral to the procedure and is not coded separately, according to guideline B3.1b.

> **Focus Point**
> When the root operation Replacement is used, the excision of the body part is included in the Replacement definition.

Urethropexy (Retropubic Urethral Suspension)

Body System
Urinary System

PCS Root Operation
Reposition

Root Operation Table
ØTS   Urinary System, Reposition

Body Part
Urethra

Approach
Open
Percutaneous Endoscopic

Description
Urethropexy, the surgical procedure used to treat stress incontinence in male or female patients, involves suturing the urethra to parts of the pubic bone or ligaments that serve as an anchor and provide stability. This type of procedure is also commonly referred to as retropubic suspension surgery.

Using a Percutaneous Endoscopic approach, a small incision is made just below the umbilicus through which a fiberoptic laparoscope is inserted. A second incision is made on the left or right side of the abdomen, and a second instrument is passed into the abdomen. The tools are manipulated so that the pelvic organs can be observed through the laparoscope. The bladder is suspended by placing several sutures through the tissue surrounding the urethra and into support structures. The sutures are pulled tight so that the urethra is elevated and moved forward. The instruments are removed, and incisions are closed with sutures.

Urethropexy may also be performed via an Open approach. A horizontal incision is made in the abdomen above the symphysis pubis, otherwise known as a "bikini line incision." The bladder is suspended by placing several sutures through the tissue surrounding the urethra and into support structures. The sutures are pulled tight, and the urethra is moved forward. The incision is closed by suturing.

The Burch and Marshall-Marchetti-Krantz (MMK) are two retropubic urethropexy procedures commonly performed. The Burch technique involves suturing the urethra and bladder to the pectineal ligaments; the MMK procedure attaches these organs to the pubic bone or fascia behind the pubic bone.

Focus Point

The objective of this Reposition procedure is to move the urethra back into its normal anatomic position.

© 2018 Optum360, LLC

Uvulopalatopharyngoplasty

See also Tonsillectomy with Adenoidectomy

Body System
Mouth and Throat

PCS Root Operation
Excision

Resection

Root Operation Table
ØCB   Mouth and Throat, Excision

ØCT   Mouth and Throat, Resection

Body Part
Soft Palate

Uvula

Pharynx

Approach
Open

External

Description
Uvulopalatopharyngoplasty (UPPP) is a surgical procedure used to treat breathing issues, snoring, and obstructive sleep apnea. It involves removing excess tissue in the throat to make the airway wider. Tissues removed during this procedure may include all or part of the uvula, soft palate (roof of mouth), and pharyngeal tissue on the sides of throat and may include adenoids and tonsils.

During the procedure, which is performed under general anesthesia, the physician removes elongated and excessive tissues of the uvula, soft palate, and pharynx. Using an Open approach, incisions are made in the soft palate mucosa, and a wedge of mucosa is excised. Excessive submucosal tissue is removed. Using an External approach, the uvula is partially or completely excised, after which the midline at the uvula is sutured closed. The physician closes the remaining mucosa in a single layer, reapproximating the soft palate and thus increasing the diameter of the oropharynx. If tonsils and adenoids have not been previously removed, they may also be removed during this same operative episode.

> **Focus Point**
> *A code is needed for each body part excised or resected as noted in guideline B3.2a.*

> **Focus Point**
> *Resection is used as the root operation when the entire body part is excised; Excision is used when part of the body part is removed.*

> **Focus Point**
> *The External approach is performed directly on the skin or mucous membrane. Open approach is used when cutting through the mucous membrane and any other body layers necessary to expose the site of the procedure. The excision or resection of the submucosal (below the mucosa) tissue via an incision is therefore an Open approach.*

Medical and Surgical

Valvotomy (Valvulotomy)

Body System
Heart and Great Vessels

PCS Root Operation
Dilation
Release

Root Operation Table
027   Heart and Great Vessels, Dilation
02N   Heart and Great Vessels, Release

Body Part
Aortic Valve
Mitral Valve
Pulmonary Valve
Tricuspid Valve

Approach
Open
Percutaneous
Percutaneous Endoscopic

Device
Intraluminal Device, Drug-eluting (Dilation)
Intraluminal Device (Dilation)
No Device

Description
Valvotomy is an operation used to restore blood flow through a valve that is abnormally narrowed due to stenosis, scarring, inflammation, or congenital deformity. A percutaneous balloon dilation procedure is most commonly performed.

Dilation
The root operation Dilation is coded when the objective of the procedure is to enlarge the diameter of a tubular body part or orifice. Dilation includes intraluminal or extraluminal methods. A device placed to maintain the new diameter that remains at the conclusion of the procedure is an integral part of the Dilation procedure and is coded to a sixth-character device value in the Dilation procedure code.

Dilation of the heart valve is performed percutaneously using a balloon-tipped catheter that is guided into the heart from an artery in the arm or the groin. Once in the opening of the valve, the balloon is inflated to enlarge the opening.

Release
Release is the freeing of fused leaflets by incising along the edges of the leaflets or by separating the leaflets with the force of a finger.

Release procedures are coded to the body part being freed and can be performed on the area around a body part, on the attachments to a body part, or between subdivisions of a body part that are causing the abnormal constraint.

> **Focus Point**
> Typically, balloon dilation is documented as valvuloplasty in an operative report; however, the objective of the procedure is the same.

> **Focus Point**
> Release should not be confused with Division. Division involves incising and separating a body part, while Release involves incising restraining tissue such as scar tissue or adhesions.

> **Focus Point**
> Commissurotomy (surgical incision of the junction between cusps of a cardiac valve) performed with the objective of dilating the valve is integral to the Dilation procedure and is not reported separately.

Coding Guidance
AHA: 2016, 1Q, 16

© 2018 Optum360, LLC

Medical and Surgical

Valvuloplasty

See also Wedge Resection, Mitral Valve Leaflet

Body System
Heart and Great Vessels

PCS Root Operation
Dilation
Repair
Replacement
Supplement

Root Operation Table
027   Heart and Great Vessels, Dilation
02Q   Heart and Great Vessels, Repair
02R   Heart and Great Vessels, Replacement
02U   Heart and Great Vessels, Supplement

Body Part
Aortic Valve
Mitral Valve
Pulmonary Valve
Tricuspid Valve
Chordae Tendineae

Approach
Open
Percutaneous
Percutaneous Endoscopic

Device
Intraluminal Device, Drug-eluting (Dilation)
Intraluminal Device (Dilation)
No Device (Dilation, Repair)
Autologous Tissue Substitute (Replacement, Supplement)
Zooplastic Tissue (Replacement, Supplement)
Synthetic Substitute (Replacement, Supplement)
Nonautologous Tissue Substitute (Replacement, Supplement)

Qualifier
Transapical (Replacement, Aortic Valve, Mitral Valve, Pulmonary Valve, Percutaneous)
Truncal Valve (Repair, Supplement, Aortic Valve)
Atrioventricular Valve, Left (Repair, Supplement, Mitral Valve)
Atrioventricular Valve, Right (Repair, Supplement Tricuspid Valve)
No Qualifier

Description
The terminology of valvuloplasty is broadly used to describe different procedures that involve repairing or even replacing a heart valve or its components.

Valvuloplasty is used to treat damaged, leaky, prolapsed, enlarged, or elongated valves or to enlarge the opening of a stenotic valve.

Related procedures may be performed as an open heart surgery with open sternotomy and direct visualization of the heart valve (Open approach), or as a minimally invasive (Percutaneous) procedure through a smaller incision in the chest wall with direct catheter access through the ascending aorta or transapical through the bottom of the heart or via a transcatheter (Percutaneous) approach.

Dilation
Dilation of the heart valve due to stiff or calcified leaflets is performed using a Percutaneous approach. The physician inserts a catheter into the femoral artery in the groin or radial artery in the arm and advances it through the aorta to the opening of the stenotic valve. A balloon at the tip of the catheter is inflated, which pushes aside the stiff or calcified leaflets and dilates the opening of the valve.

Repair
The physician uses an Open approach with a small incision into the sternum. Various suturing techniques are employed on the damaged leaflets, ruptured chordae tendineae, or around the valve opening to reduce or repair the diameter of the opening.

The root operation Repair is a "not elsewhere classified" value and is used only when the procedure performed is not reported with one of the other root operations in the Medical and Surgical section.

Replacement
A replacement procedure involves resecting the entire diseased heart valve and putting in a replacement valve (device).

Performing an Open sternotomy, the physician resects the diseased heart valve and replaces it with a device made of human tissue (Autologous Tissue Substitute or Nonautologous Tissue Substitute), animal tissue (Zooplastic Tissue), or a valve that was manufactured (Synthetic Substitute). The resection of the valve is integral to the Replacement procedure.

Alternatively, the physician may employ a Percutaneous transcatheter approach, which involves destroying the native heart valve tissue by balloon deployment in the valve with subsequent insertion of a replacement valve (device) that is of human tissue (Autologous Tissue Substitute or Nonautologous Tissue Substitute), animal tissue (Zooplastic Tissue), or a valve that was manufactured (Synthetic Substitute). Many valves use both animal and synthetic materials, these are considered Zooplastic devices.

Valvuloplasty (continued)

Supplement

The ring around the heart valve can stretch out and lose shape, which results in enlargement of the opening with improper valve closing. To rectify this, the physician, using either an Open sternotomy incision or a minimally invasive or Percutaneous transcatheter approach, sews a ring (device) around the valve. The device supplements the leaflets and brings them together. This is also known as "annuloplasty." Depending on the valve involved, other techniques include anchored pledgets connected by string, or clips.

Focus Point

A mitral valve wedge resection is another technique designed to reverse closure defects of the mitral valve. This procedure, performed with an Open approach, excises part of the redundant leaflet tissue. This is referred to as a mitral valve wedge resection but may be included in the broad terminology of valvuloplasty. See also Wedge Resection, Mitral Valve Leaflet.

Focus Point

The balloon dilation in a Percutaneous Replacement procedure would not be reported separately as this procedure must be performed for the replacement valve to be placed.

Focus Point

Decalcification of a valve may be reported separately as Extirpation when it is the only procedure performed. When decalcification is performed in preparation for another definitive surgery, report only the definitive surgery.

Coding Guidance

AHA: 2016, 2Q, 25, 26; 2015, 4Q, 22; 2015, 2Q, 23; 2013, 3Q, 3

© 2018 Optum360, LLC

Medical and Surgical

Vasectomy

Body System
Male Reproductive System

PCS Root Operation
Excision

Root Operation Table
ØVB   Male Reproductive System, Excision

Body Part
Vas Deferens, Right
Vas Deferens, Left
Vas Deferens, Bilateral

Approach
Open
Percutaneous
Percutaneous Endoscopic

Description
Vasectomy is a permanent contraceptive procedure in which a segment of the vas deferens is excised to prevent spermatozoa from being released during ejaculation. The vas deferens is also called the ductus deferens.

The testes are suspended in the scrotum by the spermatic cord, which contains nerves, blood vessels, lymphatics, and the vas deferens. The cord is encased in fascia. The vas deferens continues from the scrotum over the superior public ramus to above and behind the urinary bladder, where it enters the prostate and forms the ejaculatory duct.

Spermatozoa are manufactured in the bilateral testes and stored in the epididymides, where they mature. Spermatozoa enter the vas deferens during sexual arousal. During ejaculation, spermatozoa mix with fluid from the seminal vesicles and the prostate gland. This fluid is released from the ejaculatory duct into the urethra. After vasectomy, the patient still produces semen, but the semen contains no spermatozoa.

In an Open vasectomy, an incision is made through the scrotal wall to expose the tubular structures within, and another incision is made to expose the vas deferens, which is dissected free of adjacent structures. The isolated vas deferens is cut in two places, and the intervening section of vas deferens is removed. The cut ends of the vas deferens are cauterized and sutured closed. The operative site is closed in layers. The same procedure is performed on the contralateral vas deferens to effect the sterilization of the patient.

A Percutaneous vasectomy is often called the no-scalpel vasectomy (NSV). In NSV, the surgeon uses fingertips to find the spermatic cord within the scrotum and positions the vas deferens against the scrotal skin, where it is clamped with an open ring clamp. The vas deferens is pinched by the clamp, and the skin overlying it is incised. The vas deferens is pulled out of the skin, and a segment is excised. The remaining ends may be cauterized. The cauterized ends are allowed to retract back into the scrotum. The small incision usually does not require suture. The same procedure is performed on the contralateral vas deferens to effect the sterilization of the patient.

In a Percutaneous Endoscopic vasectomy, the vasa deferentia of the patient are severed during a separate laparoscopic procedure; for example inguinal hernia repair. The patient's abdomen is insufflated, and several portals through the skin provide access for surgical tools, lighting, and camera. The vasa deferentia are isolated in the inguinal ring or abdominal cavity, and a segment of each is removed. The remaining ends may be cauterized. No scrotal incisions are made.

Focus Point
A vasectomy performed during a separate laparoscopic procedure would be reported in addition to the code for the primary procedure. Any procedure that meets the reporting criteria for a separate procedure is coded separately in ICD-10-PCS.

Focus Point
A vasectomy is normally done on both sides and would be reported with the body part Vas Deferens, Bilateral.

Ventriculostomy

See also Monitoring, Intracranial Pressure, under "Measurement and Monitoring" in the Medical and Surgical-Related section

Body System
Central Nervous System and Cranial Nerves

PCS Root Operation
Bypass
Drainage

Root Operation Table
001 Central Nervous System and Cranial Nerves, Bypass
009 Central Nervous System and Cranial Nerves, Drainage

Body Part
Cerebral Ventricle

Approach
Percutaneous
Percutaneous Endoscopic

Device
Autologous Tissue Substitute (Bypass)
Synthetic Substitute (Bypass)
Nonautologous Tissue Substitute (Bypass)
Drainage Device (Drainage)
No Device

Qualifier
Nasopharynx (Bypass)
Mastoid Sinus (Bypass)
Atrium (Bypass)
Blood Vessel (Bypass)
Pleural Cavity (Bypass)
Intestine (Bypass)
Peritoneal Cavity (Bypass)
Urinary Tract (Bypass)
Bone Marrow (Bypass)
Cerebral Cisterns (Bypass)
Diagnostic (Drainage)
No Qualifier (Drainage)

Description
A ventriculostomy procedure is performed to alleviate the buildup of cerebral spinal fluid (CSF) such as in hydrocephalus or blood from trauma or hemorrhagic stroke. These fluids can be drained with either an intracranial artificial opening (ostomy), which drains the excess into the intracranial space, or an extracranial shunt, which involves the creation of a transcatheter shunt between the ventricle and elsewhere in the body or to an external collection system (bag).

Intracranial Ventriculostomy

Bypass
One type of intracranial ventriculocisternostomy uses a shunt and may also be referred to as an anastomosis or a Torkildsen operation. This procedure is reported with the root operation Bypass because it uses a shunt (Synthetic Substitute) to alter the route of the passage of the CSF from the lateral ventricles to the cistern magna to drain the excess CSF into the spinal canal. The cistern magna is a subarachnoid cistern between the cerebellum and medulla oblongata and is reported in ICD-10-PCS with the body part Cerebral Cisterns. In this procedure, the scalp is incised and retracted posterior to the ear. A burr hole is drilled, and the proximal portion of the shunt is inserted toward the lateral ventricles, with or without the aid of an endoscope. The distal end of the shunt is directed toward the cisterna magna until CSF flows through the shunt. The two ends are connected and tested. The dura is sutured closed, and the scalp is reapproximated and closed in sutured layers.

Drainage
Drainage is the appropriate root operation used to describe endoscopic third ventriculostomy or third ventriculocisternostomy (ETV), which is used in many hydrocephalus cases. To perform ETV, the physician uses a neuroendoscopic, or Percutaneous Endoscopic, technique to create a perforation, or communication, between the third ventricle and the cisterna magna subarachnoid space to allow the CSF to drain internally. No shunt or drainage device is used in this procedure. A small incision is made in the scalp, and a small burr hole is made in the skull just large enough to allow passage of the endoscopic instrument. Computerized tomography (CT) guidance for stereotactic positioning is used and may be reported separately. The neuroendoscope is inserted through the burr hole into the third ventricle. A contact laser fiber is inserted through the endoscope onto the floor of the third ventricle, and the contact tip perforates the intracranial tissue at different points, avoiding arteries. The newly opened communication is verified when the circulation of CSF is unobstructed. Hemostasis is achieved, the instruments are removed, and the incision is closed.

Extracranial Ventriculostomy

Bypass
When longer term drainage is needed, this anastomosis or shunt procedure drains the CSF to a location within the body and is reported with the root operation Bypass. The altered route of the CSF begins in the lateral ventricle, reported as body part value Cerebral Ventricle, and is generally terminated in the Peritoneal Cavity (referred to as ventriculoperitoneal [VP]) or the right Atrium of the heart (referred to as

© 2018 Optum360, LLC

Ventriculostomy (continued)

ventriculoatrial [VA]). Other locations and body part values that are less often used are Mastoid Sinus (ventriculomastoid), Nasopharynx, Pleural Cavity (ventriculopleural), Intestine, Urinary Tract, or Bone Marrow. These various locations are represented by the seventh character value.

During this procedure, the scalp is incised and retracted posterior to the ear. A burr hole is drilled and the proximal portion of the catheter or shunt is inserted toward the lateral ventricles with or without the aid of an endoscope until CSF flows through the shunt. The catheter is connected to a valve system that opens when the ventricle pressure increases. The distal end of the shunt is directed and tunneled subcutaneously toward the selected drain site. The two ends are connected (anastomosed) and tested. The dura is sutured closed, and the scalp is reapproximated and closed in sutured layers. If an incision is required at the distal end, the operative incision is closed in sutured layers.

Drainage
The root operation Drainage describes extraventricular drainage, which involves the insertion of a shunt or catheter, reported with Drainage Device, into the ventricle to drain the excess CSF directly to an external collection system or bag outside of the body. This is typically placed for shorter term use.

The scalp is incised and retracted at the affected site. A burr hole is drilled through the skull, and a catheter or shunt tube is inserted into the ventricle until CSF flows through the catheter to a container outside the body. External ventricular drainage may be performed by neuroendoscopic technique, reported with Percutaneous Endoscopic, where an endoscopic

instrument is inserted through the burr hole. Computerized tomography (CT) guidance for stereotactic positioning may also be used. When a neuroendoscope is inserted through the burr hole into the ventricle, a contact laser fiber is inserted through the endoscope onto the floor of the ventricle. The contact tip perforates the intracranial tissue at different points, avoiding arteries. The newly opened communication is verified when the circulation of CSF is unobstructed.

Focus Point
Ventriculostomies are also performed to monitor intracranial pressure. Monitoring of this pressure is coded separately (see also Monitoring, Intracranial Pressure).

If a laparoscope was used to inspect and identify the proposed distal site of the shunt and not to place the device, root operation Inspection of the proposed site location would be coded separately.

Focus Point
Particularly in trauma cases, a ventriculostomy may also be performed with an Open approach. Careful review of the operative report is necessary.

Focus Point
Bypass procedures are coded by identifying the body part bypassed "from" and the body part bypassed "to," which is captured by the qualifier. See guideline B3.6a.

Coding Guidance
AHA: 2015, 3Q, 12; 2013, 2Q, 36

Ventriculostomy, Reopening, Endoscopic Third (ETV)

See also Ventriculostomy

Body System
Central Nervous System and Cranial Nerves

PCS Root Operation
Dilation

Root Operation Table
007 Central Nervous System and Cranial Nerves, Dilation

Body Part
Cerebral Ventricle

Approach
Percutaneous Endoscopic

Device
No Device

Qualifier
No Qualifier

Description

In obstructive hydrocephalus, endoscopic third Ventriculostomy (ETV) is performed to create an opening, or communication, between the third Ventricle and the subarachnoid space to allow the cerebrospinal fluid (CSF) to drain internally, relieving pressure on the brain without need for a shunt. The result is decreased intracranial pressure (ICP) and stable or decreased ventricular size.

In some patients, the opening becomes narrowed and/ or blocked due to stoma narrowing, a secondary membrane, or scar tissue, resulting in a need for surgical intervention to restore the opening and drainage of CSF.

Similar to the original ETV procedure, the physician uses a neuroendoscopic (Percutaneous Endoscopic) technique to dilate the previously created perforation, or communication, between the third ventricle and the cisterna magna subarachnoid space to allow the CSF to drain internally. No shunt or drainage device is used in this procedure.

A small incision is made in the area of the previous incision in the scalp, and a small burr hole is made in the skull just large enough to allow passage of the endoscopic instrument. The dura is incised and a catheter placed into the ventricle to measure the intracranial pressure. Computerized tomography (CT) guidance for stereotactic positioning is used and may be reported separately. The catheter is removed, and the neuroendoscope is inserted through the burr hole into the third ventricle. The stoma is entered with a guidewire, and dilation is performed with a balloon catheter, inserted through the endoscope into the opening of the third ventricle. The newly reopened communication is verified when the circulation of CSF is unobstructed. Hemostasis is achieved, the instruments are removed, and the incision is closed.

Coding Guidance
AHA: 2017, 4Q, 39

© 2018 Optum360, LLC

Vertebroplasty

See also Kyphoplasty (Percutaneous Vertebral Augmentation)

Body System
Upper Bones
Lower Bones

PCS Root Operation
Supplement

Root Operation Table
ØPU   Upper Bones, Supplement
ØQU   Lower Bones, Supplement

Body Part
Cervical Vertebra
Thoracic Vertebra
Lumbar Vertebra

Approach
Percutaneous

Device
Synthetic Substitute

Description
The ICD-10-PCS root operation Supplement is used to report vertebroplasty, which is a single-step procedure for treating pain due to vertebral compression fractures from trauma or conditions such as neoplasm or osteoporotic pathological fractures. Vertebroplasty involves injecting a cement-like material into the collapsed bone to stabilize the fracture.

A trocar is inserted into the vertebral bone, and sterile biomaterial such as methyl methacrylate is injected from one or both sides into the damaged vertebral body to act as a bone cement to reinforce the fractured or collapsed vertebra. CT or fluoroscopy is used to guide percutaneous placement of the needle during the procedure and to monitor the injection process.

Based on guideline B6.1a, the cement mixture is reported with a device value Synthetic Substitute because it is left in the body at the end of the procedure. The procedure does not restore the original shape to the vertebra, but it does stabilize the bone, preventing further fracture or collapse. Following the procedure, the patient may experience significant, almost immediate, pain relief.

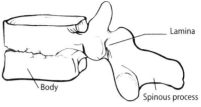

Lamina

Body

Spinous process

Lateral view of fractured body of thoracic vertebra

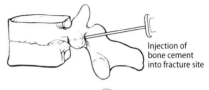

Injection of bone cement into fracture site

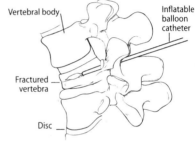

Vertebral body

Inflatable balloon catheter

Fractured vertebra

Disc

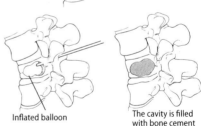

Inflated balloon

The cavity is filled with bone cement

> **Focus Point**
> *To ensure accurate code assignment, carefully review the medical record documentation for specific information regarding the procedure performed. Vertebral augmentation, or kyphoplasty, is a two-step procedure using various techniques and devices to mechanically augment vertebral body height followed by injection of the cement filler. Both conventional vertebroplasty and vertebral augmentation are Percutaneous procedures performed to treat fractured or diseased vertebrae using cement.*
>
> See also *Kyphoplasty (Percutaneous Vertebral Augmentation)*.

Coding Guidance
AHA: 2014, 2Q, 12

Vitrectomy

See also Buckling, Scleral (with Implant)

Body System
Eye

PCS Root Operation
Drainage

Excision

Resection

Root Operation Table
Ø89   Eye, Drainage

Ø8B   Eye, Excision

Ø8T   Eye, Resection

Body Part
Vitreous, Right

Vitreous, Left

Approach
Percutaneous

Qualifier
Diagnostic

No Qualifier

Description

A vitrectomy is the surgical extraction of the contents of the vitreous chamber (posterior chamber) of the eye. Vitreous is the clear, gel-like substance that fills the posterior of the eye, posterior to the lens and anterior to the retina. It contributes to the structural stability of the globe and also maintains pressure so that the retina is pressed against the blood-rich macula beneath it. Vitreous is also known as vitreous humor.

Vitreous contributes insignificantly to refraction, but because it lies in the visual pathway, any opacity in the vitreous can potentially cause a visual defect. A retinal hemorrhage, for example, may leak blood into the vitreous and partially or totally obscure vision. A vitrectomy in this case would be performed as a therapeutic measure to restore vision. Vitrectomy may also be performed so that the gel can undergo diagnostic pathologic examination. All or a portion of the vitreous may be excised or, alternatively, removed by syringe in what is commonly called a vitreous tap.

The approach for any vitrectomy is Percutaneous (entry by puncture or minor incision of instrumentation), either through the limbus (junction of sclera and cornea) or through the pars plana, an anatomical ring of ciliary body tissue just beyond the limbus. A pars plana vitrectomy (PPV) may sometimes be called a posterior sclerotomy vitrectomy.

In vitrectomy, the physician makes three small incisions at the limbus or pars plana. One incision is for a light cannula, one for an infusion cannula, and one for the cutting or suction instruments. The physician extracts the vitreous, using a mechanical cutting and suctioning process that may involve a rotoextractor or vitreous infusion suction cutter (VISC). Injections of a vitreous substitute reestablish intraocular pressure.

Resection
A complete vitrectomy involves removal of all of the vitreous and is coded to the root operation Resection.

Excision
A partial vitrectomy involves removal of a portion of the vitreous, in which case the root operation is Excision.

Drainage
In a vitreous tap, the root operation is Drainage. The physician inserts a needle into a site along the pars plana and aspirates fluid/gel from the posterior segment. This is usually a diagnostic procedure.

Focus Point
Vitrectomy is often performed in conjunction with retinal surgery; for example, prior to repair of a retinal detachment or removal of the subretinal membrane to treat choroidal neovascularization. Report the vitrectomy procedure code in addition to codes for related procedures that meet the reporting criteria for a separate procedure.

Replacement of the removed vitreous with a gas or liquid is integral to any vitrectomy and would not be reported. The gas or liquid acts as a temporary placeholder that is later absorbed and replaced with natural fluids, so the operation Replacement would be inappropriate.

Coding Guidance
AHA: 2015, 2Q, 24; 2014, 4Q, 35-36

© 2018 Optum360, LLC

Washing, Bronchial

See also Lavage, Bronchoalveolar (BAL)

See also Suctioning, Bronchial (For Removal of Mucus Plug)

Body System
Respiratory System

PCS Root Operation
Drainage

Root Operation Table
ØB9   Respiratory System, Drainage

Body Part
Main Bronchus, Right
Upper Lobe Bronchus, Right
Middle Lobe Bronchus, Right
Lower Lobe Bronchus, Right
Main Bronchus, Left
Upper Lobe Bronchus, Left
Lingula Bronchus
Lower Lobe Bronchus, Left

Approach
Via Natural or Artificial Opening Endoscopic

Device
No Device

Qualifier
Diagnostic

Description
Bronchial washing is a diagnostic procedure that uses repeated instillation and aspiration of lavage fluid to obtain cells and noncellular components such as airway secretions from the epithelial surface of the lower respiratory tract for microbiological, cytological, or immunological analysis.

The physician views the airway using a flexible fiberoptic or rigid bronchoscope (a long, thin tube that has a close-focusing telescope on the end for viewing) introduced Via Natural or Artificial Opening Endoscopic approach through the nasal or oral cavity, or tracheostomy stoma. The airway is anesthetized with a topical anesthetic. The bronchoscope is inserted and advanced through the nasal or oral cavity, or tracheostomy stoma past the larynx to inspect the bronchus. This procedure may employ fluoroscopic guidance.

After visualizing the bronchus, the physician samples the bronchial tissue by irrigating with saline in small aliquots or subsets of the total fluid volume, followed by carefully suctioning the fluid. The bronchoscope is removed.

Focus Point
Bronchial washing refers to the aspiration of secretions or small amounts of instilled saline from the larger airways within the lumen of the bronchus, while bronchoalveolar lavage involves washing out and sampling the alveoli of the lung.

Focus Point
An additional code for fluoroscopic guidance may be reported, when performed.

Coding Guidance
AHA: 2017, 1Q, 51; 2016, 1Q, 26, 27

Medical and Surgical

Wedge Resection, Mitral Valve Leaflet

See also Valvuloplasty

Body System
Heart and Great Vessels

PCS Root Operation
Excision

Root Operation Table
02B Heart and Great Vessels, Excision

Body Part
Mitral Valve

Approach
Open

Device
No Device

Qualifier
No Qualifier

Description
A mitral valve wedge resection is done to improve the ability of the mitral valve to close completely when the ventricle contracts. It is done in patients whose mitral valve has lost the ability to close normally. In most cases, this is the result of mitral valve prolapse, in which the mitral leaflets and sometimes the cords that tether them on the ventricle have become elongated.

Valve evaluation is done with a preoperative transesophageal echocardiography (TEE) to plan the procedure. The patient is positioned, prepped, and draped, and cardiopulmonary bypass is initiated. Using an Open approach, exposure is obtained through a full median sternotomy. The left atrium is opened, and the mitral valve is exposed. A wedge of redundant leaflet tissue is excised, and the defect in the valve leaflets is closed with sutures. The cords are also shortened with sutures. Valve closure is assessed after the repair. In a separately reportable procedure, the mitral valve diameter may be enlarged, requiring placement of an annuloplasty prosthetic ring. At the conclusion of the procedure, the left atrium is closed and cardiopulmonary bypass is discontinued when heart function returns. Valve closure is assessed with TEE after the repair and determined to be adequate. The surgical incisions and the sternum are closed and dressings are applied. Chest tubes and mediastinal drainage tubes may be left in place following the procedure.

Focus Point
Assign an additional code for ring annuloplasty, if performed, from table 02U Heart and Great Vessels, Supplement. See also Valvuloplasty.

Focus Point
Cardiopulmonary bypass is reported separately with 5A1221Z Performance of Cardiac Output, Continuous. See also Bypass, Cardiopulmonary.

Focus Point
TEE may also be reported with a code from Imaging, Heart, Ultrasonography, table B24. See also Echocardiography, Transesophageal (TEE).

Coding Guidance
AHA: 2015, 2Q, 23

© 2018 Optum360, LLC

Medical and Surgical

Whipple

Body System
Gastrointestinal System
Hepatobiliary System and Pancreas

PCS Root Operation
Excision
Resection

Root Operation Table
ØDB Gastrointestinal System, Excision
ØDT Gastrointestinal System, Resection
ØFB Hepatobiliary System and Pancreas, Excision
ØFT Hepatobiliary System and Pancreas, Resection

Body Part
Gallbladder
Pancreas
Common Bile Duct
Stomach
Duodenum
Jejunum

Approach
Open
Percutaneous Endoscopic

Description

A pancreaticoduodenectomy, also known as the Whipple procedure, involves excising multiple abdominal organs such as the head of the pancreas, duodenum, stomach pylorus, common bile duct, and often gallbladder and proximal jejunum. Anastomosis or reconstruction involves attaching the hepatic duct to the jejunum and the stomach to the jejunum. It is performed to treat pancreatic cancer in lieu of a total pancreatectomy.

The physician performs excision of the proximal pancreas, duodenum, distal bile duct, gallbladder, and distal stomach with reconstruction. Under general anesthesia, using an Open approach, the physician makes an abdominal incision and explores the abdomen. The duodenum, proximal pancreas, and bile duct are mobilized. The distal bile duct, distal stomach, and distal duodenum are divided. The pancreas is transected at the junction of the head and body, and the pancreatic head, duodenum, distal stomach, and distal bile duct are removed en bloc. The anatomy is reconstructed by performing sequential anastomoses between the proximal jejunum and the distal bile duct and distal stomach. The edge of the remaining distal pancreas is closed with sutures or staples. The incision is closed. The Whipple procedure can also be performed using a Percutaneous Endoscopic (laparoscopic) approach using several small incisions and a laparoscope.

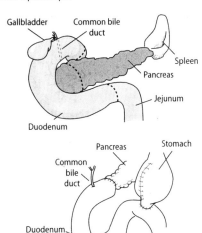

Each of the organs removed is reported separately with root operation Excision (partial) or Resection (complete). Many Whipple procedures involve gallbladder resection and distal jejunum excision, which are also reported. Because there are different versions of the Whipple, such as the pyloric sparing Whipple, the operative report must be reviewed carefully to determine the correct body part values and approach to report.

Focus Point
Assign individual codes when the same procedure is performed on separate body parts. See guideline B3.2a.

Focus Point
The anastomoses are considered inherent in the Excision and Resection procedures and are not coded separately. See guideline B3.1b.

Coding Guidance
AHA: 2014, 3Q, 32

Z-plasty, Skin (Scar Revision)

Body System
Skin and Breast

PCS Root Operation
Release

Root Operation Table
ØHN   Skin and Breast, Release

Body Part
Refer to the ICD-10-PCS tabular list for a complete list of body parts.

Approach
External

Description
Z-plasty is a surgical repositioning of a scar to ease discomfort associated with contracture and improve aesthetics. This technique allows contracted scars to be lengthened. The physician transfers or rearranges adjacent tissue to repair and release a scar or contracture of the skin. Surgical technique may vary.

Under local anesthesia, the scar is excised and surgical incisions are made on each side, creating small triangular flaps of skin. The flaps are rearranged to cover the wound at a different angle, resulting in a "Z" pattern.

Example of common Z-plasty.

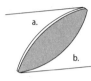

Two additional incisions (a. and b.) intersect the area

The skin of each incision is reflected back

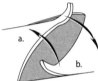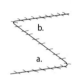

The flaps are then transposed and the repair is closed

© 2018 Optum360, LLC

Medical and Surgical Related

Obstetrics

Abortion

Body System
Pregnancy

PCS Root Operation
Abortion

Root Operation Table
10A   Obstetrics, Pregnancy, Abortion

Body Part
Products of Conception

Approach
Open
Percutaneous
Percutaneous Endoscopic
Via Natural or Artificial Opening

Qualifier
Vacuum
Laminaria
Abortifacient
No Qualifier

Description
Abortion is the medical or surgical termination of a pregnancy. All products of conception are removed from the uterus. Abortion may be performed to protect the health of the mother because the fetus is defective, or as an elective procedure.

ICD-10-PCS root operation Abortion is specific to the Obstetrics section, Pregnancy body system, and Products of Conception body part. Abortion is reported for termination of pregnancy only. It is defined as "artificially terminating a pregnancy." The abortion table is subdivided by approach, whether a device such as a laminaria or abortifacient is used, or whether the abortion was performed by mechanical means.

If a laminaria or an abortifacient is used, the approach is Via Natural or Artificial Opening. All other abortion procedures are those done by mechanical means (the products of conception are physically removed using instrumentation), and the device value is No Device.

Vacuum suction aspiration curettage is the most frequently performed type of abortion. It involves evacuation of the products of conception through a thin plastic or metal tube (cannula) that is attached to a vacuum source. The doctor inserts a speculum into the vagina and then inserts the tube through the cervix into the uterus. The tube is then is attached to a suction or vacuum pump, which removes the products of conception. Electric vacuum aspiration (EVA) employs an electric vacuum pump, while in manual vacuum aspiration (MVA), the vacuum is created using a hand-held syringe. Vacuum aspiration is performed through the vagina and is therefore reported with the approach Via Natural or Artificial Opening and the qualifier Vacuum.

Dilation and curettage (D&C) involves dilating the cervix with a series of mechanical dilators, gradually increasing the size of the opening, after which the physician passes a sharp metal curette into the uterus. The sharp curette is used to scrape the uterine lining and remove the tissue in the uterus. Dilation and curettage (D&C) is an obsolete method of surgical abortion and generally has been replaced by vacuum aspiration and/or medical methods. Dilation and curettage is performed through the vagina and is therefore reported with the approach Via Natural or Artificial Opening and the qualifier No Qualifier.

If the curettage or aspiration procedure is performed via a vaginal approach using a hysteroscope to visualize the site of the procedure (uterus), report the approach as Via Natural or Artificial Opening Endoscopic with No Qualifier selected.

A laminaria is a stick of dried and sterile sea kelp, L digitate, which expands exponentially with moisture. To instigate abortion in a vaginal (Via Natural or Artificial Opening) approach, the physician may insert a spindle of laminaria into the patient's endocervix, where it remains for six to 12 hours, absorbing body fluids. The laminaria expands to dilate the cervix, initiating the abortion by inducing labor. Laminaria may be used alone to induce abortion, or may be used in combination with other methods. This is reported with the qualifier Laminaria.

Dilation and evacuation (D&E) requires preparation of the cervix using osmotic dilators (laminaria) or pharmacological agents and evacuating the uterus using electric vacuum aspiration (EVA) and forceps. Abortion by dilation and evacuation following laminaria insertion is reported with the approach Via Natural or Artificial Opening and the qualifier Laminaria.

In a Percutaneous approach, the physician removes the products of conception by inducing labor with amniocentesis and intra-amniotic injections.

Abortion (continued)

This method is usually used after the first trimester (13 weeks or more). The physician inserts an amniocentesis needle into the abdomen to obtain a free flow of clear amniotic fluid. A hypertonic solution is administered by gravity drip. The hypertonic solution results in fetal death, and labor usually results. The products of conception are delivered through the vagina. This may be documented as injection of prostaglandin or saline for abortion, or termination of pregnancy by intrauterine injection. Report this with No Qualifier.

Prostaglandin or misoprostol, alone or combined with mifepristone or methotrexate, is administered orally or as a vaginal suppository to induce abortion. Report the approach Via Natural or Artificial Opening. The administration of the substance and its efficacy are monitored through multiple physician encounters, and more than one dose is usually required. The medication works by interfering with growth of the chorionic villi or by causing uterine contractions. Report the use of these drugs with the qualifier Abortifacient.

In extremely rare cases, the products of conception are accessed via hysterotomy (incision of the uterus). This technique is limited to unusual clinical presentations, such as patients with multiple or large leiomyomata, uterine septum, or double uterus. In an Open approach, the physician makes a horizontal or vertical incision in the skin of the abdomen, through the fascia and muscle to the uterus. The physician removes all products of conception and may perform curettage. The physician closes the abdominal and uterine incisions by suturing. In a Percutaneous Endoscopic approach, the physician removes the products of conception using laparoscopy. A trocar is inserted periumbilically, and the abdomen is insufflated with gas. Additional trocars are placed in the right and left

lower quadrants. The uterus is incised, and the products of conception are aspirated from the uterus. The physician may perform curettage. The uterine incision is repaired, and the trocars are removed. Operative incisions are closed. The qualifier No Qualifier is reported for these procedures.

Focus Point
A manually assisted spontaneous abortion (miscarriage) is reported with root operation Delivery. Use the operation Abortion only to report medically or surgically induced abortions for termination of pregnancy.

Focus Point
Report removal of retained products of conception following an abortion with the Obstetrics section, using the body part Products of Conception, Retained, and root operation Extraction.

Focus Point
Report removal of nonviable products of conception (blighted ova, hydatidiform mole, or early fetal death) with the Obstetrics section, using the body part Products of Conception and the operation Extraction.

Focus Point
The "morning after pill" is not an abortifacient; it is a drug to prevent conception after unprotected intercourse. This oral medication is considered effective if taken within five days of unprotected intercourse and may contain levonorgestrel, ulipristal acetate, estrogen with progestin, or progestin only. This drug may result in delayed ovulation, inhibited mobility of the egg or sperm, or a uterus hostile to implantation. The use of this oral medication is not reported.

© 2018 Optum360, LLC

Amniocentesis

Body System
Pregnancy

PCS Root Operation
Drainage

Root Operation Table
1Ø9   Obstetrics, Pregnancy, Drainage

Body Part
Products of Conception

Approach
Percutaneous

Qualifier
Amniotic Fluid, Therapeutic
Amniotic Fluid, Diagnostic

Description
Amniocentesis is the aspiration of fluid from the amniotic sac, achieved by inserting a needle through the skin of the abdomen of a pregnant patient using a Percutaneous approach. The needle enters the uterus and is guided into the amniotic sac. The root operation is Drainage, which involves taking or letting out fluids and/or gases from a body part. The physician aspirates fluid under separately reported ultrasonic guidance. For a diagnostic amniocentesis, the amniotic fluid collected undergoes further analysis and is reported with the qualifier Amniotic Fluid, Diagnostic. In therapeutic amniocentesis, the physician performs amnioreduction to reduce volume. This is reported with the qualifier Amniotic Fluid, Therapeutic. In some cases, serial amniotic fluid volume reductions are required. Amniocentesis is coded to the Products of Conception body part in the Obstetrics section. In the Obstetrics section, there is only one body system, Pregnancy.

The physician aspirates amniotic fluid (AF) for therapeutic reasons in a patient with polyhydramnios, (abnormal increase in AF volume). Polyhydramnios may be caused by gestational diabetes, fetal anomalies, or fetal infections. Polyhydramnios is associated with increased perinatal morbidity because it can lead to premature rupture of membranes, abnormal fetal presentation, and cord prolapse.

The physician aspirates AF for diagnostic purposes because the fluid contains fetal skin cells, urine, and pulmonary fluid. The fluid's composition changes as the fetus ages, and analysis may determine fetal karyotype, fetal lung maturity, presence of fetal stress or infection, neural tube defects, and fetal blood incompatibilities. The test may be ordered to further understand a previous abnormal finding, for example an abnormal alpha-fetoprotein (AFP) level or a suspected anomaly on a fetal ultrasound. Amniocentesis may be ordered because the patient has a personal or family history of a genetic disorder. Patients older than 35 years may undergo amniocentesis as there is an increased risk of birth defects in older patients.

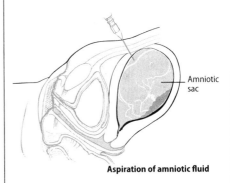

Aspiration of amniotic fluid

Focus Point

In amniocentesis, fluid is removed from the amniotic sac. When fluid is injected into the amniotic sac, report Introduction, Products of Conception, E3Ø.

Focus Point

According to ICD-10-PCS guideline C1, procedures performed on the products of conception are coded in the Obstetrics section. Procedures performed on the pregnant female that do not involve the products of conception are coded to the appropriate root operation in the Medical and Surgical section. Amniotic fluid is classified as a product of conception.

Cesarean Section (C-section)

Body System
Pregnancy

PCS Root Operation
Extraction

Root Operation Table
10D Obstetrics, Pregnancy, Extraction

Body Part
Products of Conception

Approach
Open

Qualifier
High
Low
Extraperitoneal

Description
Cesarean section (C-section) involves a surgical incision through the mother's abdomen and uterus to deliver a baby. Cesarean sections are usually performed when the mother or infant is at risk, or when a vaginal delivery is otherwise contraindicated, such as:

- Cephalopelvic disproportion
- Failure of labor to progress
- Complicating medical conditions or diseases
- Labor complications or trauma
- Fetal distress

Under spinal or other anesthesia, the abdomen is prepped with antiseptic solution. Using an Open approach, the physician most commonly makes a small, horizontal incision in the skin above the pubic bone (low transverse incision). The physician dissects the underlying tissue to the uterus. The abdominal muscles are separated and spread to expose the contents of the pelvis. Upon visualization of the uterus,

the physician usually makes a horizontal incision in the lower uterine section (Low Cervical). However, the physician may elect to perform a vertical (Classical) incision depending on the nature of the uterus or pregnancy at the time of cesarean section.

The physician manually removes the baby from the uterine incision. If the uterus has ruptured, the physician removes the baby from the peritoneal or extraperitoneal cavity. In such cases, the physician may perform an associated and separately reportable emergency hysterectomy. An Extraperitoneal C-section involves an Open incision into the lower uterine segment without actually entering the peritoneal cavity, through the paravesical space.

The baby may be placed on the mother's abdomen directly or passed to a pediatrician or nurse for examination. The physician removes the placenta and closes the abdominal incision in layers with sutures and staples.

Focus Point
In ICD-10-PCS, the infant is included in the term Products of Conception. Procedures performed on the products of conception, such as delivery, are coded to the Obstetrics section.

Cesarean section delivery is coded to the root operation Extraction; Delivery applies only to manually assisted vaginal delivery. Procedures performed on the pregnant female, such as repair of perineal tear, are coded to the appropriate root operation in the Medical and Surgical section.

Focus Point
Vacuum assistance in a C-section delivery is not reported.

Coding Guidance
AHA: 2018, 2Q, 17; 2014, 4Q, 43

© 2018 Optum360, LLC

Medical and Surgical Related

Delivery, Assisted with Instrumentation

See also Delivery, Assisted, Manually

Body System
Pregnancy

PCS Root Operation
Extraction

Root Operation Table
10D Obstetrics, Pregnancy, Extraction

Body Part
Products of Conception

Approach
Via Natural or Artificial Opening

Qualifier
Low Forceps
Mid Forceps
High Forceps
Vacuum
Internal Version
Other

Description
Routine prenatal examinations assist in planning and preparing for the best possible method of delivery. Identifying certain conditions before labor and delivery greatly reduces complications associated with birth trauma of the mother and baby. Delivery may be without complications, occur spontaneously, and require only minimal assistance. However, unforeseen events, insufficient prenatal care, and other situations may arise during the labor and birth process that require specialized intervention, such as:

- Malposition of fetus
- Obstructed labor
- Maternal fatigue
- Failed uterine contractions (e.g., uterine inertia)
- Complications related to anesthetics, sedation, or other iatrogenic causes

An assisted delivery may include the use of forceps or vacuum extraction to expel the fetus when maternal efforts alone may fail. These procedures often require the administration of some type of anesthesia, whether epidural, spinal, or other. Extraction is the appropriate root operation to use when instrumentation is used to deliver an infant Via Natural or Artificial Opening approach.

Forceps are generally specialized, spoon-like paired instruments designed to aid the delivery of the infant by applying traction to the head of the fetus. Forceps are most commonly used when the baby is in the lower portion of the birth canal (vaginal vault), which may be described as low or low outlet forceps

application. Due to the risk to the mother and baby associated with the application of mid or high forceps, forceps are rarely used and have been largely replaced by vacuum extraction or cesarean delivery.

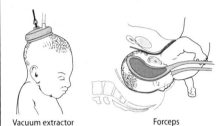

Vacuum extractor   Forceps

In a Low Forceps delivery, the physician assists a vaginal delivery by applying forceps instrumentation to the head of the fetus after it has descended into the lower portion of the vagina. In a Mid Forceps delivery, the forceps instrumentation is applied to the head of the fetus after it has descended into the middle portion of the vagina. High Forceps delivery involves applying forceps instrumentation to the head of the fetus before it has descended into the middle portion of the vagina by placing the instrumentation high in the vaginal vault.

The physician uses a vacuum assistance device for certain labor complications, such as fetal distress, poor maternal pushing efforts, or failure to progress in the second stage of labor. In Vacuum Extraction, a plastic cup is inserted into the vagina and applied to the baby's head. The cup is generally placed as far posteriorly as possible to maintain flexion of the fetal head and avoid traction over the anterior fontanel. The physician places the fingers of one hand against the suction cup and grasps the handle of the instrument with the other hand. Once vacuum is applied, the cup should not be twisted. Suction keeps the cup in place, and the doctor provides gentle traction, pulling the baby through the birth canal by a handle attached to the cup. Traction may be coordinated with maternal contractions, whereby the traction is repeated with each contraction until the head is crowned. Once the head is delivered, suction is released and the cup is removed. This procedure may also be performed with episiotomy.

Version may be described as the manual corrective repositioning of the fetus to facilitate optimal presentation for delivery. Version procedures are classified as external, internal, or combined. Internal Version involves rotation or manipulation of the fetus by inserting the hand or fingers through the dilated cervix. The physician performs corrective rotation or repositioning of the fetus with subsequent extraction

© 2018 Optum360, LLC

Medical and Surgical Related

Delivery, Assisted with Instrumentation (continued)

(delivery) of the fetus during the same operative episode.

Focus Point

In ICD-10-PCS, the infant is included in the term Products of Conception. Procedures performed on the products of conception, such as delivery, are coded to the Obstetrics section. Procedures performed on the pregnant female, such as repair of perineal tear, are coded to the appropriate root operation in the Medical and Surgical section.

Focus Point

A manually assisted delivery without the use of instrumentation is coded using the root operation Delivery (see also Delivery, Assisted, Manually).

Focus Point

Vacuum-assisted labor is not reported as Extraction and would not be reported as a separate procedure.

Focus Point

Code additional procedures performed that meet the multiple procedures guidelines, such as repair of obstetric tears, or episiotomy with repair.

Focus Point

Manually assisted spontaneous abortion is reported as Delivery of Products of Conception since this is the objective of the procedure. ICD-10-PCS codes do not include diagnoses; the spontaneous abortion diagnosis is captured with the ICD-10-CM code(s).

Coding Guidance

AHA: 2016, 2Q, 34; 2016, 1Q, 9

© 2018 Optum360, LLC

Delivery, Assisted, Manually

Body System
Pregnancy

PCS Root Operation
Delivery

Root Operation Table
1ØE   Obstetrics, Pregnancy, Delivery

Body Part
Products of Conception

Approach
External

Description
In ICD-10-PCS, the infant is included in the term Products of Conception. Procedures performed on the products of conception, such as delivery, are coded to the Obstetrics section. The root operation Delivery applies only to a manually assisted vaginal delivery with no qualifiers. During a manually assisted vaginal delivery, the physician delivers an infant and placenta through the uterus and vagina.

Using an External approach, the physician assists in the spontaneous delivery of an infant through the uterus and vagina by the application of hands to support the infant and provide gentle traction when necessary, without the need of instrumentation such as forceps or vacuum extraction.

Focus Point
Code additional procedures performed that meet the multiple procedures guidelines, such as repair of obstetric tears or episiotomy with repair.

Focus Point
Cesarean section delivery is coded to the root operation Extraction.

Focus Point
If instrumentation is used in the delivery, code only the procedures used in the actual extraction of the baby using root operation Extraction.

Focus Point
Manually assisted spontaneous abortion is reported as a Delivery of Products of Conception since this is the objective of the procedure. ICD-10-PCS codes do not include diagnoses; the spontaneous abortion diagnosis is captured with the ICD-10-CM code(s).

Coding Guidance
AHA: 2016, 2Q, 34; 2016, 1Q, 9

Delivery, Vaginal, Breech

Body System
Pregnancy

PCS Root Operation
Delivery

Root Operation Table
10E   Obstetrics, Pregnancy, Delivery

Body Part
Products of Conception

Approach
External

Description
Breech is the malposition of the fetus where the buttocks and/or the feet are the presenting parts. Although most breech presentations are delivered by cesarean section, vaginal delivery may occur.

An anesthesiologist and pediatrician should be present for delivery if possible. The physician may leave the fetal membranes intact as long as possible to ensure adequate dilation and prevent umbilical cord prolapse. An episiotomy may be performed to widen the birth canal outlet and prevent dystocia. Specialized maneuvers may be performed to facilitate delivery of the legs, but no traction should be applied until the fetal umbilicus is past the perineum. Maternal pushing efforts should be coordinated with gentle downward and outward traction (assisted by wrapping the hips of the infant in a dry towel) until the shoulders are visible. An assistant should apply transfundal pressure from above to keep the fetal head flexed. Upon visualizing

the scapula, the provider may need to perform a series of maneuvers to deliver the arms and then the fetal head.

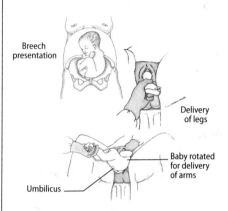

Breech presentation

Delivery of legs

Baby rotated for delivery of arms

Umbilicus

In ICD-10-PCS, the infant is included in the term Products of Conception. Procedures performed on the products of conception, such as delivery, are coded to the Obstetrics section.

Focus Point
Code additional procedures performed that meet the multiple procedures guidelines, such as repair of obstetric tears or episiotomy with repair.

Focus Point
The diagnosis code captures the breech position.

Medical and Surgical Related

© 2018 Optum360, LLC

Extraction, Retained Placenta, Manual

Body System
Pregnancy

PCS Root Operation
Extraction

Root Operation Table
10D Obstetrics, Pregnancy, Extraction

Body Part
Products of Conception, Retained

Approach
Via Natural or Artificial Opening

Qualifier
Manual
No Qualifier

Description
Following delivery, the uterus begins a series of systematic contractions that are essential to closing off the flow of blood that had nourished the fetus during gestation. Retention of the placenta in the uterus after delivery interferes with normal uterine contractions and can lead to maternal hemorrhage or, later, infection.

The normal third stage of labor begins with the complete delivery of the baby. It ends with the complete delivery of the entire placenta and attached membranes.

A retained placenta is generally defined as lack of expulsion of the placenta within 30 minutes to one hour after the completion of the second stage of labor (delivery of the baby).

To remove a retained placenta, the physician places one hand on the fundus of the uterus while guiding the other hand into the patient's vagina and uterus, following the umbilical cord to locate the placenta. The placental edge is found, and it is slowly pulled away from the uterine wall. The placenta is removed through the vagina and examined to ensure it is intact.

Focus Point

A normal delivery of the products of conception includes delivery of the placenta. This procedure is reported separately only in cases in which the placenta did not deliver normally.

Medical and Surgical Related

Insertion, Monitoring Electrode

See also Monitoring, Fetal Heart Rate, Transvaginal (Internal), under "Measurement and Monitoring" in the Medical and Surgical Related section

Body System
Pregnancy

PCS Root Operation
Insertion

Root Operation Table
10H   Obstetrics, Pregnancy, Insertion

Body Part
Products of Conception

Approach
Via Natural or Artificial Opening

Device
Monitoring Electrode

Description
Fetal heart rate monitoring is performed to assess the health of the fetus during the stresses of labor and delivery. Normally the fetal heart rate is monitored using an external transducer that is strapped to the mother's abdomen. When the provider wants more accurate and consistent data on the status of the fetus and the patient has sufficiently progressed in her labor to allow access to the fetus through the cervix, an internal monitor may be used.

A wire electrode is threaded into the vaginal orifice and through the external os of the cervix. The fetal head, in preparation for delivery, is pressed against the internal os of the cervix. A small scalp electrode is secured to the fetal scalp to sense the fetal heart rate. A lead transmits the electrode's information to an external device.

Focus Point
The body part value of Products of Conception refers to the fetus in ICD-10-PCS.

Focus Point
For transvaginal fetal heart rate monitoring, two codes are required. In addition to the code for the insertion of the electrode reported with the root operation Insertion, a second code should be reported for fetal heart rate monitoring. This is reported with a code from root operation table 4A1 Monitoring, Physiological Systems.

Medical and Surgical Related

© 2018 Optum360, LLC

Removal, Ectopic Pregnancy

Body System
Pregnancy

PCS Root Operation
Resection

Root Operation Table
1ØT   Obstetrics, Pregnancy, Resection

Body Part
Products of Conception, Ectopic

Approach
Open
Percutaneous Endoscopic
Via Natural or Artificial Opening Endoscopic

Description
Ectopic pregnancy occurs when the site of embryo implantation is in the fallopian tube, ovary, abdomen, or cervix and is a potentially life-threatening emergency in early pregnancy. Tubal pregnancy is the implantation of a fertilized ovum in the fallopian tube, more often on the right than the left. This condition is more common in women who have had previous tubal disease, such as endometriosis of the fallopian tube, tubal surgeries, or infertility due to tubal disease.

The physician treats a tubal ectopic pregnancy by removing the embryo from the tube. Using an Open approach, through an incision in the lower abdomen, the physician explores the pelvic cavity, inspects the gestation site for bleeding, and removes all products of conception, clots, and free blood. If the embryo is implanted in the fallopian tube, the physician may do one of the following: manually remove the embryo from the tube, make an incision to remove the embryo, or excise the section of the tube containing the embryo. The pelvis is lavaged with saline solution, and the incision is closed with sutures.

Using a Percutaneous Endoscopic approach, the physician treats an ectopic pregnancy by laparoscopy with separately reportable salpingectomy and/or oophorectomy. The physician inserts an instrument through the vagina to grasp the cervix while passing another instrument through the cervix and into the uterus to manipulate the uterus. The physician makes a 1 cm incision in the umbilicus through which the abdomen is inflated and a fiberoptic laparoscope is inserted. A second incision is made on the left or right side of the abdomen. After locating the site of the gestation, another small incision is made above the site. Instruments are passed into the abdomen through the incisions. The physician removes the tube and/or ovary containing the embryo and closes the abdominal incisions with sutures.

Alternatively, the physician may treat an ectopic pregnancy by laparoscopy without salpingectomy and/or oophorectomy. The physician inserts an instrument through the vagina to grasp the cervix while passing another instrument through the cervix and into the uterus to manipulate the uterus. The physician makes a 1 cm incision in the umbilicus through which the abdomen is inflated and a fiberoptic laparoscope is inserted. A second incision is made on the left or right side of the abdomen. After locating the site of gestation, another small incision is made above the site. Instruments are passed into the abdomen through the incisions. The physician removes the ectopic pregnancy by making an incision in the tube. The abdominal incisions are closed with sutures.

Removal of ectopic pregnancy may also be done with the approach Via Natural or Artificial Opening Endoscopic in a transvaginal endoscopic procedure. Under general anesthesia, the patient is placed in Trendelenburg position, with her feet in stirrups. Through the vagina, the physician creates a 1.5 cm posterior colpotomy incision just below the cervix. A trocar is placed into the pelvic cavity through this incision. An endoscope is inserted into the vaginal port, and the cavity is insufflated. The physician inspects the uterus and bilateral adnexa and performs a salpingectomy of the fallopian tube containing the ectopic pregnancy, and the ectopic pregnancy along with the portion of fallopian tube are removed through the vaginal incision. After hemostasis is obtained, the incision in the posterior vaginal wall is sutured closed.

Focus Point
Report Excision or Resection of the fallopian tube as an additional procedure when partial or total salpingectomy is performed in conjunction with Resection of ectopic products of conception.

Focus Point
Report the root operation Excision or Resection of the ovary as an additional procedure when partial or total oophorectomy is performed in conjunction with Resection of ectopic products of conception.

Coding Guidance
AHA: 2015, 3Q, 31

Repair, In Utero Fetal Myelomeningocele

Body System
Pregnancy

PCS Root Operation
Repair

Root Operation Table
10Q   Obstetrics, Pregnancy, Repair

Body Part
Products of Conception

Approach
Open

Qualifier
Nervous System

Description
Myelomeningocele is the most severe form of spinal bifida in which the spinal cord and meninges herniate through a vertebral canal defect. This defect is a result of the spinal cord not closing properly in the fetus early in pregnancy. As a result, spinal cord damage may occur since many nerves are exposed, and brain damage may occur since fluid may be lost through the spinal opening. In utero fetal myelomeningocele repair, usually performed between 19 and 25 weeks' gestation, is a surgical procedure done to close the spinal defects while the baby is still in the womb. Further spinal cord and brain damage can be minimized by closing the spinal defects in utero.

The physician performs an in utero fetal myelomeningocele repair after the pregnant patient has been given a general anesthetic. Using an Open approach, an incision is made in the pregnant patient's abdomen and a smaller incision in the uterus. Uterine staples are used to restrict the blood vessels, and continuous fluids are infused into the uterus to protect the amniotic fluid levels. The positions of the placenta and fetus are confirmed with imaging and the baby rotated if needed so the back is in view. The physician removes the myelomeningocele sac and closes the spinal cord opening. Layered closure of the uterus and the abdominal wall is then completed.

Focus Point
According to ICD-10-PCS guideline C1, procedures performed on the products of conception are coded in the Obstetrics section.

Version, External Cephalic (ECV)

See also Reposition, Uterus, Transvaginal in the Medical and Surgical section

Body System
Pregnancy

PCS Root Operation
Reposition

Root Operation Table
10S   Obstetrics, Pregnancy, Reposition

Body Part
Products of Conception

Approach
External

Device
No Device

Qualifier
No Qualifier

Description
External cephalic version (ECV) is typically performed as an elective procedure to turn a fetus from a breech (buttocks, legs, or feet first) or transverse (side-lying) position into a vertex (head-down) position in women at or near term, before labor begins, to improve the chance of having a normal vaginal birth.

ECV is performed by manipulating the fetus using an External approach from the outside of the abdominal wall. Fetal ultrasound is performed to confirm fetal position and the amount of amniotic fluid. Fetal monitoring is done before and sometimes during the procedure. The physician places both hands on the patient's abdomen and locates each pole of the fetus (head and buttocks) by palpation. The fetus is shifted so that the breech or rear end of the fetus is moved upward and the head downward. The physician may elect to use tocolytic drug therapy to relax the uterus and suppress uterine contractions during the manipulation.

Focus Point
If a uterine reposition procedure is performed on a pregnant patient without repositioning of the fetus, report a code from table 0US Female Reproductive System. No code is assigned from the obstetrics section because the intent is to reposition the mother's uterus, not the fetus (Products of Conception). ICD-10-PCS guideline C1 states: "Procedures performed on the pregnant female other than the products of conception are coded to the appropriate root operation in the Medical and Surgical section."

Coding Guidance
AHA: 2016, 1Q, 9

© 2018 Optum360, LLC

Medical and Surgical Related

Placement

Application, Stereotactic Head Frame

See also Radiation Therapy, Stereotactic Radiosurgery, Brain, under "Radiation Therapy" in the Ancillary section

Body System
Anatomical Regions

PCS Root Operation
Immobilization

Root Operation Table
2W3 Placement, Anatomical Regions, Immobilization

Body Region
Head

Approach
External

Device
Other Device

Description

A stereotactic head frame is used along with stereotactic radiotherapy to treat conditions such a brain tumor with high-dose radiation. The head frame immobilizes the head during the radiation treatment, allowing the beams to be precisely targeted at the diseased areas. A stereotactic head frame is also used for brain biopsies, deep brain stimulator implantation, and other neurological procedures.

Using an External approach, local anesthesia is administered to the four areas on the scalp where the pins are inserted. The frame is then attached with pins, two on the forehead and two on the back of the head. The head frame is removed after the radiation has been administered.

Focus Point
An additional code is needed for the stereotactic radiosurgery. See also Radiation Therapy, Stereotactic Radiosurgery.

Compression, Lymphedema, Intermittent Pneumatic

Body System
Anatomical Regions

PCS Root Operation
Compression

Root Operation Table
2W1 Placement, Anatomical Regions, Compression

Body Region
Upper Extremity, Right
Upper Extremity, Left
Upper Arm, Right
Upper Arm, Left
Hand, Right
Hand, Left
Lower Extremity, Right
Lower Extremity, Left
Lower Leg, Right
Lower Leg, Left
Foot, Right
Foot, Left

Approach
External

Device
Intermittent Pressure Device

Description

Lymphatic fluid circulates throughout the body, and a blockage in the lymphatic channels can lead to lymphedema, a swelling of the extremity, usually unilateral, due to a pooling of lymphatic fluid in that extremity. This is most commonly seen following surgery for cancer in which local lymph nodes are removed, causing scarring in the lymphatic system, such as lymphedema in the ipsilateral arm following mastectomy or lymphedema in the leg following prostatectomy.

Intermittent pneumatic compression (IPC) is a mechanical strategy for reducing the edema. In IPC, a sleeve filled with air bladders is placed around the patient's swollen extremity. The air bladders are attached to a device that regularly inflates and deflates them. The pressure placed upon the lymphatic system of the extremity during inflation hastens the flow of lymphatic fluid from the extremity by rhythmic and systemic compression, like milking the limb.

IPCs are also called sequential compression devices (SCDs).

Focus Point
Choose the most specific body system based upon documentation.

Medical and Surgical Related

Immobilization (Cast/Splint)

Body System
Anatomical Regions

PCS Root Operation
Immobilization

Root Operation Table
2W3 Placement, Anatomical Regions, Immobilization

Body Region
Refer to the ICD-10-PCS tabular list for a complete list of body regions.

Approach
External

Device
Splint
Cast

Description
Immobilization may be performed for conditions such as fractures, sprains, joint dislocations, and joint or tendon injuries and inflammatory conditions.

Fractures that are potentially unstable may be splinted while awaiting definitive care such as casting and orthopaedic referral. Splints are usually used for simple or stable fractures, sprains, and tendon injuries. Casting is used more often for more complex injury/ fracture management.

Immobilization involves the application of a rigid device used to stabilize and limit or prevent motion of a body region such as a joint structure or fractured bones to promote healing, maintain bone alignment, or protect an injury site. Anatomic site of application and type of splint device may vary, as described below:

Short arm splint: The physician applies a splint from the forearm to the hand. A short arm splint is used to immobilize the wrist. Cotton padding is applied from midforearm to the midpalm region. Plaster strips or fiberglass splint material applied along the palm side of the hand, extending to mid-forearm, maintains the wrist in the desired position. The physician applies an Ace wrap to hold the splint material in position.

Short leg splint: The physician applies a short leg splint from calf to foot. A short leg splint is used to immobilize the ankle. The physician wraps cotton bandaging from just below the knee to the toes. Plaster strips or fiberglass splinting material is applied to the posterior of the calf, around the heel, and along

the bottom of the foot to the toes. The splint material is allowed to dry. The splint is secured into place with an Ace wrap.

Cast application is similar to splinting. The extremity is prepared with a stockinette and padding and placed in the desired position. It is important in casting to use the appropriate amount and type of padding in the bony prominences and high-pressure areas. Plaster or fiberglass casting material is applied by wrapping it circumferentially, each layer overlapping the previous layer by 50 percent. Care is also taken to avoid placing too little or too much tension on the wrapping. If the cast is too loose, the patient may experience rubbing, friction, and skin injuries such as abrasions or friction blisters. If the wrapping is too tight, it can create constriction, resulting in damage to the skin or neurovascular structures. Before the final layer of casting material is applied, the physician folds back the stockinette and padding, followed by application of the final layer. The cast is then molded before the casting material hardens upon drying. Following cast application, the patient's neurovascular status is rechecked and documented.

Focus Point
Placement of casts and/or splints is integral to any fracture or dislocation treatment (open or closed) or surgical procedure performed and is not reported separately. Casting and splinting are reported only when no other definitive fracture treatment, including reduction, is performed. ICD-10-PCS code assignment is based upon the intent of the procedure performed and should follow the Multiple Procedures guidelines.

Focus Point
Procedures to fit static or dynamic orthoses, such as splints and braces or application of an inhibitory cast (inhibitory cast is included in the equipment reference table under E Orthosis), in the rehabilitation setting are described in codes F0DZ6EZ and F0DZ7EZ and apply only to the rehabilitation setting. Splints and braces placed in other inpatient and outpatient settings are coded to Immobilization, table 2W3 in the Placement section.

Focus Point
The approach to splinting and casting is always External. The root operations in the Placement section include only procedures performed without making an incision or a puncture.

© 2018 Optum360, LLC

Medical and Surgical Related

Packing

Body System
Anatomical Regions
Anatomical Orifices

PCS Root Operation
Packing

Root Operation Table
2W4 Placement, Anatomical Regions, Packing
2Y4 Placement, Anatomical Orifices, Packing

Body Region
Head
Face
Neck
Abdominal Wall
Chest Wall
Back
Inguinal Region, Right
Inguinal Region, Left
Upper Extremity, Right
Upper Extremity, Left
Upper Arm, Right
Upper Arm, Left
Lower Arm, Right
Lower Arm, Left
Hand, Right
Hand, Left
Thumb, Right
Thumb, Left
Finger, Right
Finger, Left
Lower Extremity, Right
Lower Extremity, Left
Upper Leg, Right
Upper Leg, Left
Lower Leg, Right
Lower Leg, Left
Foot, Right
Foot, Left
Toe, Right
Toe, Left
Mouth And Pharynx
Nasal
Ear
Anorectal
Female Genital Tract
Urethra

Approach
External

Device
Packing Material

Description
Packing is putting material in a body region or orifice without first making an incision or a puncture. The physician first examines the area and may perform suction or debridement before beginning the packing. The physician then pushes absorbent packing into a wound or orifice to control bleeding or to facilitate healing. The packing may be coated with a vasoconstrictor such as phenylephrine 0.25 percent or topical anesthetic. It may be impregnated with petroleum jelly or may include an inflatable balloon used for pressure to assist hemostasis. Packing is temporary.

Focus Point
There is only one code for nasal packing in ICD-10-PCS. There is no differentiation between anterior and posterior nasal packing for epistaxis.

Medical and Surgical Related

Traction

Body System
Anatomical Regions

PCS Root Operation
Traction

Root Operation Table
2W6   Placement, Anatomical Regions, Traction

Body Region
Head
Face
Neck
Abdominal Wall
Chest Wall
Back
Inguinal Region, Right
Inguinal Region, Left
Upper Extremity, Right
Upper Extremity, Left
Upper Arm, Right
Upper Arm, Left
Lower Arm, Right
Lower Arm, Left
Hand, Right
Hand, Left
Thumb, Right
Thumb, Left
Finger, Right
Finger, Left
Lower Extremity, Right
Lower Extremity, Left
Upper Leg, Right
Upper Leg, Left
Lower Leg, Right
Lower Leg, Left
Foot, Right
Foot, Left
Toe, Right
Toe, Left

Approach
External

Device
Traction Apparatus
No Device

Description
There are several types of traction treatment modalities, and multiple anatomic sites may be treated. Traction may be defined as the act of drawing or pulling, associated with forces applied to the body to stretch or separate certain anatomic sites or parts. Traction may be used in treatment of fractures, spinal disorders, and other musculoskeletal or joint maladies to relieve pain and immobility.

Traction is exerting a pulling force on a body region in a distal direction using an External approach. The physician applies sustained or intermittent mechanical traction to a body part by applying manual or mechanical forces that relieve pain or increase tissue flexibility. Traction may require the use of a device, reported with Traction Apparatus, or may be manual, reported as No Device.

Focus Point
When traction is applied in conjunction with fracture reduction to stabilize the fracture, both procedures are reported.

Focus Point
The traction device may be applied to a body part that is not the site targeted for traction. For example, a halo device may be secured to the skull for a patient requiring neck traction. Report the site (body part) targeted for traction.

Focus Point
The approach value for the root operation Traction is External. When traction is performed using another approach, such as in conjunction with an Open surgical procedure with the intent to reposition, the root operation is reported as Reposition.

Coding Guidance
AHA: 2015, 2Q, 35; 2013, 2Q, 39

© 2018 Optum360, LLC

Medical and Surgical Related

Administration

Dialysis, Peritoneal (PD)

See also Hemodialysis under "Extracorporeal Assistance and Performance" in the Medical and Surgical Related section

Body System
Physiological Systems and Anatomical Regions

PCS Root Operation
Irrigation

Root Operation Table
3E1 Administration, Physiological Systems and Anatomical Regions, Irrigation

Body System/Region
Peritoneal Cavity

Approach
Percutaneous

Substance
Dialysate

Description
Kidneys function to filter waste, minerals, and excess fluid from the bloodstream, to be eliminated as urine. When kidneys no longer function effectively, dialysis can be performed to clean the blood. The two main types of dialysis are hemodialysis and peritoneal dialysis (PD). Only peritoneal dialysis is reported with codes in the Administration section.

In peritoneal dialysis, which is performed within the body (intracorporeal), fluid (dialysate) is pumped or introduced into the patient's abdomen and the dialysate absorbs the waste and excess fluid. The dialysate is drained and replaced multiple times during the day. The dialysate is infused through a percutaneously inserted catheter that provides access to the peritoneum through a skin site near the umbilicus.

There are two types of peritoneal dialysis. In automated peritoneal dialysis (APD), a machine called a cycler performs the fluid exchanges continuously during the night while the patient is sleeping. In continuous ambulatory peritoneal dialysis (CAPD), the patient fills the abdomen through the catheter with dialysate and drains it out after 4 to 6 hours with gravity. This type of dialysis involves several exchanges during the course of each day. Between exchanges, the patient can continue everyday activities.

Focus Point
Care must be taken to avoid contamination of the peritoneal fluid during the dialysis process. Peritonitis is a potential major complication of peritoneal dialysis, caused by the introduction of bacteria into the peritoneal cavity.

Focus Point
For creation of the peritoneal dialysis port or percutaneous cutaneo/peritoneal fistula, see root operation table ØWHG Insertion, Anatomical Regions, General, Peritoneal Cavity, and report device Infusion Device.

Coding Guidance
AHA: 2015, 2Q, 36; 2013, 4Q, 126

Medical and Surgical Related

Induction of Labor, Medical

Body System
Physiological Systems and Anatomical Regions

PCS Root Operation
Introduction

Root Operation Table
3EØ Administration, Physiological Systems and
     Anatomical Regions, Introduction

Body System/Region
Peripheral Vein
Female Reproductive

Approach
Percutaneous (Peripheral Vein)
Via Natural or Artificial Opening (Female Reproductive)

Substance
Hormone (Peripheral Vein)
Other Therapeutic Substance (Female Reproductive)

Qualifier
Other Hormone (Peripheral Vein)
Other Substance (Female Reproductive)

Description
In some cases, the end of the pregnancy may be hastened for the safety of the baby or the mother, and labor is started artificially by the provider. Labor can be induced in two ways: through medical intervention or through manual intervention. Manual induction of labor involves incising the bag of waters surgically (amniotomy) or separating the amniotic sac from the wall of the uterus (stripping of membranes) with a gloved finger.

In medical induction, the physician induces labor by administering medications to initiate dilation of the cervix and uterine contractions. Route of administration may vary according to the type of medication. The physician may insert a small tablet or tampon in the vagina up against the cervix. The insert melts or elutes drugs in response to the body's temperature once in place and releases the medication that softens and thins the cervix. After the medication is administered, the patient may start to have gentle labor contractions. This is reported with the root operation Introduction, with the body region Female Reproductive. The approach is Via Natural or Artificial Opening, substance is Other Therapeutic Substance, and qualifier Other Substance.

Alternatively, the physician may order and supervise the administration of a drug such as oxytocin (Pitocin). Although a woman's body makes oxytocin naturally, the synthetic form may be injected or infused intravenously, which strengthens the intensity of uterine contractions to induce labor. This is reported with the root operation Introduction, with the body region Peripheral Vein. The approach is Percutaneous substance is Hormone, and qualifier is Other Hormone.

Coding Guidance
AHA: 2014, 4Q, 17; 2014, 2Q, 8

Medical and Surgical Related

© 2018 Optum360, LLC

Infusion, Vasopressor Agent

Body System
Physiological Systems and Anatomical Regions

PCS Root Operation
Introduction

Root Operation Table
3E0 Administration, Physiological Systems and Anatomical Regions, Introduction

Body Part
Peripheral Vein
Central Vein

Approach
Percutaneous

Substance
Vasopressor

Description
Vasopressor infusion therapy is used to treat low blood pressure and shock, typically in gravely ill patients. Vasopressor infusion therapy is reserved for cases that do not respond to conventional medical treatment protocol.

Shock is defined as a state in which blood flow to and perfusion of peripheral tissue or organs is restricted due to inadequate cardiac output or inadequate systemic blood flow. Shock cases that are unresponsive to general medical management protocol are at high risk for progressing along the continuum of illness to multiple organ dysfunction syndrome (MODS) and ultimately death. Medical treatment options include restoration of normal intravascular blood volume and treatment of the underlying cause or condition. For patients who do not respond to initial treatment of IV fluids, vasopressor drugs are administered to improve systemic blood pressure. Vasopressors raise blood pressure by tightening (contracting) the blood vessels.

Using a Percutaneous approach, a physician or an assistant under direct physician supervision injects or infuses a vasopressor agent via an intravenous route. Vasopressors can be administered through an intravenous catheter inserted by needle into a patient's vein or by injection or infusion through an existing indwelling intravascular access catheter or port. Careful monitoring is required throughout the infusion therapy.

Medical and Surgical Related

Injection, Epidural Steroid

Body System
Physiological Systems and Anatomical Regions

PCS Root Operation
Introduction

Root Operation Table
3EØ Administration, Physiological Systems and Anatomical Regions, Introduction

Body System/Region
Spinal Canal

Approach
Percutaneous

Substance
Anti-inflammatory

Description
A spinal epidural steroid injection is a minimally invasive procedure that is typically administered to patients with chronic pain due to conditions such as lumbar disc herniation, degenerative disc disease, or lumbar spinal stenosis, which cause inflammation or pressure on the spinal nerve roots.

The spinal epidural space is the area between the dura, or covering of the spinal cord, and the bony vertebrae and is filled with fat and small blood vessels. Corticosteroids injected into the spinal epidural space provide an anti-inflammatory action, decreasing pain and allowing patients improved function as a conservative alternative to surgery. The injection may also include a local anesthetic and/or a saline solution.

The patient is placed in a sitting or lateral decubitus position so the physician can insert a needle into the vertebral interspace of the cervical, thoracic, lumbar, or sacral spine. The site to be entered is sterilized, local anesthesia is administered, and the needle is inserted. Contrast media may be injected to confirm proper needle placement under fluoroscopy. The physician injects a steroid solution to provide a therapeutic outcome. The solution is injected, reported with root operation Introduction, into the spinal epidural space. In some cases, the injection is administered on a tilting table so that after administration, the table can be tilted a few degrees to direct the flow of the injected steroid into the site of inflammation. When the procedure is complete, the needle is removed and the wound is dressed. The approach value reported is Percutaneous as the instrumentation (needle) is inserted via a puncture through the skin and other body layers necessary to reach the site of the procedure—in this case the spinal canal.

Focus Point
According to the ICD-10-PCS Body Part Key, the appropriate body part for the spinal epidural space is Spinal Canal.

Focus Point
If a local anesthetic is injected in combination with the steroid, separate coding of the anesthetic is allowed but is optional, according to the policies of the facility.

Coding Guidance
AHA: 2014, 4Q, 45

Medical and Surgical Related

© 2018 Optum360, LLC

Injection, Sclerosing Agent for Esophageal Varix

Body System
Physiological Systems and Anatomical Regions

PCS Root Operation
Introduction

Root Operation Table
3EØ   Administration, Physiological Systems and Anatomical Regions, Introduction

Body System/Region
Upper GI

Approach
Via Natural or Artificial Opening Endoscopic

Substance
Destructive Agent

Description
Esophageal varices are swollen varicose veins in the esophageal lining. The presence of esophageal varices is a complication of hypertension, which is caused by liver disease. Portal hypertension is increased blood pressure in the portal vein, which causes a buildup of pressure in vessels, including the esophageal veins.

Esophageal varices put the patient at risk for esophageal hemorrhage.

In sclerotherapy, an irritating solution (sclerosant) is injected into the vein. The sclerosant causes swelling and the vessel is occluded, blocking blood flow.

The physician passes a rigid or flexible esophagoscope through the patient's mouth and into the esophagus to identify and treat dilated, enlarged, and tortuous veins. The physician passes a sclerotherapy needle through the scope to the site of the varices and injects an agent that stops any bleeding by coagulating the blood and shrinking the vessel, causing scarring. Over time, this results in the reabsorption of the vein or veins by the local tissue.

Focus Point
The introduction of the sclerosing agent into a varicose vein causes the aberrant vessel to shrink and scar without actually destroying it. The sclerosing agent dissolves over time, and the vessel is absorbed by the body. Therefore, the root operation Destruction would not be appropriate for injection of a sclerosing agent.

Coding Guidance
AHA: 2013, 1Q, 27

Introduction, Antineoplastic Agent, Hepatic Artery

See also Chemoembolization, Hepatic Artery, in the Medical and Surgical section

See also Insertion, Hepatic Artery Infusion Device

Body System
Physiological Systems and Anatomical Regions

PCS Root Operation
Introduction

Root Operation Table
3E0   Administration, Physiological Systems and Anatomical Regions, Introduction

Body System/Region
Peripheral Artery

Approach
Percutaneous

Substance
Antineoplastic

Qualifier
Other Antineoplastic

Description
Liver cancer may be treated by delivering antineoplastic substances directly to the tumor site via a catheter inserted into the hepatic artery. This delivery method minimizes side-effects, like nausea and vomiting, and maximizes the cancer-killing properties of the drugs. Antineoplastic substances may be combined with embolic material that not only destroys cancer cells but also cuts off the blood supply to the tumor. Delivery of an antineoplastic substance alone is referred to as hepatic artery infusion (HAI), while delivery of both an antineoplastic and embolic material is referred to as chemoembolization. Chemoembolization requires two codes, one from the Administration section to report the introduction of the antineoplastic and embolic material and a second from the Medical/Surgical section to report the

embolization procedure. The Introduction component is described here. Introduction is defined as putting in or on a therapeutic, diagnostic, nutritional, physiological, or prophylactic substance except blood or blood products.

Prior to the HAI procedure, a separate procedure is performed in which a catheter is placed in the hepatic artery via an open or laparoscopic approach and a subcutaneous pump is placed to deliver the antineoplastic substance.

Before the chemoembolization procedure, diagnostic tests are performed to demonstrate patency of the portal vein to ensure the patient will have an adequate blood supply to the liver after treatment. With the patient under local anesthesia and mild intravenous sedation, the physician inserts a catheter percutaneously via the femoral artery and threads it into the hepatic artery. Angiography is then performed to identify the branches of the hepatic artery that supply blood to the tumor. Smaller catheters are then threaded into these branches, followed by injection of the antineoplastic or embolic chemotherapy mixture. Embolic material may consist of tiny microbeads or microspheres, a viscous collagen agent, gelatin sponges, or polyvinyl alcohol (PVA) particles.

Focus Point

The insertion of the hepatic artery infusion device is reported with the root operation Insertion from the Medical and Surgical Section. For a description of the insertion procedure for HAI, see Insertion, Hepatic Artery Infusion Device.

The embolization component of the procedure is reported with the root operation Occlusion from the Medical and Surgical Section. For a description of the embolization component, see Chemoembolization, Hepatic Artery.

Coding Guidance
AHA: 2015, 1Q, 38; 2014, 3Q, 26

Medical and Surgical Related

© 2018 Optum360, LLC

Irrigation, Joint

Body System
Physiological Systems and Anatomical Regions

PCS Root Operation
Irrigation

Root Operation Table
3E1 Administration, Physiological Systems and Anatomical Regions, Irrigation

Body System/Region
Joints

Approach
Percutaneous

Substance
Irrigating Substance

Qualifier
Diagnostic
No Qualifier

Description
Irrigation is putting in or on a cleansing substance. To irrigate a joint, the physician uses a syringe to inject a large volume of irrigation fluid into a diseased joint, such as one infected with septic arthritis. Fluid flushing the joint by Percutaneous injection (irrigation) is removed by aspiration or using irrigation and drainage catheters.

Focus Point
If the purpose of the irrigation is to retrieve samples from the joint for study, the Diagnostic qualifier is reported. If the purpose of the irrigation is to clean or flush the joint, No Qualifier is reported.

Focus Point
Irrigation done to clean a wound as part of another procedure, such as open reduction internal fixation (ORIF) of a fracture, would not be separately coded.

Coding Guidance
AHA: 2014, 4Q, 32

Medical and Surgical Related

Pleurodesis, Talc

See also Thoracoscopy (Diagnostic) in the Medical and Surgical section

Body System
Physiological Systems and Anatomical Regions

PCS Root Operation
Introduction

Root Operation Table
3EØ Administration, Physiological Systems and Anatomical Regions, Introduction

Body System/Region
Pleural Cavity

Approach
Percutaneous
Percutaneous Endoscopic

Substance
Other Therapeutic Substance

Qualifier
Other Substance

Description

Each lung is covered in two protective layers of pleural tissue. The visceral layer of pleura is the inner layer, and the parietal pleura is the outer layer. Between the layers of pleurae and lungs is a small amount of fluid to reduce any rub that might occur in the thorax during respiration. Excess fluid can build up in the pleural space as a result of disease, and air can collect in the pleural space if it leaks from the lung (pneumothorax). When extra fluid or air builds in the pleural space, normal respiration is compromised. Talc pleurodesis may be performed to reduce or eliminate the problem.

Pleurodesis is defined as the obliteration of the pleural space. In a talc pleurodesis, talc acts as a sclerosing agent, irritating the lining of the pleura and causing the parietal and visceral walls to heal with adhesions that effectively close the space between them, preventing the reaccumulation of pleural fluid or air.

Talc pleurodesis is also called pleural sclerosis. The physician delivers or introduces talc via a percutaneously inserted chest tube or catheter (Percutaneous approach) inserted through the skin, between the ribs, and into the pleural space. To enter the pleural space, the physician passes a trocar over the top of a rib, punctures through the parietal pleura, and enters the pleural cavity. With the end of the trocar in the chest cavity, the physician advances a plastic tube into the pleural cavity. The sharp instrument is removed, leaving one end of the plastic catheter in place within the pleural cavity. A syringe is attached to the outside of the catheter, and the talc is injected into the pleural cavity. The patient is instructed to change positions periodically for several hours, so that the talc is distributed throughout the pleural space. The talc is suctioned from the pleural space, the tube is removed, and the site is closed. The irritated tissue of the parietal and visceral pleurae will heal and adhere secondarily, obliterating the pleural space. Report the substance as Other Therapeutic Substance with qualifier Other Substance for talc pleurodesis.

In some cases, the pleurodesis is performed using video-assisted thoracoscopic surgery (VATS) so that the physician may visualize the operative site. The approach for VATS is Percutaneous Endoscopic.

Coding Guidance
AHA: 2015, 2Q, 31

Medical and Surgical Related

© 2018 Optum360, LLC

Thrombolysis (Injection of Thrombolytic) (Tissue Plasminogen Activator [tPA][r-tPA])

Body System
Physiological Systems And Anatomical Regions

PCS Root Operation
Introduction

Root Operation Table
3E0   Administration, Physiological Systems and Anatomical Regions, Introduction

Body System/Region
Peripheral Vein
Central Vein
Peripheral Artery
Central Artery
Coronary Artery

Approach
Percutaneous

Substance
Thrombolytic

Qualifier
Other Thrombolytic

Description
Thrombolytic therapy is the Introduction (administration) of drugs called lytics to dissolve blood clots that acutely block major arteries or veins. Ideally, the therapy should be initiated as soon as possible after the acute event to prevent permanent damage. Thrombolytic therapy may be administered to reverse or reduce the effects of stroke, myocardial infarction, pulmonary embolism, deep vein thrombosis (DVT), acute arterial thrombosis/ischemia of the extremities, blocked bypass grafts, dialysis grafts and fistulas, or indwelling vascular catheters. A thrombolytic agent is a substance that dissolves a thrombus, a localized clot formation that impairs circulation. Thrombolytics may be documented as:

- Alteplase
- Anistreplase
- Reteplase
- Streptokinase
- Tenecteplase
- Tissue plasminogen activator (tPA)(r-tPA)
- Urokinase

Thrombolytics can be administered systematically via a peripheral or central catheter, or can be delivered directly via catheter-directed thrombolysis (CDT) into the area of the thrombus. The type of thrombolytic, method of administration, and duration of treatment depend upon the size and location of the clot.

In a catheter-directed thrombolysis, a small Percutaneous incision is made at the site of insertion. The physician places a hollow catheter and, using fluoroscopic guidance, the physician advances the catheter tip to the clot location in the vessel and confirms the presence of thrombus (blood clot) using contrast media and imaging. The physician infuses a thrombolytic agent into the affected vessel to dissolve the thrombus. The physician may perform contrast injections to assess the size and extent of the thrombus after infusion of the thrombolytic agent. The catheter may be left in place, and the length of treatment varies, depending on the underlying cause. When treatment is complete, the catheter is removed from the patient's body. Pressure is placed over the incision for 20 to 30 minutes to stem bleeding, and the patient is observed afterward.

Coding Guidance
AHA: 2014, 4Q, 19; 2013, 4Q, 124

Medical and Surgical Related

Transfusion, Fresh Frozen Plasma (FFP)

Body System
Circulatory

PCS Root Operation
Transfusion

Root Operation Table
302 Administration, Circulatory, Transfusion

Body System/Region
Peripheral Vein
Central Vein

Approach
Percutaneous

Substance
Frozen Plasma

Qualifier
Autologous
Nonautologous

Description

Fresh frozen plasma (FFP) is a source of all clotting factors in normal concentration, excluding platelets, that is centrifuged, separated, and frozen solid at 0° F or colder when "fresh" (within eight hours of collection).

As it maintains clotting factors in the frozen state, FFP is used to treat coagulation factor deficiencies that are congenital, or acquired deficiencies that are secondary to liver disease, warfarin anticoagulation, disseminated intravascular coagulation (DIC), etc., with active bleeding or risk of active bleeding such as prior to a surgical procedure with potential for blood loss.

FFP may also be used for plasma exchanges to treat diseases like thrombotic thrombocytopenic purpura (TTP), Raynaud's disease, and glomerulonephritis.

The procedure involves thawing the plasma, after which the physician or clinician transfuses the FFP by establishing venous access with a sterile needle and catheter through which the plasma is infused into the recipient patient's circulatory system.

Focus Point

Use substance value Frozen Plasma for both frozen and fresh frozen plasma. This substance value indicates that the plasma has been frozen. The substance value Fresh would be reported for liquid plasma that is separated and prepared from whole blood and stored in a liquid state that has never been frozen. Plasma in a liquid state can be stored refrigerated for approximately 26 days and is ready for immediate administration as it does not require thawing before use.

Medical and Surgical Related

© 2018 Optum360, LLC

Transplant, Bone Marrow (BMT)

See also Harvest, Graft, Autologous Bone Marrow in the Medical and Surgical section

See also Therapy, Bone Marrow Cell, Autologous, Intramuscular in the New Technology section

Body System
Circulatory

PCS Root Operation
Transfusion

Root Operation Table
3Ø2 Administration, Circulatory, Transfusion

Body System/Region
Peripheral Vein
Central Vein

Approach
Percutaneous

Substance
Bone Marrow

Qualifier
Autologous
Allogeneic, Related
Allogeneic, Unrelated
Allogeneic, Unspecified

Description
Bone marrow is the soft, spongy, fatty tissue inside bones that produces the immature blood-forming cells that can grow into red or white blood cells, or platelets.

A bone marrow transplant replaces unhealthy bone marrow with healthy bone marrow to regenerate bone marrow and immune systems destroyed by chemotherapy and/or radiation therapy. An autologous transplant uses the patient's own bone marrow for the transplant, while an allogeneic transplant uses a donor's bone marrow. The harvested bone marrow is usually obtained from a large bone of the donor.

Harvested bone marrow that has been previously processed to remove blood and bone fragments and cryopreserved is thawed and is infused into the bloodstream of the recipient through an intravenous catheter. This is reported with root operation Transfusion in the Administration section.

Focus Point
Administration procedures should not be confused with Transplantation procedures. Instilling autologous or allogeneic bone marrow is coded to Administration, whereas implanting a functioning, living body part from another individual is coded to the root operation Transplantation in the Medical and Surgical section. Bone marrow transplant procedures are coded in the Administration section with the root operation Transfusion.

Focus Point
Intramuscular injection of concentrated bone marrow aspirate is reported with ICD-10-PCS code XKØ23Ø3 Introduction of Concentrated Bone Marrow Aspirate into Muscle, Percutaneous Approach, New Technology Group 3.

Medical and Surgical Related

Transplant, Stem Cell

Body System
Circulatory

PCS Root Operation
Transfusion

Root Operation Table
3Ø2   Administration, Circulatory, Transfusion

Body System/Region
Peripheral Vein
Central Vein

Approach
Percutaneous

Substance
Stem Cells, Embryonic
Stem Cells, Cord Blood
Stem Cells, Hematopoietic

Qualifier
Autologous
Allogeneic, Related
Allogeneic, Unrelated
Allogeneic, Unspecified

Description
Hematopoietic or blood-derived progenitor cells, or stem cells, harvested for transplantation are used to regenerate bone marrow and immune systems destroyed by chemotherapy and/or radiation therapy. These progenitor cells are present not only in bone marrow, but also in peripheral blood collected by apheresis.

The recipient's immune system is first suppressed using radiation or chemotherapy. The patient is prepared much the same way as when giving a regular blood transfusion. The stem cells, which were frozen until needed for transplant, are thawed. The processed stem cells are infused into the bloodstream of the recipient through an intravenous catheter much like a blood transfusion. This is reported with root operation Transfusion in the Administration section.

Focus Point
Administration procedures should not be confused with Transplantation root operations. Instilling autologous or allogeneic stem cells is coded to Administration, whereas implanting a functioning, living body part from another individual is coded to the root operation Transplantation in the Medical and Surgical section. Stem cell transplant procedures are coded in the Administration section with the root operation Transfusion.

© 2018 Optum360, LLC

Medical and Surgical Related

Measurement and Monitoring

Angiography, Intraoperative Fluorescence Vascular

Body System
Physiological Systems

PCS Root Type
Monitoring

Root Operation Table
4A1 Measurement and Monitoring, Physiological Systems, Monitoring

Body Part
Cardiac
Gastrointestinal
Skin and Breast

Approach
External

Function/Device
Vascular Perfusion

Qualifier
Indocyanine Green Dye

Description

Intraoperative fluorescence vascular angiography (IFVA) is an imaging technology that assesses blood flow through vascular tissue (perfusion). Used during breast and skin reconstruction, and coronary or gastrointestinal procedures, IFVA allows the physician to visualize blood flow and make intraoperative procedural adjustments, resulting in greater graft and patent anastomosis success.

During IFVA, indocyanine green (IC-Green™) dye is injected into the bloodstream and rapidly binds to plasma proteins in blood. An external imaging system generates fluorescence excitation with a light source. Using a camera, real-time images showing vascular perfusion are displayed.

Focus Point
No additional code is needed from the Imaging section; a code from table 4A1 is considered a complete code when perfusion is assessed with fluorescence vascular angiography.

Coding Guidance
AHA: 2016, 4Q, 114

Medical and Surgical Related

Catheterization, Cardiac

See also Angiography, Cardiac (Coronary Arteriography) (Angiocardiography) under "Imaging" in the Ancillary section

Body System
Physiological Systems

PCS Root Operation
Measurement

Root Operation Table
4A0 Measurement and Monitoring, Physiological Systems, Measurement

Body System
Cardiac

Approach
Percutaneous

Function/Device
Sampling and Pressure

Qualifier
Right Heart
Left Heart
Bilateral

Description
Diagnostic cardiac catheterizations are performed to evaluate conditions such as valve disease, coronary artery disease, and pulmonary hypertension and include:

- Recording of intracardiac and intravascular pressures
- Tracings
- Obtaining blood samples for measurement of blood gases
- Measuring cardiac output

Cardiac angiography is most often performed with cardiac catheterization. *See also* Angiography, Cardiac (Coronary Arteriography) (Angiocardiography).

Left Heart Cardiac Catheterization
Diagnostic left cardiac catheterization performed via an arterial route is more commonly performed than right heart or bilateral catheterizations. Operative reports often refer to the procedure as left heart cath or LHC. Left heart cardiac catheterization includes the study of the left atrium and ventricle, the mitral and aortic valves, the ascending left aorta, and possibly the pulmonary veins.

A catheter is threaded to the heart through an introducing sheath placed percutaneously into the femoral, brachial, or axillary artery. The catheter passes through the aortic valve into the left ventricle. Blood

samples, pressure and electrical recordings, and/or other tests are performed. ECG monitoring for the entirety of the procedure is included. The PCS root operation Measurement is reported along with the function value of Sampling and Pressure as it includes the pressure measurements along with any blood samples. The root operation Measurement is defined as determining the level of a physiological or physical function at a point in time. The qualifier value of Left Heart indicates that the catheterization was performed only in the left heart.

Right Heart Cardiac Catheterization
Diagnostic right heart catheterization is performed via a venous route and is often referred to as right heart cath, RHC, or Swan-Ganz catheterization. Right heart cardiac catheterization includes the study of the right atrium and ventricle, the tricuspid and pulmonic valves, the main pulmonary artery and its branches, and the superior and inferior vena cava.

The physician threads a catheter to the heart through an introducing sheath placed percutaneously into the femoral vein. However, the physician may elect to use the subclavian, internal jugular, or antecubital vein instead. The catheter is threaded into the right atrium, through the tricuspid valve into the right ventricle, and across the pulmonary valve into the pulmonary arteries. ECG monitoring for the entirety of the procedure is included. Blood samples, pressure and electrical recordings, and/or other tests are performed through the catheter. The PCS root operation Measurement is reported along with the function value of Sampling and Pressure, as it includes the pressure measurements along with any blood samples. The qualifier value of Right Heart indicates that the catheterization was performed only in the right heart.

Combined Right and Left Heart Cardiac Catheterization (Bilateral)
This procedure is performed to evaluate both right and left heart function. For right heart catheterization, the physician threads a catheter through an introducing sheath placed percutaneously into the femoral, subclavian, internal jugular, or antecubital vein. The catheter is threaded into the right atrium, through the tricuspid valve into the right ventricle, and across the pulmonary valve into the pulmonary arteries. Left heart catheterization is also performed in this case using retrograde technique. The catheter is inserted through an introducing sheath placed percutaneously into the femoral, brachial, or axillary artery. The catheter is passed through the aortic valve into the left ventricle. ECG monitoring for the entirety of the procedure is included. Blood samples, pressure and electrical recordings, and/or other tests are performed through the catheter. The PCS root operation Measurement is reported along with the function

Medical and Surgical Related

© 2018 Optum360, LLC

Catheterization, Cardiac (continued)

value of Sampling and Pressure, as it includes the pressure measurements along with any blood samples.

Combined right and left heart cardiac catheterization is a single procedure with study and evaluation of both right and left heart. The qualifier value of Bilateral indicates that the catheterization was performed in both the left and right heart.

Focus Point
Report in addition any concurrent, separately reportable procedures such as cardiac angiography (Fluoroscopy, Heart, Coronary Arteries, Single or Multiple) or left ventriculography (Fluoroscopy, Heart, Left). See also Angiography, Cardiac (Coronary Arteriography) (Angiocardiography); and Ventriculography, Cardiac.

Coding Guidance
AHA: 2016, 3Q, 37

Electrocorticography (Intraoperative)

Body System
Physiological Systems

PCS Root Operation
Measurement

Monitoring

Root Operation Table
4A0   Measurement and Monitoring, Physiological Systems, Measurement

4A1   Measurement and Monitoring, Physiological Systems, Monitoring

Body System
Central Nervous

Approach
Open

Function/Device
Electrical Activity

Qualifier
Intraoperative

Description
Intraoperative electrocorticography (ECoG) is used in surgical management of medically refractory epilepsy as an aid in identifying the epileptic focus and area of resection in a cerebral lobectomy.

During an Open craniotomy surgical procedure, part of the skull is removed to expose a large area of the brain surface. Approximately 16 electrocorticography electrodes or sensors are placed directly on the brain's cortical surface in a grid formation to measure and/or monitor and record the brain's electrical activity. Brain waves are captured on paper or electronic medium for study to be used in a separately reported procedure such as a cerebral excision for tumor or epilepsy.

Focus Point
Measurement and Monitoring root operations differ in only one respect: Measurement defines one procedure, and Monitoring defines a series of procedures.

Medical and Surgical Related

Fractional Flow Reserve (FFR), Coronary

See also Angiography, Cardiac (Coronary Arteriography) (Angiocardiography), under "Imaging" in the Ancillary section

Body System
Physiological Systems

PCS Root Operation
Measurement

Root Operation Table
4AØ Measurement and Monitoring, Physiological Systems, Measurement

Body System
Arterial

Approach
Percutaneous

Function/Device
Pressure

Qualifier
Coronary

Description
Fractional flow reserve (FFR), or intravascular pressure measurement, is a type of intracoronary pressure measurement used to evaluate blood flow using comparative pressure measurements of the blood flow across a coronary lesion or stenosis. Fractional flow reserve is used to evaluate the severity of coronary artery stenosis and complex disease such as multivessel disease. Intravascular pressure measurement may be used in addition to coronary angiography to provide a more complete assessment of the severity of coronary disease. *See also* Angiography, Cardiac (Coronary Arteriography) (Angiocardiography), in the Imaging section of the Ancillary section.

A pressure-sensitive guidewire is inserted distal to the native coronary lesion to compare the coronary pressure with the aortic pressure proximal to the lesion to assess the severity of the lesion in terms of limitation of blood flow. Since this pressure is being determined at a point in time rather than over a period of time, the root operation used to report this procedure is Measurement. The pressure of blood flow being measured is within the coronary arteries and therefore the body system Arterial is reported. The qualifier Coronary identifies the location of the arteries.

Focus Point
Additional codes should be assigned for any synchronous diagnostic or therapeutic procedures such as angiography, ventriculography, or PTCA.

Coding Guidance
AHA: 2016, 3Q, 37

Medical and Surgical Related

© 2018 Optum360, LLC

Interrogation, Device, Cardiac Rhythm Related

Body System
Physiological Devices

PCS Root Operation
Measurement

Root Operation Table
4BØ Measurement and Monitoring, Physiological Devices, Measurement

Body System
Cardiac

Approach
External

Function/Device
Pacemaker
Defibrillator

Qualifier
No Qualifier

Description
Cardiac pacemaker devices are used to control the rate of the heart by electrical stimulation and response mechanism. Implantable cardioverter-defibrillators (ICDs) are devices that administer an electric shock to control cardiac arrhythmias and restore a normal heartbeat.

Patients with previously implanted cardiac pacemakers and defibrillators require periodic analysis of device function. Many devices can be checked in the home with a remote monitoring system connected by telephone or internet that records the data and transmits the information to the provider for review.

Frequently, device interrogation is performed in the physician's office by a manufacturer representative or specially trained providers who bring the appropriate device readers and perform the interrogation. In some cases, emergency device interrogation may be performed in the emergency department for diagnostic management. Interrogation includes evaluating the device functions and battery status, and checking for any significant events the device has stored and its response.

Before the interrogation, the type of device and manufacturer are confirmed. Device interrogation machines differ by manufacturer and are not interchangeable. During the interrogation, the cardiac device is connected in an External approach, noninvasively outside the body, to a device interrogation/programming machine using a special radiofrequency telemetry wand placed on the skin over the pacemaker or ICD. The data are transmitted from the device to the programmer and evaluated, and a report is created. The interrogation machine checks battery voltage and measures lead impedance, threshold and sensing, percentage of time paced and sensed, underlying rhythm, mode switch episodes, events, and pacing mode output. Care must be taken during interrogation to avoid inadvertent reprogramming or disabling the device entirely. Any necessary reprogramming of the device is done at the time of interrogation under controlled conditions.

Focus Point
A check/interrogation of an automatic implantable cardioverter defibrillator (AICD) differs from an electrophysiology study (EPS) because the interrogation is performed on the AICD device. An EPS study is performed on the patient's heart.

© 2018 Optum360, LLC

Measurement, Portal Venous Pressure

Body System
Physiological Systems

PCS Root Operation
Measurement

Root Operation Table
4A0 Measurement and Monitoring, Physiological Systems, Measurement

Body System
Venous

Approach
Percutaneous

Function/Device
Pressure

Qualifier
Portal

Description
This procedure, reported with root operation Measurement, is performed to calculate portal hypertension. It is also referred to as Hepatic Venous Pressure Gradient (HVPG) since it employs percutaneous venous catheterization to determine the pressure difference between free hepatic venous pressure (FHVP) and the wedged hepatic venous pressure (WHVP) of the hepatic vein.

Under mild conscious sedation, using fluoroscopy, a catheter with a balloon tip is inserted into the right jugular vein and through the right atrium into the inferior vena cava (IVC), and then advanced to the hepatic vein. The pressure is measured with the catheter in the hepatic vein and again after using the balloon to occlude the hepatic vein. Normal HVPG is between 1 mmHg and 5 mmHg with varices developing when the HVPG is over 10 mmHg. Further increases in pressure can lead to variceal bleeding, ascites, portal hypertensive gastropathy, and a multitude of other complications.

Focus Point
Root operation Measurement determines a physiological or physical function at a point in time while Monitoring determines the function over a period of time.

© 2018 Optum360, LLC

Monitoring, Central Venous Pressure

Body System
Physiological Systems

PCS Root Operation
Monitoring

Root Operation Table
4A1 Measurement and Monitoring, Physiological Systems, Monitoring

Body Systems
Venous

Approach
Percutaneous

Function/Device
Pressure

Qualifier
Central

Description
Central venous pressure (CVP) monitoring is used to quantify changes in the pressure of blood returning to the heart. This procedure involves monitoring of venous pressure using a sensor introduced through an intravenous catheter. CVP monitoring is often used to assess fluid volume status.

Using a Percutaneous approach, the physician inserts a venous catheter into an upper extremity or subclavian vein and advances it just superior to the right atrium of the heart. Positioning is verified by x-ray. The catheter is attached to monitoring systems that record and display the data. Venous pressure is detected by the sensor at the tip of the catheter, which travels through the fluid-filled catheter to the transducer, where it is transformed into a signal that is recorded by the CVP recording unit. Once the procedure is complete, the catheter is removed.

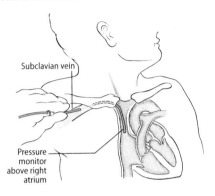

Subclavian vein

Pressure monitor above right atrium

Focus Point
Root operation Measurement determines a physiological or physical function at a point in time while Monitoring determines the function over a period of time.

Focus Point
Insertion of the Monitoring Device, Pressure Sensor, is a separately reportable procedure, using the Percutaneous approach and the table for the appropriate body part value based on the documented position of the catheter tip.

Medical and Surgical Related

Monitoring, Fetal Heart Rate, Transvaginal (Internal)

See also Insertion, Monitoring Electrode, under "Obstetrics" in the Medical and Surgical Related section

Body System
Physiological Systems

PCS Root Operation
Monitoring

Root Operation Table
4A1   Measurement and Monitoring, Physiological Systems, Monitoring

Body System
Products of Conception, Cardiac

Approach
Via Natural or Artificial Opening

Function/Device
Rate

Description
Fetal heart rate monitoring is performed to assess the health of the fetus during the stresses of labor and delivery. Normally fetal heart rate monitoring is done using an external transducer that is strapped to the mother's abdomen. When the provider wants more accurate and consistent data on the status of the fetus, and the patient's water has broken and the cervix is sufficiently dilated to allow access to the fetus through the cervix, an internal monitor may be used.

The physician evaluates fetal heart rate response to contractions in the mother. The fetal head, in preparation for delivery, is pressed against the internal os of the cervix. A wire electrode is threaded into the vaginal orifice, through the external os of the cervix and a transducer is secured to the fetal scalp to sense the fetal heart rate. A lead transmits the electrode's information to an external recording device. The fetal heart rate and uterine contractions are monitored and recorded for 20 minutes to determine the effect of contractions on the fetus. This procedure is usually performed during the third trimester.

Alternatively, the physician evaluates fetal heart rate response to its own activity. The patient reports fetal movements as an internal monitor records fetal heart rate changes. If the fetus is not active, an acoustic device may be used to stimulate activity.

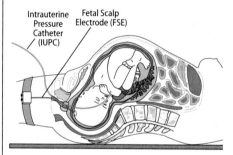

Intrauterine Pressure Catheter (IUPC)   Fetal Scalp Electrode (FSE)

Focus Point

For transvaginal fetal heart rate monitoring, two codes are required. In addition to the code for the monitoring, a second code should be reported for the insertion of the monitoring electrode transducer onto the fetal scalp.. This is reported with a code from root operation table 10H Insertion.

© 2018 Optum360, LLC

Medical and Surgical Related

Monitoring, Intracranial Pressure

See also Ventriculostomy in the Medical and Surgical section

Body System
Physiological Systems

PCS Root Operation
Monitoring

Root Operation Table
4A1 Measurement and Monitoring, Physiological Systems, Monitoring

Body System
Central Nervous

Approach
Percutaneous

Function/Device
Pressure

Qualifier
Intracranial

Description
Intracranial pressure monitoring devices are used to manage cerebrovascular injury, traumatic brain injury, and other disorders of the brain that result in increased intracranial pressure. This increased pressure can cause a decrease in the tissue oxygenation levels in the brain. Intracranial pressure can be monitored by placing a device inside the head that measures the pressure inside the brain cavity and then sends those

measurements to a recording device. Monitoring may be performed in various ways.

A burr hole is drilled through the skull through which an intraventricular catheter (a thin, flexible tube) is threaded into one of the two lateral ventricles. The catheter passes through the brain matter and into the lateral ventricle, which normally contains the cerebrospinal fluid (CSF) that protects the brain and spinal cord. The intracranial pressure can be monitored and also lowered if necessary by draining the CSF out via the catheter. This is felt to be the most accurate method of measurement.

Alternatively, a bolt or screw may be placed just through the skull into the subarachnoid space (the space between the arachnoid membrane and the cerebral cortex). The subarachnoid bolt is typically used if immediate access is necessary. This device consists of a hollow screw that is inserted through an opening made in the skull and through the dura mater (the outermost membrane protecting the brain and spinal cord).

An epidural sensor, which is less invasive than the previous two methods, may also be used. Placed through a burr hole drilled into the skull just over the epidural covering, the epidural sensor cannot remove excess CSF since no hole is created in the epidural lining. Rather, it is inserted between the skull and the epidural tissue.

Coding Guidance
AHA: 2016, 2Q, 29

Monitoring, Neurophysiological, Intraoperative

Body System
Physiological Systems

PCS Root Operation
Monitoring

Root Operation Table
4A1 Measurement and Monitoring, Physiological Systems, Monitoring

Body System
Central Nervous
Peripheral Nervous

Approach
Open
Percutaneous
External

Function/Device
Electrical Activity

Qualifier
Intraoperative

Description
The objective of intraoperative neurophysiological monitoring is to protect the function of the central and peripheral nervous systems from injuries during surgery that cause deficits such as muscle weakness, paralysis, hearing loss, and other loss of normal body functions after the operation.

Electromyography
Electromyography (EMG) is often used during posterior spinal procedures, particularly during insertion of pedicle screws to identify changes from the spinal cord to the peripheral nervous system. This assists with the correct placement of the screw into the bony pedicle in relationship to the exiting nerve root. Several EMG needles are placed in various peripheral muscles to monitor, along with the use of a sterile stimulating probe used intraoperatively during the surgery. Recording feedback may be sent visually and audibly. Other examples of uses for EMG monitoring include cranial nerve monitoring during surgery for acoustic neuroma, parotid gland or temporal bone surgery, and rhizotomy surgery for conditions causing spasticity.

Somatosensory Evoked Potentials
Somatosensory evoked potentials (SSEP) recordings use external recording electrodes placed on the scalp, cervical spine, lumbosacral spine or Erb's point to monitor electrical activity in central and peripheral nerves. Stimulation sites vary depending on the target for monitoring such as medial nerve for upper extremity monitoring or posterior tibial nerve for lower extremity monitoring. Complex SSEP recordings for changes in latency and amplitude are monitored and interpreted for use in various surgical settings such as spinal, cerebral, carotid, and vascular procedures.

Neurosensory monitoring is reported with a code from the Measurement and Monitoring section of ICD-10-PCS. Since the measurements are being taking repetitively over a period of time, Monitoring is used with Electrical Activity function.

Focus Point
Erb's point, named after Wilhelm Heinrich Erb, is a site in the brachial plexus in the upper trunk where six types of nerves meet.

Focus Point
Facilities may or may not choose to report neuromonitoring performed during surgical procedures.

Coding Guidance
AHA: 2015, 2Q, 14; 2015, 1Q, 26

Medical and Surgical Related

© 2018 Optum360, LLC

Stress Test, Cardiac (Myocardial Perfusion Scan)(Cardiovascular Stress Test)

Body System
Physiological Systems

PCS Root Operation
Monitoring

Root Operation Table
4A1 Measurement and Monitoring, Physiological Systems, Monitoring

Body System
Cardiac

Approach
External

Function/Device
Total Activity

Qualifier
Stress

Description
Cardiac stress testing is performed to evaluate and manage patients with known or suspected heart disease. It is performed using exercise with a treadmill or bicycle, or a pharmacological agent (e.g., Persantine [dipyridamole], Adenosine) may be used as an alternative to exercise when the patient is unable to perform the adequate level of exertion. During a stress test, the patient exercises either until symptoms occur or the patient reaches a maximum heart rate (85 percent of predicted heart rate based on age). It can be done with exercise and electrocardiography without imaging, or exercise or pharmacologic stress combined with imaging such as stress echocardiography or radionuclide myocardial perfusion imaging (MPI).

Monitoring
An assistant supervised by a qualified health care professional continuously records the electrical activity of the heart while the patient is exercising on a treadmill or bicycle and/or given medicines. The stress on the heart during the test is monitored.

Echocardiography may be performed in conjunction with the stress test. In echocardiography, high-frequency sound waves record the structure and blood flow of the heart, including heart chamber size, contraction, wall motion and thickness, as well as valve structure. Most commonly performed is the transthoracic echocardiogram (TTE). During this procedure, an ultrasonic transducer is moved over the chest to capture ultrasound images of the heart.

Radionuclide, which adheres to the patient's red blood cells, may be injected intravenously for cardiac blood pool imaging, and is a separately reportable procedure. Multiple images of the heart, synchronized with the electrocardiographic RR interval (ECG gated), are taken several minutes later, after the radionuclide has spread through the blood pool. A computer synthesizes these images and generates data to produce a video display of cardiac wall motion, calculations of left ventricular ejection fractions, and images based on computer manipulation of the data received.

Focus Point
Measurement and Monitoring root operations differ in only one respect: Measurement defines one procedure, and Monitoring defines a series of procedures.

Focus Point
Codes for imaging such as echocardiogram and/or thallium nuclear medicine scans may be reported in addition to the monitoring procedure, if desired.

Medical and Surgical Related

Extracorporeal or Systemic Assistance and Performance

Balloon Pump, Intra-aortic (IABP)

Body System
Physiological Systems

PCS Root Operation
Assistance

Root Operation Table
5A0 Extracorporeal or Systemic Assistance and Performance, Physiological Systems, Assistance

Body System
Cardiac

Duration
Intermittent
Continuous

Function
Output

Qualifier
Balloon Pump

Description
Implantation of an intra-aortic pulsation balloon pump (IABP) consists of placing a balloon catheter into the descending thoracic aorta that inflates and deflates with the patient's heartbeat. This pump assists in circulating the blood to the heart and the body, allowing the heart to rest or recover from heart failure, MI, injury, trauma, or shock. This procedure is done to help support the function of the left ventricle of the heart and can also be used during interventional cardiac procedures such as arthrectomies and angioplasties, particularly in high-risk patients.

The left or right femoral artery is exposed in the groin. After the vessel is occluded above and below the proposed insertion site, the artery is opened transversely. Occasionally, the end of a small tube of Gore-Tex may be sewn to the side of the artery. The tip of the balloon catheter is inserted into the artery (or Gore-Tex tube). The clamp occluding the artery upstream is released, and the balloon catheter is advanced to the femoral artery and into the aorta above the level of the kidney arteries, but not beyond the left arm artery. It is connected to a pump, and the pump is turned on. The pump inflates and deflates the balloon during each heartbeat cycle. Inflation of the balloon can be set to trigger intermittently according to the patient's ECG or blood pressure or continuously by a cardiac pacemaker or a pre-set continuous internal rate. The pump may be used for a few hours or up to two weeks.

Focus Point
IABP, like cardiopulmonary bypass, is an exception to the usual practice of not reporting supporting procedures that are components of a larger operation. When a surgical procedure is performed with IABP, it is coded as an additional procedure.

Focus Point
An IABP is neither classified nor coded as a device in ICD-10-PCS. It is not appropriate to assign a code with root operation Insertion when the balloon pump is placed or with the root operation Removal when the pump is disconnected. The use of an IABP is appropriately reported using the root operation Assistance.

Coding Guidance
AHA: 2018, 2Q, 3; 2013, 3Q, 18

© 2018 Optum360, LLC

Medical and Surgical Related

Bypass, Cardiopulmonary

Body System
Physiological Systems

PCS Root Operation
Performance

Root Operation Table
5A1 Extracorporeal or Systemic Assistance and Performance, Physiological Systems, Performance

Body System
Cardiac

Duration
Continuous

Function
Output

Description
Cardiopulmonary bypass, also known as artificial heart and lung or pump oxygenator, is a form of extracorporeal (situated or occurring outside the body) circulation utilized to temporarily perform the complete functions of the heart and lungs during surgery and maintain the circulation of blood and the oxygen content of the body.

In cardiopulmonary bypass (CPB), venous blood is diverted to a heart-lung machine, which mechanically pumps and oxygenates the blood on a continuous basis temporarily so the heart can be bypassed while an open procedure on the heart or coronary arteries is performed. Roller or centrifugal pumps push the patient's venous blood through a membrane oxygenator to perform the gas exchange usually performed by the lungs, and then the blood is returned to the patient's arterial flow. During bypass, the lungs are deflated and immobile, and the heart is motionless and bloodless. CPB is performed under systemic hypothermia, reducing the risk of ischemia.

Focus Point
Cardiopulmonary bypass is an exception to the usual practice of not reporting supporting procedures that are components of a larger operation. When a surgical procedure is performed with cardiopulmonary bypass, it is coded as an additional procedure.

Coding Guidance
AHA: 2016, 1Q, 27; 2015, 4Q, 22; 2014, 3Q, 16, 20; 2014, 1Q, 10; 2013, 3Q, 18

Cardioversion and Defibrillation, External

Body System
Physiological Systems

PCS Root Operation
Restoration

Root Operation Table
5A2 Extracorporeal or Systemic Assistance and Performance, Physiological Systems, Restoration

Body System
Cardiac

Duration
Single

Function
Rhythm

Description
External cardioversion is used to administer an electronic shock to a patient's chest to regulate heartbeats considered dangerously irregular. Large patches called electrodes are placed on the outside of the patient's chest and/or back and connected to a defibrillator. A defibrillator machine delivers a measured electric shock through the chest to the heart. This shock briefly disturbs all electrical activity to the heart and, if successful, converts the heartbeat to a regular rhythm.

Medical and Surgical Related

Hemodialysis

Body System
Physiological Systems

PCS Root Operation
Performance

Root Operation Table
5A1 Extracorporeal or Systemic Assistance and Performance, Physiological Systems, Performance

Body System
Urinary

Duration
Intermittent, Less than 6 Hours Per Day
Prolonged Intermittent, 6-18 hours Per Day
Continuous, Greater than 18 Hours Per Day

Function
Filtration

Description
Hemodialysis describes a replacement method for nonfunctioning kidneys that artificially removes waste products such as free water, urea, and potassium from the blood and restores proper balance of electrolytes in the blood. Dialysis may be performed in a hospital, clinic, or home environment. The procedure involves a previously placed catheter in an artery or vein to withdraw the patient's blood, mechanically circulating the blood through a dialysis machine to remove the toxins and wastes, and transfusing the blood back to the patient.

The dialysis machine operates on the principle of diffusion of solutes across a semipermeable membrane using counter-current flow; whereby the dialysate flows in the opposite direction of the blood flow. This counter-current flow keeps the concentration gradient across the membrane at a consistent maximum by hydrostatic pressure, which helps filter the waste products.

This procedure may also be documented as artificial kidney, hemofiltration, hemodiafiltration, or renal dialysis.

Focus Point
Hemodialysis consists of a set of dialysis treatments of varying lengths of continuity. The Duration qualifiers are assigned based upon the documentation of the length of each dialysis treatment session. Intermittent Hemodialysis (IHD) is administered for less than 6 hours per day. Prolonged Intermittent Renal Replacement Therapy (PIRRT) is administered between 6 and 18 hours per day, as compared with Continuous Renal Replacement Therapy (CRRT), which is administered for longer than 18 hours per day.

Focus Point
Peritoneal dialysis differs from hemodialysis as the filtering process takes place in the patient's own body instead of externally. A solution is instilled via a catheter into the peritoneal cavity, where it remains over a determined amount of time to filter out the waste. It is then drained out into a bag and disposed of. This cycle is called an exchange and is repeated several times either during the day or overnight. It is reported with a code from the Irrigation table of the Administration section (3E1).

Coding Guidance
AHA: 2016, 1Q, 29

© 2018 Optum360, LLC

Oxygen Therapy, Supersaturated

Body System
Physiological Systems

PCS Root Operation
Assistance

Root Operation Table
5AØ Extracorporeal or Systemic Assistance and Performance, Physiological Systems, Assistance

Body System
Circulatory

Duration
Intermittent
Continuous

Function
Oxygenation

Qualifier
Supersaturated

Description
Supersaturated oxygenation therapy (SSO2) involves the creation of super-oxygenated arterial blood, which is infused directly to oxygen-deprived myocardial tissue in acute myocardial infarction patients. Infusion of supersaturated oxygen into the infarct area results in a significant reduction in infarct size and preserves myocardial tissue. SSO2 is used as an adjunct to other procedures that restore coronary artery blood flow, such as percutaneous transluminal coronary angioplasty (PTCA), coronary atherectomy, and coronary artery stent insertion.

Immediately following the intervention procedure, super oxygenated saline is mixed with the patient's blood to produce super oxygenated blood, which is delivered to the oxygen-deficient tissue via a catheter. No additional access site is needed as the blood is circulated through the existing access site used for the procedure.

This therapy may also be documented as superoxygenation, superoxygenation infusion therapy, SSO2, or aqueous oxygen (AO) therapy.

Focus Point
The duration value Intermittent versus Continuous, is assigned based on documentation of the level of circulatory assistance required. Intermittent assistance is started and stopped as needed, while Continuous assistance is performed without interruption as long as the patient requires it.

Focus Point
SSO2 should not be confused with other oxygen therapy, which is a respiratory therapy procedure or vascular perfusion, which is the infusion of other substances into the vessel.

Focus Point
Report separately any percutaneous coronary intervention performed such as percutaneous transluminal coronary angioplasty (PTCA), coronary atherectomy, or insertion of coronary artery stents.

Medical and Surgical Related

Oxygenation, Extracorporeal Membrane (ECMO)

Body System
Physiological Systems

PCS Root Operation
Performance

Root Operation Table
5A1 Extracorporeal or Systemic Assistance and Performance, Physiological Systems, Performance

Body System
Circulatory

Duration
Continuous

Function
Oxygenation

Qualifier
Membrane, Central
Membrane, Peripheral Veno-arterial
Membrane, Peripheral Veno-venous

Description

Extracorporeal membrane oxygenation (ECMO) is a simplified form of cardiopulmonary bypass (extracorporeal circulation) that may be used as life support for patients awaiting organ transplantation or for newborns with serious birth complications or defects. ECMO provides both cardiac and respiratory support to oxygenate severely ill patients whose heart and lungs cannot function without assistance.

In ECMO, the patient's blood is pumped to a machine, oxygenated, and returned to the patient, similar to a cardiopulmonary bypass but modified for prolonged use (days to weeks) at the bedside. Its purpose is to provide mechanical support for the heart and lungs to allow time for recovery. Patients receiving ECMO require daily management to monitor for infections of the skin along cannulas and to identify any evidence of clotting in the legs or any deposits visualized within the pump.

Oxygenation, Hyperbaric, Wound

Body System
Physiological Systems

PCS Root Operation
Assistance

Root Operation Table
5A0 Extracorporeal or Systemic Assistance and Performance, Physiological Systems, Assistance

Body System
Circulatory

Duration
Intermittent
Continuous

Function
Oxygenation

Qualifier
Hyperbaric

Description
Adequate blood supply is essential to wound healing. Chronic diseases like atherosclerosis and diabetes can reduce the blood supply to extremities, as can conditions like poor nutrition and radiation therapy.

When a skin wound is slow to heal, it is at risk for infection and necrosis. Hyperbaric oxygen therapy (HBOT) may be administered to the patient whose blood supply is compromised, in an attempt to increase tissue oxygenation at the site of the wound and improve healing.

Hyperbaric oxygen therapy is administered inside a specialized pressure chamber. Within the chamber, the atmospheric pressure is elevated two to three times higher than normal air pressure and pure oxygen is pumped into the chamber. This increases oxygen saturation in the tissue of the patient, who is lying down entirely within the chamber.

This is reported with root operation Assistance, as the hyperbaric oxygen therapy is supporting the oxygenation performed by the circulatory system. The duration may be Intermittent or Continuous.

Focus Point
Report qualifier Supersaturated when the therapy includes placing a high concentration of oxygen into blood plasma and delivering it directly to the area of treatment—for example, the site of an acute myocardial infarct.

© 2018 Optum360, LLC

Performance, Extracorporeal Hepatic (Liver Dialysis)

Body System
Physiological Systems

PCS Root Operation
Performance

Root Operation Table
5A1 Extracorporeal or Systemic Assistance and Performance, Physiological Systems, Performance

Body System
Biliary

Duration
Single
Multiple

Function
Filtration

Description
There are two types of extracorporeal assistance devices, classified by artificial or biological methods. The artificial system based on filtration most commonly used is the molecular adsorbent recirculating system (MARS). Bioartificial cell-based liver support systems use human or animal cells; an example is extracorporeal liver assist device (ELAD).

Both MARS and ELAD involve devices outside the body that perform the detoxification function of the liver. Liver dialysis is used to treat patients in acute hepatic failure, as a bridge to transplantation for patients in end-stage liver disease (ESLD) or temporarily for filtration assistance in patients with alcoholic hepatitis or other liver decompensation. Currently liver dialysis has Food and Drug Administration approval in the United States only for treatment of acute hepatic encephalopathy due to intoxication and/or poisoning.

Using a mobile bedside device that is similar in function to a hemodialysis machine, blood is alternately withdrawn, passed through a hemodiafilter with albumin dialysate and returned to the patient, with toxins removed, through an access catheter. Liver dialysis is designed to remove toxins from blood and help maintain metabolic balance.

Focus Point
The duration value (single vs multiple) is assigned based on documentation of a continuous (single) treatment or separate (multiple) treatments.

Removal, Carbon Dioxide, Extracorporeal (ECCO$_2$R) (Respiratory Dialysis)

Body System
Physiological Systems

PCS Root Operation
Assistance

Root Operation Table
5A0 Extracorporeal or Systemic Assistance and Performance, Physiological Systems, Assistance

Body System
Respiratory

Duration
Continuous

Function
Filtration

Qualifier
No Qualifier

Description
Extracorporeal carbon dioxide removal (ECCO$_2$R) is minimally invasive partial respiratory support that is designed to remove carbon dioxide (CO$_2$) from the body in patients with acute hypercapnic respiratory failure or needing respiratory support while awaiting lung transplant. Oxygen is supplied and CO$_2$ is removed from blood circulated through the system. The intent is to reduce or eliminate the need for mechanical ventilation, or as an alternative to extracorporeal membrane oxygenation (ECMO).

Similarly to dialysis, CO$_2$ is filtered from the blood through a low blood flow (0.4–1 L/min) extracorporeal circuit.

In a separately reportable procedure, a large-bore, dual-lumen, central venous catheter, which provides both inflow and outflow, is inserted under imaging guidance. The catheter lumens are connected via tubing to the gas exchanger. From the drainage (outflow), lumen blood is passed through a blood inlet tubing into an external centrifugal pump, where a membrane filters out excess CO$_2$. The filtered blood is then returned to the body through the blood outlet tubing of the system to the infusion (inflow) lumen of the central catheter. The controller system controls the pump speed and gas flow and provides real-time continuous measurement of CO$_2$ levels in the blood.

Coding Guidance
AHA: 2017, 4Q, 71

Ventilation, Mechanical, Assistance (Respiratory)

See also Ventilation, Mechanical, Performance (Respiratory)

Body System
Physiological Systems

PCS Root Operation
Assistance

Root Operation Table
5A0   Extracorporeal or Systemic Assistance and Performance, Physiological Systems, Assistance

Body System
Respiratory

Duration
Less than 24 Consecutive Hours
24-96 Consecutive Hours
Greater than 96 Consecutive Hours

Function
Ventilation

Qualifier
Continuous Positive Airway Pressure
Intermittent Positive Airway Pressure
Continuous Negative Airway Pressure
Intermittent Negative Airway Pressure
No Qualifier

Description
Mechanical (respiratory) assisted ventilation involves respiratory assistance (root operation Assistance) when the patient's spontaneous breathing is supplemented by a mechanical device; it does not completely replace the physiological function of breathing.

Assistance and Performance are two variations of the same kinds of procedures, varying only in the degree of control exercised over the physiological function. Assistance mechanical ventilation is usually delivered using a noninvasive interface such as a face mask, nasal mask, nasal pillow, oral mouthpiece, or oronasal mask. *See also* Ventilation, Mechanical, Performance (Respiratory).

Positive airway pressure ventilation can be either intermittent or continuous. The most common types of positive pressure ventilation are continuous positive airway pressure (CPAP) and bilevel positive airway pressure (BPAP).

CPAP generally delivers, through a nasal or face mask, a continuous fixed level of positive airway pressure. CPAP is commonly used to treat hypoxemia and obstructive sleep apnea.

BPAP, most commonly referred to as BiPAP (BiPAP is a registered trademark held by Respironics, Inc.), is a two-level, or bilevel, pressure mode of positive pressure ventilation that delivers a preset inspiratory positive airway pressure (IPAP) and an expiratory positive airway pressure (EPAP). The inspiratory level is greater than the expiratory level to avoid making the patient exhale against pressure. Indications for BPAP include respiratory failure, chronic obstructive pulmonary disease (COPD), pulmonary edema, atelectasis, pulmonary embolisms, and pneumonia.

Negative pressure ventilation can also be either continuous or intermittent and is generally used in patients with progressive neuromuscular diseases, central hypoventilation, or chest wall deformities that inhibit breathing. This type of mechanical ventilation uses various devices outside the patient's chest that generate negative pressure to expand the lungs with air. The release of the negative pressure allows the chest to relax and the lungs to exhale. Some examples of these types of ventilators are the "iron lung," cuirass, tortoise shell, or body suit. The most commonly used negative-pressure ventilator is a "jacket" ventilator, an airtight, impermeable nylon jacket suspended by a rigid piece that fits over the chest and abdomen. These ventilators are lightweight but must be connected to negative-pressure generators that can weigh 30 to 60 pounds.

Focus Point
The number of hours of ventilation assistance must be calculated to assign the appropriate Duration. To calculate the number of hours, begin the count from the start of the mechanical ventilation. The duration ends when the machine is turned off.

Focus Point
If a patient is on mechanical ventilation only at night, count the duration of time the patient is actually on the ventilator. Assign a code for each episode, counting the duration for each individual episode. If the duration includes weaning time, the weaning period is included until the ventilator is turned off.

Coding Guidance
AHA: 2017, 1Q, 29; 2014, 4Q, 3-11

Medical and Surgical Related

© 2018 Optum360, LLC

Ventilation, Mechanical, Performance (Respiratory)

See also Intubation, Endotracheal in the Medical and Surgical section

See also Ventilation, Mechanical, Assistance (Respiratory)

Body System
Physiological Systems

PCS Root Operation
Performance

Root Operation Table
5A1 Extracorporeal or Systemic Assistance and Performance, Physiological Systems, Performance

Body System
Respiratory

Duration
Less than 24 Consecutive Hours
24-96 Consecutive Hours
Greater than 96 Consecutive Hours

Function
Ventilation

Qualifier
No Qualifier

Description

Mechanical (respiratory) ventilation represents the root operation of Performance when it completely controls the patient's physiological function of breathing with a mechanical device. The major indication for this type of mechanical ventilation is acute respiratory failure. The goal of mechanical ventilation is to relieve respiratory distress, decrease the patient's work of breathing, improve pulmonary gas exchange, reverse respiratory muscle fatigue, and permit lung healing in patients with no spontaneous breathing or to prevent the patient from having to perform the work of breathing.

Assistance and Performance are two variations of the same kinds of procedures, varying only in the degree of control exercised over the physiological function. Performance mechanical ventilation is usually delivered using an invasive interface such as an orally or nasally placed endotracheal tube or a tracheostomy (artificial opening in the trachea) tube. *See also* Ventilation, Mechanical, Assistance (Respiratory).

Ventilators offer a variety of modes. The mode controlling how and when breaths are to be delivered is determined by the physician based on the needs of the patient. Most modern ventilators use intermittent positive-pressure ventilation (IPPV), which inflates the lungs by generating and applying positive pressure. In controlled mechanical ventilation (CMV), the ventilator delivers a preset number of breaths per minute of a preset volume, rather than breaths triggered by the patient. Mechanically ventilated patients may be placed in a drug-induced coma or paralyzed using paralytic drugs.

Patients are weaned off of ventilation slowly, as clinical and physiological criteria are met. This ensures that the patient can gradually build respiratory efforts and breathing independence as strength is regained.

Focus Point
The number of hours of ventilation must be calculated to assign the appropriate duration. To calculate the number of hours of continuous mechanical ventilation, begin the count from the start of the (endotracheal) intubation. The duration ends with (endotracheal) extubation. If a patient is intubated prior to admission, begin counting the duration from the time of the admission. If a patient is transferred (discharged) while intubated, the duration would end at the time of transfer (discharge).

For patients who begin on (endotracheal) intubation and subsequently have a tracheostomy performed for mechanical ventilation, the duration begins with the (endotracheal) intubation and ends when the mechanical ventilation is turned off (after the weaning period). The entire weaning period during the process of withdrawing the patient from ventilatory Performance is included in calculating the duration of mechanical ventilation, whether endotracheal or with tracheostomy.

Focus Point
An additional code for endotracheal tube insertion may generally be reported. However, if mechanical ventilation and endotracheal intubation are used only during a surgical procedure, they are usually considered inherent and not reported. If the patient remains on mechanical ventilation for an extended period (several days) after surgery, the mechanical ventilation can be reported.

Coding Guidance
AHA: 2017, 1Q, 29; 2014, 4Q, 3-11

Medical and Surgical Related

Extracorporeal or Systemic Therapies

Oxygenation, Hyperbaric (Decompression)

Body System
Physiological Systems

PCS Root Operation
Decompression

Root Operation Table
6A1 Extracorporeal or Systemic Therapies,
Physiological Systems, Decompression

Body System
Circulatory

Duration
Single
Multiple

Description
Patients who have carbon monoxide (CO) poisoning or decompression (DCS) sickness are treated with hyperbaric oxygenation to return their blood oxygen

levels to normal. The pure oxygen in a hyperbaric chamber is pressurized and assimilated more readily into the bloodstream. Patients with DCS have nitrogen bubbles in their bloodstream. These bubbles form from changing altitude too quickly, as seen in divers, mountain climbers, and astronauts.

Hyperbaric oxygen is administered inside a hyperbaric chamber that combines high atmospheric pressure with pure oxygen. Normal room air is only about 20 percent oxygen. For hyperbaric oxygenation, the root operation is Decompression, as the oxygen chamber's high pressure is what returns the patient's blood oxygen levels to normal. The duration may be Single or Multiple.

Focus Point
Hyperbaric oxygen treatment (HBOT) for nonhealing wounds is reported with root operation table 5ØA.

Medical and Surgical Related

© 2018 Optum360, LLC

Perfusion, Respiratory Donor Organ (EVLP) (ex-vivo lung perfusion)

See also Transplant, Lung, in the Medical and Surgical section

Body System
Physiological Systems

PCS Root Operation
Perfusion

Root Operation Table
6AB Extracorporeal or Systemic Therapies, Physiological Systems, Perfusion

Body Part
Respiratory System

Duration
Single

Qualifier
Donor Organ

Qualifier
No Qualifier

Description
Lung transplants replace diseased lungs with healthy lungs from an organ donor. Most donated lungs are taken from deceased donors; preserving the donor lung for transplantation is essential. The lungs can sustain cell damage after brain death before they can be removed for donation. This means that only one in five lungs may be safe for transplantation and thus suitable for donation.

Previously, the maximum acceptable time donor lungs could remain outside the body was six to eight hours. Respiratory donor organ perfusion, also known as ex-vivo lung perfusion (EVLP), is a new technique that involves removing the lungs from the donor body and evaluating, preparing, and preserving them for transplantation into the recipient body.

ELVP can double the time the donor lungs can remain outside the body, making lungs that used to be marginally acceptable now viable transplantable organs. The increased time can also allow retrieval of donor lungs across greater geographical areas, improving outcome and reducing costs.

The donor lungs are first cooled to slow down further deterioration and tissue injury, then treated and evaluated with the EVLP system for three to six hours. The EVLP system is a specialized sterile protective dome attached to a ventilator, pump, and filters, through which a solution of oxygen, proteins, and nutrients is continuously pumped into the lungs, simulating normal physiological function. This helps repair damage to the donor lungs, which are assessed for acceptable function. After the lungs are determined to be suitable for transplant, they are cooled again for transport to the recipient site.

Coding Guidance
AHA: 2016, 4Q, 115

Medical and Surgical Related

Pheresis

Body System

Physiological Systems

PCS Root Operation

Pheresis

Root Operation Table

6A5 Extracorporeal or Systemic Therapies,
Physiological Systems, Pheresis

Body System

Circulatory

Duration

Single

Multiple

Qualifier

No Qualifier

Qualifier

Erythrocytes

Leukocytes

Platelets

Plasma

Stem Cells, Cord Blood

Stem Cells, Hematopoietic

Description

In pheresis, whole blood is removed from the patient
(extracorporeal), filtered so that a targeted element is
extracted, and then the blood is returned to the
patient. Pheresis is also known as hemipheresis and
apheresis. Pheresis is usually performed in a centrifuge.
In some cases, a filtration system is used.

The qualifier in pheresis describes the blood product
that is therapeutically removed from the blood before

it is returned to the patient. Leukapheresis, which
removes leukocytes, is a common treatment for
chronic myeloid leukemia and some other leukemias.
Plateletpheresis (thrombocytapheresis), which
removes thrombocytes, is a therapeutic treatment for
thrombocytosis. In plasmapheresis, plasma is replaced
with a plasma substitute, usually to eliminate
antibodies that may be causing an autoimmune
disorder. In hematopoietic stem cell (HSC) pheresis,
blood is collected from a peripheral blood vessel and
the stem cells are removed and may be stored for
transplant. Stem cells can also be retrieved from the
blood in the umbilical cord. After the birth of a baby
and after the umbilical cord has been cut, the cord is
frozen so that blood can be retrieved from the cord for
future needs.

Therapeutic pheresis is the removal of some specific
circulating blood component, cells, or plasma solute.
The patient is prepared much the same as giving a
regular blood donation. Whole blood is drawn out of
one arm and into an instrument called a separator,
which uses a microprocessing technique to draw the
blood, anticoagulate it, and separate the component
to be removed by centrifugal spinning, filtration, or
column adsorption with the help of computerized
calibration. The cells to be removed are collected while
the remainder of the blood is recombined and
returned to the patient through a tube and needle in
the other arm.

Focus Point

*Photopheresis, in which blood is infused with a
photosensitive substance, withdrawn from the patient,
exposed to light, and returned to the patient, is reported
with root operation table 6A6 Phototherapy,
Physiological Systems.*

© 2018 Optum360, LLC

Medical and Surgical Related

Phototherapy

Body System
Physiological Systems

PCS Root Operation
Phototherapy

Root Operation Table
6A6 Extracorporeal or Systemic Therapies, Physiological Systems, Phototherapy

Body System
Skin
Circulatory

Duration
Single
Multiple

Description
Phototherapy is extracorporeal treatment performed by directing light rays of various concentrations at tissue or blood. It can be applied topically to the skin, or it can be used as a circulatory treatment.

The most common type of phototherapy is the treatment of hyperbilirubinemia in newborns. Fluorescent light breaks down the bilirubin deposits in the newborn's skin. These deposits give the skin its yellow tint. Once broken down, the bilirubin deposits can be eliminated as waste.

For treatment of hyperbilirubinemia, the infant is placed in the incubator with only its eyes and genitals covered, and lights are focused on the infant's skin for several days.

Phototherapy can also be directed at a patient's blood (photopheresis). In photopheresis, the patient is injected with a photoactive substance that targets certain elements in the bloodstream; for example, leukocytes in a patient with graft-versus-host disease. The blood is removed from the patient (extracorporeal) and exposed to light that destroys the cells to which the injected substance has bonded. Extracorporeal photopheresis (ECP) uses different wavelengths, depending on the targeted cells and the light being used.

Focus Point
In some cases, to sensitize the skin to the ultraviolet rays, the patient may take a psoralen pill. This is called photochemotherapy. Ultraviolet light directed at the skin can reduce psoriatic plaque or eczema by treating inflammation in the skin on the skin. The light is directed only at the affected skin. This type of phototherapy is also called actinotherapy. This is reported from table 6A8 Ultraviolet Light Therapy, Physiological Systems.

Therapy, Shock Wave, Extracorporeal (ESWT), Musculoskeletal (Orthotripsy)

Body System
Physiological Systems

PCS Root Operation
Shock Wave Therapy

Root Operation Table
6A9   Extracorporeal or Systemic Therapies, Physiological Systems, Shock Wave Therapy

Body System
Musculoskeletal

Duration
Single

Multiple

Qualifier
No Device

Qualifier
No Qualifier

Description
Musculoskeletal extracorporeal shock wave therapy (ESWT), also known as orthotripsy, uses noninvasive pulses of high- or low-energy shock waves applied from outside the body directly to specific areas of the body to reduce chronic pain and promote healing of injuries and calcifications that have not responded to conservative treatment measures.

Examples of conditions treated with orthotripsy are chronic plantar fasciitis, chronic medial and/or lateral epicondylitis, and chronic tendonitis.

ESWT is generally performed as an outpatient procedure and may require from one to five treatments, depending on the level of energy administered.

The patient is placed in a supine position. The physician examines and palpates the affected site, marking the targeted most painful area with a surgical pen. The patient is then given a local or regional anesthetic. Ultrasound gel is applied to the site. The affected body part is placed close against the treatment head. The treatment head has a plastic dome filled with water with a spark plug inside, which creates the shock waves that pass through the dome into the body part.

> **Focus Point**
> *The duration value (single vs multiple) is assigned based on documentation of a continuous (single) treatment or separate (multiple) treatments.*

Medical and Surgical Related

© 2018 Optum360, LLC

Ultrasound, Therapeutic

Body System
Physiological Systems

PCS Root Operation
Ultrasound Therapy

Root Operation Table
6A7 Extracorporeal or Systemic Therapies, Physiological Systems, Ultrasound Therapy

Body System
Circulatory

Duration
Single
Multiple

Qualifier
Head and Neck Vessels
Heart
Peripheral Vessels
Other Vessels

Description
Therapeutic ultrasound, or intravascular sonotherapy, is an interventional treatment modality that uses lower frequency and higher intensity levels of ultrasound energy than those employed in diagnostic ultrasound. Utilizing nonablative energy to reduce intimal hyperplasia or restenosis associated with atherosclerotic vascular disease, therapeutic ultrasound permits healing of the vessels following stent implantation.

Therapeutic Ultrasound of Vessels of Head and Neck
A needle is inserted percutaneously into a blood vessel of the head and neck. A guidewire is threaded through the needle into the blood vessel, and the needle is removed. An intravascular ultrasound catheter is placed over the guidewire. The ultrasound catheter is used to administer nonablative energy to reduce intimal hyperplasia or restenosis associated with atherosclerotic vascular disease. The catheter and guidewire are removed, and pressure is applied over the puncture site to stop bleeding.

Therapeutic Ultrasound of Heart
A needle is inserted percutaneously into a blood vessel of the groin and threaded through the vessel to the heart. A guidewire is threaded through the needle into the blood vessel, and the needle is removed. An intravascular ultrasound catheter is placed over the guidewire. The ultrasound catheter is used to administer nonablative treatment inside the vessel. The catheter and guidewire are removed, and pressure is applied over the puncture site to stop bleeding.

Therapeutic Ultrasound of Peripheral Vascular Vessels
A needle is inserted percutaneously into a peripheral blood vessel. A guidewire is threaded through the needle into the blood vessel, and the needle is removed. An intravascular ultrasound catheter is placed over the guidewire. The ultrasound catheter is used to administer nonablative treatment inside the vessel. The catheter and guidewire are removed, and pressure is applied over the puncture site to stop bleeding.

Focus Point
The duration value (single vs multiple) is assigned based on documentation of a continuous (single) treatment or separate (multiple) treatments.

Coding Guidance
AHA: 2014, 4Q, 19

Osteopathic

Manipulative Treatment, Osteopathic

Body System
Anatomical Regions

PCS Root Operation
Treatment

Root Operation Table
7W0 Osteopathic, Anatomical Regions, Treatment

Body Region
Head
Cervical
Thoracic
Lumbar
Sacrum
Pelvis
Lower Extremities
Upper Extremities
Rib Cage
Abdomen

Approach
External

Method
Articulatory-Raising
Fascial Release
General Mobilization
High Velocity-Low Amplitude
Indirect
Low Velocity-High Amplitude
Lymphatic Pump
Muscle Energy-Isometric
Muscle Energy-Isotonic
Other Method

Description

This category describes osteopathic manipulative treatment (OMT), a method of therapy that employs the use of the hands to diagnose, treat, and prevent illness or injury. The physician, who is a specially trained Doctor of Osteopathic Medicine (D.O.), uses the hands to move muscles and joints using techniques including stretching, gentle pressure, and resistance to ease pain, promote healing, and increase mobility.

OMT is performed to reduce or eliminate somatic dysfunction and related disorders. Somatic dysfunction is an osteopathic term that describes asymmetry, edema, fibrosis, restriction, hypertonicity, or atrophy of related components in a patient's musculoskeletal system, affecting range of motion and sometimes neurological or circulatory function.

Terms used to describe specific forces of osteopathic manipulative therapies include:

- Velocity—speed of motion, swiftness
- Amplitude—magnitude, breadth, or range
- Isotonic—involving muscular contraction in which the muscle remains under relatively constant tension while its length changes
- Isometric—involving muscular contraction in which tension increases while length remains constant

Osteopathic services rely heavily on the physical examination of the joints and muscles before diagnosis and treatment. The provider uses fingertips to sense areas of dysfunction and administers treatment by manual manipulation. OMT includes isolating and reducing tensions and malalignments in the soft tissues, bones, and joints. OMT techniques vary depending on the nature of the presenting problem and focus of therapy: counterstrain, cranial, muscle energy, myofascial release (MFR), and high velocity-low amplitude (HVLA) thrust, among others.

The therapy methods are not explicitly defined in ICD-10-PCS; use the standard definitions used in this specialty.

The articulatory technique uses manipulation of the range of motion within a joint to restore joint mobility. This is a low-velocity/moderate- to high-amplitude technique where a joint is carried through its full motion, using repetitive springing motions or concentric movements through the restrictive barrier.

In fascial release (myofascial release [MFR]), muscle and fascia are massaged through pressure on the skin to increase mobility, relax contracted muscles, and increase circulation. Myofascial release involves palpating a restriction in the myofascial tissue. In direct MFR, the restrictive barrier is engaged with constant force until the tissue is released. In indirect MFR, the myofascial tissues are moved away from the restrictive barrier, freeing movement.

In general manipulation, as tolerated by the patient, the provider gently and repeatedly forces the joint to the point of resistance, reducing the restrictive barrier to improve range of motion.

High velocity-low amplitude (HVLA) method is designed to restore the symmetry of joint movements with short, fast manipulations of a joint to improve range of motion. HVLA is also called a thrust technique. The provider slowly eases the joint in the direction of resistance. At the point of resistance, the physician

© 2018 Optum360, LLC

Manipulative Treatment, Osteopathic (continued)

pulls gently against the restraint while applying a quick force to affect a "pop" in the joint, resulting in immediate increased range and freedom of motion.

Low velocity-high amplitude (LVHA) method is designed to achieve the same goal as HVLA but uses pressure that is delivered more slowly but with somewhat greater force. Both are direct techniques. LVHA is a form of articulatory treatment (ART) in which the joint is carried through its full range of motion to increase range of motion. The provider may engage the restrictive barrier repeatedly to produce increased freedom of motion.

In the indirect method, the provider treats pain, fascial and connective tissue strains, or malalignments by exerting pressure or tension on opposing parts to cause an indirect release. Techniques may vary and include facilitated positional release (FPR). In FPR, the provider performs myofascial treatment. The body is placed into a neutral position, diminishing tissue and joint tension in all planes. A force such as compression or torsion may be added. This provides therapeutic results without direct manipulation of the affected region.

Lymphatic pump treatment (LPT) is directional massage that pushes lymphatic fluids along the lymphatic system to therapeutically alter circulation of lymph fluid.

In isometric and isotonic muscle energy, the physician conducts manipulations using the force of muscle contractions in a specific way to release pain in an affected area and increase range of motion. Isometric manipulations consist of the force applied by the physician on a particular muscle or muscle group that is equal to the force exerted by the patient. Isotonic manipulations consist of a force applied by the physician on a particular muscle or muscle group that is less than the force exerted by the patient.

Focus Point

ICD-10-PC Osteopathic codes may be reported by any provider using the ostreopathic manipulative therapies.

Focus Point

Multiple codes are reported when multiple body sites or techniques are involved.

Medical and Surgical Related

Other Procedures

Acupuncture

Body System
Physiological Systems and Anatomical Regions

PCS Root Type
Other Procedures

Root Operation Table
8E0   Other Procedures, Physiological Systems and Anatomical Regions, Other Procedures

Body Region
Integumentary System and Breast

Approach
Percutaneous

Method
Acupuncture

Qualifier
Anesthesia
No Qualifier

Description
Acupuncture is a method of producing analgesia by inserting tiny needles into specific sites on the body along channels, called meridians, and twirling, energizing, or warming the needles. It may be used to reduce pain and discomfort in a number of conditions, including headaches, labor pain, chemotherapy-induced nausea and vomiting, and back and neck pain.

Using a Percutaneous approach, the health care provider applies acupuncture therapy by inserting one or more fine needles into the patient as dictated by acupuncture meridians for the relief of pain or anesthesia. Five to 20 needles may be inserted during a single session. The needles are twirled or manipulated by hand to generate therapeutic stimulation, remaining in place for 10 to 20 minutes. At the end of the session, the needles are removed.

> **Focus Point**
> *When the intent of the procedure is for anesthesia, the qualifier Anesthesia is used.*

Medical and Surgical Related

© 2018 Optum360, LLC

Assistance, Computer

Body System
Physiological Systems and Anatomical Regions

PCS Root Operation
Other Procedures

Root Operation Table
8E0   Other Procedures, Physiological Systems and
      Anatomical Regions, Other Procedures

Body Region
Head and Neck Region
Trunk Region
Upper Extremity
Lower Extremity

Approach
External

Method
Computer Assisted Procedure

Qualifier
With Fluoroscopy
With Computerized Tomography
With Magnetic Resonance Imaging
No Qualifier

Description
Computer-assisted surgery (CAS) expands the surgeon's abilities by augmenting them with real-time radiographic imagery that adds precision at the surgical site. Common methods of computer assistance include intraoperative fluoroscopic computer guidance, computed tomography (CT) computer guidance, and magnetic resonance imaging (MRI) computer guidance.

Computer assistance is reported in addition to the main surgery with a code from the Other Procedures section and operation, and the body system Physiological Systems and Anatomical Regions. Because computer-assisted surgery is augmenting traditional surgery with radiographic imaging, it is performed using an External approach. Computer assistance is more than traditional guidance because the computer interprets the images and provides guidance for surgical direction.

CAS is used in intracranial, ENT, orthopaedic, and spinal surgeries and involves image-guided navigation, markers, reference frames, and intraoperative sensing. Planning, registration, and navigation are the key activities of computer-assisted surgery. The planning part is based on imaging. Preoperative 3D images may be taken, as well as intraoperative images using MRI, CT, and fluoroscopy in different combinations.

Registration occurs at the start of the procedure to set up spatial relationships between the points on the images taken and those same corresponding points on a patient's actual anatomy. Landmarks are the key to properly aligning image to actual anatomy. A landmark is a particular point on the anatomy that can be readily identified both in the actual surgical field and within the image. The landmark must be completely stationary with respect to the surrounding anatomy so that the relative position does not change. Natural anatomical structures or artificial markers, like a pin within bone, may be used.

To maintain the spatial relationship throughout the computer-assisted surgery, dynamic referencing is used. Dynamic referencing utilizes a reference frame fixed to the anatomy that allows infrared, electromagnetic, or radiowave sensors to detect and follow movement of the patient, which the computer measures and compensates for.

Navigation is the intraoperative tracking of tools and instruments, together with the surgical field in real time with display of this movement shown laid over the images and 3D models of the anatomy. This ensures safe progression of invasive surgical procedures with increased precision and accuracy.

These types of computer-assisted surgery, also called image-guided surgery (IGS) or image-guided navigation (IGN), are used for intracranial and ENT procedures, as well as for orthopaedic procedures such as hip replacements, where angle calculations are critical. CAS is an important adjunct to complicated surgery or surgery performed where normal anatomic reference points have been destroyed by disease or previous surgeries.

In some instances, using direct imageless applications, landmarks are established on a "universal" limb model. This application requires touch-pointing the anatomic landmarks, which are then registered on the computer for use in accurate navigation and measurement in relation to any bone or instrument movement as the surgery is performed. This application establishes coordinates as an aid for precisely locating anatomical structures for Open or Percutaneous procedures without the use of preoperative or intraoperative images. Imageless computer assistance is reported with No Qualifier.

Preoperative images of patient-specific bone geometry are obtained for the surgical plan. The patient-specific surgical plan and images of the individual's anatomy are used during surgery to help guide the surgeon by combining these with intraoperative navigation capabilities. Optical targets, or trackers, such as digitizing or LED-equipped probes, are attached to points on the bone anatomy or to surgical tools. An optical camera tracks the position of these for accurate navigation and measurement in relation to any bone or instrument movement as the

Assistance, Computer (continued)

surgery is performed. The software in these navigational systems matches, or "registers," the position of the patient on the operating table to the geometric description of the bony surface derived from the images already used to plan the surgery. Multiple images are simultaneously displayed on the monitor. The virtual tool trajectory that corresponds to the tracked tool movements is displayed over the

previously saved views in real-time as the surgeon operates.

Focus Point

Reporting of computer assistance is always secondary to the intended root operation being performed.

Assistance, Robotic

Body System
Physiological Systems and Anatomical Regions

PCS Root Operation
Other Procedures

Root Operation Table
8E0   Other Procedures, Physiological Systems and Anatomical Regions, Other Procedures

Body Region
Head and Neck Region
Trunk Region
Upper Extremity
Lower Extremity

Approach
External
Open
Percutaneous
Percutaneous Endoscopic

Method
Robotic Assisted Procedure

Description
Robotic-assisted surgery expands the surgeon's abilities by augmenting them with miniaturized instruments combined with the use of robotic arms and high-definition 3D cameras that add precision at the surgical site. Common brands of robotic instrumentation are the da Vinci Surgical System® and the Cyberknife®.

Because robotic-assisted surgery is augmenting traditional surgery, it can be performed using various approaches, depending upon the intended root operation being performed. Report the code for the primary procedure first, followed by the appropriate robotic-assisted surgery code. Robotic assistance is reported with a code from the Other Procedures

section in the body system Physiological Systems and Anatomical Regions.

Robotic-assisted surgery was first used with general laparoscopic surgeries such as gallbladder removal and for treating severe heartburn. Since then, use of robotic-assisted surgical systems has expanded into several other surgical areas, including gynecological laparoscopic procedures such as hysterectomy and myomectomy; radical prostatectomy; certain procedures of the heart, such as coronary artery bypass surgery and mitral valve repair; and procedures involving the lungs, esophagus, and internal thoracic artery.

Three stainless steel rods are inserted into the operative site. One of the rods is equipped with a 3D camera, and the other two are fitted with surgical instruments. The rods are held in place by three robotic arms. Sitting at the computer control console a few feet from the operating table, the physician views a magnified, three-dimensional image of the surgical site and manipulates the surgical instruments using two fingertip controls. The physician guides the arms of the robot that hold the surgical tools, and the surgery is performed using the robotic arms and instruments. At the end of the procedure, all instrumentation is removed and the incisions are closed.

Focus Point

Reporting of robotic assistance is always secondary to the intended root operation being performed. The approach value for the robotic assistance should match that of the primary procedure, unless the intended root operation is attempted using one approach but must be converted to a different approach during the procedure.

Coding Guidance
AHA: 2015, 1Q, 33; 2014, 4Q, 33; 2014, 1Q, 20

© 2018 Optum360, LLC

Collection, Cerebrospinal Fluid from Indwelling Device

See also Ventriculostomy in the Medical and Surgical section

Body System
Indwelling Device

PCS Root Operation
Other Procedures

Root Operation Table
8CØ   Other Procedures, Indwelling Device, Other Procedures

Body Region
Nervous System

Approach
External

Method
Collection

Qualifier
Cerebrospinal Fluid

Description
The cerebrospinal fluid (CSF) is a clear, watery liquid that circulates around the spinal cord and brain, acting as a protective cushion and supplying nutrients. CSF testing is performed to evaluate substances in the CSF to diagnose certain diseases or conditions affecting the central nervous system (brain and spinal cord) such as infections (meningitis), bleeding or stroke, brain or spinal cord damage, autoimmune disorders, tumors, or demyelinating diseases such as multiple sclerosis. In some cases, serial CSF sampling is required for these diagnostic studies.

The CSF is collected from a previously inserted lumbar or ventricular catheter that is connected to a collecting system with an external sampling and injection ports outside the body and is used to obtain CSF and inject therapeutic fluid or medications. This system is inserted and left in place to avoid the need for repeated catheter insertions in the central nervous system for sample collection.

Under strict sterile techniques, the external ports are soaked in an alcohol solution and the caps are discarded. The physician inserts a needle into the external sampling port. The CSF pressure is measured, and a sample of CSF is aspirated through the needle into a sterile test tube. Three or more separate tubes of CSF may be collected, depending on the tests to be performed, and multiple tests may be performed on the different samples. After the CSF sample collection, the volume removed is measured, and an amount of sterile isotonic saline equivalent to the volume of CSF removed may be injected through the external injection port with another needle. The ports are flushed multiple times with sterile saline to prevent infection. New sterile port caps are applied.

Medical and Surgical Related

Chiropractic

Manipulation, Chiropractic, Mechanically Assisted

Body System
Anatomical Regions

PCS Root Operation
Manipulation

Root Operation Table
9WB   Chiropractic, Anatomical Regions, Manipulation

Body Region
Head
Cervical
Thoracic
Lumbar
Sacrum
Pelvis
Lower Extremities
Upper Extremities
Rib Cage
Abdomen

Approach
External

Method
Mechanically Assisted

Description
Chiropractic manipulations are delivered manually or with the use of a mechanical instrument. The force applied using a mechanical instrument provides for less variation and, therefore, more consistency than a manual manipulation, which can vary from manipulation to manipulation as well as among practitioners. Mechanical manipulation also allows for variable force and speed.

Two types of mechanically assisted manipulation devices include spring-loaded and electromechanical devices. The spring-loaded device is a hand-held device that delivers precise force from the spring into the joint. The amount of force can be adjusted as needed. With an electromechanical adjusting device, force is applied to the painful area, and a response is recorded and analyzed after each application. The device continues to produce a series of repetitive applications if the response indicates improvement.

Medical and Surgical Related

© 2018 Optum360, LLC

Ancillary

Imaging

Angiography, Cardiac (Coronary Arteriography) (Angiocardiography)

See also Catheterization, Cardiac under "Measurement and Monitoring" in the Medical and Surgical-Related section

See also Ventriculography, Cardiac in the "Imaging" section of the Ancillary section

Body System
Heart

PCS Root Type
Fluoroscopy

Root Operation Table
B21   Imaging, Heart, Fluoroscopy

Body Part
Coronary Artery, Single
Coronary Arteries, Multiple
Coronary Artery Bypass Graft, Single
Coronary Artery Bypass Grafts, Multiple
Internal Mammary Bypass Graft, Right
Internal Mammary Bypass Graft, Left
Bypass Graft, Other

Contrast
High Osmolar
Low Osmolar
Other Contrast

Qualifier
Laser
None

Qualifier
Intraoperative
None

Description

A diagnostic cardiac angiography is the x-ray visualization of the heart and coronary arteries after injection of a radiopaque contrast medium. Cardiac angiography is useful for diagnosing and evaluating cardiovascular disease and cardiac abnormalities. Technique and extent of exam may vary. The physician may employ the Sones technique, using a single catheter, or the Judkins, Abrams, or Ricketts technique, which uses two catheters. Testing for patient hypersensitivity to the iodine content of the medium is advised before the radiopaque substance is used.

A local anesthetic is applied over the site where the catheter is to be introduced, and the access vein or artery is percutaneously punctured with a needle. A catheter is threaded over a guide wire into an artery (usually the femoral or brachial artery) for a left heart catheterization or into a peripheral vein (usually the femoral or brachial vein), for a right heart catheterization. The guide wire is then removed. When the catheter is in place, using fluoroscopy to guide placement, the physician injects the contrast medium, and images (angiograms) are recorded as the dye moves through the vessels, providing images of the heart structures and coronary arteries that are displayed on a monitor and recorded for evaluation. The physician may use a laser-aiming device attached to a C-arm to aid in accuracy and reduce radiation exposure during intraoperative fluoroscopy.

At this time, imaging of the heart ventricles is often performed in conjunction with angiography (see also Ventriculography, Cardiac). Any required repositioning of catheters or use of automatic power injectors is included in this procedure. The catheter is removed and pressure applied to the wound, or a closure device is used.

> **Focus Point**
> *Report in addition any concurrent, separately reportable procedures such as cardiac catheterization (4A02 Measurement and Monitoring, Cardiac). See also Catheterization, Cardiac.*

> **Focus Point**
> *Assign the coronary artery and bypass graft body part values, single or multiple, based on the numbers visualized.*

Coding Guidance
AHA: 2016, 3Q, 36

© 2018 Optum360, LLC

Arteriography, Renal (Renal Angiography) (Angiography, Renal Arteries)

Body System
Lower Arteries

PCS Root Type
Plain Radiography
Fluoroscopy

Root Operation Table
B4Ø Imaging, Lower Arteries, Plain Radiography
B41 Imaging, Lower Arteries, Fluoroscopy

Body Part
Renal Artery, Right
Renal Artery, Left
Renal Arteries, Bilateral

Contrast
High Osmolar
Low Osmolar
Other Contrast
None

Qualifier
Laser (Fluoroscopy)
None

Qualifier
Intraoperative (Fluoroscopy)
None

Description
Renal arteriography, also known as renal angiography, is performed to visualize the blood vessels of the kidneys. This is typically performed for problems with the blood vessels that feed the kidneys such as blood clots, blockages, abnormal structures, spasms, neoplasms, high blood pressure, abnormally narrowed (stenosed) or widened vessels (aneurysms), fistulas, or bleeding. Renal arteriography may also be performed to examine kidney donors and recipients before transplant surgery.

The access area is prepped and anesthetized. A vascular access catheter is inserted through a small incision, usually an artery in the groin region. The catheter is guided by passage of a guide wire and using fluoroscopic imaging, and it is threaded through the pelvic vessels and the aorta to the renal artery. When the catheter is in place, dye is injected. X-ray images are recorded as the dye moves through the vessels. The physician may use a laser-aiming device attached to a C-arm to aid in accuracy and reduce radiation exposure during intraoperative fluoroscopy. After images are recorded, the needle and catheter are removed. Pressure may be applied to the site to stop bleeding, or a closure device may be used.

Focus Point
When an imaging service is provided secondary to a principal procedure, the imaging service may be reported separately.

Coding Guidance
AHA: 2016, 3Q, 36

© 2018 Optum360, LLC

Echocardiography, Intracardiac

See also Echocardiography, Transesophageal (TEE)

Body System
Heart

PCS Root Type
Ultrasonography

Root Operation Table
B24   Imaging, Heart, Ultrasonography

Body Part
Heart, Right
Heart, Left
Heart Right and Left
Pediatric Heart

Contrast
None

Qualifier
Intravascular

Description
Diagnostic ultrasound is an imaging technique bouncing sound waves far above the level of human perception through interior body structures. The sound waves pass through different densities of tissue and reflect back to a receiving unit at varying speeds. The unit converts the waves to electrical pulses that are immediately displayed in picture form on screen. Real-time scanning displays structure images and movement with time.

Intracardiac echocardiography (ICE) uses real-time, intravascular ultrasound imaging systems in the cardiac chambers to provide direct endocardial visualization. ICE is performed during separately reportable electrophysiologic evaluation, percutaneous closure of patent foramen ovale (PFO) and atrial septal defects (ASD), or intracardiac catheter ablation of arrhythmogenic focus. ICE is replacing the use of transesophageal echocardiography (*see* Echocardiography, Transesophageal [TEE]) due to its many advantages, which include the use of local versus general anesthesia, excellent image quality, reduced procedure times, and lower radiation exposure.

Using local anesthesia, a single rotating transducer that provides a 360-degree field of view in a plane transverse to the long axis of the catheter is introduced through a long vascular sheath. Access is typically via the femoral vein. The transducer is directed to various sites within the heart. The definitive procedure being performed takes place through a separate venous sheath. During electrophysiologic evaluation, ICE is used to guide placement of mapping and stimulating catheters. ICE is used during PFO or ASD closures to measure the defects and to facilitate optimal device placement. For intracardiac ablation procedures, ICE allows for precise anatomic localization of the ablation catheter tip in relation to endocardial structures. At the end of the procedure, the transducer and catheter are removed.

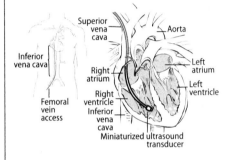

Focus Point
ICE is coded in the Imaging section of ICD-10-PCS as Ultrasonography. The qualifier Intravascular differentiates the ICE from other methods of ultrasonography.

Focus Point
Other procedures performed with the ICE are coded separately according to multiple procedures guideline B3.2c.

Focus Point
ICE is not the same as an Echocardiogram which is also an ultrasound of the heart structures but is performed using an external transducer. The code is differentiated by the qualifier value, which in the case of the Echocardiogram is None.

Ancillary

Echocardiography, Transesophageal (TEE)

Body System
Heart

PCS Root Type
Ultrasonography

Root Operation Table
B24   Imaging, Heart, Ultrasonography

Body Part
Coronary Artery, Single
Coronary Arteries, Multiple
Heart, Right
Heart, Left
Heart, Right and Left
Heart with Aorta
Pericardium
Pediatric Heart

Qualifier
Transesophageal

Description
Diagnostic ultrasound is an imaging technique bouncing sound waves far above the level of human perception through interior body structures. The sound waves pass through different densities of tissue and reflect back to a receiving unit at varying speeds. The unit converts the waves to electrical pulses that are immediately displayed in picture form on screen. Real-time scanning displays structure images and movement with time.

Transesophageal echocardiography (TEE) specifically produces pictures of the heart muscles, chambers, and valves; the coronary arteries; and pericardium. The images from a TEE are used to determine the presence of conditions such as valve disease, coronary artery disease, myocardial disease, congenital disorders, masses, or infective processes of the heart. TEE provides detailed images of the heart without interference from the lungs or ribs because they are taken from the esophagus, which is next to the heart chambers. The echo transducer for the TEE is passed down the throat into the esophagus via an endoscope. This procedure is coded in the Imaging section as Ultrasonography. The qualifier Transesophageal differentiates the TEE from other methods of ultrasonography.

© 2018 Optum360, LLC

Endoscopic Retrograde Cholangiopancreatography (ERCP)

Body System
Hepatobiliary System and Pancreas

PCS Root Type
Fluoroscopy

Root Operation Table
BF1 Imaging, Hepatobiliary System and Pancreas, Fluoroscopy

Body Part
Biliary and Pancreatic Ducts

Contrast
High Osmolar
Low Osmolar
Other Contrast

Description
An endoscopic retrograde cholangiopancreatography (ERCP) is an imaging procedure that uses a lighted endoscope and fluoroscopy to visualize the bile and pancreatic ducts and is used for both diagnostic and therapeutic purposes. When it is used to help in the performance of a specific therapy, it is considered inherent in the procedure and not coded separately.

When used for diagnostic purposes, it is reported with a code from the Imaging section.

The physician performs a diagnostic ERCP, which involves an endoscopic and radioscopic exam of the pancreatic and common bile ducts, with contrast material injected in the opposite direction of normal flow through the catheter. The physician passes the endoscope through the patient's oropharynx, esophagus, stomach, and into the small intestine. The ampulla of Vater is cannulated and filled with contrast. The common bile duct and the whole biliary tract, including the gallbladder, are visualized.

Focus Point
This procedure differs from endoscopic retrograde cholangiography (ERC) and endoscopic retrograde pancreatography (ERP) in the extent of the examination performed. ERCP is a comprehensive procedure in which the entire biliary tract is examined. ERC and ERP provide a limited examination of certain structures as specified in their names.

Coding Guidance
AHA: 2016, 3Q, 27,36

Fluoroscopy

Body System

Central Nervous System

Heart

Upper Arteries

Lower Arteries

Veins

Ear, Nose, Mouth and Throat

Respiratory System

Gastrointestinal System

Hepatobiliary System and Pancreas

Skull and Facial Bones

Non-Axial Upper Bones

Non-Axial Lower Bones

Axial Skeleton, Except Skull and Facial Bones

Urinary System

Female Reproductive System

Male Reproductive System

Anatomical Regions

PCS Root Type

Fluoroscopy

Root Operation Table

BØ1 Imaging, Central Nervous System, Fluoroscopy

B21 Imaging, Heart, Fluoroscopy

B31 Imaging, Upper Arteries, Fluoroscopy

B41 Imaging, Lower Arteries, Fluoroscopy

B51 Imaging, Veins, Fluoroscopy

B91 Imaging, Ear, Nose, Mouth and Throat, Fluoroscopy

BB1 Imaging, Respiratory System, Fluoroscopy

BD1 Imaging, Gastrointestinal System, Fluoroscopy

BF1 Imaging, Hepatobiliary System and Pancreas, Fluoroscopy

BN1 Imaging, Skull and Facial Bones, Fluoroscopy

BP1 Imaging, Non-Axial Upper Bones, Fluoroscopy

BQ1 Imaging, Non-Axial Lower Bones, Fluoroscopy

BR1 Imaging, Axial Skeleton, Except Skull and Facial Bones, Fluoroscopy

BT1 Imaging, Urinary System, Fluoroscopy

BU1 Imaging, Female Reproductive System, Fluoroscopy

BV1 Imaging, Male Reproductive System, Fluoroscopy

BW1 Imaging, Anatomical Regions, Fluoroscopy

Body Part

Refer to the ICD-10-PCS tabular list for a complete list of body parts.

Contrast

High Osmolar

Low Osmolar

Other Contrast

None

Description

Fluoroscopy is a radiology technique that allows visual examination of part of the body or a function of an organ using a device that projects an x-ray image on a fluorescent screen. In the Imaging section of ICD-10-PCS, the root operation Fluoroscopy is defined as a single plane or biplane real-time display of an image developed by capturing external ionizing radiations on a fluorescent screen. The image may also be stored by either digital or analog means. The Food and Drug Administration (FDA) describes fluoroscopy as a type of imaging employing an x-ray beam that passes through the body and tracks the movement of the body part, or an instrument or contrast dye within the body, which is transmitted to a monitor showing the body in detail.

Fluoroscopy is used in various diagnostic procedures. Some of these include:

- Catheter insertion and manipulation to guide through blood vessels, bile ducts, or other tubular body parts
- Angiograms using contrast to visualize blood vessels and organs
- Guidance and visualization for placement of devices in the body such as stents or leads
- Visualization of the GI tract using barium enemas
- Guidance during joint replacement and fracture repairs
- Placement of lumbar punctures
- Placement and guidance of central venous catheters
- Location and removing foreign bodies

Fluoroscopy does involve a certain amount of radiation exposure so it is not recommended for use on pregnant women. The use of contrast can also be a risk factor, especially for those with a history of kidney failure or kidney disease. Fluoroscopy is regulated by the FDA and must meet specific criteria to be considered safe and effective.

Focus Point

Fluoroscopy is more often reported for outpatient procedures. For inpatient coding, reporting imaging is typically a facility decision as it is generally considered inherent in many inpatient procedures. If the facility decides to report it, a code from the Imaging section is used.

Coding Guidance

AHA: 2016, 3Q, 36

© 2018 Optum360, LLC

Ancillary

MRI, Fetal, Central Nervous System

See also Ultrasonography, Fetal

Body System
Fetus and Obstetrical

PCS Root Type
Magnetic Resonance Imaging (MRI)

Root Operation Table
BY3 Imaging, Fetus and Obstetrical, Magnetic Resonance Imaging (MRI)

Body Part
Fetal Head

Contrast
None

Description
Magnetic resonance imaging (MRI) is a radiation-free, noninvasive technique for producing high-quality sectional images of the inside of the body in multiple planes. MRI uses the natural magnetic properties of the hydrogen atoms in our bodies that emit radiofrequency signals when exposed to radio waves within a strong electromagnetic field. A computer processes and converts these signals into high-resolution, three-dimensional, tomographic images. Contrast material may be administered for image enhancement.

Used in conjunction with fetal ultrasound, MRI can be used to identify and evaluate fetal abnormalities. The preferred time to complete a fetal MRI is after 18 weeks' gestation. Evaluation for central nervous system (CNS) abnormalities is the most common reason a fetal MRI is performed since ultrasonography cannot fully evaluate the fetal scalp, neck, and airway.

After ultrasound has verified fetal position, the pregnant patient lies supine on an exam table that slides into the tube-shaped MRI machine. No sedation or contrast is used, but the pregnant patient is usually told not to eat anything four hours before and is made as comfortable as possible to minimize fetal motion during the examination. A receiver coil is placed on the mother's abdomen or pelvis in the area where the fetal head is located. If the fetus moves, it may be repositioned. Images are obtained using ultrafast MRI techniques. Total scan time is usually 30 to 40 minutes. A microphone inside the scanner allows the pregnant patient to communicate with MRI staff during the procedure.

Focus Point
Any accompanying fetal ultrasound is coded separately, according to multiple procedure guideline B3.2c. See also Ultrasonography, Fetal.

Ultrasonography, Fetal

Body System
Fetus and Obstetrical

PCS Root Type
Ultrasonography

Root Operation Table
BY4   Imaging, Fetus and Obstetrical, Ultrasonography

Body Part
Fetal Umbilical Cord

Placenta

First Trimester, Single Fetus

First Trimester, Multiple Gestation

Second Trimester, Single Fetus

Second Trimester, Multiple Gestation

Third Trimester, Single Fetus

Third Trimester, Multiple Gestation

Contrast
None

Description
Diagnostic ultrasound is an imaging technique that bounces sound waves far above the level of human perception through interior body structures. Using a transducer, sound waves pass through different densities of tissue and reflect back to a receiving unit at varying speeds. The unit converts the waves to electrical pulses that are immediately displayed in picture form on screen. Real-time scanning displays structure images and movement with time.

Fetal ultrasounds may be performed to determine gestational age, number of fetuses, fetal position, fetal growth, placenta, and amniotic fluid levels and to indicate abnormalities. A fetal ultrasound may be done using a transvaginal or transabdominal approach; both approaches are best performed when the pregnant patient has a full bladder.

A standard ultrasound creates two-dimensional images using sound waves. A Doppler ultrasound shows the movement of blood through the umbilical cord, in the fetal heart, or between the placenta and the fetus.

3-D and sometimes 4-D ultrasounds are sometimes performed but are optional, rather than standard, prenatal tests. They are normally indicated only when needed to show certain birth defects that might not show up on a standard ultrasound; otherwise, they are done only as a courtesy to parents. A 3-D ultrasound creates a three-dimensional image of the baby, and a 4-D ultrasound creates a video effect.

A transvaginal ultrasound is typically done in the early stages of pregnancy and for obese patients. During a transvaginal ultrasound, with the pregnant patient in supine position and feet in stirrups, an ultrasound transducer that has been appropriately prepped with a latex sleeve and lubricant, is inserted into the patient's vagina.

For a transabdominal ultrasound, with the pregnant patient in supine position, gel is applied to the patient's stomach and an ultrasound transducer is moved over the stomach. The gel is removed at the conclusion of the procedure.

Focus Point
Report the appropriate body part based upon the focus or objective of the ultrasound procedure.

© 2018 Optum360, LLC

Ultrasound, Intravascular, Coronary Arteries (IVUS)

Body System
Heart

PCS Root Type
Ultrasonography

Root Operation Table
B24 Imaging, Heart, Ultrasonography

Body Part
Coronary Artery, Single
Coronary Artery, Multiple

Qualifier
Intravascular

Description

Intravascular ultrasound (IVUS) is three-dimensional visualization of the interior arterial walls from the inside of the artery as compared with conventional angiographic techniques, which are two-dimensional external visualization of vessels. IVUS is also significantly different from noninvasive ultrasound, since noninvasive ultrasonographic angiography produces only two-dimensional images of vessels from outside the body. IVUS produces detailed, three-dimensional images of the interior walls of vessels that allow the physician to make real-time decisions about treatment options. After intervention, IVUS can be used to assess the efficacy of the treatment.

Compared with IVUS, images produced with conventional radiographic angiography have several limitations, as noted below:

- Images are only two-dimensional and do not afford real-time decision-making.
- The images provide no information about the actual condition of the interior walls of the vessel.
- Conventional radiography is insensitive to the severity of plaque build-up in remodeled vessel walls and is unable to detect any vessel wall disruption during angioplasty.

The ICD-10-PCS table for IVUS is found in the Imaging section, Heart body system, and root type Ultrasonography. The body part value options are Coronary Artery, Single or Coronary Artery, Multiple, depending on the number of arteries viewed. The qualifier Intravascular is what differentiates this code from noninvasive ultrasonography. The IVUS technique is similar to conventional balloon angioplasty. A 6 to 8 French access sheath and guiding catheter are used to introduce a conventional angioplasty guidewire to distal artery sites. The intravascular ultrasound catheter, available as over-the-wire or monorail configuration, is introduced after administration of intracoronary nitroglycerin to avoid vessel spasm, as well as the administration of an anticoagulant such as heparin. The IVUS catheter contains a miniature transducer that emits ultrasounds that bounce off irregularities, which are sent back as images. There are two types of IVUS transducers: the mechanical rotating transducer and the electronically switched multi-element array system. A high-resolution image is produced consisting of three layers around the lumen. These images are used to determine measurements of the severity of plaque build-up, plaque composition, stability of the plaque, and blood flow adequacy.

After the therapeutic procedure such as balloon angioplasty is performed, IVUS can be used to determine blood flow adequacy of the lumen in remodeled vessels. The completeness of the opposition of a stent against the vessel wall after a stent insertion can be determined, as well. If a stent is inserted and the stent is not up against the vessel walls, the risk of restenosis is increased. Once a stent is in place, IVUS can be used to determine whether the lumen opening has been made large enough to allow adequate blood flow.

> **Focus Point**
>
> *Other applications of IVUS include assessment of vasculopathy after transplant surgery, regression/progression of lumen patency after antilipemic therapy, noncoronary artery disease, interventional target lesion, restenosis vein graft disease, serial stent studies for mechanism of restenosis process, and restenosis after brachytherapy.*

> **Focus Point**
>
> *Codes should also be assigned for any synchronous diagnostic or therapeutic procedures such as angiography, ventriculography, or PTCA.*

> **Focus Point**
>
> *IVUS can be performed in blood vessels in other parts of the body. These are reported based on their respective body systems and body part values.*

Ancillary

Ventriculography, Cardiac

See also Angiography, Cardiac (Coronary Arteriography) (Angiocardiography)

See also Catheterization, Cardiac under "Measurement and Monitoring" in the Medical and Surgical Related section

Body System
Heart

PCS Root Type
Fluoroscopy

Root Operation Table
B21   Imaging, Heart, Fluoroscopy

Body Part
Heart, Right
Heart, Left
Heart, Right and Left

Contrast
High Osmolar
Low Osmolar
Other Contrast

Description
A ventriculogram or ventriculography is commonly performed in conjunction with a coronary angiogram. These procedures are reported separately as each involves visualizations of different body part values (*See also* Angiography, Cardiac [Coronary Arteriography] [Angiocardiography]). Both are performed in real time with fluoroscopy with contrast media; however, the diagnostic cardiac angiography visualizes coronary arteries whereas the ventriculography visualizes the left or right ventricles of the heart. Ventriculography is reported with the root operation Fluoroscopy in the Imaging section. Ventriculography is used most often to evaluate the function of the left heart ventricle but can be performed in the right heart or both. With recent advances in noninvasive methods to achieve the same purpose, the use of this diagnostic procedure is becoming less frequent.

A local anesthetic is applied over the site where the catheter is to be introduced, and the access vein or artery is percutaneously punctured with a needle. A catheter is threaded over a guide wire into an artery (usually the femoral or brachial artery). After the coronary artery angiogram is performed, contrast medium (dye) is injected into the right ventricle or atrium and/or the left ventricle or atrium to evaluate the right (pulmonary valve, right atrium, right ventricle [outflow tract]) and/or left (aortic valve, left atrium, left ventricle [outflow tract]) heart structures with fluoroscopy. Any required repositioning of catheters or use of automatic power injectors is included in this procedure. The catheter is removed and pressure applied to the wound, or a closure device is used.

Focus Point
Left ventriculography (LV) is performed along with left heart catheterization (LHC), which measures the left ventricular pressure, and is reported separately. See also Catheterization, Cardiac.

Focus Point
Contrast media can be high osmolar (ionic—e.g., isopaque), low osmolar (nonionic—e.g., Isovue), or other contrast (nonionic, iso-osmolar—e.g., Visipaque).

Coding Guidance
AHA: 2016, 3Q, 36

© 2018 Optum360, LLC

Videofluoroscopy, Esophageal (Modified Barium Swallow)

Body System
Gastrointestinal System

PCS Root Type
Fluoroscopy

Root Operation Table
BD1 Imaging, Gastrointestinal System, Fluoroscopy

Body Part
Esophagus

Contrast
Other Contrast

Description
Esophageal videofluoroscopy of swallowing (VFS) is a diagnostic method for determining the cause and effects of a swallowing disorder. It is also called a videofluoroscopic swallowing study (VFSS), modified barium swallow (MBS), or esophagram. The test allows the provider to visualize food entering the airway instead of the pharynx, esophagus, and stomach as well as peristalsis and stricture defects in the esophagus. It is used primarily to evaluate swallowing function and look for evidence of aspiration of food or liquid into the trachea.

In the test, the patient is given various food products and drinks to swallow, with various instructions on head positioning, force of each swallow, and amount to swallow. These swallowed items have been treated with barium, which is radiopaque. The patient's swallowing is recorded using fluoroscopy cineradiography, or video recording, as the physiologic event of swallowing occurs too rapidly for normal fluoroscopic viewing. High-speed frame rates are used to evaluate swallowing and are later reviewed and interpreted by the radiologist.

Ancillary

Nuclear Medicine

Adenosine Sestamibi Planar Scan, Heart Muscle (Technetium)

Body System
Heart

PCS Root Type
Planar Nuclear Medicine Imaging

Root Operation Table
C21   Nuclear Medicine, Heart, Planar Nuclear Medicine Imaging

Body Part
Myocardium

Radionuclide
Technetium 99m (Tc-99m)
Indium 111 (In-111)
Thallium 201 (Tl-201)
Other Radionuclide

Description

Planar nuclear medicine imaging describes the introduction of radioactive materials into the body for single plane display of images developed from the capture of radioactive emissions. Technetium 99m (Tc-99m) emits gamma rays that aid in radiographic visualization. In a planar scan of the heart muscle, the perfusion of blood into the heart muscle is evaluated to determine the level of ischemia. When the heart muscle is ischemic, it fails to contract properly, and arterial circulation is compromised.

The physician injects a solution containing technetium into the patient's bloodstream to evaluate regional myocardial perfusion and function. The anatomy of the heart is viewed on the screen, without the need for computer 3D reconstruction. A planar scan of the heart muscle of patients can be performed bedside using portable equipment, while the 3D imagery (tomography) requires transport of the patient to the imaging lab.

For planar myocardial perfusion imaging at stress conditions, stress is induced with the standard treadmill exercise test or pharmacologically with the infusion of a vasodilator. The patient receives an intravenous injection of a radionuclide, usually thallium or technetium-99m, which localizes only in nonischemic tissue. Planar images of the heart are scanned immediately with a gamma camera that detects the radiation in the heart tissue to identify areas of infarction. In the nonstress version of the procedure, radionuclide is injected and images are taken without stress induction. A single study may be performed, at rest or stress. Multiple procedures may be performed at rest and/or at stress with a second injection of radionuclide given again in the redistribution or resting phase just before resting images being taken.

Ancillary

© 2018 Optum360, LLC

Cisternography, Cerebrospinal Fluid Flow Imaging

Body System
Central Nervous System

PCS Root Type
Planar Nuclear Medicine Imaging
Tomographic (Tomo) Nuclear Medicine Imaging

Root Operation Table
C01 Nuclear Medicine, Central Nervous System, Planar Nuclear Medicine Imaging
C02 Nuclear Medicine, Central Nervous System, Tomographic (Tomo) Nuclear Medicine Imaging

Body Part
Cerebrospinal Fluid

Radionuclide
Indium 111 (In-111)
Other Radionuclide

Description
Diagnostic nuclear medicine uses small amounts of gamma-emitting radioactive materials, or tracers, to determine the cause of the medical problem based on the function, or chemistry, of the organ or tissue. Cisternography is done to determine whether there is any abnormal cerebral spinal fluid (CSF) flow occurring in or around the brain. It is often used to detect CSF leaks and normal pressure hydrocephalus, and to evaluate CSF shunts.

Following localized anesthesia of the lower back, the radiotracer (radionuclide) is introduced intrathecally by lumbar puncture into the lower spinal canal region. The patient may be asked to lie flat after the lumbar puncture. A few hours later, a scintillation or gamma camera takes images that show how the radiotracer flows through the cerebrospinal fluid. The camera detects gamma radiation from the radiopharmaceutical in the body tissue as it "scintillates," or gives off energy, when coming in contact with the camera's detector. An additional scan is taken 24 hours after the injection and possibly at 48 and 72 hours.

Focus Point
Planar imaging refers to a single plane display of images while tomographic (tomo) refers to three-dimensional displays.

Focus Point
Substances such as contrast, radionuclide, and radioisotope injected to support the objective of procedures in the Imaging, Nuclear Medicine, and Radiation Therapy sections are included in the definitive procedure code and should not be separately reported with substances in the Administration section, in which the procedure's objective is to administer the substance.

© 2018 Optum360, LLC

Scan, Pulmonary, Ventilation and Perfusion

Body System
Respiratory System

PCS Root Type
Planar Nuclear Medicine Imaging
Tomographic (Tomo) Nuclear Medicine Imaging

Root Operation Table
CB1 Nuclear Medicine, Respiratory System, Planar Nuclear Medicine Imaging
CB2 Nuclear Medicine, Respiratory System, Tomographic (Tomo) Nuclear Medicine Imaging

Body Part
Lungs and Bronchi

Radionuclide
Technetium 99m (Tc-99m)
Krypton (Kr-81m)
Xenon 127 (Xe-127) (Planar Nuclear Medicine Imaging)
Xenon 133 (Xe-133) (Planar Nuclear Medicine Imaging)
Other Radionuclide

Description
Often performed together, ventilation and perfusion tests are a pair of nuclear scans. Radioactive material is injected into the patient's veins and the patient is scanned to measure the movement of blood (perfusion), and the patient inhales radioactive gas and is scanned to measure the movement of air throughout the lungs (ventilation). Ventilation and perfusion scans are most often used to identify pulmonary emboli. A significant difference between the ventilation and perfusion scan results can be indicative of pulmonary emboli. Ventilation and perfusion imaging of the lungs may also be done for the evaluation of other lung conditions.

During the perfusion scan, a radioactive albumin (radionuclide), generally Technetium 99m macroaggregated albumin (MAA) (Tc-99m), is injected into the patient's vein and the patient is placed under a machine that scans the lungs. Where there is abnormal flow of blood in the lungs, the radionuclide collects and the scanner detects radiation emitted by the radionuclide.

A nuclear ventilation image is obtained to complement the perfusion image. As the patient inhales a radioactive gas, such as Krypton or Xenon 127 or Xenon 133, an image is obtained that detects the radioactivity from the gas in the lungs, showing well-ventilated areas having uniform activity and poorly ventilated areas with decreased or absent radioactivity. If there is no obstruction, the air spaces of the lungs have a consistent appearance and no evidence of radioactive gas.

A chest X-ray is typically performed before and after the ventilation and perfusion scans.

Focus Point
Two codes may be required to report ventilation and perfusion scans, one to report the perfusion portion with injected radionuclide and one to report the ventilation portion with inhaled gas radionuclide.

Focus Point
Planar imaging refers to a single plane display of images, while Tomographic (Tomo) refers to three-dimensional displays.

Ancillary

© 2018 Optum360, LLC

Radiation Therapy

Brachytherapy, Prostate

Body System
Male Reproductive System

PCS Modality
Brachytherapy

Root Operation Table
DV1 Radiation Therapy, Male Reproductive System, Brachytherapy

Treatment Site
Prostate

Modality Qualifier
High Dose Rate (HDR)
Low Dose Rate (LDR)

Isotope
Cesium 137 (Cs-137)
Iridium 192 (Ir-192)
Iodine 125 (I-125)
Palladium 103 (Pd-103)
Californium 252 (Cf-252)
Other Isotope

Description
Transperineal placement of needles or catheters into the prostate gland for interstitial radioelement application is a form of brachytherapy. Brachytherapy is the application of radioactive isotopes for internal radiation, which delivers the dose of radiation in a more direct fashion to the tissue being treated.

There are two types of brachytherapy for prostate cancer treatment: temporary high dose and permanent low dose. Low dose rate (LDR), also called permanent seed implants, uses radioactive pellets, permanently imbedded in rows within the prostate. These seeds or pellets continuously emit radiation for several weeks until depleted and are harmlessly left in place after treatment.

Temporary, high dose rate (HDR) brachytherapy uses several extremely tiny catheters together with a single, high-intensity radioactive material (isotope) to produce the desired radiation distribution pattern around the tumor area. The catheters are fixed in place around the tumor and connected to the treatment machine. These catheters, or applicators, usually do not require surgical manipulation to set them in place. Once the catheters are in position, the machine loads its radioactive pellets into each catheter, placing them at predetermined positions for previously calculated treatment time. The catheters are removed at the end of the treatment.

Focus Point
Brachytherapy treatment of the prostate also requires a code for the Insertion of the brachytherapy seeds. This is reported with a code in the Male Reproductive System in the Medical and Surgical section. The root operation is Insertion, into the Prostate body part with the device value of Radioactive Element.

Oncology Treatment, Hyperthermia

Body System

Central and Peripheral Nervous System
Lymphatic and Hematologic System
Eye
Ear, Nose, Mouth and Throat
Respiratory System
Gastrointestinal System
Hepatobiliary System and Pancreas
Endocrine System
Skin
Breast
Musculoskeletal System
Urinary System
Female Reproductive System
Male Reproductive System
Anatomical Regions

PCS Modality

Other Radiation

Root Operation Table

D0Y Radiation Therapy, Central and Peripheral Nervous System, Other Radiation
D7Y Radiation Therapy, Lymphatic and Hematologic System, Other Radiation
D8Y Radiation Therapy, Eye, Other Radiation
D9Y Radiation Therapy, Ear, Nose, Mouth and Throat, Other Radiation
DBY Radiation Therapy, Respiratory System, Other Radiation
DDY Radiation Therapy, Gastrointestinal System, Other Radiation
DFY Radiation Therapy, Hepatobiliary System and Pancreas, Other Radiation
DGY Radiation Therapy, Endocrine System, Other Radiation
DHY Radiation Therapy, Skin, Other Radiation
DMY Radiation Therapy, Breast, Other Radiation
DPY Radiation Therapy, Musculoskeletal System, Other Radiation
DTY Radiation Therapy, Urinary System, Other Radiation
DUY Radiation Therapy, Female Reproductive System, Other Radiation
DVY Radiation Therapy, Male Reproductive System, Other Radiation
DWY Radiation Therapy, Anatomical Regions, Other Radiation

Treatment Site

Refer to the ICD-10-PCS tabular list for a complete list of treatment sites.

Modality Qualifier

Hyperthermia

Description

Hyperthermia (adjunct therapy to radiation) is induced by microwave, ultrasound, low-energy radio frequency, probes (interstitial), or other means to treat cancer. Hyperthermia uses heat in conjunction with radiation in an attempt to speed cell metabolism, which increases potential cell destruction. This aids in the treatment of a malignancy by making tumors more susceptible to the therapy. The heat can be generated by various sources, including microwave, ultrasound, and radio frequency conduction. Hyperthermia may be externally generated, superficial (i.e., heating to a depth of 4 cm or less), or deep (i.e., heating to depths greater than 4 cm). Alternatively, heat may be generated by interstitial probes acting like small antennae or microwave radiators placed directly into the tumor area or a body cavity.

© 2018 Optum360, LLC

Radiation Therapy, External Beam

Body System

Central and Peripheral Nervous System
Lymphatic and Hematologic System
Eye
Ear, Nose, Mouth and Throat
Respiratory System
Gastrointestinal System
Hepatobiliary System and Pancreas
Endocrine System
Skin
Breast
Musculoskeletal System
Urinary System
Female Reproductive System
Male Reproductive System
Anatomical Regions

PCS Modality

Beam Radiation

Root Operation Table

DØØ Radiation Therapy, Central and Peripheral Nervous System, Beam Radiation

D7Ø Radiation Therapy, Lymphatic and Hematologic System, Beam Radiation

D8Ø Radiation Therapy, Eye, Beam Radiation

D9Ø Radiation Therapy, Ear, Nose, Mouth and Throat, Beam Radiation

DBØ Radiation Therapy, Respiratory System, Beam Radiation

DDØ Radiation Therapy, Gastrointestinal System, Beam Radiation

DFØ Radiation Therapy, Hepatobiliary System and Pancreas, Beam Radiation

DGØ Radiation Therapy, Endocrine System, Beam Radiation

DIIØ Radiation Therapy, Skin, Beam Radiation

DMØ Radiation Therapy, Breast, Beam Radiation

DPØ Radiation Therapy, Musculoskeletal System, Beam Radiation

DTØ Radiation Therapy, Urinary System, Beam Radiation

DUØ Radiation Therapy, Female Reproductive System, Beam Radiation

DVØ Radiation Therapy, Male Reproductive System, Beam Radiation

DWØ Radiation Therapy, Anatomical Regions, Beam Radiation

Treatment Site

Refer to the ICD-10-PCS tabular list for a complete list of treatment sites.

Modality Qualifier

Photons <1MeV
Photons 1-10 MeV
Photons >10 MeV
Heavy Particles (Protons, Ions)
Neutrons
Neutron Capture
Electrons

Description

External beam radiation treatment involves the delivery of a beam of radioactive electromagnetic energy onto cancerous cells within the body from a treatment machine distanced from the treatment area. Radiation therapy damages the DNA of the tumor cells by directing a focused beam of radiation to the tumor, disrupting the cells' ability to divide and reproduce, either destroying or effectively shrinking the tumor.

External beam radiation is often delivered by machines called linear accelerators (also called LINAC), which can deliver x-rays (photon radiation) or electrons (particle radiation) to a targeted area. Photons can target deeper-lying tumor tissue, while electrons are used for the maximum dose of radiation near the skin surface. High-energy neutron radiation treatment is used to treat larger tumors and is particularly effective in treating inoperable salivary gland tumors, bone cancers, and certain types of advanced malignancies of the pancreas, bladder, lung, prostate, and uterus. Due to the high potency of neutron radiation, the required dose is much less than other radiotherapy. Proton radiation treatment is particularly beneficial in treating malignancies and other neoplastic abnormalities near sensitive structures such as the optic nerve and spinal cord since there is less damage to surrounding tissue.

The initial step in external beam radiation involves marking the targeted site with either a permanent marker or tattoo. Imaging verifies the site and size of tumor to plan radiation treatment. A complex process is used to determine the exact amount of radiation to be delivered. During radiation therapy, the patient is asked to remain very still during the procedure, which typically lasts up to 30 minutes. Radiation is directed at the targeted site and repeated over a number of weeks in order to be most effective while minimizing damage to normal tissue.

Ancillary

Radiation Therapy, Plaque Radiation, Eye

Body System
Eye

PCS Modality
Other Radiation

Root Operation Table
D8Y   Radiation Therapy, Eye, Other Radiation

Treatment Site
Eye

Modality Qualifier
Plaque Radiation

Description
Radioactive plaque therapy is used to treat small to medium-sized ocular melanomas. This procedure uses eye plaques that contain radioactive seeds placed into a soft, plastic template and covered with gold. The plaque is implanted over the tumor and emits low-energy photons that cause the diseased cells to die and the tumor to shrink. By directly aiming the radiation at the tumor, there is minimal damage to the surrounding tissues. The eye plaques are specifically tailored to the size of the tumor. The length of time the plaque needs to remain in place to emit an effective amount of radiation depends on the size and type of tumor.

After appropriate anesthesia has been administered, an incision is made in the conjunctiva. The physician sutures the radioactive plaque over the tumor on the outside of the eye (sclera). The conjunctiva is then sutured over the plaque. Prior to the patient leaving the hospital, usually three to five days after the initial procedure, the plaque is removed.

© 2018 Optum360, LLC

Radiation Therapy, Stereotactic Radiosurgery, Brain

Body System
Central and Peripheral Nervous System

PCS Modality
Stereotactic Radiosurgery

Root Operation Table
D02 Radiation Therapy, Central and Peripheral
Nervous System, Stereotactic Radiosurgery

Treatment Site
Brain
Brain Stem

Modality Qualifier
Stereotactic Other Photon Radiosurgery
Stereotactic Particulate Radiosurgery
Stereotactic Gamma Beam Radiosurgery

Isotope
None

Description
Stereotactic radiosurgery (SRS) uses 3-D imaging to
administer high doses of radiation to treat tumors and
other diseased areas of the brain. Unlike traditional
surgery, this is a noninvasive procedure that does not
require incision or drilling into the skull. The targeted
radiation damages the DNA of the affected cells,
reducing the ability to reproduce and shrinking the
tumor(s).

Prior to imaging and radiation treatment, a stereotactic
head frame is applied to immobilize the patient's head
and enable accurate, precision delivery. Using
stereotactic techniques, a precise 3-D location of the
brain lesion is identified using computed tomography
(CT), magnetic resonance imaging (MRI), or
angiogram. The physician uses the coordinates
obtained from the images to focus photons, gamma
ray or particulate (charged particle or proton beam)
energy onto the lesion, thereby destroying it.
Treatment is often a single session or multiple sessions
for larger tumors.

Focus Point
*Qualifier Stereotactic Other Photon Radiosurgery refers
to the use of linear accelerator (LINAC) machines that
use x-rays (photons) to treat the diseased area. LINAC
machines are known by brand names, such as
CyberKnife, Novalis Tx, XKnife, and Axesse TrueBeam.
Stereotactic Particulate Radiosurgery refers to proton
beams and is the newest type of stereotactic
radiosurgery performed in only a few facilities.
Stereotactic Gamma Beam Radiosurgery refers to the
use of gamma rays (Gamma Knife) to treat the diseased
area.*

Focus Point
*Robotic assistance may be employed and is coded
additionally with a code from Other Procedures table
(8E0).*

Ancillary

Radiation Therapy, Superficial Dermatologic

See also Radiation Therapy, External Beam

Body System
Skin

PCS Modality
Other Radiation

Root Operation Table
DHY   Radiation Therapy, Skin, Other Radiation

Treatment Site
Skin, Face
Skin, Neck
Skin, Arm
Skin, Chest
Skin, Back
Skin, Abdomen
Skin, Buttock
Skin, Leg

Modality Qualifier
Contact Radiation

Description
Superficial radiation therapy (SRT) is a procedure that uses low-energy radiation to treat nonmelanoma skin cancers (basal cell and squamous cell carcinomas). Radiation is applied directly to the lesion, penetrating the top surface layer of the skin and avoiding deep tissue. Otherwise known as contact radiation, this type of radiation therapy causes less scarring and yields more favorable aesthetic (cosmetic) results than surgical approaches. By targeting abnormal skin cells, the low-energy radiation damages the tumor cells and disrupts the cells' ability to divide and reproduce, either destroying or effectively shrinking the tumor.

After the targeted lesion has been identified and properly marked, an applicator cone is placed over the lesion. Radiation is applied through the cone to the lesion for approximately 90 minutes. No anesthesia is needed as this a nonsurgical procedure. Following treatment, the skin turns red and forms a scab under which new skin grows. Multiple sessions may be needed.

> **Focus Point**
> See also *Radiation Therapy, External Beam* for high-energy radiation applications.

© 2018 Optum360, LLC

Therapy Treatment, Laser Interstitial (LITT) (Brain)

Body System
Central and Peripheral Nervous System

PCS Modality
Other Radiation

Root Operation Table
DØY Radiation Therapy, Central and Peripheral
     Nervous System, Other Radiation

Treatment Site
Brain
Brain Stem

Modality Qualifier
Laser Interstitial Thermal Therapy

Description
Treatment options for patients with brain cancer
typically include a combination of surgical resection,
stereotactic radiosurgery, external beam or intracranial
radiation, and chemotherapy. Laser interstitial thermal
therapy (LITT) under real-time MRI guidance has been
developed for ablation of brain tumors. LITT for tumor
ablation uses a laser probe that focuses the laser's
energy on the targeted tumor tissue, reducing or
avoiding damage to surrounding tissue. LITT under
guidance, such as MRI or ultrasound, has been
effective at destroying or reducing the size of tumors in
the brain, head and neck, thyroid, lung, breast, liver,
bone, prostate, uterus, and rectum. LITT has also
proven to be an effective treatment for drug-resistant
epilepsy.

The treating physician visualizes the procedure in real
time using an MRI scanner with software and controls
to remotely monitor and position devices allowing
precise control of the thermal ablation in real time. A
thin, side-firing laser combined with gas cooling
within the probe tip is inserted through a small burr
hole in the skull. The laser energy discharged heats the
targeted tissue while cooling all surrounding tissue,
allowing the physician to selectively treat the targeted
tissue without damaging other tissue.

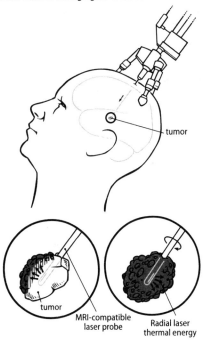

tumor

tumor

MRI-compatible
laser probe

Radial laser
thermal energy

Ancillary

Physical Rehabilitation and Diagnostic Audiology

Assessment, Cochlear Implant

See also Implant, Cochlear in the Medical and Surgical section

Qualifier
Diagnostic Audiology

PCS Root Type
Hearing Aid Assessment

Root Operation Table
F14 Physical Rehabilitation and Diagnostic Audiology, Diagnostic Audiology, Hearing Aid Assessment

Body System/Region
None

Type Qualifier
Cochlear Implant

Equipment
Cochlear Implant

Description
A diagnostic analysis of a cochlear implant, including programming, is done postoperatively to fit the previously placed external devices, connect to the implant, and program the stimulator. Cochlear implants are equipped with software that allows for different programming specific to the patient's daily activities. Threshold levels, volume, pulse widths, live-voice speech adjustments, input dynamic range, and frequency-shaping templates are evaluated and set according to individual needs.

Following implantation of the cochlear device, an audiologist activates the implant by attaching a headset that includes the transmitter, a microphone, and speech processor. Sound signals are sent across the skin to the implant via the transmitter. All components of the implant are checked, and the speech processor is programmed. Once the speech programmer is activated, the patient can hear through the cochlear implant. The audiologist provides instruction on how to wear the speech processor and verifies that a range of sounds are heard. Additional visits may be needed to fine-tune the device.

> **Focus Point**
> The insertion of the implant is coded separately. See also *Implant, Cochlear in the Medical and Surgical section.*

Ancillary

© 2018 Optum360, LLC

Electrocochleography, Transtympanic (ECOG)

Section Qualifier
Diagnostic Audiology

PCS Root Type
Hearing Assessment

Body System/Region
None

Root Operation Table
F13 Physical Rehabilitation and Diagnostic Audiology, Diagnostic Audiology, Hearing Assessment

Type Qualifier
Electrocochleography

Equipment
Electrophysiologic

Description
Electrocochleography (ECOG) is a specialized test used to assess hearing loss in children who are unable to be tested by conventional audiometry or to evaluate endolymphatic hydrops, such as in Ménière's disease. During an electrocochleography, an electrode is placed through the tympanic membrane into the promontory of the inner ear. The ear is stimulated and recordings are made of the electrical response of the cochlear nerve. By placing the electrode as close as possible to the inner ear, the electrical potentials or signals generated in response to sound can be measured.

After appropriate anesthesia and with the patient lying down in a sound booth, the physician places the electrode through the eardrum and positions it next to the inner ear. An audiologist performs a sound test. The electrode is removed at the conclusion of the procedure.

Ancillary

Mental Health

Biofeedback

Body System
None

PCS Root Type
Biofeedback

Root Operation Table
GZC   Mental Health, Biofeedback

Type Qualifier
Other Biofeedback

Description
Biofeedback involves a person learning to influence autonomic or involuntary nervous system responses and physiologic responses that are normally regulated voluntarily because his or her control has been affected by trauma or disease. The patient learns through monitoring to associate body responses with related stimuli and how to control those responses. Biofeedback helps regulate body processes such as heart rate, blood pressure, temperature, and muscle tension, and is considered effective in the treatment of migraine headaches, high blood pressure,

incontinence, Raynaud's syndrome, and anticipatory nausea due to chemotherapy.

Common forms of biofeedback therapy include electromyography (EMG) for muscle tension measurement, thermal biofeedback for skin temperature measurement, and electroencephalography (EEG) for brain wave activity measurement.

The clinician prepares the patient with electrodes attached to the skin or handheld sensors. The electrodes or sensors measure information (feedback) about the body (bio) such as skin temperature, blood pressure, muscle tension, or brain wave activity and send signals that are displayed on a monitor. The clinician then leads the patient through mental exercises that teach the patient how certain thought processes, stimuli, and actions affect these physiological responses. The treating clinician works with the patient to learn to recognize and manipulate these responses through relaxation and awareness techniques. Through trial and error, biofeedback helps the patient to use thoughts to control the body.

Electroconvulsive Therapy

Body System
None

PCS Root Type
Electroconvulsive Therapy

Root Operation Table
GZB   Mental Health, Electroconvulsive Therapy

Type Qualifier
Unilateral-Single Seizure
Unilateral-Multiple Seizure
Bilateral-Single Seizure
Bilateral-Multiple Seizure
Other Electroconvulsive Therapy

Description
Electroconvulsive therapy (ECT), formerly known as electroshock therapy or shock treatment, is the intentional initiation of a seizure used to treat certain mental illnesses. ECT is often used to combat chronic or profound major depression, especially psychotic or intractable manic forms, and for people who cannot take antidepressants. Electric current is used to trigger

a seizure, which causes changes in the brain that improve symptoms related to mental health conditions.

Following administration of a general anesthetic and a muscle relaxant, electrodes are placed on one or both sides of the patient's head. Bilateral electrode placement passes the electric current across the whole brain. Unilateral electrode placement passes the current across one hemisphere of the brain. Using an ECT machine, a measured electrical dose is applied for about a second to commence either single or multiple seizures, with the seizures typically lasting 30 seconds to a minute. EEG and EKG monitors follow the seizure activity and heart rhythm while the patient sleeps through the therapy. The patient awakens a few minutes later. Multiple sessions may be needed to complete treatment.

Focus Point
An additional code for the EEG or EKG should be appended according to multiple procedures guideline B3.2c.

© 2018 Optum360, LLC

Intervention, Crisis

Body System
None

PCS Root Type
Crisis Intervention

Root Operation Table
GZ2 Mental Health, Crisis Intervention

Type Qualifier
None

Description
Crisis intervention (therapy) provides supportive therapy to help a patient overcome assault, violence, or other trauma. Crisis intervention is aimed at reducing the intensity of the reaction to the crisis, developing more effective coping skills, and helping the patient recover from the crisis.

The therapist provides individual psychotherapy in an office or outpatient facility using supportive interactions, suggestion, persuasion, reality discussions, re-education, behavior modification techniques, reassurance, and occasionally medication. These interactions are done with the goal of gaining further insight and affecting behavior change or support through understanding. The technique and type of therapy may vary in accordance with the patient's circumstances.

Narcosynthesis

Body System
None

PCS Root Type
Narcosynthesis

Root Operation Table
GZG Mental Health, Narcosynthesis

Type Qualifier
None

Description
Narcosynthesis, or narcoanalysis, is a procedure by which a hypnotic sedative, Amytal, is used to diagnose dissociative disorders and to treat trauma victims by accessing repressed memories, emotions, or events to facilitate healing. This is often used after other measures have failed and/or when identifying a definitive diagnosis is medically essential.

A hypnotic drug known as Amytal or sodium amobarbital is infused into the patient via an intravenous drip for psychiatric diagnostic or psychotherapeutic treatment purposes. A sodium Amytal interview is often conducted in an inpatient setting, to monitor the effects of the drug. The patient, under the influence of a narcotic, is in a hypnotic state where memories, as the patient perceives them, are more confidently reviewed. These interviews are often videotaped for later discussion.

Ancillary

Substance Abuse Treatment

Detoxification, Substance Abuse

Body System
None

PCS Root Type
Detoxification Services

Root Operation Table
HZ2 Substance Abuse Treatment, Detoxification Services

Type Qualifier
None

Description
Detoxification is a program designed to treat the physical symptoms experienced during withdrawal from alcohol or drug dependence. Typical withdrawal symptoms may include nausea, vomiting, anxiety, tremors, seizures, and mood swings. The detoxification process involves cessation of use and prevention of withdrawal symptoms.

A patient is treated for physical symptoms during withdrawal from alcohol or drug dependence. During this medically supervised period of withdrawal, medications may be administered to reduce symptoms, the patient is monitored, and additional services may be recommended. Detoxification can take a few days to several weeks.

Focus Point

Drug and/or alcohol rehabilitation, which focuses on the psychological components of addictive behaviors by providing psychotherapeutic counseling and support strategies for the patient, is coded separately using the Substance Abuse Treatment section, type Individual Counseling.

Ancillary

© 2018 Optum360, LLC

New Technology

Application, Wound Matrix

Body System
Skin, Subcutaneous Tissue, Fascia and Breast

PCS Root Operation
Replacement

Root Operation Table
XHR New Technology, Skin, Subcutaneous Tissue, Fascia and Breast, Replacement

Body Part
Skin

Approach
External

Device/Substance/Technology
Skin Substitute, Porcine Liver Derived

Qualifier
New Technology Group 2

Description
MIRODERM is a new acellular wound matrix that is derived from porcine (pig) liver. Unlike other acellular biologic wound substitute products, which are derived from dermis, urinary bladder, or small intestine submucosa, making them thin, dense, and relatively avascular, the porcine liver is a highly vascularized substrate. The result is a more rapid wound remodeling process.

MIRODERM may be used in the management of wounds such as partial- and full-thickness wounds, pressure ulcers, venous ulcers, chronic vascular ulcers, diabetic ulcers, trauma wounds, drainage wounds, and surgical wounds (donor sites/grafts, post-Mohs surgery, post-laser surgery, podiatric, wound dehiscence).

Using an External approach, the physician applies the porcine acellular wound matrix to contact the entire surface of the wound bed and extend slightly beyond all wound margins. The physician anchors the biologic wound matrix to the wound with sutures or another method. After anchoring, a nonadherent wound dressing is applied over the matrix. A secondary dressing is applied to manage the wound exudate, to keep the MIRODERM matrix moist, and to secure the layers. Additional applications may be applied as needed until the wound has closed.

Focus Point
The root operation Replacement is used since the MIRODERM functions as skin during the wound remodeling process.

Focus Point
Qualifier New Technology Group 2 indicates that this code was in the second group of new-technology codes to be implemented.

Coding Guidance
AHA: 2016, 4Q, 116

New Technology

Atherectomy, Orbital

Body System
Cardiovascular System

PCS Root Operation
Extirpation

Root Operation Table
X2C   New Technology, Cardiovascular System, Extirpation

Body Part
Coronary Artery, One Artery
Coronary Artery, Two Arteries
Coronary Artery, Three Arteries
Coronary Artery, Four or More Arteries

Approach
Percutaneous

Device/Substance/Technology
Orbital Atherectomy Technology

Qualifier
New Technology Group 1

Description
An atherectomy procedure involves the removal of atherosclerosis from an artery, typically via a sharp blade on the end of a catheter or using rotational atherectomy. Orbital atherectomy also removes severely calcified atherosclerosis via a new technology using a diamond-coated crown on a coil placed in the plaque-filled artery and spun at variable rpms to debride the plaque from the arterial walls. The unique crown can be advanced forward and backward once in the artery, which provides for advantages over rotational atherectomy. Only one part of the vessel is in contact with the crown at any given time, which results in less heat generation and thus minimizes the potential for restenosis. The abrasive surface "sands" the plaque, and microscopic particulate matter is continuously flushed into the blood stream as the crown is pressed against the lesion with centrifugal force.

As a new technology, orbital atherectomy is not classified within the regular PCS tables but can be accessed in the New Technology section. The body part identifies the number of coronary arteries that were revascularized. The qualifier identifies the year in which a particular new technology is added to this section. As this procedure was placed into the first group of new-technology codes to be implemented, the qualifier character is New Technology Group 1.

Coding Guidance
AHA: 2015, 4Q, 8, 13

New Technology

© 2018 Optum360, LLC

Filtration, Cerebral Embolic

See also Replacement, Transcatheter Aortic Valve (TAVR), in the Medical and Surgical section

Body System
Cardiovascular System

PCS Root Type
Assistance

Root Operation Table
X2A New Technology, Cardiovascular System, Assistance

Body Part
Innominate Artery and Left Common Carotid Artery

Approach
Percutaneous

Device/Substance/Technology
Cerebral Embolic Filtration, Dual Filter

Qualifier
New Technology Group 2

Description
Embolic debris can be dislodged during transcatheter aortic valve replacements (TAVR) and other endovascular procedures, resulting in increased risk of stroke, dementia, and cognitive impairment. The Claret Medical Sentinel Cerebral Protection System protects the brain from this debris by filtering and removing it during the TAVR or other endovascular procedure.

Via a Percutaneous approach, two conically shaped polyurethane filters mounted onto self-expanding wire frames are delivered through a catheter sheath placed in the right radial artery. The proximal filter is deployed in the brachiocephalic artery, and the distal filter is delivered to the left common carotid artery at the beginning of the TAVR procedure. Debris released during the procedure is collected in the filters, preventing the debris from traveling to the brain. At the completion of the TAVR procedure, the filters and captured debris are withdrawn into the catheter and removed from the patient.

Focus Point
New Technology codes are stand-alone codes. The use of the filtration during a TAVR necessitates the use of multiple codes since two distinct objectives are being met. Both the filtration code (X2A5312) and a code for the TAVR should be reported. See also Replacement, Transcatheter Aortic Valve (TAVR).

Focus Point
In the ICD-10-PCS Body Part key, the brachiocephalic artery is included in the Innominate Artery body part.

Focus Point
Qualifier New Technology Group 2 indicates that this code was in the second group of new-technology codes to be implemented.

Coding Guidance
AHA: 2016, 4Q, 115

Fusion, Spinal, Interbody Fusion Device, Radiolucent Porous

See also Fusion, Cervical Spine, Anterior (ACF) in the Medical and Surgical section

See also Fusion, Lumbar, Anterior Interbody (ALIF) (Anterior Lumbar Vertebral Arthrodesis) in the Medical and Surgical section

Body System
Joints

PCS Root Operation
Fusion

Root Operation Table
XRG   New Technology, Joints, Fusion

Body Part
Occipital-cervical Joint
Cervical Vertebral Joint
Cervical Vertebral Joints, 2 or more
Cervicothoracic Vertebral Joint
Thoracic Vertebral Joint
Thoracic Vertebral Joints, 2 to 7
Thoracic Vertebral Joints, 8 or more
Thoracolumbar Vertebral Joint
Lumbar Vertebral Joint
Lumbar Vertebral Joints, 2 or more
Lumbosacral Joint

Approach
Open

Device
Interbody Fusion Device, Radiolucent Porous

Qualifier
New Technology Group 3

Description
This type of spinal fusion fuses together one or more cervical, thoracic, or lumbar vertebral joints with a radiolucent, porous interbody fusion device made from polyether-ether-ketone (PEEK) polymer. The porous material in this interbody device promotes bone ingrowth to enhance the fusion and because the device is radiolucent, it does not generate artifacts on imaging, allowing early postsurgical assessment of the fusion and improved patient outcomes. Spinal fusion may be performed to treat conditions such as degenerative, traumatic, or congenital lesions or herniated discs; or to stabilize fractures or dislocations of the spine.

Under general anesthesia, the patient is placed supine. Using an Open approach, depending on the vertebral

level fused, an incision is made in the front of the neck beside the trachea, or a transverse or oblique incision is made on the left side of the abdomen. The muscles and other structures are retracted carefully to one side and retractors placed. Bone and degenerated or herniated intervertebral disc material are removed at the levels to be decompressed using rongeurs or curettes. Distractor instruments are used to restore the normal height of the disc space and to determine the appropriate sized spacer to be placed. A radiolucent, porous interbody fusion device, also called a spacer or cage, is inserted into the disc space. A bone graft is placed into and sometimes in front of the cage. Fluoroscopic x-rays are used to confirm that the device is in the correct position.

After the spine is stabilized, the wound area is irrigated with sterile water containing antibiotics. The retractors are removed, restoring the retracted tissues to normal anatomic position, and the incision is closed in layers with sutures. The skin is closed with sutures or staples. Temporary drains may be inserted in the surgical wound to prevent fluid buildup. A sterile bandage is applied.

> **Focus Point**
> Discectomy is usually performed with spinal fusion surgery. Report an additional code for the discectomy procedure, using root operation Excision for a partial discectomy and Resection for a total discectomy.

> **Focus Point**
> The codes in table XRG are complete, and no additional codes are assigned from tables ØRG Upper Joints, Fusion, and ØSG Lower Joints, Fusion. Fixation with plates and screws is included in the fusion root operation, and no additional codes are assigned.

> **Focus Point**
> Nanotextured surface interbody fusion device is also found in the New Technology Fusion (XRG) table. This nanoLOCK ™device by Titan Spine uses a proprietary manufacturing process that produces surface features at a macro, micro, and nano level that generates a response at the cellular level promoting osteoblasts, which build bone. This technology is said to eliminate challenges of other conventional fusion devices such as surface deterioration, which creates debris and inflammation.

Coding Guidance
AHA: 2017, 4Q, 76

© 2018 Optum360, LLC

Immunotherapy, Engineered Autologous Chimeric (KTE-C19) (axicabtagene ciloleucel)

Body System
Anatomical Regions

PCS Root Operation
Introduction

Root Operation Table
XWØ New Technology, Anatomical Regions, Introduction

Body Part
Peripheral Vein
Central Vein

Approach
Percutaneous

Substance
Engineered Autologous Chimeric Antigen Receptor T-cell Immunotherapy

Qualifier
New Technology Group 3

Description

Engineered autologous chimeric antigen receptor T-cell immunotherapy with KTE-C19, also known as axicabtagene ciloleucel, is an immunotherapy consisting of chimeric antigen receptor (CAR) construct T lymphocytes (T-cells) that recognize tumor antigen CD19-expressing cancer cells and normal B-cells. It is used to treat patients with relapsed or refractory aggressive B-cell non-Hodgkin lymphoma who, for various reasons, are not eligible for autologous stem cell transplant. The patient's own T-cells are harvested and genetically engineered using a disarmed virus to produce receptors on their surfaces and turning them into chimeric antigen receptors, or CARs. After being infused back into the patient, the new CAR T-cells recognize, target, activate, and kill the target cancer cells throughout the body.

Engineered autologous CAR T-cell immunotherapy is an autologous, single-infusion immunotherapy performed as an inpatient procedure to allow monitoring of potential patient adverse events. It involves an approximately 30-minute gravity infusion without an IV pump of an entire bag of previously harvested and prepared, patient-specific cell suspension through a central venous access such as a Port-A-Cath or a peripherally inserted central catheter.

Focus Point
The codes in table XWØ are complete, and no additional codes are assigned from table 3EØ Administration, Physiological Systems and Anatomical Regions, Introduction.

Coding Guidance
AHA: 2017, 4Q, 77

Insertion, Intraoperative Knee Replacement Sensor

See Also Joint Replacement, Knee in the Medical and Surgical section

Body System
Joints

PCS Root Operation
Monitoring

Root Operation Table
XR2   New Technology, Joints, Monitoring

Body Part
Knee Joint, Right
Knee Joint, Left

Approach
Open

Device/Substance/Technology
Intraoperative Knee Replacement Sensor

Qualifier
New Technology Group 1

Description

An intraoperative knee replacement sensor is a sterile, disposable tibial insert used to aid orthopaedic surgeons in placing prosthetic joint components during knee replacement surgery.

During knee replacement surgery, the surgeon first evaluates the appropriate size and thickness of the standard tibial trial insert. The surgeon takes the leg through a full range of motion and once unobstructed motion is confirmed, replaces the standard tibial trial insert with an intraoperative knee replacement sensor device of the same size and thickness that is placed directly on the tibial tray. It is not secured to the bone, but the knee capsule is temporarily clipped closed. Once placed within the knee capsule, it provides the surgeon with monitoring and tracking of the balance of the articulation of the femur to the tibial implant components, allowing the assessment of knee function during the surgical procedure. During the knee replacement procedure, the surgeon uses the data provided by the monitoring device to make the most effective surgical adjustments, resulting in improved knee implant stability and articulation. The separately reportable knee replacement procedure is then completed. *See also* Joint Replacement, Knee.

Focus Point
Effective October 1, 2015, new "Section X New Technology" codes were created to report placement of intraoperative knee replacement sensors. The new section provides a place for codes that uniquely identify procedures requested via the new-technology application process. When section X contains a code title that describes a specific new-technology procedure, only that X code is reported for the procedure. See ICD-10-PCS New Technology section, general guidelines D1.

Coding Guidance
AHA: 2015, 4Q, 8-12

New Technology

Placement, Magnetic Growth Rods

Body System
Bones

PCS Root Operation
Reposition

Root Operation Table
XNS New Technology, Bones, Reposition

Body Part
Lumbar Vertebra
Cervical Vertebra
Thoracic Vertebra

Approach
Open

Device/Substance/Technology
Magnetically Controlled Growth Rod(s)

Qualifier
New Technology Group 2

Description
Scoliosis is a condition characterized by spinal curvature that makes the patient's spine look like an "S" or "C" rather than a straight line. Magnetically controlled growing rod (MCGR) insertion is a relatively new procedure to treat spinal deformities that consists of one or two sterile, single-use adjustable spinal rods implanted as fixation devices, and an external remote controller (ERC). MCGRs are surgically implanted like traditional growing rods but do not require additional surgery for expansion; the MCGR rods are magnetically lengthened in a noninvasive procedure that can take place in a physician's office.

After general anesthesia has been administered, the patient is placed in prone position, and an Open approach is used with an incision through the skin, fascia, and paravertebral muscles, which are retracted to expose the vertebrae. Rods are placed on either side of the spine and secured with pedicle screws and surgical hooks above and below the curve to adequately brace the spine during growth, minimizing the progression of scoliosis. The incision is closed by layered sutures.

During follow-up visits, the external controller is placed over the patient's spine. The implanted magnet in the rod is then activated, causing it to rotate and lengthen or shorten the rod. At the completion of the treatment, the rods are removed.

Focus Point
Reposition is used as the root operation since the intent of the procedure is to move the vertebrae into normal position.

Coding Guidance
AHA: 2016, 4Q, 117

New Technology

Replacement, Rapid Deployment Aortic Valve (RDAVR)

Body System
Cardiovascular System

PCS Root Operation
Replacement

Root Operation Table
X2R New Technology, Cardiovascular System, Replacement

Body Part
Aortic Valve

Approach
Open

Device/Substance/Technology
Zooplastic Tissue, Rapid Deployment Technique

Qualifier
New Technology Group 2

Description
Traditional aortic valve replacement can involve a full sternotomy, excising the diseased aortic valve, and placing between 12 and 15 sutures through the aortic annulus and sewing the ring of the valve into place. Rapid deployment aortic valve replacement (RDAVR) uses a minimally invasive technique with a balloon expandable stent that allows precise positioning of the new valve with only three sutures, rather than the normal 12 to 15. The system uses a flexible deployment arm that allows the surgeon optimal access to anatomy for valve deployment and suturing. This technique allows rapid deployment of the valve, reducing the duration of cardiopulmonary bypass, and by simplifying the steps required to implant the valve, allowing the use of smaller, less-invasive incisions.

The patient is placed under general anesthesia and cardiopulmonary bypass. Using an Open approach, either through a standard sternotomy or a mini-thoracotomy incision with or without thoracoscopic assistance, the physician opens the aorta after cross-clamping. The damaged leaflets from the annulus are removed. Using a sizer barrel, the replacement valve size is determined. Three equally spaced sutures are placed through the annulus. The valve is deployed and positioned in the annulus using a specialized delivery system. The replacement valve is placed into the annulus, and the position is confirmed and secured with sutures. Using a catheter, the new valve is deployed by inflating the balloon to the appropriate pressure. The balloon is then deflated and the delivery system and valve holder are retracted as a single unit. The suture snares are removed, the guiding sutures are tied, and the aortotomy and chest incisions are closed in the usual fashion.

Focus Point
Qualifier New Technology Group 2 indicates that this code was in the second group of new-technology codes to be implemented.

Focus Point
A mini-thoracotomy, while less invasive, is still considered an Open approach. A mini-thoracotomy with thoracoscopic assistance is also still considered an Open approach, according to ICD-10-PCS guideline B5.2.

Focus Point
The ICD-10-PCS Device Key currently lists the EDWARDS INTUITY Elite valve system and the Perceval sutureless valve under the PCS value Zooplastic Tissue, Rapid Deployment Technique in New Technology.

Coding Guidance
AHA: 2017, 1Q, 36; 2016, 4Q, 116

© 2018 Optum360, LLC

Therapy, Aquablation, Prostate (Robotic Water Resection of the Prostate)

Body System
Male Reproductive System

PCS Root Operation
Destruction

Root Operation Table
XV5 New Technology, Male Reproductive System, Destruction

Body Part
Prostate

Approach
Via Natural or Artificial Opening Endoscopic

Device/Substance/Technology
Robotic Waterjet Ablation

Qualifier
New Technology Group 4

Description
Aquablation therapy is delivered using the AquaBeam system, an ultrasound image-guided waterjet system that uses a robotically controlled and targeted high-velocity saline stream to ablate obstructive prostate tissue in males suffering from lower urinary tract symptoms (LUTS) due to benign prostatic hyperplasia (BPH). The therapy, which does not use heat, is provided after endoscopic visualization and planning with surgical mapping by the surgeon. The AquaBeam system is made up of three main elements: the conformal planning unit (CPU), robotic hand-piece, and a console.

With the patient placed in the dorsal lithotomy position and under appropriate anesthesia, the transrectal ultrasound (TRUS) device is mounted into position. The bladder is accessed using a Via Natural or Artificial Opening Endoscopic approach using a cystoscope, and the robotic hand-piece is introduced via the cystoscope and stabilized using an articulating arm attached to the operating table. When optimal position is confirmed, the system software is activated to adjust the alignment as necessary. The surgeon, using measurements from the TRUS image, uses mapping to plan the required depth and angle of resection of prostate tissue and manually inputs the dimensions into the console software. The high-velocity sterile saline is then applied using the robotic hand piece at various flow rates based on the depth required. The flow is controlled by the console pump using a foot pedal control.

Once the aquablation is complete, hemostasis is obtained by applying a thin layer of cautery to the resected area of the prostate using a low-power laser or a rollerball. The articulating arm is unlocked, and the device is removed. A three-way Foley catheter is placed.

Focus Point
There is currently only one guideline for coding New Technology section X procedures, guideline D1, which states, "Section X codes are standalone codes. They are not supplemental codes. Section X codes fully represent the specific procedure described in the code title, and do not require any additional codes from other sections of ICD-10-PCS. When section X contains a code title which describes a specific new technology procedure, only that X code is reported for the procedure. There is no need to report a broader, non-specific code in another section of ICD-10-PCS."

Therapy, Bone Marrow Cell, Autologous, Intramuscular

See also Transplant, Bone Marrow (BMT) in the Medical and Surgical Related section, Administration

See also Harvest, Graft, Autologous Bone Marrow in the Medical and Surgical section

Body System
Muscles, Tendons, Bursae and Ligaments

PCS Root Operation
Introduction

Root Operation Table
XKØ   New Technology, Muscles, Tendons, Bursae and Ligaments, Introduction

Body Part
Muscle

Approach
Percutaneous

Substance
Concentrated Bone Marrow Aspirate

Qualifier
New Technology Group 3

Description
Peripheral artery disease (PAD) is a chronic disorder that is defined by atherosclerotic narrowing and blocking of arteries in the extremities, typically the legs.

Intramuscular autologous bone marrow cell therapy is a new technique that involves the collection, concentration, and direct application of mononuclear stem cells originating in the patient's own bone marrow to promote the formation of new blood vessels (angiogenesis, arteriogenesis, and/or vasculogenesis). The new blood vessels revascularize the affected limbs.

In a separately reportable procedure, the bone marrow is harvested, usually from the iliac crest. The bone marrow is extracted into an anticoagulant-coated syringe and then prepared using a special concentration and separation system such as the MarrowStim™ system, to create a concentrated bone marrow stem cell aspirate (cBMA). The cBMA is then injected at multiple locations along a muscle in the affected limb, such as the gastrocnemius muscle.

Focus Point
Bone marrow transplant procedures are coded using table 302, found in the Medical and Surgical Related section, Administration, with the root operation Transfusion. See also Transplant, Bone Marrow (BMT).

Focus Point
Bone marrow graft harvested from the local incision or operative site is not reported separately. However, if a separate incision in a different body part/location is required to harvest the graft, such as from the pelvis or iliac crest, this may be reported in addition to the primary procedure. This is consistent with ICD-10-PCS guideline B3.9. See also Harvest, Graft, Autologous Bone Marrow in the Medical and Surgical section.

Coding Guidance
AHA: 2017, 4Q, 74

New Technology

© 2018 Optum360, LLC

Treatment, Intraoperative, Vascular Grafts (Intraoperative Administration of Endothelial Damage Inhibitor)

See also Bypass Graft, Coronary Artery (CABG) in the Medical and Surgical section

Body System
Extracorporeal

PCS Root Operation
Introduction

Root Operation Table
XYØ New Technology, Extracorporeal, Introduction

Body Part
Vein Graft

Approach
External

Substance
Endothelial Damage Inhibitor

Qualifier
New Technology Group 3

Description
Intraoperative administration of endothelial damage inhibitor is an intraoperative treatment of vascular grafts for the prevention of vein graft disease (VGD) and vein graft failure following coronary artery bypass surgery or peripheral artery bypass surgery.

Autologous vascular grafts such as saphenous vein grafts are used frequently as bypass grafts in coronary artery bypass and peripheral bypass surgeries. These vein grafts are susceptible to VGD, which can affect the durability and patency of the graft via pathophysiologic changes that occur in vein grafts after they are harvested and grafted to the new location. These changes can lead to thrombus formation, intimal hyperplasia, and atherosclerosis, resulting in graft stenosis, occlusion, and loss of patency of the graft.

Intraoperative vascular graft treatment takes place during a bypass procedure; the tissue preservation solution is prepared using a kit containing two solutions that are mixed in the surgical suite immediately before use. After the vein graft is harvested, it is flushed with the tissue preservation solution that contains an endothelial damage inhibitor designed to inhibit damage to the endothelial cells lining the graft lumen. After it is flushed with the solution, the harvested vein graft is then placed in the solution to soak until immediately before the final bypass anastomosis takes place. The bypass procedure is completed as usual.

Focus Point
The bypass and harvesting of vein graft procedures are coded separately.

Coding Guidance
AHA: 2017, 4Q, 78

Alphabetic Index

A

abdomen 454, 460
abdomen muscle
    left 130, 298
    right 130, 298
abdominal aorta 96, 116, 314
abdominal artery 117
abdominal wall 81, 205, 285, 415, 416
abdominoplasty 81
ablation
    cardiac 82
    endometrial 83
ablation, vein, thermal, endovenous 84
abortifacient 401
abortion 401
acupuncture 456
adenoidectomy (without tonsillectomy) 85
adenoids 85, 369
adenosine sestamibi planar scan, heart muscle
    (technetium) 472
adjustment, cardiac pacemaker lead 86
administration 417
    dialysis, peritoneal (PD) 417
    induction of labor, medical 418
    infusion, vasopressor agent 419
    injection, epidural steroid 420
    injection, sclerosing agent for esophageal varix 421
    introduction, antineoplastic agent, hepatic artery
        422
    irrigation, joint 423
    pleurodesis, talc 424
    thrombolysis (injection of thrombolytic) (tissue
        plasminogen activator) 425
    transfusion, fresh frozen plasma (FFP) 426
    transplant, bone marrow (BMT) 427
    transplant, stem cell 428
adrenal gland 87
    left 87
    right 87
allogeneic 376, 378, 379
allogenic 377
alteration 81, 109, 111, 194, 266, 341
alveoloplasty 88
alveolotomy 89
amniocentesis 403
amniotic fluid
    diagnostic 403
    therapeutic 403
ampulla of vater 260, 261, 353
amputation
    below knee 90
    foot and toe ray 91
    toe 92
amygdalohippocampectomy 93
anal sphincter 171, 173, 325
anastomosis, billroth I 94
    see also anastomosis, billroth II 94

anastomosis, billroth II 95
    see also anastomosis, billroth I 95
    see also gastrectomy 95
anatomical orifices 415
anatomical regions 81, 90, 91, 92, 111, 151, 158,
        166, 193, 194, 202, 203, 205, 285, 286,
        325, 362, 363, 373, 413, 414, 415, 416,
        417, 418, 419, 420, 421, 422, 423, 424,
        425, 454, 456, 457, 458, 460, 466, 476,
        477
    general 81, 111, 151, 158, 166, 193, 194, 205,
        285, 286, 325, 362, 363
    lower extremities 90, 91, 92, 202, 203
ancillary 461
aneurysmectomy, abdominal aortic, with replacement
    96
angiography, cardiac (coronary arteriography)
    (angiocardiography) 461
angiography, intraoperative fluorescence vascular 429
angioplasty, percutaneous transluminal coronary
    (PTCA) 97
angioplasty, percutaneous transluminal coronary
    (PTCA) with stent(s) 98
ankle joint 179
    left 179
    right 179
anorectal 415
anterior chamber 370, 371
    left 370, 371
    right 370, 371
anti-inflammatory 420
antineoplastic 422
anus 171, 173, 325, 336
aorta 117
aortic valve 329, 334, 388, 389, 494
application, stereotactic head frame 413
    see also radiation therapy, stereotactic radiosurgery
        413
application, wound matrix 487
arterial 432
arteriography, renal (renal angiography) (angiography,
    renal arteries) 462
arterioplasty (bovine patch) 99
artificial sphincter 209
assessment, cochlear implant 482
    see also implant, cochlear in the medical and
        surgical section 482
assistance 440, 444, 446, 489
assistance, computer 457
assistance, robotic 458
atherectomy, orbital 488
atrial appendage 127
    left 127
atrial septum 317
atrioventricular valve 389
    left 389
atrium 127, 217, 392

© 2018 Optum360, LLC

Alphabetic Index

© 2018 Optum360, LLC

Alphabetic Index

Alphabetic Index

© 2018 Optum360, LLC

perfusion, respiratory donor organ (EVLP) (ex-vivo lung perfusion) **449**

pheresis **450**

phototherapy **451**

therapy, shock wave, extracorporeal (ESWT), musculoskeletal (orthotripsy) **452**

ultrasound, therapeutic **453**

extraction **102, 143, 147, 161, 257, 289, 310, 404, 405, 409**

extraction, extracapsular cataract with intraocular lens implantation **167**

extraction, retained placenta, manual **409**

extraluminal device **101, 122, 127, 133, 258, 259**

extraocular muscle **296**

    left **296**

    right **296**

extraperitoneal **404**

eye **109, 112, 156, 167, 212, 251, 296, 370, 371, 396, 476, 477, 478**

    left **112, 156, 212**

    right **112, 156, 212**

F

face **111, 415, 416**

facial muscle **320**

fallopian tube **259, 265**

    bilateral **259, 265**

    left **259, 265**

    right **259, 265**

fasciectomy, plantar **168**

fasciotomy, palmar (dupuytren's contracture) **169**

feeding device **134, 239**

female genital tract **415**

female reproductive **418**

female reproductive system **83, 122, 129, 132, 147, 172, 206, 259, 265, 269, 273, 325, 466, 476, 477**

femoral arteries

    bilateral **116**

femoral artery **120, 202**

    left **120**

    right **120**

femoral region **202**

    bilateral **202**

    left **202**

    right **202**

femoral shaft **229**

    left **229**

    right **229**

fetal head **467**

fetal umbilical cord **468**

fetus and obstetrical **467, 468**

fibula **229**

    left **229**

    right **229**

filtration, cerebral embolic **489**

    See also Replacement, Transcatheter Aortic Valve (TAVR), in the medical and Surgical Section **489**

finger **415, 416**

    left **415, 416**

    right **415, 416**

first trimester

    multiple gestation **468**

    single fetus **468**

fistula, arteriovenous (AV) **170**

fistulectomy, anal **171**

fistulectomy, vesicovaginal **172**

fistulotomy, anal **173**

fluoroscopy **461, 462, 465, 466, 470, 471**

fontan stage I (norwood procedure) **174**

    see also blalock-taussig shunt procedure, modified **174**

    see also conduit, right ventricle to pulmonary artery (RV-PA) (sano shunt) **174**

    see also fontan stage ii (glenn procedure) (caval-pulmonary artery anastomosis) **174**

    see also fontan stage iii, completion **174**

fontan stage II (glenn procedure) (caval-pulmonary artery anastomosis) **175**

    see also blalock-taussig shunt procedure, modified **175**

    see also fontan stage i (norwood procedure) **175**

    see also fontan stage iii, completion **175**

fontan stage III, completion **176**

    see also fontan stage i (norwood procedure) **176**

    see also fontan stage ii (glenn procedure) (caval-pulmonary artery anastomosis) **176**

foot **91, 413, 415, 416**

    left **91, 413, 415, 416**

    right **91, 413, 415, 416**

foot tendon **115**

    left **115**

    right **115**

foot vein **257**

    left **257**

    right **257**

fractional flow reserve (FFR), coronary **432**

    see also angiography, cardiac (coronary arteriography) (angiocardiography), in the imaging section of the ancillary chapter. **432**

fragmentation **260, 261, 277**

frenectomy, labial **177**

frenotomy, labial **177**

frontal sinus **351**

    left **351**

    right **351**

frozen plasma **426**

fundoplication, gastroesophageal **178**

fusion **179, 180, 182, 184, 186**

fusion, ankle (arthrodesis) **179**

fusion, cervical spine, anterior (ACF) **180, 181**

    see also fusion, cervical spine, posterior (PCF) **180**

fusion, cervical spine, posterior (PCF) **182**

    see also fusion, cervical spine, anterior (ACF) **182**

fusion, lumbar, anterior interbody (ALIF) (anterior lumbar vertebral arthrodesis) **184**

    see also fusion, lumbar posterior (PLF) **184**

see also fusion, spinal, interbody fusion device,
  radiolucent porous **184**
fusion, lumbar, posterior (PLF) **186**
  see also fusion, lumbar anterior interbody (ALIF)
    (anterior lumbar vertebral arthrodesis) **186**
fusion, spinal, interbody fusion device, radiolucent
  porous **490**
  see also fusion, cervical spine, anterior (ACF) **490**
  see also fusion, lumbar, anterior interbody (ALIF)
    (anterior lumbar vertebral arthrodesis) **490**

G

gallbladder **124, 260, 261, 399**
gastrectomy **188**
  see also anastomosis, billroth ii **188**
  see also gastrectomy, vertical sleeve (VSG) **188**
gastrectomy, vertical sleeve (VSG) **189**
  see also switch, duodenal (biliopancreatic diversion)
    189
Gastrointestinal **477**
gastrointestinal **429**
gastrointestinal system **94, 101, 128, 134, 137,
  138, 148, 155, 159, 160, 161, 171, 173,
  178, 188, 189, 190, 191, 192, 200, 239,
  264, 291, 293, 309, 325, 336, 338, 359,
  399, 466, 471, 476, 477**
gastrointestinal tract **166**
gastrojejunostomy, roux-en-y (gastric bypass for
  morbid obesity) **190**
gastroplasty, collis **191**
  see also fundoplication, gastroesophageal **191**
gastrostomy, percutaneous endoscopic (PEG) **192**
gender reassignment surgery **193**
genioplasty, augmentation **194**
glenoid surface **248**
graft, arteriovenous (AV) **195**
graft, dura mater, intracranial **196**
  see also decompression, posterior fossa (chiari
    malformation) **196**
graft, skin, split-thickness (STSG) **197**

H

hand **413, 415, 416**
  left **413, 415, 416**
  right **413, 415, 416**
hard palate **321**
harvest, graft, autologous bone marrow **198**
  see also biopsy, bone marrow **198**
  see also therapy, bone marrow cell, autologous
    intramuscular **198**
  see also transplant, bone marrow (BMT) **198**
harvesting, knee chondrocytes **199**
  see also implantation, autologous chondrocyte
    (ACI), knee **199**
head **413, 415, 416, 454, 460**
head and facial bones **88, 89, 142, 143, 152, 227,
  301, 302, 311, 312, 321**

mandible, left **88, 89**
mandible, right **88, 89**
maxilla **88, 89**
head and neck region **457, 458**
head and neck vessels **453**
hearing aid assessment **482**
hearing assessment **483**
hearing device **208**
  multiple channel cochlear prosthesis **208**
  single channel cochlear prosthesis **208**
heart **86, 237, 376, 430, 453, 461, 463, 464, 466,
  469, 470, 472**
  bilateral **430**
  left **430, 463, 464, 470**
  right **430, 463, 464, 470**
  right and left **463, 464, 470**
Heart and Great Vessels **97**
heart and great vessels **82, 86, 98, 108, 117, 127,
  131, 174, 175, 211, 217, 221, 237, 267,
  294, 317, 322, 329, 330, 334, 360, 364,
  376, 388, 389**
heart with aorta **464**
hemicolectomy **200**
hemodialysis **442**
hemorrhoidal plexus **201**
hemorrhoidectomy **201**
hepatic artery **123, 225**
hepatic duct **260, 261**
  common **260, 261**
  left **260, 261**
  right **260, 261**
hepatobiliary duct **166**
hepatobiliary system **103, 124**
hepatobiliary system and pancreas **166, 260, 261,
  353, 378, 399, 465, 466, 476, 477**
herniorrhaphy, femoral **202**
herniorrhaphy, inguinal **203**
herniorrhaphy, paraesophageal (diaphragmatic) **204**
herniorrhaphy, ventral, incisional (hernia repair) **205**
high dose rate (HDR) **475**
high forceps **405**
hip joint **240, 241, 243, 244**
  acetabular surface
    left **240, 243, 244**
    right **240, 243, 244**
  femoral surface
    left **240, 243, 244**
    right **240, 243, 244**
  left **241, 243, 244**
  right **241, 243, 244**
humeral surface **248**
hyperthermia **476**
hysterectomy **206**

I

ileocutaneous **150**
ileum **138, 359**
imaging **461**

© 2018 Optum360, LLC

© 2018 Optum360, LLC

see also replacement, intervertebral disc, artificial
253
large intestine **128, 200**
  left **200**
  right **200**
laser **461**
laser (fluoroscopy) **462**
laser interstitial thermal therapy **481**
lavage, bronchoalveolar (BAL) **254**
  see also suctioning, bronchial (for removal of mucus
    plug) **254**
  see also washing, bronchial **254**
lengthening, tendon **255**
lens **167**
  left **167**
  right **167**
leukocytes **450**
ligamentoplasty, interspinous **256**
ligation and stripping, varicose veins **257**
ligation, esophageal varices **258**
ligation, tubal (sterilization) **259**
lingula bronchus **223, 319**
lithotripsy, direct intracorporeal **260**
  see also lithotripsy, extracorporeal, shock wave
    (ESWL) **260**
lithotripsy, extracorporeal shock wave (ESWL) **261**
  see also lithotripsy, direct intracorporeal **261**
liver **103, 378**
  left lobe **103**
  right lobe **103**
lobectomy, lung **262**
lobectomy, temporal, brain (epilepsy) **263**
  see also electrocorticography (intraoperative),
    under measurement and monitoring in the
    medical and surgical related section. **263**
low cervical **404**
low dose rate (LDR) **475**
low forceps **405**
low osmolar **461, 465**
lower arm **415, 416**
  left **415, 416**
  right **415, 416**
lower arm vein **170, 195**
lower arteries **96, 99, 116, 120, 123, 153, 225,
314, 364, 462, 466**
lower bones **113, 114, 142, 143, 215, 229, 252,
284, 301, 302, 311, 343, 395**
lower extremities **454, 460**
lower extremity **413, 415, 416, 457, 458**
  left **413, 415, 416**
  right **413, 415, 416**
lower eyelid **109**
  left **109**
  right **109**
lower femur **229**
  left **229**
  right **229**
lower jaw **194**
lower joints **100, 125, 149, 179, 184, 186, 210,
231, 240, 241, 243, 244, 246, 272, 301,**

303, 332, 380
lower leg **90, 413, 415, 416**
  left **90, 413, 415, 416**
  right **90, 413, 415, 416**
lower leg tendon
  left **305**
  right **305**
lower lip **177**
lower lobe bronchus **223, 319**
  left **223, 319**
  right **223, 319**
lower spine bursa and ligament **256**
lower vein **201, 257**
lower veins **201, 224, 257, 258, 347, 364**
lumbar **454, 460**
lumbar nerve **147, 253, 342**
lumbar spinal cord **253**
lumbar vertebra **252, 395, 493**
lumbar vertebral disc **149, 332**
lumbar vertebral joint **184, 186, 231**
lumbar vertebral joints **184, 186**
  2 or more **184, 186**
lumbosacral disc **149, 332**
lumbosacral joint **184, 231**
lung **105, 146, 262, 290, 379**
  bilateral **105, 146, 290, 379**
  left **105, 146, 290, 379**
  lower lobe
    left **105, 146, 262, 290, 379**
    right **105, 146, 262, 290, 379**
  middle lobe
    right **105, 146, 262, 290, 379**
  right **105, 146, 290, 379**
  upper lobe
    left **105, 146, 262, 290, 379**
    right **105, 146, 262, 290, 379**
lung lingula **105, 146, 262, 290, 379**
lungs and bronchi **474**
lymphatic and hematologic system **476, 477**
lymphatic and hemic systems **102, 106, 337, 355,
356**
lymphatic, aortic **106, 337**
lymphatic, head **106, 337**
lymphatic, internal mammary, left **106, 337**
lymphatic, internal mammary, right **106, 337**
lymphatic, left axillary **106, 337**
lymphatic, left inguinal **106, 337**
lymphatic, left lower extremity **106, 337**
lymphatic, left neck **106, 337**
lymphatic, left upper extremity **106, 337**
lymphatic, mesenteric **106, 337**
lymphatic, pelvis **106, 337**
lymphatic, right axillary **106, 337**
lymphatic, right inguinal **106, 337**
lymphatic, right lower extremity **106, 337**
lymphatic, right neck **106, 337**
lymphatic, right upper extremity **106, 337**
lymphatic, thorax **106, 337**
lysis, adhesions, abdominal (abdominal adhesiolysis)
264

Alphabetic Index

lysis, adhesions, female pelvic (pelvic adhesiolysis) 265

M

magnetic resonance imaging (MRI) 467
magnetically controlled growth rod(s) 493
main bronchus 223, 319
  left 223, 319
  right 223, 319
male reproductive system 126, 230, 282, 283, 292, 307, 391, 466, 475, 476, 477
mammoplasty, reduction 266
mandible, left 88, 89
mandible, right 88, 89
manipulation 460
manipulation, chiropractic, mechanically assisted 460
manipulative treatment, osteopathic 454
map 267, 268
mapping 267, 268
  cardiac 267
  cortical 268
marsupialization, bartholin's gland cyst 269
marsupialization, pilonidal cyst 270
mastectomy 271
mastoid sinus 392
maxilla 88, 89, 321
maxillary sinus 351
  left 351
  right 351
measurement 430, 431, 432, 434
measurement and monitoring 429
  angiography, intraoperative fluorescence vascular 429
  catheterization, cardiac 430
  electrocorticography (intraoperative) 431
  fractional flow reserve (FFR), coronary 432
  interrogation, device, cardiac rhythm related 433
  measurement, portal venous pressure 434
  monitoring, central venous pressure 435
  monitoring, fetal heart rate, transvaginal (internal) 436
  monitoring, intracranial pressure 437
  monitoring, neurophysiological, intraoperative 438
  stress test, cardiac (myocardial perfusion scan)(cardiovascular stress test) 439
measurement, portal venous pressure 434
mechanically assisted chiropractic manipulation 460
median nerve 306
medical and surgical related 401
meniscectomy, knee 272
mental health 484
  biofeedback 484
  electroconvulsive therapy 484
  narcosynthesis 485
metatarsal 113, 114
  left 113, 114
  right 113, 114
mid forceps 405
middle lobe bronchus 223, 319
  right 223, 319

minor salivary gland 348, 350
mitral valve 322, 388, 389
monitoring 429, 431, 435, 436, 437, 438, 439, 492
monitoring electrode 410
monitoring, central venous pressure 435
monitoring, fetal heart rate, transvaginal (internal) 436
  see also insertion, monitoring electrode, under "obstetrics" in the medical and surgical related section 436
monitoring, intracranial pressure 437
  see also ventriculostomy in the medical and surgical chapter 437
monitoring, neurophysiological, intraoperative 438
mouth and pharynx 415
mouth and throat 85, 157, 163, 177, 320, 321, 348, 349, 350, 367, 368, 369, 387
MRI, fetal, central nervous system 467
  see also ultrasonography, fetal 467
muscles 130, 142, 143, 298, 320, 325
musculoskeletal system 476, 477
myocardium 472
myomectomy, uterine 273
myringotomy with tubes (tympanostomy) 274

N

narcosynthesis 485
nasal 415
nasal mucosa and soft tissue 341, 342
nasal septum 344
nasal turbinate 383
nasopharynx 392
neck 373, 415, 416
nephrolithotomy, percutaneous 275
  see also nephrolithotripsy, percutaneous 275
nephrolithotripsy, percutaneous 276
  see also nephrolithotomy, percutaneous 276
  see also nephrostomy (with fragmentation), percutaneous 276
nephrostomy (with fragmentation), percutaneous 277
  see also nephrolithotripsy, percutaneous 277
nephrostomy (without fragmentation), percutaneous 277
nephroureterectomy 278
nervous system 412
neurolysis, trigeminal (trigeminal nerve decompression) 279
neuroplasty, peripheral 280
neurostimulator generator 227, 312
neurostimulator lead 228, 313
new technology 487
nipple 271
  left 271
  right 271
nonautologous tissue substitute 81, 88, 96, 99, 108, 109, 116, 117, 131, 137, 138, 174, 179, 180, 182, 193, 194, 197, 204, 251, 280, 294, 299, 300, 317, 321, 322, 329, 330, 341, 380, 385, 389, 392

© 2018 Optum360, LLC

Alphabetic Index

compression, lymphedema, intermittent pneumatic 413

immobilization (cast/splint) 414

packing 415

traction 416

placement, magnetic growth rods 493

placenta 468

plain radiography 462

planar nuclear medicine imaging 472, 473, 474

plaque radiation 478

plasma 450

platelets 450

pleura

left 289

right 289

pleural cavity 362, 363, 392, 424

left 362, 363

right 362, 363

pleurectomy, parietal, with decortication 289

pleurodesis, talc 424

see also thoracoscopy (diagnostic) in the medical and surgical chapter 424

plication, emphysematous bleb 290

portal vein 347

pregnancy 401, 403, 404, 405, 407, 408, 409, 410, 411, 412

prepuce 126

pressure 434, 435

proctectomy 291

see also resection, abdominoperineal (APR) 291

products of conception 401, 403, 404, 405, 407, 409, 410, 411, 412

ectopic 411

retained 409

products of conception, cardiac 436

prolonged intermittent

6-18 hours per day 442

prostate 292, 475

prostatectomy 292

pulmonary artery 108, 175

left 108

right 108, 175

pulmonary trunk 108, 131, 294, 360

pulmonary valve 294, 388, 389

pyloromyotomy 293

R

radial artery 170, 195

left 170, 195

right 170, 195

radiation therapy 475

brachytherapy, prostate 475

oncology treatment, hyperthermia 476

radiation therapy, external beam 477

radiation therapy, plaque radiation, eye 478

radiation therapy, stereotactic radiosurgery, brain 479

radiation therapy, superficial dermatologic 480

therapy treatment, laser interstitial (LITT) (brain) 481

radiation therapy, external beam 477

radiation therapy, plaque radiation, eye 478

radiation therapy, stereotactic radiosurgery, brain 479

radiation therapy, superficial dermatologic 480

see also radiation therapy, external beam 480

rastelli procedure (right ventricular-pulmonary artery conduit) 294

see also repair, ventricular septal defect (VSD) 294

ravitch procedure (repair of pectus deformity) 295

see also nuss procedure 295

reattachment 335

recession, extraocular muscle 296

reconstruction

breast (transverse rectus abdominis myocutaneous (TRAM) free flap) 297

breast (transverse rectus abdominis myocutaneous (TRAM) pedicle flap) 298

lateral ulnar collateral ligament (LUCL) 299

urethra, male (urethroplasty)

see also release, chordee 300

see also repair, hypospadias 300

reconstruction, urethra, male (urethroplasty) 300

rectum 291, 325, 336, 338

reduction

fracture, closed with percutaneous pinning 301

fracture, open, with internal fixation (ORIF) 302

joint dislocation 303

reimplantation, parathyroid (autotransplantation) 304

see also parathyroidectomy 304

release 130, 146, 177, 253, 264, 265, 279, 305, 306, 307, 308, 343, 388, 400

achilles' tendon (achillotenotomy) (achillotomy) 305

carpal tunnel 306

chordee 307

see also repair, hypospadias 307

coracoacromial ligament 308

see also decompression, subacromial, rotator cuff tendon 308

see also repair, rotator cuff (shoulder) 308

removal 309, 310, 311, 312, 313, 333

esophageal foreign body 309

ingrown toenail 310

internal fixation device, bone 311

intracranial responsive neurostimulator (RNS) generator 312

see also removal, intracranial responsive neurostimulator (RNS) or deep brain stimulator (DBS) lead 312

intracranial responsive neurostimulator (RNS) or deep brain stimulator (DBS) lead 313

see also insertion, deep brain stimulator (dbs) 313

see also removal, intracranial responsive neurostimulator (RNS) generator 313

removal, carbon dioxide, extracorporeal (ECCO2R) (respiratory dialysis) 445

removal, ectopic pregnancy 411

© 2018 Optum360, LLC

renal arteries
  bilateral **462**
renal artery
  left **462**
  right **462**
Repair **320**
repair **81, 109, 111, 129, 172, 202, 203, 204, 205, 256, 280, 283, 290, 314, 315, 316, 317, 319, 320, 321, 322, 323, 324, 325, 326, 327, 328, 329, 330, 349, 351, 353, 389, 412**
  aneurysm, abdominal aorta, endovascular with stent graft (EVAR) **314**
  aneurysm, cerebral, craniotomy with clipping **315**
  aneurysm, cerebral, endovascular **316**
  atrial septal defect (ASD) (atrioseptoplasty) (repair of foramen ovale (patent)) **317**
  bronchopleural fistula, autologous graft, omentum **319**
  cleft lip (cheiloplasty) **320**
    see also repair, cleft palate, alveolar **320**
  cleft palate, alveolar **321**
    see also repair, cleft lip (cheiloplasty) **321**
  complete common atrioventricular canal defect **322**
    see also repair, atrial septal defect (ASD) (atrioseptoplasty) (repair of foramen ovale patent) **322**
    see also repair, ventricular septal defect (VSD) **322**
  hypospadias **323**
    see also reconstruction, urethra, male (urethroplasty) **323**
    see also release, chordee **323**
  labral tear (shoulder) **324**
  obstetrical laceration/episiotomy extension **325**
  rotator cuff (shoulder) **326**
    see also decompression, subacromial, rotator cuff tendon **326**
    see also joint replacement, shoulder (partial) **326**
    see also joint replacement, shoulder (total) **326**
    see also joint replacement, shoulder, reverse (reverse shoulder arthroplasty) **326**
  superior labrum anterior and posterior (SLAP) **327**
    see also repair, labral tear (shoulder) **327**
  tendon (tenorrhaphy) **328**
  truncus arteriosus with aortic valve creation **329**
    see also rastelli procedure (right ventricular-pulmonary artery conduit) **329**
    see also repair, ventricular septal defect (VSD) **329**
  ventricular septal defect (VSD) **330**
repair, in utero fetal myelomeningocele **412**
replacement **88, 96, 109, 156, 167, 197, 211, 240, 241, 244, 246, 248, 249, 250, 251, 297, 332, 334, 357, 380, 385, 389, 494**
replacement, intervertebral disc, artificial **332**
replacement, pacemaker generator (end of life) **333**
  see also insertion, cardiac pacemaker generator **333**
replacement, rapid deployment aortic valve (RDAVR) **494**

replacement, transcatheter aortic valve (TAVR) **334**
  see also filtration, cerebral embolic, the new technology section **334**
replantation, scalp **335**
reposition **109, 114, 152, 157, 252, 281, 283, 284, 295, 296, 301, 303, 344, 352, 360, 382, 386, 493**
reposition, uterus, transvaginal **335**
  see also version, external cephalic (ECV) **335**
resection **85, 94, 124, 126, 128, 139, 149, 159, 160, 188, 200, 206, 262, 271, 278, 282, 288, 291, 292, 310, 336, 337, 348, 356, 365, 368, 369, 387, 396, 399, 411**
resection, abdominoperineal (APR) **336**
  see also creation, colostomy **336**
resection, lymph node **337**
resection, stapled transanal rectal (STARR) (rectorectostomy) **338**
respiratory **446, 447**
respiratory system **105, 146, 204, 223, 238, 262, 289, 290, 319, 372, 374, 379, 449, 466, 474, 476, 477**
restriction **101, 178, 314, 315, 316**
resurfacing device **243**
revision **86**
revision, graft, arteriovenous (AV) **339**
  see also graft, arteriovenous (AV) **339**
revision, shunt, transjugular intrahepatic portosystemic (TIPS) **340**
  see also shunt, transjugular intrahepatic portosystemic (TIPS) **340**
rhinoplasty, augmentation **341**
rhinoscopy **342**
rhizotomy, spinal nerve root **342**
rib cage **454, 460**
right ventricle **294**
robotic assisted procedure **458**
rupture, shoulder joint adhesions (arthrolysis) (manual) **343**

S

sacral nerve **147, 253, 342**
sacroplasty **343**
sacrum **343, 454, 460**
saphenous vein
  left **257**
  right **257**
scan, pulmonary, ventilation and perfusion **474**
sclera **370**
second trimester
  multiple gestation **468**
  single fetus **468**
see also conversion, gastrostomy to jejunostomy (PEG-PEJ)
  see also conversion, gastrostomy to jejunostomy (PEG-PEJ) **239**
septoplasty, deviated nasal septum **344**
septostomy, percutaneous, atrial balloon (rashkind procedure) **345**

© 2018 Optum360, LLC

intervention, crisis **485**
suctioning, bronchial (for removal of mucus plug) **358**
  see also lavage, bronchoalveolar (BAL) **358**
  see also washing, bronchial **358**
superior vena cava **175, 221**
supernumerary breast **271**
supplement **81, 88, 99, 109, 112, 174, 202, 203, 204, 205, 210, 243, 280, 299, 300, 317, 319, 329, 330, 343, 389**
supracervical (uterus) **206**
switch procedure, arterial **360**
switch, duodenal (biliopancreatic diversion) **359**
  see also gastrectomy, vertical sleeve (VSG) **359**
sympathectomy, thoracic endoscopic (ETS) **361**
syngeneic **376, 377, 378, 379**
synthetic substitute **81, 88, 96, 108, 109, 116, 117, 131, 137, 138, 179, 180, 182, 193, 194, 204, 205, 240, 241, 244, 246, 251, 280, 294, 300, 317, 321, 322, 329, 330, 341, 343, 385, 389, 392**
  ceramic **240, 241, 244**
  ceramic on polyethylene **241, 244**
  metal **240, 241, 244**
  metal on polyethylene **241, 244**
  oxidized zirconium on polyethylene **241, 244, 246**
  polyethylene **240, 244**

T

temporal artery **119**
  left **119**
  right **119**
tendons **115, 142, 143, 145, 255, 305, 326, 328**
testes **282, 283**
  bilateral **282, 283**
testis **282, 283**
  left **282, 283**
  right **282, 283**
therapy treatment, laser interstitial (LITT) (brain) **481**
therapy, aquablation, prostate (robotic water resection of the prostate) **495**
therapy, bone marrow cell, autologous, intramuscular **496**
  see also harvest, graft, autologous bone marrow **496**
  see also transplant, bone marrow (BMT) **496**
therapy, shock wave, extracorporeal (ESWT), musculoskeletal (orthotripsy) **452**
third trimester
  multiple gestation **468**
  single fetus **468**
thoracentesis **362**
thoracic **454, 460**
thoracic aorta **174, 329, 360**
  ascending/arch **174, 329, 360**
  descending **329**
thoracic artery **117**
thoracic nerve **147, 253, 342**
thoracic spinal cord **253**
thoracic vertebra **252, 395, 493**

thoracic vertebral disc **149**
thoracic vertebral joint **231**
thoracolumbar vertebral disc **149**
thoracolumbar vertebral joint **231**
thoracoscopy (diagnostic) **363**
thoracostomy, tube **363**
thrombectomy, percutaneous mechanical (pharmacomechanical) (PMT) **364**
thrombolysis (injection of thrombolytic) (tissue plasminogen activator) **425**
thrombolytic **425**
thumb **415, 416**
  left **415, 416**
  right **415, 416**
thyroid gland
  isthmus **365**
thyroid gland (resection) **365**
thyroid gland lobe **365**
  left **365**
  right **365**
thyroidectomy **365**
tibia **229, 284**
  left **229, 284**
  right **229, 284**
tissue expander **233, 234**
toe **415, 416**
  left **415, 416**
  right **415, 416**
toe nail **310**
toe phalanx **114**
  left **114**
  right **114**
tomographic (Tomo) nuclear medicine imaging **473, 474**
tonsillectomy (without adenoidectomy) **368**
tonsillectomy with adenoidectomy **369**
tonsillectomy, lingual **367**
  see also epiglottopexy, transoral endoscopic **367**
  see also excision, lingual, submucosal minimally invasive (SMILE) **367**
tonsils **368, 369**
trabeculectomy ab externo **370**
trabeculoplasty, laser **371**
trachea **372, 374**
tracheostomy **372**
tracheostomy revision (stomaplasty) **373**
  see also tracheostomy **373**
  see also tracheostomy tube change **373**
tracheostomy tube change **374**
  see also tracheostomy **374**
  see also tracheostomy revision (stomatoplasty) **374**
traction **416**
traction apparatus **416**
transapical **334, 389**
transesophageal **464**
transfer **115, 191, 298, 320**
transfer, lymph node (LNT) **375**
transfusion **426, 427, 428**
transfusion, fresh frozen plasma (FFP) **426**
transplant **376, 377, 378**

heart 376
kidney 377
liver 378
transplant, bone marrow (BMT) 427
  see also therapy, bone marrow cell, autologous,
    intramuscular in the new technology section
    427
transplant, lung 379
  see also transplant, heart 379
transplant, meniscus 380
  see also meniscectomy, knee 380
transplant, stem cell 428
transplant, uterus 381
transplantation 376, 377, 378, 379
transposition, nerve 382
transverse rectus abdominis myocutaneous flap 297,
  298
treatment 454
treatment, intraoperative, vascular grafts
  (intraoperative administration of endothelial
  damage inhibitor) 497
  see also bypass graft, coronary artery (CABG) 497
tricuspid valve 322, 388, 389
trigeminal nerve 279
truncal valve 329, 389
trunk region 457, 458
turbinectomy, submucous resection 383
tympanic membrane
  left 274
  right 274

U

ultrasonography 463, 464, 468, 469
ultrasonography, fetal 468
ultrasound therapy 453
ultrasound, intravascular, coronary arteries (IVUS) 469
ultrasound, therapeutic 453
uncemented 240, 244
unilateral-multiple seizure 484
unilateral-single seizure 484
upper arm 413, 415, 416
  left 413, 415, 416
  right 413, 415, 416
upper arm vein 170, 195
upper arteries 99, 119, 133, 154, 165, 170, 195,
  315, 316, 364, 466
upper bones 142, 143, 215, 252, 281, 295, 301,
  302, 311, 395
upper extremities 454, 460
upper extremity 413, 415, 416, 457, 458
  left 413, 415, 416
  right 413, 415, 416
upper eyelid 109
  left 109
  right 109
upper femur 229
  left 229
  right 229
upper GI 421

upper joints 100, 149, 180, 182, 231, 248, 249,
  250, 301, 303, 324, 327, 332, 343
upper leg 415, 416
  left 415, 416
  right 415, 416
upper lip 177, 320
upper lobe bronchus 223, 319
  left 223, 319
  right 223, 319
upper spine bursa and ligament 256
upper veins 165, 364
Ureter 385
ureter 141, 150, 260, 261, 278, 384, 385
  bilateral 150, 384
  left 150, 260, 261, 278, 384, 385
  right 150, 260, 261, 278, 384, 385
ureteroneocystostomy 384
ureteroplasty 385
urethra 107, 209, 260, 261, 300, 325, 352, 386,
  415
urethropexy (retropubic urethral suspension) 386
urinary 442
urinary system 107, 139, 140, 141, 150, 172, 209,
  260, 261, 275, 276, 277, 278, 300, 325,
  352, 377, 384, 385, 386, 466, 476, 477
urinary tract 392
uterine artery 153
  left 153
  right 153
uterine supporting structure 265
uterus 206, 265, 273
uvula 387
uvulopalatopharyngoplasty 387
  see also tonsillectomy with adenoidectomy 387

V

vacuum 401, 405
vagina 129, 172, 193, 325
valvotomy (valvulotomy) 388
valvuloplasty 389
  see also wedge resection, mitral valve leaflet 389
vas deferens 391
  bilateral 391
  left 391
  right 391
vascular access device 235
  totally implantable 235
  tunneled 235
vascular perfusion 429
vasectomy 391
vasopressor 419
veins 466
venous 434, 435
ventilation 447
ventilation, mechanical, assistance (respiratory) 446
  see also ventilation, mechanical, performance
    (respiratory) 446
ventilation, mechanical, performance (respiratory) 447

© 2018 Optum360, LLC

see also intubation, endotracheal in the medical and surgical chapter **447**
see also ventilation, mechanical, assistance (respiratory) **447**
ventricle **131, 211, 217**
   left **211, 217**
   right **131, 211, 217**
ventricular septum **330**
ventriculography, cardiac **470**
   see also angiography, cardiac (coronary arteriography) (angiocardiography) **470**
   see also catheterization, cardiac under measurement and monitoring in the medical and surgical-related chapter. **470**
ventriculostomy **392**
   see also monitoring, intracranial pressure, under "measurement and monitoring" in the medical and surgical-related chapter. **392**
ventriculostomy, reopening, endoscopic third (ETV) **394**
   see also ventriculostomy **394**
version, external cephalic (ECV) **412**
   see also reposition, uterus, transvaginal **412**
vertebral artery **165**
   left **165**
   right **165**
vertebral vein **165**
   left **165**
   right **165**
vertebroplasty **395**

see also kyphoplasty (percutaneous vertebral augmentation) **395**
vestibular gland **269**
videofluoroscopy, esophageal (modified barium swallow) **471**
vitrectomy **396**
   see also buckling, scleral (with implant) **396**
vitreous **396**
   left **396**
   right **396**
vulva **325**

W

washing, bronchial **397**
   see also lavage, bronchoalveolar (BAL) **397**
   see also suctioning, bronchial (for removal of mucus plug) **397**
wedge resection, mitral valve leaflet **398**
   see also valvuloplasty **398**
whipple **399**

Z

zooplastic **376, 378, 379**
zooplastic tissue **108, 117, 131, 294, 317, 322, 329, 330, 334, 389, 494**
   rapid deployment technique **494**
z-plasty, skin (scar revision) **400**